Recreational Therapy
for
Specific Diagnoses
and Conditions

Heather R. Porter, Ph.D., CTRS

Idyll Arbor's Recreational Therapy Practice Series

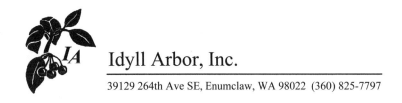

Idyll Arbor, Inc.

39129 264th Ave SE, Enumclaw, WA 98022 (360) 825-7797

Idyll Arbor's Recreational Therapy Practice Series Editor: Heather R. Porter, Ph.D., CTRS
Idyll Arbor, Inc. Editor: Thomas M. Blaschko
Cover design: Curt Pliler

ISBNs 9781882883967 paper 9781611580556 e-book

Contents

Contributing Authors

Jared Allsop, M.S., CTRS
Lecturer
School of Public Health
Department of Recreation, Park, & Tourism Studies
Indiana University
Bloomington, IN

Andrew P. Bogenschutz, M.S., CTRS
Recreational Therapist
Shepherd Center
Atlanta, GA

John Campbell, Psy.D.
Chief, Psychology Service
Central Alabama Veterans Health Care System
Tuskegee, AL

Jodie Charters, M.S., CTRS
Recreational Therapist
Addictions and Mental Health Program
Capital District Health Authority
Halifax, NS, Canada

Jo Ann Coco-Ripp, Ph.D., LRT/CTRS
Associate Professor
Therapeutic Recreation Program Coordinator
School of Education and Human Performance
Winston-Salem State University
Winston-Salem, NC

Dawn R. DeVries, DHA, MPA, CTRS
Assistant Professor
Therapeutic Recreation Program
College of Health Professions
Grand Valley State University
Grand Rapids, MI

Kathryn D. Elokdah, Ed.M., CTRS, ATP
Recreational Therapist
National Institutes of Health
Clinical Research Center
Rehabilitation Medicine Department
Recreational Therapy Section
Bethesda, MD

Donna L. Gregory, MBA, CTRS
Chief, Recreation Therapy
National Institutes of Health
Clinical Research Center
Rehabilitation Medicine Department
Recreational Therapy Section
Bethesda, MD

Lei Guo, Ph.D., LRT/CTRS
Assistant Professor
Department of Physical Education and Recreation
North Carolina Central University
Durham, NC

Brenda L. Hart, M.S., M.Ed., CTRS
Independent Contractor
Therapeutic Recreation Services
Wesley Enhanced Living in Doylestown
New Hope, PA

Natalie Haynes, M.Ed., M.S., CTRS
Branch Manager of Therapeutic Recreation Services
Fairfax County Neighborhood and Community Services
Fairfax, VA

Julie Hoehl, B.S., CTRS, HF/S, BFC
Lead Recreation Therapist
National Institutes of Health
Clinical Research Center
Rehabilitation Medicine Department
Recreational Therapy Section
Bethesda, MD

Laurie Jake, BS, CTRS
Private Practice
Phoenix, AZ 85045

Ruthie Kucharewski, Ph.D., CTRS
Professor, Division Coordinator
Director, Recreation and Recreational Therapy
College of Health Sciences
University of Toledo
Toledo, OH

Joy Lauerer, DNP, MSN, PMHCNS-BC, RN
Psychiatric Advance Practice Nurse
Instructor of Nursing
Medical University of South Carolina
College of Nursing
Charleston, SC

Stephen Lewis, Ph.D., CTRS
Recreational Therapy Lecturer
Clemson University
Department of Parks, Recreation, and Tourism Management
Clemson, SC

Donna L. Long, M.Ed., CTRS
Clubhouse Manager
MossRehab
Philadelphia, PA

Susan E. Lynch, Ph.D., CTRS
Associate Professor
Longwood University
Department of Health, Athletic Training, Recreation, and Kinesiology
Farmville, VA

Kenneth E. Mobily, Ph.D., CTRS
Professor, Leisure Studies
Department of Health and Human Physiology
University of Iowa
Iowa City, IA

Kathy Neely, Re.D., CTRS
Associate Professor
Department of Health, Physical Education & Recreation
Alabama State University
Montgomery, AL

Barbara L. Parker, B.S., CTRS
Chief, Therapeutic Recreation Services
Bay Pines Veterans Administration Healthcare System
Bay Pines, FL

Dean Parker, M.S., CTRS
Recreational Therapist
Brandywine Hospital
Coatesville, PA

Margalyn P. Payne, M.S. Ed., CTRS
Recreational Therapist
Willows Way, Inc.
St. Charles, MO

Tara L. Perry, Ph.D.
Former Professor (Recreation/Recreation Therapy) &
Current Outdoor Recreation Planner
Federal Energy Regulatory Commission
Washington, DC

Heather R. Porter, Ph.D., CTRS
Assistant Professor
Department of Rehabilitation Sciences
Temple University
Philadelphia, PA

Mary Lou Schilling, Ph.D., CTRS
Associate Professor
Department of Recreation, Parks, & Leisure Services
Administration
Central Michigan University
Mt. Pleasant, MI

Arlene A. Schmid, Ph.D., OTR
Associate Professor
Colorado State University
Department of Occupational Therapy
Fort Collins, CO

Karen Smith, M.L.S.
Clinical Informationist
National Institutes of Health Library
Bethesda, MD

Rachel L. Smith, M.S.
Doctoral Student
Indiana University
Department of Recreation, Park, & Tourism Studies
Bloomington, IN

Gretchen Snethen, Ph.D., CTRS
Assistant Professor
Department of Rehabilitation Sciences
Temple University
Philadelphia, PA

Anne-Marie Sullivan, Ph.D., CTRS
Associate Professor
School of Human Kinetics & Recreation
Memorial University of Newfoundland
St John's, NL, Canada

Juan Tortosa-Martínez, Ph.D.
Assistant Professor
Department of General and Specific Didactics
University of Alicante
Alicante, Spain

Jasmine Townsend, Ph.D., CTRS
Assistant Professor
Department of Parks, Recreation, & Tourism Management
Clemson University
Clemson, SC

Marieke Van Puymbroeck, Ph.D., CTRS
Associate Professor
Department of Parks, Recreation, & Tourism Management
Clemson University
Clemson, SC

Nannette M. Vliet, Ed.M., CTRS
Assistant Dean
Jefferson School of Health Professions
Thomas Jefferson University
Philadelphia, PA

Karen C. Wenzel, M.A., CTRS
Major Donor Acquisition Director
Ability Connection Colorado
Denver, CO
Adjunct Instructor
Department of Health Professions
Metropolitan State University of Denver
Denver, CO
Former Executive Director
Rocky Mountain Multiple Sclerosis Center
Westminster, CO

Brenda P. Wiggins, Ph.D.
Associate Professor and Graduate Co-Coordinator
School of Recreation, Health, and Tourism
George Mason University
Manassas, VA

Stephanie Wood, M.A., CTRS
Coordinator, Primary Health Care
Capital District Health Authority
Halifax, NS, Canada

J. Randal Wyble, M.S., CTRS
Assistant Professor & Therapeutic Recreation Program
Director
Therapeutic Recreation Program
College of Health Professions
Grand Valley State University
Grand Rapids, MI

Heewon Yang, Ph.D., CTRS
Professor
Department of Health Education and Recreation
Southern Illinois University — Carbondale
Carbondale, IL

Daniel G. Yoder, Ph.D.
Professor and Interim Chair of the Recreation, Park, &
Tourism Administration Department
Western Illinois University
Macomb, IL

Reviewers

Thanks to the individuals who graciously gave their time to review the 2006 edition and provide feedback for re-shaping this edition.

Jo Ann Coco-Ripp, Ph.D., LRT/CTRS
Associate Professor
Therapeutic Recreation Program Coordinator
School of Education and Human Performance
Winston-Salem State University
Winston-Salem, NC

Jennifer A. Piatt, Ph.D., CTRS
Assistant Professor
Department of Recreation, Park, & Tourism Studies
School of Public Health
Indiana University
Bloomington, IN

Thomas K. Skalko, Ph.D., LRT/CTRS
Professor
Recreational Therapy
College of Health and Human Performance
East Carolina University
Greenville, NC
and
Honorary Professor
College of Health Sciences
University of KwaZulu-Natal
Durban, South Africa

Research and Editing Assistants

The following individuals volunteered their time to be Research & Editing Assistants. Their dedication to assist with Recreational Therapy research is highly commendable.

Rebecca Baro
Recreational Therapy Student
Temple University

Genee Bower
Recreational Therapy Student
Temple University

Joshua Cino
Recreational Therapy Student
Temple University

Morgan Ferrante
Recreational Therapy Student
Temple University

Tonya D. Fromm
Recreational Therapy Student
Temple University

Kristen Hartman
Recreational Therapy Student
Temple University

Tracy Ann Jastrzab
Recreational Therapy Student
Temple University

Lea Peterson
Recreational Therapy Student
Temple University

Erin Kate MacElroy
Recreational Therapy Student
Temple University

Yekaterina Mishin
Recreational Therapy Student
Temple University

Hannah R. Porter
Honor Student
New Foundations Charter High School

Marianella Sanchez
Recreational Therapy Student
Temple University

Alexa Szal
Psychology Student
Temple University

Mandi Shearer
Recreational Therapy Student
Temple University

Rachel L. Thomas
Recreational Therapy Student
Temple University

Foreword

The chapter authors and I are excited to provide this updated set of diagnoses and conditions. Since the first edition of the book we have been able to add eleven new chapters. We have been able to update the chapters that are based on the fifth edition of the *Diagnostic and Statistical Manual of Mental Disorders* (*DSM-5*), which means that recreational therapists who read this volume will have the latest information when they are working in the field of mental health. We plan to add information on the tenth edition of the *International Statistical Classification of Diseases and Related Health Problems* (*ICD-10*) in the next edition.

Looking at the field of recreational therapy, it is wonderful to see how many places we can document the efficacy of the practices described in this volume. There are still many things recreational therapists do that have not yet been proven through research, but, compared to the first edition, this volume takes a large step forward in presenting information on the work researchers and professionals in the field have done to make recreational therapy an efficacy-based practice. Because this is a book of recreational therapy *practice*, rather than a book about recreational therapy *efficacy*, we have included areas of recreational therapy practice that have not been demonstrated to be efficacious yet. We hope that by the next edition many more of them will be proven to be effective.

Lastly, we are most excited to be able to describe our practice in terms of the *International Classification of Functioning, Disability, and Health* (ICF). We believe that being able to do this demonstrates that what we do is at the cutting edge of healthcare practice. When we provide treatment to those who have the diagnoses in this volume, we are doing so much more than treating their medical condition. We are finding ways to restore their minds, bodies, and spirits to the best possible levels of personal, interpersonal, societal, and environmental well-being. No other field takes on such a meaningful set of challenges.

— *Heather Porter*

Introduction

There are two trends related to treatment that need to be understood by anyone providing services in the current healthcare environment. The first is that any treatment provided must be efficacious. Many studies are being done to find best practice for any given diagnosis. It is no longer the case that insurance reimburses providers for whatever treatment they choose to provide. Many reimburse set amounts for a given diagnosis and the provider needs to treat the condition in a way that will let them stay in business. Recreational therapy has conducted and is continuing to conduct research to demonstrate that its practice is efficacious in order to strengthen its place in the modern healthcare environment.

The second trend has to do with accurate documentation. In current healthcare practice, it is vitally important to thoroughly document all of the client's health conditions. It is not enough to say, for example, that a client has an eating disorder. If there are comorbid conditions of depression, osteoporosis, and significant damage to the heart, they need to be documented, too. In fact, everything that needs to be treated in a client needs to be documented.

More complicated clients require more resources. Healthcare insurers, whether they are governmental or private, recognize the need to pay more for complicated cases, but it is the responsibility of the provider to write up thorough descriptions of each client's condition using a classification system that is recognized by the insurer and other healthcare providers.

The first reason that providers must document the client's condition accurately is so that all of the providers working with the client understand the client's condition. The second and equally important reason is that each aspect of the treatment must be tied to the client's condition. In the example above, the cost of treatment for osteoporosis will not be reimbursed unless the diagnosis of osteoporosis is in the client's chart. This is a big change which has recently hit many providers. The documentation required for demonstrating the need for a particular treatment is much greater than is was just a few years ago.

Recreational therapists, in general, do not use the same language as the people reimbursing the costs of treatment, and may not adequately tie interventions to specific diagnoses and conditions. This situation needs to change, as insurers are increasingly demanding it. This book provides the information required to make this change.

Let's look first at the diagnostic languages used by insurers and other providers in the healthcare professions. There are currently two diagnostic systems in widespread use in healthcare: the *Diagnostic and Statistical Manual of Mental Disorders* (DSM) published by the American Psychiatric Association (APA, 2013) and the International Statistical Classification of Diseases and Related Health Problems, more commonly known as the International Classification of Diseases (ICD), from the World Health Organization (World Health Organization, 2010).

Currently the DSM is in the fifth edition (*DSM-5*). The ICD has had the tenth edition (*ICD-10*) out since 1992. While most of the world has adopted this edition, the United States is still using the ninth edition (*ICD-9*). The U.S. Department of Health and Human Services (HHS) issued a rule on July 31, 2014, that finalized October 1, 2015, as the new compliance date for healthcare providers, health plans, and healthcare clearinghouses to transition to *ICD-10* (Centers for Medicare and Medicaid Services, 2014d). The *ICD-10* includes 69,000 diagnosis codes compared to 14,000 codes in the *ICD-9*. It allows the clinician to capture a greater level of detail with changes that include laterality, severity parameters, and combination codes to better capture complexity.

In addition to these two diagnostic systems, there are specific prospective payments systems that are tied to reimbursement. Long-term care providers are required to provide the federal government with the Minimum Data Set from the Resident Assessment

Instrument for each resident (Centers for Medicare and Medicaid Services, 2014b). This instrument is a way to calculate the complexity of care required for a particular resident and the resulting rate of reimbursement. The result is a per diem prospective payment system that is adjusted for case mix and geographic variation in wages and covers all costs related to the furnishing of covered services (Centers for Medicare and Medicaid Services, 2013c). Inpatient rehabilitation facilities are required to complete the Inpatient Rehabilitation Facility Patient Assessment Instrument (IRF-PAI). This instrument classifies clients into distinct groups based on clinical characteristics and expected resource needs. The classification is then used to calculate reimbursement rates (Centers for Medicare and Medicaid Services, 2013a). Outpatient hospital services are reimbursed through payments weights and conversion factors for specific services rendered (Centers for Medicare and Medicaid Services, 2014c). Inpatient psychiatric facilities are reimbursed a reasonable cost per case, limited by a hospital's specific target amount per discharge, which is calculated based on the hospital's cost per discharge in a base year (Centers for Medicare and Medicaid Services, 2013b).

In addition to the diagnosis classification systems (*DSM-5, ICD-9*), the World Health Organization developed the International Classification of Functioning, Disability, and Health (ICF) to complement the DSM and ICD. It provides a unified and standard language and framework for the description of health and health-related states (Word Health Organization, 2002). It is recognized throughout the world as a system for classifying and documenting body structure and function impairments, activity limitations, participation restrictions, and contextual factors that hinder and facilitate health and functioning. While the ICF is not currently recognized as a basis for reimbursement by insurers in the United States, it is recognized by other healthcare providers as an effective system for recording the current condition of a client. The trend in healthcare is to look more at the whole person and many feel that the ICF will be the instrument used to achieve that goal. The World Health Organization (2002) says

> Studies show that diagnosis alone does not predict service needs, length of hospitalization, level of care or functional outcomes. Nor is the presence of a disease or disorder

an accurate predictor of receipt of disability benefits, work performance, return to work potential, or likelihood of social integration. This means that if we use a medical classification of diagnoses alone we will not have the information we need for health planning and management purposes. What we lack is data about levels of functioning and disability. ICF makes it possible to collect those vital data in a consistent and internationally comparable manner (p. 5).

Diagnosing a client with a specific disease or health problem using the ICD and DSM codes is most often done through a team approach with the final decision made by the treating physician or psychiatrist. With the ICF however, recreational therapists will be able to provide diagnostic information to the rest of the healthcare team in an internationally recognized format. It will also enable recreational therapists to tie treatment interventions to specific ICF items, which are linked to specific health conditions. When ongoing efficacy studies are added into the mix, recreational therapists will meet the requirements of the current healthcare trends.

Using ICF Codes Correctly

It's not enough to use the ICF; it's important to understand how to use ICF codes correctly. The companion book specifically on the ICF (*Recreational Therapy and the International Classification of Functioning, Disability, and Health*) explains how to score each code. This book identifies the ICF codes connected to specific health conditions and related treatment interventions. Let's look at a code that is easy to misunderstand (d132 Acquiring Information) as a way of describing the correct process.

A common misunderstanding is that the code d132 Acquiring Information is used when you are providing information to a client about, for example, recreation opportunities. This seems reasonable because the client is, in fact, acquiring information. However, a diagnostic code of d132 Acquiring Information does not say that the client needs to acquire information. It says, instead, that the client has a deficit in his/her ability to acquire information. Teaching the client more effective ways to acquire information would be documented with this code.

Giving information to a client, on the other hand, should be documented based on what the information is about. It could be d920 Recreation and Leisure, if the client has been diagnosed with a deficit in leisure participation. It could just as easily be d240 Handling Stress and Other Psychological Demands if the information is related to issues with handling a stressful condition. The ICF code is used to document the part of the health condition that is being treated.

This can be put another way: Don't code what the treatment is. Code what the treatment does. A recreation program should usually not be coded as any part of d920 Recreation and Leisure. If it is being done to reduce depression, it could be coded as b126 Temperament and Personality Functions. If it is intended to improve physical condition, it would be coded as b455 Exercise Tolerance Functions, b730 Muscle Power Functions, or something similar. It could also be for improving social interactions with friends and be coded as treatment for d750 Informal Social Relationships.

The important point to remember is that the diagnosis covers the conditions that need to be addressed in the client. The treatment codes need to be tied to items in the diagnosis and need to describe how the treatment makes a documented deficit better. There is a chain of connection in this process. Health condition is tied to the issues related to health condition, which is then tied to ICF codes that reflect the issues related to the health condition. The ICF codes are then tied to interventions found to be efficacious for treatment of the issue related to the health condition.

The list of codes provided in this book for a particular diagnosis is often quite long. Remember that it isn't necessary to write something for each code, but it is useful to think about each code when conducting an assessment. The goal is to provide a complete picture of the client's condition. Leaving any part out makes it much harder to decide what is needed for effective treatment. It also leaves the therapist in a position where specific aspects of treatment may be difficult to explain. It is better to provide a thorough assessment of the client's health condition at the beginning, which will then lead to effective treatment and the best possible care for the client.

Other Notes

Quality of life is often mentioned as a criterion for deciding the efficacy of a treatment. The ICF does not specifically address quality of life. Instead, some components of quality of life, although not all, can be evaluated in the ICF with codes such as b1265 Optimism. Specific aspects of a client's life that may make a high quality of life difficult, such as pain (b280 Sensation of Pain), can also be documented.

Recreational therapists need to consider using ICF codes in their efficacy studies to demonstrate the benefits of treatment within a consistent system of diagnosis.

References

American Psychiatric Association. (2013). *Diagnostic and statistical manual of mental disorders, fifth edition.* Washington, DC: American Psychiatric Publishing.

Centers for Medicare and Medicaid Services. (2013a). Inpatient rehabilitation facility PPS. http://www.cms.gov/Medicare/Medicare-Fee-for-Service-Payment/InpatientRehabFacPPS/

Centers for Medicare and Medicaid Services. (2013b). Inpatient psychiatric facility PPS. http://www.cms.gov/Medicare/Medicare-Fee-for-Service-Payment/InpatientPsychFacilPPS/index.html

Centers for Medicare and Medicaid Services. (2013c). Skilled nursing facility PPS. http://www.cms.gov/Medicare/Medicare-Fee-for-Service-Payment/SNFPPS/index.html

Centers for Medicare and Medicaid Services. (2014a). ICD-10. http://www.cms.gov/Medicare/Coding/ICD10/index.html?redirect=/icd10.

Centers for Medicare and Medicaid Services. (2014b). MDS 3.0 RAI Manual. http://www.cms.gov/Medicare/Quality-Initiatives-Patient-Assessment-Instruments/NursingHomeQualityInits/MDS30RAIManual.html.

Centers for Medicare and Medicaid Services. (2014c). Hospital outpatient PPS. http://www.cms.gov/Medicare/Medicare-Fee-for-Service-Payment/HospitalOutpatientPPS/Hospital-Outpatient-Regulations-and-Notices-Items/CMS-1601-FC-.html?DLPage=1&DLSort=2&DLSortDir=descending

Centers for Medicare and Medicaid Services. (2014d). Road to 10: The small physician's practice route to ICD-10. www.roadto10.org

World Health Organization. (2002). *Towards a common language for functioning, disability and health: ICF.* http://www.who.int/classifications/icf/training/icfbeginners-guide.pdf

World Health Organization. (2010). ICD-10 Version: 2010. http://apps.who.int/classifications/icd10/browse/2010/en.

World Health Organization. (2014). ICF browser. http://apps.who.int/classifications/icfbrowser/Default.aspx.

1. Amputation and Prosthesis

Kathryn Elokdah and Heather R. Porter

Amputation is the complete loss of all limb elements below a certain point. Amputations may be performed because of limb disease, trauma, or congenital malformations. Limb disease generally falls into three categories: (1) peripheral arterial disease (e.g., a complication of diabetes), (2) cancer, or (3) sudden blockage of an artery (embolus) causing a lack of oxygenated blood to the tissue. When tissue is deprived of oxygen, bacterial infections follow and tissue dies. The decay of tissue is called gangrene. Gangrene is not curable and the dead, infected tissue must be removed before healing can occur. Amputations are often described by the level of excision at which the normal anatomy does not exist and may include the percentage of the limb remaining. Classifications for lower extremity and upper extremity amputations are shown below.

Lower Extremity Amputation

Partial toe: Excision of any part of one or more toes.

Toe disarticulation: Disarticulation at the metatarsal phalangeal joint.

Partial foot: Amputation of the metatarsals and digits including ray amputations, transmetatarsal amputations, tarsometatarsal disarticulation (Lisfranc), and transtarsal disarticulation (Chopart).

Symes: Ankle disarticulation with attachment of heel pad to distal end of tibia, with or without removal of malleoli and distal tibial/fibular flares.

Transtibial (below-knee): Amputation through the tibia and fibula, standard length is 35-50% of tibial length. Typically described as long or short if outside standard lengths.

Knee disarticulation (transcondylar/supracondylar): Amputation through the knee joint; femoral condyles intact, with or without the patella.

Transfemoral (above-knee): Amputation through the femur, standard length is 35-60% of femoral length. Typically described as long or short if outside standard lengths.

Hip disarticulation: Amputation through hip joint; pelvis intact.

Hemipelvectomy: Resection of lower half of the pelvis.

Hemicorporectomy: Amputation of both lower limbs and pelvis below L4/5 level.

Adapted from: Braddom, R. L. & Chan, L. (2011). *Physical Medicine and Rehabilitation* (4th ed.). Philadelphia: Elsevier Saunders.

Upper Extremity Amputation

Hand

Fingertip: The most common type of amputation. Removes part or all of fingertip.

Thumb: Partial or complete, resulting in loss of palmer grip, side-to-side pinch, and tip-to-tip pinch.

Radial: Involves the thumb and index finger.

Transverse digit: Occurs at one or more digits.

Ulnar: Involves digits four and five, loss of hook grasp.

Central: Involves digits three and four.

Below-Elbow

Styloid/wrist disarticulation: 90-100% preservation of length.

Transcarpal: Amputation through the wrist.

Long transradial: 55-90% preservation of length with up to 60 degrees of supination and pronation with a prosthesis and strong elbow flexion.

Medium transradial: 35-50% preservation of length with loss of pronation and supination.

Short transradial: Less than 35% preservation of length with the loss of full range of motion at the elbow.

Above-Elbow

Elbow disarticulation: 90-100% of humeral length preserving humeral rotation to the prosthesis.

Long transhumeral: 50-90% of humeral length with glenohumeral motions preserved.

Short transhumeral: 30-50% of humeral length with glenohumeral motion loss due to socket encompassing the acromion.

Forequarter and shoulder disarticulation: Less than 30% of humeral length with loss of glenohumeral motions of flexion, extension, and abduction.

Adapted from: Sheehan, T. P. (2011). Rehabilitation and prosthetic restoration in upper limb amputation. In R. L. Braddom (Ed.), *Physical Medicine and Rehabilitation* (4th ed., pp. 257-276). Philadelphia: Elsevier Saunders.

Prosthetics

Healthcare professionals who prescribe and manufacture prostheses consider comfort, ease of donning (putting on) and doffing (taking off), weight (the lighter the better), durability, required maintenance (e.g., cleaning), visual cosmetic appeal, and functionality of the unit when choosing an appropriate prosthesis for a client. The average life of a prosthesis for an adult is two years with daily use. Teenagers and children may require more frequent prostheses due to growth. The weight of the prosthesis is usually about half the weight of the body segment it replaces, from three to seven pounds for a below-knee prosthesis, and from seven to twelve pounds for an above-knee prosthesis. Lightweight and sport prosthetics may also be considered (Kottke & Lehmann, 1990).

Lower Extremity Prosthesis

Lower extremity prosthesis components:

- *Socket*: The socket is a bucket-like component that slides onto the residual limb. It is designed to protect the residual limb, as well as to disperse the forces associated with standing and walking. The client's residual limb is measured by making a plaster mold from the limb or through computer-assisted technology. The socket should be wiped out daily with a damp cloth and mild soap. When not wearing the prosthetic, it should be laid down on its side on the floor so that it does not fall over and crack.

- *Sock or gel liner*: Socks of various plies are worn on the stump to make up for the gap between the limb and the prosthesis to ensure a good fit. See Prosthetic Socks below for more information.

- *Suspension system*: This is how the prosthesis stays on the limb without falling off. It may consist of a variety of belts and straps that bolt onto the socket and connect to a waist strap or it may be a suction suspension. The most common type of suction suspension is silicon suction. A silicon-based sock is worn over the residual limb and then is inserted into the socket. It forms an airtight seal that stabilizes the prosthesis.

- *Articulating joint* (if needed): This is the knee joint. The prosthetic knee must provide support during the swing phase and maintain unrestricted motion for sitting and kneeling. The prosthetic knee can have a single axis with a simple hinge and a single pivot point, or it may have a polycentric axis with multiple centers of rotation (Bodeau & Mipro, 2002b).

- *Pylon*: This is the metal shaft that attaches to the socket and the terminal device. It is the replacement for the femur and/or the tibia and fibula. Once all of the adjustments are made to the prosthesis as a whole so that it fits the client correctly, the pylon is covered in soft foam contoured to match the other limb with a hard laminated shell (exoskeleton) or covered with a cosmetic soft covering (endoskeleton).

- *Terminal device*: This is the foot, but it may take other forms for athletic activities, such as running. The ankle joint is typically part of the terminal device. However, like the foot, separate ankle joints that incorporate more complex motion and strength can be fitted for physically demanding work or physically demanding recreational pursuits (e.g., rock climbing).

Upper Extremity Prosthesis

There are two types of upper extremity prostheses referred to as body-powered prostheses and myoelectric prostheses. Bodeau & Mipro (2002a) explain the difference between the two units:

- The body-powered prostheses are manipulated using cables and straps. They are the most durable prostheses and have higher sensory feedback. However, body powered prostheses are less cosmetically pleasing than a myoelectric unit and they require more gross limb movement.

- Myoelectric prostheses, operated by myoelectricity, may give more proximal function and increased cosmetic appeal, but they can be heavy and expensive. They have less sensory feedback and require more maintenance. They function by sensing electrical activity on the residual limb muscles and transmitting the information to electric motors that operate the prosthesis.

Components depend on the amputation site. Below elbow amputations (BEA) have a voluntary opening (VO) split hook, a friction wrist, a double-walled plastic laminate socket, a flexible elbow hinge, a single-control cable system, a biceps or triceps cuff, and a figure-of-eight harness. Above elbow amputations (AEA) are the same as below elbow amputation except for three things. There is an internal-locking elbow for the flexible elbow hinge. The prosthesis uses a dual control cable instead of a single control and it does not have a biceps or triceps cuff.

The upper extremity prosthesis tries to replicate hand functions of the missing hand. The five relevant grips are

- *Precision grip* (e.g., pincher grip): The pad of the thumb and index finger are in opposition to pick up or pinch a small object (e.g., small bead, grain of rice).
- *Tripod grip* (e.g., palmar grip, three-jaw chuck pinch): The pad of the thumb is against pads of the index and middle finger.
- *Lateral grip*: The pad of the thumb is in opposition to the lateral aspect of the index finger to manipulate a small object (e.g., turning a key in a lock).
- *Hook power grip*: The distal interphalangeal (DIP) joint and proximal interphalangeal (PIP) joint are flexed with the thumb extended (e.g., carrying a briefcase by the handle).
- *Spherical grip*: Tips of fingers and thumb are flexed (e.g., screwing in a light bulb or opening a doorknob).

Prosthetic Socks

Prosthetic socks are made from nylon, cotton, wool, or synthetic material and are placed over an amputated limb to fill up the gap and ensure a good fit between the residual limb and the prosthetic. Prosthetic socks come in various lengths, widths, and plies. The length and width of socks are prescribed by the prosthetist (a professional who designs, makes, and fits prosthetics). The number of plies is determined by the therapist. A ply refers to the number of threads knitted together to make the sock. Some prosthetic socks have a gel insert to provide added cushioning. Prosthetic socks come in four plies.

- Nylon stocking (0 ply/thickness)
- White trim (1 ply/thickness)
- Yellow trim (3 ply/thickness)
- Green trim (5 ply/thickness)

A client's sock ply is determined by adding up all of the sock plies that the client needs to wear to fill the gap (e.g., one green sock (5 ply) + one yellow sock (3 ply) = 8 ply). Generally, more than 10 plies are too much. If more than 10 plies are needed, the socket may need to be redesigned or modified. A poor fit can cause secondary skin problems.

Prior to applying socks, the stump shrinker or ace wrap must be removed. The stump should always be clean and dry prior to applying socks. The skin should be inspected for signs of ulceration or infection every time socks are put on and every time the prosthetic and socks are removed. Any change in skin color that lasts more than 30 minutes deserves medical attention prior to further use of the prosthetic.

The nylon sock is put on first (0 ply), followed by the prosthetic socks initially recommended by the physical therapist and prosthetist. Each sock should fit smoothly without any wrinkles. The seams along the bottom of the sock are worn on the outside (not against the skin). The stump will continue to shrink as a result of atrophied muscles, pressure from the prosthesis, and wrapping. As a result, the client will need to have readjustments to the sock plies and, less often, the prosthesis. Residual limbs also change in volume throughout a day, so the client must always have extra socks readily available and make changes as needed.

If the residual limb fits snugly (not too tight or loose), then no pain is felt, no ulceration or bruising is evident after wearing the prosthesis, and the pressure mark from wearing the prosthesis is not on a bony area (e.g., knee cap, elbow). For the person with a below-knee amputation, if the pressure mark is located below the kneecap and above the top of the shinbone then the number of sock plies is correct. If the pressure mark is on the kneecap, add one sock ply. If the pressure mark is on the shinbone, take off one sock ply. Continue modifying the number of plies until the pressure mark is in the correct location.

Skin checks are done before donning the prosthesis and after doffing the prosthesis. The client will be put on a wearing schedule by the physical therapist.

When the client is walking (lower extremity prosthesis) or using the prosthesis (upper extremity prosthesis), the therapist should be attentive to the fit of the prosthesis. Socks should be worn thick enough so that they do not slide up or down when in the socket of the prosthesis.

Cotton socks absorb moisture. This is a good thing because it takes moisture away from the skin. Prolonged moisture on the skin along with friction promotes skin breakdown. Because they absorb moisture, socks must be changed frequently throughout the day. The frequency of this will vary depending on the client's activity level, the weather, and perspiration. Socks must be washed by hand or on the gentle cycle daily in lukewarm water and mild soap. To dry the socks, wrap them in a towel (do not twist socks) and then lay them flat to air-dry. Socks should not be placed on a radiator, in a dryer, or in direct sunlight because that can shrink the sock. If a hole or run develops, the sock needs to be replaced. It should not be sewn or repaired. Sewing a sock may decrease the sock's dimensions or add seams that could result in a poor fit or skin irritation.

Incidence/Prevalence in U.S.

In the year 2005, 1.7 million persons in the U.S. were living with the loss of a limb (Ziegler-Graham et al., 2008). It is projected that the number of people living with the loss of a limb will more than double by the year 2050 to 3.6 million due to the rise of diabetes associated with obesity (Ziegler-Graham et al., 2008). In 2006, about 65,700 non-traumatic lower-limb amputations were performed in people with diabetes in the United States (Diseases, 2005). As of January 2010, more than 950 military service members sustained major limb amputations from the Iraq and Afghanistan war (Pasquina & Cooper, 2009). Even accounting for the incidence of war-related amputations, trends for the rates of trauma-

related and cancer-related amputations have both declined by approximately half over the past 20 years and the incidence of congenital limb difference has remained stable over the past 30 years (National Limb Loss Information Center, 2008). Despite vast improvements in limb salvage techniques, the number of amputations remains on the rise (Duwayri et al., 2012).

The distribution of amputation levels, which accounts for 31% of all traumatic limb loss in the U.S. was 31% lower limb (the majority were toes 13.9%, transtibial 7.3%, and foot 2.3%); and 68.6% upper limb (the majority were finger(s) 51.2%, transradial 2%, and transhumeral 1.5%) (Dillingham et al., 2002).

The distribution is different when looking at dysvascular limb loss, which is caused by circulation problems including those associated with diabetes. In the U.S. lower limbs account for 97% of these amputations with 25.8% at above-knee level, 27.6% at below-knee level, 31.5% at toe level, 10.5% at foot level, and the balance at other levels (Dillingham et al., 2002). The number of individuals living with amputated limbs is significant.

Predominant Age

Among all etiologies of amputation in the U.S., approximately one percent are under the age of 18, 18% between 18 and 44 years of age, 38% between 45 and 64 years of age, 21% between 65 and 74 years of age, and 22% between 75 and 100 years of age (Dillingham et al., 2002). Other areas of the world have similar distributions. Data from the United Kingdom report most lower extremity amputations occurred in individuals aged over 65 years (60.4% of diabetes-related and 68.3% of nondiabetes-related) (Vamos et al., 2010). The risk of amputation rises with age among all etiologies, including trauma, irrespective of race or gender (Dillingham et al., 2002). However, almost 70% of all traumatic amputations are of upper extremities and 75% of those amputations occurred at the finger level (Dillingham et al., 2002). The statistics from U.S. military conflicts have a different pattern. Eighty-five percent of military service members who sustained a major limb loss from the Iraq and Afghanistan wars were under the age of 35 (Pasquina & Cooper, 2009). The majority of individuals in the U.S. living with amputated limbs are adults who face the real potential to have their primary life role as a self-supporting wage earner disrupted.

Causes

It is estimated that the majority of amputations are due to vascular disease (82%) (Dillingham et al., 2002). In a United Kingdom study which looked at trends in the incidence of non-traumatic lower extremity amputations among individuals with and without diabetes, 51% occurred among people with diabetes — 59.6% of minor amputations and 42.6% of major amputations (Vamos et al., 2010). The remaining 18% of amputations are due to congenital malformation (58.5% upper limb amputation, 41.5% lower limb amputation), cancer (76.1% lower limb amputation, 23.9% upper limb amputation), and trauma (68.6% upper limb amputation, 30.4% lower limb amputation) (National Limb Loss Information Center, 2008). To not misrepresent the problem of amputation, having one amputation doesn't preclude an individual from having additional ones. A prospective study of 190 individuals with primary lower limb amputations noted the re-amputation rate was 17% (Johannesson, Larsson, & Oberg, 2004). Much research has been conducted to identify factors that lead to amputation, hoping to reduce the occurrence.

Individuals with a diagnosis of diabetes are clearly at greater risk of amputation. It has been claimed that every 30 seconds a lower limb is amputated somewhere in the world due to diabetes (Boulton et al., 2005). The pathway typically starts with "diabetic foot syndrome." The diabetic foot can be defined as ulceration associated with neurological abnormalities, infection, and various degrees of peripheral vascular disease (Gershater et al., 2009). Approximately 85% of diabetes-related amputations are preceded by a foot ulcer (IDF, 2007). The combination of neuropathy and peripheral vascular disease adds significantly to the risk for amputation among clients with diabetic foot syndrome (Moura Neto et al., 2012).

To further clarify the contributing factors for amputation, smoking diabetic clients underwent more amputations, as well as more proximal amputations than those who did not smoke. A higher amount of smoking in pack years correlated with an increasing trend of more proximal amputations as well (Anderson et al., 2012). Research literature identifies another risk factor: gender. Males are significantly more likely to have amputations for dysvascular and trauma etiologies than females, with the exception of females less than 14 years old with a dysvascular etiology (Dillingham et al., 2002). Only with cancer-related amputations do the genders have comparable frequencies across all age groups. As the overwhelming majority of amputation etiologies are not cancer-related, the increased frequency of male vs. female amputations results in significantly more males having amputations.

Life expectancy following an amputation depends upon a variety of factors; one of the most important is the etiology. An otherwise healthy individual with an amputation of traumatic etiology has a relatively standard survival rate.

The statistics for life expectancy for an individual with an amputation due to dysvascular disease are much more harsh. After a vascular amputation, the 30-day mortality rate ranges from nine percent to 21% and long-term survival has recently been found to be 48% to 69% at one year, 42% at three years, and 35% to 45% at five years (Huang, 2011). Another published source reveals similar data: there is only a two- to five-year life expectancy following amputation for chronic vascular disease for 60% of clients because of the risk of death from cardiovascular disease (Bradley & Kirker, 2006). It is no wonder that the foot complications in diabetes present a particularly troubling picture.

This underlies the importance of successful early rehabilitation to allow for an improved quality of life in their remaining years (Gitter & Bosker, 2005). A 2008 study of 82 individuals from Canada who had undergone bilateral transtibial amputations and received rehabilitation services including prosthetic fitting, revealed that, of those who survived, 85% were still wearing prostheses regularly and were walking. Most remained independent in ADLs for more than four years after discharge. They continued to do well at long-term follow-up (Mac Neill et al., 2008).

The success of prosthetic fitting is dependent upon many factors including the etiology, the level of amputation, age, and arguably the receipt of rehabilitation services. Among people with traumatic leg amputations, 95% are reported to have been fitted with a prosthesis and are using it for ambulation within three months (MacKenzie et al., 2004).

Success rates for people with dysvascular leg amputations are lower. On average, only around 40% of all people with lower limb amputations are fitted with a prosthesis (Condie et al., 2007). People with transtibial amputations have more chance of being prescribed with a prosthesis (around 60%) compared to people with transfemoral amputations (around 25%) (Condie et al., 2007). Other studies report similar findings. In a prospective study of 190 people with leg amputations, it was reported that 43% received a prosthesis after the primary amputation (Johannesson et al., 2004).

Statistics of successful prosthetic fitting of upper extremity amputations are elusive. A statement by Douglas G. Smith, MD, regarding his personal experience was, "about 80 percent of my clients with below-elbow amputations use their prosthesis daily. But while having a prosthesis is incredibly important for people with above-elbow amputations, only about 20 percent use one regularly" (Smith, 2007). A broadly grouped study of 307 people with upper extremity amputations revealed only 7.3% received rehabilitation services with less than half of them (44.7%) using their prostheses for eight or more hours a day, and 76.9% using their prostheses for regular or irregular cosmetic purposes (Jang et al., 2011). Even following prosthetic fitting, the rates of upper limb prosthesis rejection are high (Resnik et al., 2012). In the same study by Jang et al., only 30.0% of the respondents with upper extremity amputations reported satisfaction with their prostheses (Jang et al., 2011). It is proposed that these rates may be reduced with sufficient training by a highly specialized, multidisciplinary team of clinicians and a focus on client education and empowerment throughout the rehabilitation process (Resnik et al., 2012).

Systems Affected

Loss of bone, muscle, joint, and bodily tissue are related to the amputation. Other systems affected are dependent upon the type, extent, and number of amputations. Because there are so many different types of amputations, the ICF codes listed are very broad. The therapist will need to select the particular codes that apply to the particular type of amputation. For example, a person utilizing a lower extremity (LE) prosthesis requires more cardiopulmonary and muscular energy to perform tasks such as walking, household chores, and recreational activities than

someone who has all four limbs (Amputee Coalition of America, 2004; Frontera & DeLisa, 2010; Kelly, 2009). Deconditioning (b455 Exercise Tolerance Functions) is much more significant in a LE amputation than in something like a finger amputation, where the issues are centered more on d440 Fine Hand Use. Looking more at energy requirements, we see that, if using crutches instead of a prosthesis, the person will have increased energy demands for weight bearing on crutches; and, if using a prosthesis, the person will have increased energy demands from "utilizing the remaining proximal muscles to substitute for lost muscle function distal to the amputation" (Brown et al., 2012). Estimated increases in energy consumption (percentage above normal) by amputation level are as follows: unilateral transtibial 9-28%, unilateral transfemoral 40-65%, bilateral transtibial 41-100%, bilateral transfemoral 280%, transtibial plus transfemoral 75%, unilateral hip disarticulation 82%, and hemipelvectomy 125% (Wilken & Marin, 2009). Energy expenditure varies due to prosthetic malalignment, leg length discrepancies, limb-socket interface mismatches, person's age, presence of vascular disease, and gait deviations due to loss of sensory perception, shock absorbing, and propulsion properties of the foot and ankle, and loss of loading response at the knee (Wilken & Marin, 2009).

It is also common for people with LE amputations to experience musculoskeletal changes due to compensation for limb loss. For example, a person who has a right transtibial amputation (R TTA) may weight bear on his left LE more than his prosthetic right LE when standing and walking. When one leg is favored, musculoskeletal changes can cause pain in the hip and back (Amputee Coalition of America, 2004). This is a common problem for people who have had a LE amputation. It can be caused by: (1) reduced sensory input from the residual limb as compared to the intact limb, (2) fear of placing weight on the stump and/or prosthesis, (3) discomfort or pain from pressure on the stump or groin area when the prosthesis is fitting poorly, and (4) poor skill development from inadequate therapy (Amputee Coalition of America, 2004; Kaufman et al., 2012). A related problem is that prostheses do not provide a full sensory experience. The client's deficits in using other methods gathering required information for safe movement with a prosthesis can be coded with d120

Other Purposeful Sensing. Treatment interventions that focus on normalization of body mechanics during prosthetic use will positively impact the individual's musculoskeletal system.

The level of functioning, independence, and quality of life for people with amputations depends on variables such as rehabilitation received, level of acceptance and adaptation, other medical issues (including comorbidities), barriers including attitudinal and architectural, and level of support. Recreational therapists should code the effects on the body functions using codes such as b280 Sensation of Pain and all of the relevant codes under b7 Neuromusculoskeletal and Movement-Related Functions. Related issues with activities and participation will usually be recorded using the codes in d4 Mobility. Specific deficits in activities and participation may also be noted using other A&P codes.

Secondary Problems

Traumatic brain injury: Individuals who sustain a major amputation as a result of trauma may also sustain a concomitant traumatic brain injury due to the extreme forces involved during the event (Sheehan, 2011). One-third of service members who sustained a major limb loss in the Iraq and Afghanistan wars also sustained a traumatic brain injury (Pasquina & Cooper, 2009). Clinical treatment team members should routinely evaluate for concomitant injuries as a component of a comprehensive evaluation. Codes under b1 Mental Functions can be used to report the observed deficits. See the TBI diagnosis chapter for information on how to assess other deficits when a TBI is associated with an amputation.

Post-traumatic stress disorder (PTSD): Individuals who sustain a major amputation as a result of trauma are predisposed to a comorbidity of PTSD (Huang, 2011). One-fourth of service members who sustained a major limb loss in the Iraq and Afghanistan wars were also diagnosed with PTSD (Pasquina & Cooper, 2009). A retrospective study of 1369 clients with burn trauma in Ankara, Turkey, revealed 45 individuals who were subsequently diagnosed with a psychiatric disorder. Of the 45 individuals dually diagnosed, six sustained limb amputations. The psychiatric disorders, with frequency of occurrence, were listed as PTSD, 12 (26.6%); delirium, 11 (24.4%); anxiety disorder, eight (17.7%); depression,

seven (15.5%); PTSD and depression, two (4.4%); PTSD and delirium, two (4.4%); PTSD and anxiety disorder, one (2.2%); withdrawal syndrome, one (2.2%); and schizoaffective disorder, one (2.2%) (Yabanoglu et al., 2012). The whole treatment team should be aware of the increased potential for psychological complications and actively monitor individuals who have sustained an amputation. When clinical depression, anxiety disorders, or adjustment disorders are identified, a comprehensive treatment plan should be initiated, with cognitive behavioral psychotherapy and pharmacotherapy as needed (Huang, 2011). See the PTSD diagnosis chapter for information on how to assess deficits when PTSD is associated with an amputation.

Psychosocial stressors: If the amputation, regardless of the etiology, is significant enough to cause major life changes, psychosocial stressors can be expected. Identification of the psychosocial stressors has been documented in many publications. Some include coping with pain, level of disability, adequacy of cosmesis (restoration of appearance), cultural issues, presence of social supports, the reactions of caregivers and other loved ones, and a client's preamputation coping style (Bhuvaneswar et al., 2007). Some of the codes that may be affected are b280 Sensation of Pain, d2 General Tasks and Demands, d4 Mobility, d5 Self-Care, d6 Domestic Life, d7 Interpersonal Interactions and Relationships, d8 Major Life Areas, d9 Community, Social, and Civic Life, e3 Support and Relationships, and e4 Attitudes.

Good quality comprehensive healthcare systems recognize and provide education, counseling, and support for clients experiencing these stressors. A high percentage of service members who sustained a major limb loss in the Iraq and Afghanistan wars experiences "a significant number of psychosocial stresses that may complicate rehabilitation… [H]ealthcare providers must be sensitive to these needs and develop strategies to help mitigate their negative effects on recovery and community reintegration" (Pasquina & Cooper, 2009, p. xii).

Clinicians and researchers have continually attempted to identify and provide individuals with strategies and skills to mitigate psychosocial stressors. One such attempt was a research study completed with 120 individuals with transtibial and transfemoral lower limb amputations with a primary etiology of peripheral arterial disease (PAD) who had undergone an inpatient rehabilitation stay in Scotland. Research was conducted to determine if psychological variables would predict prosthetic use and activity utilizing Leventhal's Common Sense Self-Regulation Model (CS-SRM), a social cognition model in health psychology (Callaghan & Johnston 2008). Several significant CS-SRM models emerged for predicting prosthetic use and activity limitations, which may be helpful to the treatment team during the rehabilitation process. At six months post-discharge, factors influencing more prosthetic use indoors included: (1) physical symptoms that fluctuated less, (2) belief that treatment would be effective in controlling their condition, and (3) outdoor use was affected primarily by emotional and psychological factors (e.g., stress, mental attitude, personality, etc.). At six months post-discharge, factors influencing more hours per day of outdoor prosthetic use included: (1) physical symptoms that fluctuated less, (2) condition was not caused by risk factors (e.g., diet, overwork, smoking, etc.), but was caused by emotional and psychological factors (e.g., stress, mental attitude, personality, etc.). Lastly, at one month post-discharge, factors influencing mobility and independence (basic and advanced) included: people with amputations who perceived during rehabilitation (1) their physical symptoms fluctuated less, (2) their treatment would be effective in controlling their condition, (3) they had less negative emotional representations about their condition (e.g., worried, angry, afraid, etc.), and (4) their condition was caused by emotional and psychological factors (e.g., stress, mental attitude, personality, etc.) (Callaghan & Johnston, 2008). This research illuminates common areas of education clinicians can address during the rehabilitation process. Establishment and maintenance of a trusting relationship with the clinical care team is key to addressing psychosocial stressors (d7 Interpersonal Interactions and Relationships and e355 Health Professionals). Team members are encouraged to take an individualized approach with each client, as broad categories of common factors require narrowing to the specific concerns of the individual to be effectively addressed.

Pain: Pain after amputation is usually divided into four types: (1) acute post-surgical pain from the surgery itself, (2) phantom limb pain where the pain is experienced as if it were located in the amputated limb, (3) psychogenic pain in a non-amputated body part where no physical cause is found, and (4) painful residual limb where the pain in the residual limb has an identified cause (Esquenazi, 2003). The medical team addresses the first area and the prosthetic team addresses the fourth area. The second and third are addressed below. Asking the client for a definitive description of pain history, source, frequency, duration, location(s), and intensity is part of providing effective treatment. Pain issues can be documented using b280 Sensation of Pain.

Phantom sensation: The sensation that an amputated limb is still there is called phantom sensation (no pain, just sensation). In the ICF these would be described using b265 Touch Function and b270 Sensory Functions Related to Temperature and Other Stimuli. There are three theories as to why clients experience phantom limb pain and/or phantom limb sensation (Chapman, 2011). One theory is that the remaining nerves continue to generate impulses. Another is that the spinal cord nerves begin excessive spontaneous firing in the absence of expected sensory input from the limb. The third theory is that there is an altered signal transmission and modulation within the somatosensory cortex. Individuals with first-time amputations are not always educated about phantom sensation despite its common occurrence. Its incidence ranges from 50% to 90% (Ephraim et al., 2005; Kern et al., 2009). Because the origin remains unclear, many treatments are currently being utilized and researched. Some approaches include anticonvulsants (Bone et al., 2002), relaxation techniques (Ketz, 2008), contralateral local anesthesia (Casale et al., 2009), opiates (Wilder-Smith et al., 2005), injections with botulinum toxin (Jin et al., 2009), and electromagnetic stump lining (Kern et al., 2006). Neurophysiological treatments are also implemented, such as mirror visual feedback (Kim & Kim, 2012), sensory discrimination training (Moseley & Wiech, 2009), virtual integrated environment (Alphonso et al., 2012), and virtual mental exercises (Cole et al., 2009). Despite the many approaches to management of phantom limb sensation, it remains a problem for many people with amputations. It is considered a critical component of comprehensive client education during rehabilitation after an amputation.

Infection: The prevalence and incidence of infection of the amputated limb is unknown. Post-surgical wound infections of 127 patients who underwent major lower limb amputations were reported as common (34.6%) by a study in the United Kingdom (Coulston et al., 2012). When looking at individuals who have passed the acute phase of amputation in a study looking for determinants of skin problems of the stump in people with lower-limb amputations, the 805 completed questionnaires revealed six percent of the individuals had an skin infection actively or within the prior one-month period (Meulenbelt et al., 2009). Infection is a potential problem at the incision site if it is not well cleaned and cared for after surgery. Once the incision site is fully dry and healed, the entire stump site remains at an increased risk for infection as residual limbs tend to harbor more abundant bacterial flora than unaffected limbs (Braddom & Chan, 2011). The successful use of a prosthesis requires good skin integrity, yet the skin of a residual limb is not adapted to the heat, humidity, friction, and pressure resulting from prosthesis use (Munoz et al., 2008). Some skin problems, including infections following amputation, appear inevitable. Prosthetic adjustments, oral and/or topical medication, dressings, and advice to modify the use of the prosthesis can all prevent and treat skin disorders including infections (Dudek et al., 2006). This highlights the necessity of a multidisciplinary approach to the ongoing care of people with amputations. Problems with the skin would be coded with s8 Skin and Related Structures and b8 Functions of the Skin and Related Structures.

Edema: Edema (or swelling) is a natural occurrence after any trauma to tissue, including surgery. Following an amputation, the residual limb will be swollen. The degree of swelling can be recorded using b435 Immunological System Functions or s410 Structure of Cardiovascular System and s420 Structure of Immune System. The residual limb will benefit from effective edema management with resulting expedited healing time (Pasquina & Cooper, 2009). Management of the edema is critical to successful management of the pain and the eventual shape of the limb. Creating a "good shape" facilitates a good fit of a prosthesis, which in turn facilitates good functional use (Latlief et al., 2012). Beyond use of medication and properly elevated positioning of the limb, management of edema is commonly done in two ways: application of a rigid cast immediately following surgery while in the operating room (the

less common of the two techniques) or application of an ace bandage (worn 24 hours per day) (Meier & Atkins, 2004; Pasquina & Cooper, 2009). Alternatively, an UE limb may have a double layer of Tubigrip® applied rather than an ace bandage (Meier & Atkins, 2004). Ace bandages are applied to the limb to a point above the knee for transtibial amputations, to the hip (and possibly around the entire pelvis) for transfemoral amputations, to a point above the elbow for transradial amputations, to the shoulder (and possibly around the chest) for transhumeral amputations (Meier & Atkins, 2004). The level of wrapping is critical for optimal edema management. The technique is also critical for successful shaping of the limb (Latlief et al., 2012). After the staples are removed and the skin can tolerate the pressure generated from the application, a properly fitting "stump shrinker" can be used instead of Ace wraps on a limb. Many people report this to be an easier method to manage the edema versus Ace wrapping. Some report elastic compression as superior to the use of a stump shrinker for edema management (Meier & Atkins, 2004). At the time of initial fitting and training with a pylon, edema fluctuations can be a hindrance to donning the pylon. Some techniques utilized to optimize reduction of edema include wrapping the stump with an Ace bandage and applying the socket liner over the wrap and application of a semi-rigid dressing (also referred to as Unna paste or boot) (Wong & Edelstein, 2000). P. G. Unna, a German dermatologist, developed Unna paste, a compound of zinc oxide, gelatin, glycerin, and calamine in 1850 (Barnes & Cox, 2000). "Unna-booting" is a technique utilized by a physical therapist in conjunction with a physiatrist. A small study of 21 people with amputations showed Unna semirigid dressings are more effective in fostering amputation limb wound healing and preparing the amputation limb for prosthetic fitting and those same subjects treated were more likely to be fitted with prostheses and to return home walking with a prosthesis (Wong & Edelstein, 2000).

A residual limb's volume (edema) also changes throughout the day with the largest fluctuations occurring in the early stages following the amputation. Typically, there is a pattern of reduced fluctuations as the time from surgery passes. Part of the reason a person is provided with a "pylon" or "check socket" (an easily adjustable prosthesis) is to allow for wearing and use of a prosthesis while the limb size is regulated. In fact, a positive feedback cycle is fostered with prosthetic use. The more the person uses a prosthesis, the more the residual limb attains a consistent size and volume, which in turn facilitates increased use of the prosthesis. During inpatient rehabilitation, clients are typically taught how to "manage socks" to accommodate fluctuations in residual limb volume with the goal of effective fit of the prosthesis at all times, regardless of the residual limb volume size (DeLisa et al., 2005). Once a client's volume changes are within a few sock plies throughout a day with little to no impact on the person's ability to don the prosthesis, and both the alignment and the fit of the prosthesis facilitate functional gait patterns, a permanent prosthesis is fabricated and issued to the patient (DeLisa et al., 2005). This process usually takes several months post inpatient rehabilitation (DeLisa et al., 2005). In summary, the early protection and compression of residual limbs has been shown to improve and accelerate prosthetic fit (Duwayri et al., 2012).

Contractures: Contractures of the hip and particularly the knee joint are frequent complications for people with new amputations. These can be recorded using b7 Neuromusculoskeletal and Movement-Related Functions. Contractures are usually the result of poor positioning following the amputation along with lack of movement through the full range of motion (a lack of remobilization) (Braddom & Chan, 2011). Correct positioning must be taught and implemented consistently post surgery (Braddom & Chan, 2011). Furthermore, transtibial amputation generally requires knee support to avoid flexion contracture while the wound is healing (Duwayri et al., 2012). Prone lying for people with LE amputations is a useful technique to reduce the chance of developing contractures (Braddom & Chan, 2011). Performing range of motion exercises as least once daily is another recommended technique (DeLisa et al., 2005). Inadequate range of motion caused by contractures can affect prosthetic fit and activity performance (Kelly, 2009).

Deconditioning: Deconditioning is a very common problem for people with an amputation. General deconditioning is included in b455 Exercise Tolerance Functions and b730-b749 Muscle Functions. Codes for specific problems may also need to be added. Acute rehabilitation goals for all disciplines typically include increasing muscle power, range of movement, core stability, stamina, and cardiovascular endurance for clients following an amputation (Cumming et al., 2006). Individuals with unilateral traumatic transtibial amputations use approximately 25% more energy to walk the same distance as people without amputations. People with traumatic transfemoral amputations use 63% more energy. People with vascular transtibial amputations use 40% more energy and people with transfemoral amputations use up to 120% more energy (Braddom & Chan, 2011). With the well-documented increased energy demands post amputation, optimizing an individual's overall health is a key to successful functioning with an amputation. Additionally, therapists must be aware that sustaining the increased energy demands may be difficult and result in increased sedentary behavior, further contributing to deconditioning and related issues.

Dermatologic problems: Skin breakdown (ulcers), contact dermatitis, sebaceous cysts, verrucous hyperplasia, infections, and hyperhidrosis are common skin management issues for the individual with an amputation (Braddom & Chan, 2011). Problems with the skin would be coded with s8 Skin and Related Structures and b8 Functions of the Skin and Related Structures. A six-year retrospective chart review of skin lesions diagnosed in patients with amputations examined in a specialty outpatient clinic at a regional, referral rehabilitation hospital in Ottawa, Canada, found 528 skin problems in 337 lower extremity residual limbs. Of those documented skin problems, ulcers, irritations (an area of erythema over a pressure-sensitive area that persists for at least 10 minutes after removal of the prosthetic device), inclusion (sebaceous) cysts, calluses, and verrucous hyperplasia were the five most common skin problems representing 79.5% of all documented skin disorders (Dudek et al., 2006). A study of 247 Vietnam veterans reported recurring stump site dermatoses prevalence rate ranging from 34% to 74% among individuals with major amputations occurring at least 38 years prior to the study (Yang et al., 2012). Another large retrospective study of 745 Canadian individuals with lower extremity amputations documented skin problems in 40.7% of those who functionally used a prosthesis (Dudek et al., 2005). Verrucous hyperplasia (papillomatosis cutis lymphostatica) is the development of a wart-like lesion on the end of a residual limb, mostly occurring with transtibial amputations. The pathophysiology remains unknown (Wlotzke et al., 1997). This dysplastic skin condition is thought to be due to a choking effect on the residual limb and is treated with the addition of distal pressure from the socket; resolution normally occurs in a few weeks or months (Braddom & Chan, 2011). The fabrication of a new total contact socket may be another option for resolution (Dudek et al., 2006). The liner, socks, and suspension mechanism are the usual culprits for contact dermatitis, a condition of skin inflammation and mild edema. The socket is a less likely cause. Treatment requires removal or adjustment of the offending item and appropriate treatment (e.g., topical cream). Cysts and sweating can be a sign of excessive shear forces and components that need adjustments. This should be brought to the attention of the prosthetist (Kelly, 2009). Hyperhidrosis or excessive sweating of a residual limb after amputation is one of the most common reasons for impaired prosthesis use and poorer quality of life. It affects 30-50% of all people with amputations, causing skin irritation in about 25% (Kern et al., 2012). This issue is seen with all types of prosthetic suspension and liner materials. Alleviation can be an ongoing challenge for the individual and treatment team. It can be minimized with sock changes or, when indicated, with antiperspirants like CertainDry® or prescription medications like Drysol™ (Amputee Coalition of America, 2004). One case series (Charrow et al., 2008) and a small study of nine people with amputations (Kern et al., 2012) showed promise with the use of botulinum toxin for alleviating this symptom. It is useful to note the same treatment has been studied for reduction of phantom limb pain and suboptimal frequency of prosthetic use. Skin breakdown is also referred to as ulceration. Over 80% of skin ulcers were thought to be caused by poor prosthetic fit in the Canadian study evaluating the etiology of skin problems after amputations (Dudek et al., 2006). Ulceration can be prevented or reduced by client education in proper socket fit, control of the volume of the residual limb, stump sock management, prosthetic alignment, skin disease management, wearing tolerance of the skin for the prosthesis (Braddom & Chan, 2011; Dudek et al., 2006; Sanders & Fatone, 2011), and stabilization of the individual's weight (Dudek et al., 2006). Routine follow up by a multidisciplinary treatment team to ensure good prosthetic fit and residual limb care is critical. A physician should be contacted immediately for any skin breakdown. Recurring residual limb dermatoses often prevent the regular use of the prosthesis and even lead to prosthesis abandonment (Yang et al., 2012).

Neuromas: Neuromas occur at the end of injured nerve fibers as a form of ineffective, unregulated nerve regeneration. It occurs most commonly near a scar, either superficially (skin, subcutaneous fat) or deep (e.g., after a cholecystectomy) (Huang, 2011; Murdoch & Wilson, 1996). Neuroma formation in amputation surgery is inevitable — all transected nerves form neuromas. Not all neuromas are symptomatic, but painful conditions should be reported with b280 Sensation of Pain. Persistent symptoms associated with neuromas have been reported in approximately 20% to 30% of amputations (Pasquina & Cooper, 2009), and the majority of these can be managed without revision surgery. Prosthetic socket adjustments (e.g., moving the socket wall away from the area of pain) commonly relieves neuroma pain (Huang, 2011). If this is unsuccessful, neuropathic pain medication; intralesional steroid and anesthetic injection; or neuroma ablation with phenol, alcohol, or cryoablation can provide pain relief (Huang, 2011). Ultrasound-guided phenol instillation has been shown in a small case series to provide some benefit in the treatment of neuroma pain (Gruber et al., 2008) and in two case studies treatment using dehydrated alcohol solution gave significant benefit without need for analgesics (Lim et al., 2012).

Prognosis

No overall discussion of prognosis is possible because of the wide range of causes of amputations and severities of the amputation. Discussions in other sections of this chapter point out the risk factors associated with particular etiologies.

Assessment

Typical Scope of Team Assessment

The surgical team will determine whether the person is sufficiently stable medically to undergo amputation surgery (non-traumatic cause). This is decided upon after extensive lab work, a physical exam, and testing reports. For people who have had a traumatic amputation, the emergency medical team will evaluate the current situation and respond in the appropriate manner.

Once the amputation is completed, the amputation will be formally classified, as the surgeon cannot know the extent of the amputation until the site is opened and diseased bodily tissue has been clearly seen. All attempts are made to save as many joints as possible during surgery (Pasquina & Cooper, 2009). Prosthetic joints do not function as well as natural joints, so functional skills and independence are greater for those who are able to keep major joints. Amputations are classified by the location of the amputation and the percent of the remaining limb as described at the beginning of this chapter (Esquenazi, 2004; Frontera & DeLisa, 2010; Meier & Atkins, 2004).

In some cases clients will not be candidates for a prosthesis. There are several variables to consider. The client with a lower extremity amputation must have sufficient cardiopulmonary capacity, adequate wound healing, good soft tissue coverage, good active range of motion, muscle strength, motor control, adequate learning ability to achieve successful use of a prosthesis, upper body strength, static and dynamic balance, and adequate posture to be successful with a prosthesis (Amputee Coalition of America, 2004; Kelly, 2009). Individuals with severe coronary artery disease, severe polyneuropathy, multiple-joint arthritis, short life expectancy, and/or significant fluctuations in body weight are not typically candidates for a prosthesis (Gitter & Bosker, 2005). ICF codes that may be used to document these abilities and deficits include b1 Mental Functions; b2 Sensory Functions and Pain; b4 Functions of the Cardiovascular, Hematological, Immunological, and Respiratory Systems; b7 Neuromusculoskeletal and Movement-Related Functions; and b8 Functions of the Skin and Related Structures. Body Structure codes may also be used by the treatment team.

Once basic ambulatory skills are achieved, stability, ease of movement, energy efficiency, and the appearance of a natural gait are possible (Vining Radomski & Trombly Latham, 2008). Other important areas to document include the level of amputation, the expected function of the prosthesis, the cognitive level of the client, the client's vocation, the client's recreation and leisure interests, the cosmetic importance of the prosthesis, the client's financial resources, and the client's desire to wear a prosthesis (Kelly, 2009; Meier & Atkins, 2004; Zidarov et al., 2009). ICF codes discussed in the Systems Affected and Secondary Problems sections should be used here, as appropriate.

Areas of Concern for RT Assessment

In addition to the issues described above, the initial evaluation of a person with a newly acquired amputation will most often reflect the following deficits in both the pre-prosthetic and the prosthetic training stages of rehabilitation.

Deconditioning: This may be due to comorbidities resulting in a commonly seen gradual decline in function prior to an amputation, the activity restrictions after surgery, and/or premorbid lifestyle behaviors. People who have had an amputation due to a disease process such as diabetes typically have a higher rate of sedentary behavior than the normal population. Appropriate ICF codes were discussed earlier.

Impaired sense of self: A physical piece of the person is gone after an amputation. The person does not look the same. Body-image anxiety and social discomfort have been pointed out as frequent consequences of a lower limb amputation (Senra et al., 2012). Having an altered physical appearance can be an impetus for self-identity changes related to limb loss. To explore adults' experiences of lower limb amputation, focusing on the changes in self-identity related to the impairment, a cross-sectional and qualitative study of 42 adults with lower-limb amputations was conducted in Portugal (Senra et al., 2012). Eight themes emerged from interviews: (1) reactions and feelings about having an amputation, (2) changes in own life, (3) problems in well-being, (4) relation with the prosthesis, (5) self-perceptions, (6) aims related to the rehabilitation and future plans, (7) relation with the rehabilitation, and (8) perceived social support. Understanding the types of changes in self-identity following amputation will assist the treatment team in comprehensively evaluating and treating the client with an amputation.

It is recommended that every patient who has an amputation be evaluated by an experienced psychologist including an assessment of past psychological problems, alcohol and drug use, mood, coping skills, body image issues, and sexuality (Huang,

2011). When there is a negative impact to the person's sense of self, it seems to be related to the existence of the amputation. A study comparing people with unilateral and bilateral leg amputations showed this change to body image does not seem to change with the number of amputations (i.e., two amputation were not found to cause more of an impact than one). However, quality of life scores and satisfaction with prostheses do increase in parallel with the use of prostheses (Akarsu et al., 2013).

Effective coping with the psychological changes from an amputation can be improved when the client becomes successfully engaged in activities (Amputee Coalition of America, 2004; Zidarov et al., 2009). Peer support can be invaluable to build and strengthen a healthy sense of self following an amputation (Amputee Coalition of America, 2004).

An uncommon yet serious development can be clinical depression (Machado Vaz et al., 2012) or even suicide (Llorente & Malphurs, 2008). All people who have sustained an amputation deserve assistance with the psychological recovery process, including education about coping and grief. Signs of clinical depression or suicidal ideation should be brought to the attention of the treatment team immediately.

As common as an altered sense of self may be among those with amputations, some individuals studied have reported a different experience. These clients appraised the amputation positively and reported fewer losses and changes in their self-identity domains (Senra et al., 2012). Even though they did not represent the larger portion of clients who had an amputation, there is a group of clients who tend to report less pain, more social functioning, and fewer health concerns, as the literature has stressed (Couture et al., 2011).

The ICF codes used for these issues come from Activities and Participation. Important personal ones include d2 General Tasks and Demands, d4 Mobility, d5 Self-Care, and d6 Domestic Life. Interpersonal concerns should be documented with d7 Interpersonal Interactions and Relationships; d8 Major Life Areas; and d9 Community, Social, and Civic Life.

Lack of awareness and knowledge: Individuals who are experiencing amputation for the first time will not know how to use a prosthesis or how to use it in functional tasks. Even persons with a second amputation will need to learn how to perform tasks with two prostheses — a different skill set from using

one. Knowledge that needs to be acquired usually is part of b7 Neuromusculoskeletal and Movement-Related Functions or d4 Mobility.

Challenges in the environment: If there are concerns about the environment the client will be living in, a variety of ICF codes in e1 Products and Technology; e2 Natural Environment and Human-Made Changes to Environment; e3 Support and Relationships; e4 Attitudes; or e5 Services, Systems, and Policies may additionally be used to address contextual factors related to the attainment of a healthy active lifestyle.

ICF Core Set

An ICF Core Set for Amputation is currently in development. For more information go to http://www.icf-research-branch.org/icf-core-sets-projects-sp-1641024398/other-health-conditions/icf-core-set-for-persons-following-an-amputation.

Treatment Direction

The military healthcare system is shifting from the traditional medical model of disease-specific care to a more comprehensive, systemic, and holistic model that treats the individual and the family together. The "treatment plan is individualized to address all existing issues simultaneously in an integrated fashion, rather than waiting for one problem to be resolved before addressing the next" (Pasquina & Cooper, 2009, p. xii).

The therapist is likely to see the person with an amputation in three different situations: pre-prosthetic training, prosthetic training, and community settings. The person's needs will be different in each. While the treatment is geared toward the specific functional and emotional needs of the person at each phase, the therapist also has an opportunity to provide continuity in treatment in areas such as balancing leisure activities, increasing resource awareness, and helping polish the client's problem solving skills.

Pre-Prosthetic versus Prosthetic Training

Amputation rehabilitation is typically divided into two stays:

- *Pre-prosthetic training*: During this stay, the client is taught how to care for the residual limb and how to function without the limb. The client is then discharged until the incision site is fully healed (about three months). Once the incision site is fully healed, the client is readmitted to rehabilitation for prosthetic training.

- *Prosthetic training*: At this stage the client is able to wear a prosthesis and learns how to incorporate it into functional tasks.

Pre-Prosthetic Training

The goal of pre-prosthetic training is to teach the client how to function without a limb. As listed by Sheehan (2011), the focus of the immediate post-amputation period is to control pain and edema, promote wound healing, prevent contractures, initiate remobilization, continue supportive counseling for management of expectations, and provide education, including orientation to prosthetics, as indicated.

Whole Team Approach

The client learns how to: function without the limb; perform activities of daily living such as dressing and bathing; develop the skills needed for a form of mobility (typically a wheelchair, crutches, or a standard walker for a lower extremity amputation, no device for an upper extremity amputation); develop a home exercise program that promotes and improves active range-of-motion throughout all joints, especially in the residual limb; and gain muscular and cardiopulmonary strength (Amputee Coalition of America, 2004). A program to desensitize the residual limb for the prosthesis is initiated and taught to the client (Esquenazi, 2004). The skin on the bottom of the residual limb is very sensitive to pressure. Gentle tapping on the distal end of the residual limb is helpful in desensitizing the residual limb. The client is also taught to massage the residual limb to prevent excessive scar formation and wrap the residual limb with an Ace wrap in a figure-eight pattern (Latlief et al., 2012) to control edema and promote the development of a properly shaped distal stump that will fit correctly into a prosthesis (Esquenazi, 2004; Meier & Atkins, 2004). These treatments cover problems documented with ICF codes b280 Sensation of Pain, b7 Neuromusculoskeletal and Movement-Related Functions, d4 Mobility, and d5 Self-Care.

Recreational Therapy Approach

During inpatient rehabilitation for pre-prosthetic training, the primary focus is on the development of a healthy lifestyle for the time between pre-prosthetic training and prosthetic training. If a client is not a candidate for a prosthesis, the following interventions are also appropriate. The major goals include having the client maintain an active lifestyle, so that wearing prosthesis will be physically possible. An active lifestyle also promotes emotional health (including motivation, self-confidence, and adjustment to disability), which makes it more likely that the client will choose to go to the effort of learning to use a prosthesis. RTs are addressing concerns noted in ICF codes d2 General Tasks and Demands; d4 Mobility; d5 Self-Care; d7 Interpersonal Interactions and Relationships; d8 Major Life Areas; and d9 Community, Social, and Civic Life. Environmental factors may also be addressed at this time.

Recreational Therapy Interventions — Pre-Prosthetic

The following interventions are commonly used for clients with amputations during the pre-prosthetic rehabilitation stay:

Functional Skill Development

- *Residual limb care*: Educate the client about the importance of caring for his/her residual limb within activities (e.g., being careful that the residual limb does not get bumped, scraped, or injured during activities) (d570 Looking After One's Health). Damage to the skin will lengthen the healing period and prolong the person's waiting period to wear a prosthesis. Skin openings could lead to infection. Residual limb care typically includes skin care, skin inspection, desensitization, skin mobilization, and stump wrapping (d520 Caring for Body Parts, d540 Dressing). It is also important to educate the person regarding how to identify problems and when to contact medical care providers (Esquenazi, 2004; Sanders, 1986).

- *Movement and range of motion*: The client must understand the importance of, and participate in, regular physical activities (d570 Looking After One's Health, especially d5701 Managing Diet and Fitness) that allow for the range of motion of all joints (b710 Mobility of Joint Functions, d4 Mobility). The physical activities may be a prescribed set of range of motion exercises or leisure activities (d920 Recreation and Leisure) that provide the same result. There are some special issues for lower limb amputations (Esquenazi, 2004; Ham & Cotton, 1991). When in a seated position, the residual limb should be supported with the knee straight to prevent knee contractures. When supine, the residual limb should be straight, not propped up on pillows, to prevent hip contractures. Lying in a prone position may also help prevent hip contractures. Recreational therapists can help clients to identify activities that can be performed lying prone to make the time pass more easily and increase the chance the client will perform the proper exercises.

- *Mobility*: Mobility (d4 Mobility) is an issue for all amputations. A client who has had a LE amputation will probably use a wheelchair as his/her primary mode of mobility before s/he gets a prosthesis (d450-d469 Walking and Moving). A client with an UE amputation will probably be able to walk unless other health conditions are present. Other aspects of the ICF's d4 Mobility code, such as d445 Hand and Arm Use apply to UE amputations. Address mobility skills related to play, leisure, recreation, and community engagement (e.g., community wheelchair skills, energy conservation techniques) to foster engagement in active, healthy activities post discharge for continued recovery, health promotion, and quality of life.

- *Cardiopulmonary endurance and muscle strength*: Identify forms of physical activity that are realistic for post-discharge participation and develop the skills and the desire so the client will be able to function with a prosthesis. Use activity-based interventions that enhance cardiopulmonary endurance (b455 Exercise Tolerance Functions) and muscle strength (b730 Muscle Power Functions), as these are commonly compromised due to amputation-related health conditions, hospitalization, and/or decreased physical activity.

- *Activity adaptation*: Adapt or modify play, leisure, recreation, and community activities to accommodate the client's current abilities and limitations. If the client is coming back for prosthetic training, only focus on adapting activities that will be performed between rehabili-

tation stays. (Choose ICF codes as they relate to the specific activity.)

Education and Counseling

Common topics related to optimizing health include:

- *Inactivity*: Individuals with a new amputation, especially a LE amputation, tend to significantly reduce their activity level after the pre-prosthetic rehabilitation stay for various reasons, such as fear of falling, mobility restrictions, activity participation barriers, and increased energy expenditure (b455 Exercise Tolerance Functions). Consequently, it is not uncommon for clients to self-limit activity engagement and opt for a more a sedentary lifestyle during the healing process (d570 Looking After One's Health). Significantly limiting activity engagement can have profound consequences on holistic health, as well as the person's future ability to wear a prosthetic. Sedentary behavior results in deconditioning which can impact cardiopulmonary endurance, muscle strength, and joint mobility through formation of contractures. To minimize these problems, clients are educated about the consequences of inactivity and the impact it can have on reaching personal and rehabilitation goals. Engaging in activities reduces the tendency to be inactive and keep the prosthesis fitting by maintaining or even reducing body weight (Zidarov et al., 2009) (d570 Looking After One's Health). If a person gains significant weight post fitting with a prosthesis, a common occurrence when a person stops being active, the prosthesis will eventually not fit.

- *Barriers*: Participating in an active leisure lifestyle that includes community activities is necessary for emotional health (Zidarov et al., 2009) (d7 Interpersonal Interactions and Relationships, d8 Major Life Areas, d910 Community Life). Feeling stuck in the home and staring at the same four walls every day can have a devastating effect on a client's emotional health. Social isolation is a significant problem following an acquired physical disability (Zidarov et al., 2009). Suicide is a rare yet realistic concern post amputation (Amputee Coalition of America, 2004). Development of an activity pattern that promotes cardiopulmonary health via a well-rounded leisure lifestyle contributes significantly to the promise of a healthy and happy life with a significantly reduced chance of being limited by barriers (Amputee Coalition of America, 2004).

Prosthetic Training

The goal of prosthetic training is to teach the client how to operate a prosthetic and incorporate it into life activities.

Whole Team Approach

The person begins prosthetic training once the incision site is fully dry and healed. Individuals typically receive inpatient rehabilitation for initial prosthetic training, followed by several months of outpatient or in-home therapy. Prosthetic training focuses on achieving a proper prosthetic fit and maximizing a client's ability to perform tasks using a prosthesis (d4 Mobility). Once the person is cleared to weight bear on the stump, a wearing schedule is developed that gradually increases the length of time the prosthesis is worn (e.g., one hour on, one hour off; two hours on, two hours off). This allows the stump to desensitize to the pressure and the skin to toughen (Esquenazi, 2004; Meier & Atkins, 2004). Clients are taught how to care for the prosthesis, as well as proper techniques to: don and doff prosthesis (d540 Dressing); check the residual limb for signs of skin breakdown (d570 Looking After One's Health); perform functional transfers and mobility skills (d4 Mobility); address psychosocial adjustment issues (d240 Handling Stress and Other Psychological Demands); and learn the skills and resources necessary to lead an optimally healthy, productive, and fulfilling life (d7 Interpersonal Interactions and Relationships; d8 Major Life Areas; d9 Community, Social, and Civic Life). Good skin/stump care is an essential component of maintaining independence (Huang, 2011). Should skin breakdown occur, the client may not be able to wear the prosthesis for a period of time, possibly resulting in secondary problems such as deconditioning.

Recreational Therapy Approach

The primary focus is on the development of an optimally healthy lifestyle after prosthetic training for health promotion and prevention of disability and illness. To achieve this, the person requires education, training, and counseling related to the use and functional incorporation of the prosthesis into home and community tasks (d5 Self-Care; d6 Domestic Life; d7 Interpersonal Interactions and Relationships; d8 Major Life Areas; d9 Community, Social, and Civic Life) (Esquenazi, 2004; Zidarov et al., 2009).

Recreational Therapy Interventions — Prosthetic

In addition to carrying over interventions from the pre-prosthetic stage, as appropriate, the following interventions are commonly used for individuals with amputations during the prosthetic training rehabilitation stay.

Functional Skill Development

- *Limb and prosthesis care*: Care issues include the parts of the prosthesis, how to operate and maintain a prosthesis, how to put on and take off a prosthesis, how to incorporate the prosthesis into functional activities, how to inspect the skin on the residual limb for irritation and breakdown, how to adjust the fit of a prosthesis, how to choose and apply sock plies and other liners, abilities and restrictions related to specific activities, specialized adaptive equipment to enhance activity participation, and problem solving techniques (Esquenazi, 2004; Meier & Atkins, 2004). These skills are related to ICF codes d4 Mobility, d540 Dressing, d570 Looking After One's Health, d6504 Maintaining Assistive Devices, and e1 Products and Technology.

- *Bilateral integration*: It can be difficult for a client to use a prosthesis in activities because it lacks sensory feedback about its position and cannot be controlled as easily as an intact limb. Incorporating the prosthesis into activities promotes movement of the residual limb and maintains muscle and joint integrity, as well as contributing to independence and functioning (Esquenazi, 2004; Sanders, 1986). Examples of working on bilateral integration include shooting billiards while standing and walking (using both legs) or making a craft project (using both arms). Bilateral integration includes coordination (b760 Control of Voluntary Movement Functions), balance (b755 Involuntary Movement Reaction Functions, d415 Maintaining a Body Position), shifting weight from one lower extremity to the other (d4106 Shifting the Body's Center of Gravity), and other tasks included under d4 Mobility (d430 Lifting and Carrying Objects, d440 Fine Hand Use, d445 Hand and Arm Use, d450 Walking, and specific sports movements, e.g., d4554 Swimming).

- *Postural control and alignment*: Individuals may have poor posture (d415 Maintaining a Body Position) when using a prosthesis in functional tasks as a way to compensate for comorbidities, decreased range of motion, decreased muscle strength, decreased endurance, decreased sensation, poor prosthetic fit, limb contractures, discomfort, awkwardness, and lack of skill (Esquenazi, 2004; Pasquina & Cooper, 2009). If proper body alignments and postures are not maintained, secondary problems may occur, such as back and hip pain, and functional abilities may not be fully maximized (Amputee Coalition of America, 2004). Therapists teach the person how to incorporate proper posture into activities. Treatment outcomes can be scored under one of the codes in b750-b789 Movement Functions or d4 Mobility. Therapists also teach the person about the impact of heel height on the alignment of the prosthetic leg. Clients are educated about the correct heel height for the prosthetic foot.

- *Sensory awareness and processing*: Prostheses do not provide a full sensory experience. Clients must learn to compensate for this decreased sensory input and learn how to optimize use of all of their senses to fully evaluate a situation. This includes judging the ground surface or weight of an item through sight and feeling the pressure on the residual limb warning the client of the need to readjust the fit of the prosthesis. This can be coded with d120 Other Purposeful Sensing.

- *Activity adaptation*: The person is taught how to adapt activities that will be part of the client's lifestyle after discharge. This is done for deficits noted in ICF codes under d9 Community, Social, and Civic Life, as well as other relevant Activity and Participation codes such as d5 Self-Care (e.g., changing into a swimsuit at the health club), d650 Caring for Household Objects (e.g., taking care of a pet), and d880 Engagement in Play. This may also include assisting a person with developing a deeper understanding of his/her leisure motivators. In some instances,

adaptation of the activity may not be appropriate (or acceptable to the client), in which case activity substitution and exploration of new leisure interests may be needed. Evaluation for assistive technology may also be needed (e1 Products and Technology) including device demonstrations and skill acquisition. For example long-handled gardening tools for a person with a bilateral transfemoral amputation or a mouse emulator for a person with a bilateral transhumeral amputation, may be needed (Esquenazi, 2004; Pasquina & Cooper, 2009).

Education and Counseling

Topics discussed during pre-prosthetic rehabilitation are expanded during the prosthetic training rehabilitation stay to cover the use of the prosthesis. These topics typically involve issues related to engagement in play, leisure, recreation, and community activities, such as consequences of inactivity, barriers, selecting appropriate and healthy activities, and integration back into the community. Other education and counseling topics include:

- *Energy conservation*: Since using a prosthetic increases cardiopulmonary demands, clients may find themselves becoming fatigued more quickly. Recreational therapists teach clients specific techniques for conserving energy to maximize continued activity participation. This may require clients to also monitor vital signs, adapt activities, and select methods of mobility that don't exceed their ability or compromise health, such as using a wheelchair for long community distances instead of a walker (Esquenazi, 2004; Vining Radomski & Trombly Latham, 2008). The related ICF code is d2303 Managing One's Own Activity Level.

- *Community problem solving*: This includes problem solving for activity-related skills in the community, such as making adjustments to the prosthetic and changing sock plies in a public setting, correlating activities with one's wearing schedule, problem solving for architectural barriers, and managing awkward social situations, such as shaking hands with a upper extremity prosthetic or responding to a child's question, "What happened to your leg?" (Esquenazi, 2004; Meier & Atkins, 2004). These are scored with codes in d460 Moving Around in Different Locations, d465 Moving Around Using Equipment, d470 Using Transportation, d570 Looking After One's Health, and d7 Interpersonal Interactions and Relationships.

- *Community mobility skills*: Individuals with amputations benefit from practicing community mobility skills that present unique challenges. Examples include climbing sloped surfaces and retrieving objects from low storage places with a LE amputation and pushing grocery carts and lawn mowers with an UE amputation (Esquenazi, 2004; Zidarov et al., 2009). Choose appropriate mobility-related codes such as d460 Moving Around in Different Locations, d465 Moving Around Using Equipment, and d470 Using Transportation, etc.

Community Settings

The recreational therapist is likely to see a client with an amputation in community-based sports or other recreation activities. The primary purpose of the intervention in the community is twofold: (1) ensuring adequate physical activity levels (d570 Looking After One's Health) and (2) helping to improve the client's access to leisure and recreation activities (d920 Recreation and Leisure) (Esquenazi, 2004; Pasquina & Cooper, 2009; Zidarov et al., 2009). Individuals with lower extremity amputations have a high risk of secondary complications because of inactivity (Amputee Coalition of America, 2004). Causes of this inactivity include comorbidities, lack of access to recreational therapy at the outpatient level of service causing reduced skill development and reduced knowledge of benefits and resources, and the extra energy required for mobility (Frontera & DeLisa, 2010). Recreation and leisure activity performance will be suboptimal unless the client experiences regular involvement in enjoyable physical activity promoting agility, balance, coordination, endurance, stretching, and strengthening (Ham & Cotton, 1991; Pasquina & Cooper, 2009; Sanders, 1986). Regular physical activity can increase cardiovascular endurance, mobility efficiency, and symmetry of gait (Amputee Coalition of America, 2004; James, 1973; Kelly, 2009). Access to leisure and recreation activities often involves helping the person identify activities that match the capabilities of his/her prosthesis or identifying specialty prosthetic devices required for specific activities. Many types of physical activities such as walking, riding a bike, or rowing, do not require specialized artificial limbs. Running and swimming are two common activities that may benefit from a specialized artificial limb (Esquenazi, 2004; Meier & Atkins, 2004; Pasquina & Cooper, 2009). Published literature is readily available identifying, describing, and even showing how to modify sports-related equipment and prosthetics for people with amputations (Bragaru, Dekker, & Geertzen, 2012; Bragaru, Dekker, Geertzen, & Dijkstra, 2011; Carroll, 2001). Most physical medicine and rehabilitation textbooks have a section about rehabilitation after an amputation that provides detailed descriptions and photographs of sports-related prosthetics (Braddom & Chan, 2011; DeLisa et al., 2005; Esquenazi & Meier, 1996; Pasquina & Cooper, 2009). In conclusion, manufacturers of sports-related equipment, disabled recreation and sporting associations/clubs, and recreation therapists possess critical knowledge, information, skills, and experience to assist people with amputations as they return to an active lifestyle. The physical benefits of community recreation can be demonstrated by documenting improvements in ICF codes b455 Exercise Tolerance Functions, b7 Neuromusculoskeletal and Movement-Related Functions, and d4 Mobility.

Resources

Amputee Coalition of America
9303 Center St, Suite 100
Manassas, VA 20110
888-AMP-KNOW (888-267-5669)
www.amputee-coalition.org
The Amputee Coalition is a national, non-profit amputee consumer educational organization.

OandP
3870 NW 83rd St
Gainesville, FL 32606
800-876-7740
www.oandp.com
An online information resource for orthotics and prosthetic information.

TRS, Inc. (sport prosthetics)
3090 Sterling Circle, Studio A
Boulder, Colorado 80301-2338
800-279-1865
www.trsprosthetics.com

A company that sells prosthetic adaptations for people with amputations.

References

Akarsu, S., Tekin, L., Safaz, I., Goktepe, A. S., & Yazicioglu, K. (2013). Quality of life and functionality after lower limb amputations: Comparison between uni- vs. bilateral amputee patients. *Prosthet Orthot Int, 37*(1), 9-13.

Alphonso, A. L., Monson, B. T., Zeher, M. J., Armiger, R. S., Weeks, S. R., Burck, J. M., … & Tsao, J. W. (2012). Use of a virtual integrated environment in prosthetic limb development and phantom limb pain. *Stud Health Technol Inform, 181*, 305-309.

Amputee Coalition of America. (2004). *Senior step.* Knoxville, TN: Amputee Coalition of America.

Anderson, J. J., Boone, J., Hansen, M., Spencer, L., & Fowler, Z. (2012). A comparison of diabetic smokers and non-smokers who undergo lower extremity amputation: A retrospective review of 112 patients. *Diabet Foot Ankle, 3*. doi: 10.3402/dfa.v3i0.19178.

Barnes, R. W. & Cox, B. (2000). *Amputations: An illustrated manual.* Philadelphia: Hanley and Belfus, Inc.

Bhuvaneswar, C. G., Epstein, L. A., & Stern, T. A. (2007). Reactions to amputation: Recognition and treatment. *Prim Care Companion J Clin Psychiatry, 9*(4), 303-308.

Bodeau, V. & Mipro, R. (2002a). Upper limb prosthetics. http://www.emedicine.com/pmr/ topic174.htm on 1/19/04.

Bodeau, V. & Mipro, R. (2002b). Lower limb prosthetics. http://www.emedicine.com/pmr/ topic175.htm on 1/19/04.

Bone, M., Critchley, P., & Buggy, D. J. (2002). Gabapentin in postamputation phantom limb pain: A randomized, double-blind, placebo-controlled, cross-over study. *Reg Anesth Pain Med, 27*(5), 481-486.

Boulton, A. J., Vileikyte, L., Ragnarson-Tennvall, G., & Apelqvist, J. (2005). The global burden of diabetic foot disease. *Lancet, 366*(9498), 1719-1724.

Braddom, R. L. & Chan, L. (2011). *Physical medicine and rehabilitation* (4th ed.). Philadelphia: Elsevier/Saunders.

Bradley, L. & Kirker, S. G. (2006). Secondary prevention of arteriosclerosis in lower limb vascular amputees: A missed opportunity. *Eur J Vasc Endovasc Surg, 32*(5), 491-493.

Bragaru, M., Dekker, R., & Geertzen, J. H. (2012). Sport prostheses and prosthetic adaptations for the upper and lower limb amputees: An overview of peer reviewed literature. *Prosthet Orthot Int, 36*(3), 290-296.

Bragaru, M., Dekker, R., Geertzen, J. H., & Dijkstra, P. U. (2011). Amputees and sports: A systematic review. *Sports Med, 41*(9), 721-740.

Brown, M. L., Tang, W., Patel, A., & Baumhauer, J. F. (2012). Partial foot amputation in patients with diabetic foot ulcers. *Foot Ankle Int, 33*(9), 707-716. doi: 10.3113/fai.2012.0707.

Callaghan, B., Condie, E., & Johnston, M. (2008). Using the common sense self-regulation model to determine psychological predictors of prosthetic use and activity limitations in lower limb amputees. *Prosthet Orthot Int, 32*(3), 324-336.

Carroll, K. (2001). Adaptive prosthetics for the lower extremity. *Foot Ankle Clin, 6*(2), 371-386.

Casale, R., Ceccherelli, F., Labeeb, A. A., & Biella, G. E. (2009). Phantom limb pain relief by contralateral myofascial injection with local anaesthetic in a placebo-controlled study: Preliminary results. *J Rehabil Med, 41*(6), 418-422.

Chapman, S. (2011). Pain management in patients following limb amputation. *Nurs Stand, 25*(19), 35-40.

Charrow, A., DiFazio, M., Foster, L., Pasquina, P. F., & Tsao, J. W. (2008). Intradermal botulinum toxin type A injection effectively reduces residual limb hyperhidrosis in amputees: A case series. *Arch Phys Med Rehabil, 89*(7), 1407-1409.

Cole, J., Crowle, S., Austwick, G., & Slater, D. H. (2009). Exploratory findings with virtual reality for phantom limb pain; From stump motion to agency and analgesia. *Disabil Rehabil, 31*(10), 846-854.

Condie, M. E., Scott, H., & Crosse, O. (2007). A survey of the lower limb amputee population in Scotland, 2005. Glasgow UK University of Strathclyde.

Coulston, J. E., Tuff, V., Twine, C. P., Chester, J. F., Eyers, P. S., & Stewart, A. H. (2012). Surgical factors in the prevention of infection following major lower limb amputation. *Eur J Vasc Endovasc Surg, 43*(5), 556-560.

Couture, M., Desrosiers, J., & Caron, C. D. (2011). Cognitive appraisal and perceived benefits of dysvascular lower limb amputation: A longitudinal study. *Arch Gerontol Geriatr, 52*(1), 5-11.

Cumming, J. C., Barr, S., & Howe, T. E. (2006). Prosthetic rehabilitation for older dysvascular people following a unilateral transfemoral amputation. *Cochrane Database Syst Rev, 18*(4).

DeLisa, J. A., Gans, B. M., & Walsh, N. E. (2005). *Physical medicine and rehabilitation: Principles and practice* (4th ed.). Philadelphia: Lippincott Williams & Wilkins.

Dillingham, T. R., Pezzin, L. E., & MacKenzie, E. J. (2002). Limb amputation and limb deficiency: Epidemiology and recent trends in the United States. *South Med J, 95*(8), 875-883.

Diseases. (2005). National diabetes statistics fact sheet: General information and national estimates on diabetes in the United States Retrieved January 8, 2013, from http://diabetes.niddk.nih.gov/dm/pubs/statistics/index.htm.

Dudek, N. L., Marks, M. B., & Marshall, S. C. (2006). Skin problems in an amputee clinic. *Am J Phys Med Rehabil, 85*(5), 424-429.

Dudek, N. L., Marks, M. B., Marshall, S. C., & Chardon, J. P. (2005). Dermatologic conditions associated with use of a lower-extremity prosthesis. *Arch Phys Med Rehabil, 86*(4), 659-663.

Duwayri, Y., Vallabhaneni, R., Kirby, J. P., Mueller, M. J., Volshteyn, O., Geraghty, P. J., …, & Curci, J. A. (2012). Early protection and compression of residual limbs may improve and accelerate prosthetic fit: A preliminary study. *Ann Vasc Surg, 26*(2), 242-249.

Ephraim, P. L., Wegener, S. T., MacKenzie, E. J., Dillingham, T. R., & Pezzin, L. E. (2005). Phantom pain, residual limb pain, and back pain in amputees: Results of a national survey. *Arch Phys Med Rehabil, 86*(10), 1910-1919.

Esquenazi, A. (2003). Pain management post amputation. Retrieved from http://www.aapmr.org/zdocs/assembly/03handouts/C183_5.pdf.

Esquenazi, A. (2004). Amputation rehabilitation and prosthetic restoration: From surgery to community reintegration. *Disabil Rehabil, 26*(14-15), 831-836.

Esquenazi, A. & Meier, R. H., 3rd. (1996). Rehabilitation in limb deficiency. 4. Limb amputation. *Arch Phys Med Rehabil, 77*(3 Suppl), S18-28.

Frontera, W. R. & DeLisa, J. A. (2010). *DeLisa's physical medicine & rehabilitation: Principles and practice* (5th ed.). Philadelphia: Lippincott Williams & Wilkins.

Gershater, M., Löndahl, M., Nyberg, P., Larsson, J., Thörne, J., Eneroth, M., & Apelqvist, J. (2009). Complexity of factors related to outcome of neuropathic and neuroischaemic/ischaemic diabetic foot ulcers: A cohort study. *Diabetologia, 52*(3), 398-407. doi: 10.1007/s00125-008-1226-2.

Gitter, A. & Bosker, G. (2005). Upper and lower extremity prosthetics. In J. DeLisa (Ed.), *Physical medicine and rehabilitation: Principles and practice.* Philadelphia: Lippincott Williams & Wilkins.

Gruber, H., Glodny, B., Kopf, H., Bendix, N., Galiano, K., Strasak, A., & Peer, S. (2008). Practical experience with sonographically guided phenol instillation of stump neuroma: Predictors of effects, success, and outcome. *AJR Am J Roentgenol, 190*(5), 1263-1269.

Ham, R. & Cotton, L. (1991). *Limb amputation: From aetiology to rehabilitation.* New York: Chapman and Hall.

Huang, M. E. (2011). Rehabilitation and prosthetic restoration in lower limb amputation. In R. L. Braddom & L. Chan (Eds.), *Physical medicine and rehabilitation* (4th ed., pp. xxiv, 1506 p.). Philadelphia, PA: Elsevier/Saunders.

IDF. (2007). Practical guidelines in the management and the prevention of the diabetic foot: Based upon the International Consensus on the Diabetic Foot (DVD).

James, U. (1973). Oxygen uptake and heart rate during prosthetic walking in healthy male unilateral above-knee amputees. *Scand J Rehabil Med, 5*(2), 71-80.

Jang, C. H., Yang, H. S., Yang, H. E., Lee, S. Y., Kwon, J. W., Yun, B. D., ... & Jeong, H. W. (2011). A survey on activities of daily living and occupations of upper extremity amputees. *Ann Rehabil Med, 35*(6), 907-921.

Jin, L., Kollewe, K., Krampfl, K., Dengler, R., & Mohammadi, B. (2009). Treatment of phantom limb pain with botulinum toxin type A. *Pain Med, 10*(2), 300-303.

Johannesson, A., Larsson, G. U., & Oberg, T. (2004). From major amputation to prosthetic outcome: A prospective study of 190 patients in a defined population. *Prosthet Orthot Int, 28*(1), 9-21.

Kaufman, K. R., Frittoli, S., & Frigo, C. A. (2012). Gait asymmetry of transfemoral amputees using mechanical and microprocessor-controlled prosthetic knees. *Clin Biomech (Bristol, Avon), 27*(5), 460-465. doi: 10.1016/j.clinbiomech.2011.11.011.

Kelly, B. M. (2009). Lower limb prosthetics introduction and definitions Retrieved June 16, 2011, from http://emedicine.medscape.com/article/317358-overview.

Kern, U., Altkemper, B., & Kohl, M. (2006). Management of phantom pain with a textile, electromagnetically-acting stump liner: a randomized, double-blind, crossover study. *J Pain Symptom Manage, 32*(4), 352-360.

Kern, U., Busch, V., Rockland, M., Kohl, M., & Birklein, F. (2009). [Prevalence and risk factors of phantom limb pain and phantom limb sensations in Germany. A nationwide field survey]. *Schmerz, 23*(5), 479-488.

Kern, U., Kohl, M., Seifert, U., & Schlereth, T. (2012). [Effect of botulinum toxin type B on residual limb sweating and pain. Is there a chance for indirect phantom pain reduction by improved prosthesis use?]. *Schmerz, 26*(2), 176-184.

Ketz, A. K. (2008). The experience of phantom limb pain in patients with combat-related traumatic amputations. *Arch Phys Med Rehabil, 89*(6), 1127-1132.

Kim, S. Y. & Kim, Y. Y. (2012). Mirror therapy for phantom limb pain. *Korean J Pain, 25*(4), 272-274.

Kottke, F. & Lehmann, J. (1990). *Krusen's handbook of physical medicine and rehabilitation, 4th edition.* Philadelphia: W. B. Saunders Company.

Latlief, G., Elnitsky, C., Hart-Hughes, S., Phillips, S. L., Adams-Koss, L., Kent, R., & Highsmith, M. J. (2012). Patient safety in the rehabilitation of the adult with an amputation. *Phys Med Rehabil Clin N Am, 23*(2), 377-392.

Lim, K. B., Kim, Y. S., & Kim, J. A. (2012). Sonographically guided alcohol injection in painful stump neuroma. *Ann Rehabil Med, 36*(3), 404-408.

Llorente, M. D. & Malphurs, J. (2008). Recognizing late-life depression. *InMotion, 18*(3), 14-16.

Machado Vaz, I., Roque, V., Pimentel, S., Rocha, A., & Duro, H. (2012). [Psychosocial characterization of a Portuguese lower limb amputee population]. *Acta Med Port, 25*(2), 77-82.

MacKenzie, E. J., Bosse, M. J., Castillo, R. C., Smith, D., Webb, L. X., Kellam, J. F., ... & McCarthy, M. L. (2004). Functional outcomes following trauma-related lower-extremity amputation. *J Bone Joint Surg Am*, 1636-1645.

MacNeill, H. L., Devlin, M., Pauley, T., & Yudin, A. (2008). Long-term outcomes and survival of patients with bilateral transtibial amputations after rehabilitation. *Am J Phys Med Rehabil, 87*(3), 189-196.

Meier, R. H. & Atkins, D. J. (Eds.). (2004). *Functional restoration of adults and children with upper extremity amputation.* New York: Demos Medical Publishing, Inc.

Meulenbelt, H. E., Geertzen, J. H., Jonkman, M. F., & Dijkstra, P. U. (2009). Determinants of skin problems of the stump in lower-limb amputees. *Arch Phys Med Rehabil, 90*(1), 74-81.

Moseley, G. L. & Wiech, K. (2009). The effect of tactile discrimination training is enhanced when patients watch the reflected image of their unaffected limb during training. *Pain, 144*(3), 314-319.

Moura Neto, A., Zantut-Wittmann, D. E., Fernandes, T. D., Nery, M., & Parisi, M. C. (2012). Risk factors for ulceration and amputation in diabetic foot: Study in a cohort of 496 patients. *Endocrine, 3*, 3.

Munoz, C. A., Gaspari, A., & Goldner, R. (2008). Contact dermatitis from a prosthesis. *Dermatitis, 19*(2), 109-111.

Murdoch, G. & Wilson, A. B., Jr., (Eds.). (1996). *Amputation: Surgical practice and patient management.* Oxford: Butterworth-Heinemann.

National Limb Loss Information Center. (2008). Amputation Statistics by Cause: Limb Loss in the United States. Retrieved January 10, 2013, from http://www.amputee-coalition.org/fact_sheets/amp_stats_cause.html.

Pasquina, P. F. & Cooper, R. A. (Eds.). (2009). *Care of the combat amputee.* Washington, DC: Borden Institute, Walter Reed Army Medical Center.

Resnik, L., Meucci, M. R., Lieberman-Klinger, S., Fantini, C., Kelty, D. L., Disla, R., & Sasson, N. (2012). Advanced upper limb prosthetic devices: Implications for upper limb prosthetic rehabilitation. *Arch Phys Med Rehabil, 93*(4), 710-717.

Sanders, G. (1986). *Lower limb amputations: A guide to rehabilitation.* Philadelphia: F. A. Davis Company.

Sanders, J. E. & Fatone, S. (2011). Residual limb volume change: Systematic review of measurement and management. *J Rehabil Res Dev, 48*(8), 949-986.

Senra, H., Oliveira, R. A., Leal, I., & Vieira, C. (2012). Beyond the body image: A qualitative study on how adults experience lower limb amputation. *Clin Rehabil, 26*(2), 180-191.

Sheehan, T. P. (2011). Rehabilitation and prosthetic restoration in upper limb amputation. In R. L. Braddom (Ed.), *Physical medicine and rehabilitation* (4th ed., pp. 257-276). Philadelphia: Elsevier Saunders.

Smith, D. G. (2007). Introduction to upper-limb prosthetics: Part 1. *InMotion, 17*(2), 40-44.

Vamos, E. P., Bottle, A., Edmonds, M. E., Valabhji, J., Majeed, A., & Millett, C. (2010). Changes in the incidence of lower extremity amputations in individuals with and without diabetes in England between 2004 and 2008. *Diabetes Care, 33*(12), 2592-2597.

Vining Radomski, M. & Trombly Latham, C. A. (Eds.). (2008). *Occupational therapy for physical dysfunction* (6th ed.). Philadelphia: Lippincott Williams and Wilkins.

Wilder-Smith, C. H., Hill, L. T., & Laurent, S. (2005). Postamputation pain and sensory changes in treatment-naive patients: Characteristics and responses to treatment with tramadol, amitriptyline, and placebo. *Anesthesiology, 103*(3), 619-628.

Wilken, J. & Marin, R. (2009). Gait analysis and training of people with limb loss. In P. F. Pasquina & R. A. Cooper (Eds.), *Care of the combat amputee* (pp. 535-552). Falls Church VA: Office of the Surgeon General, United States Army.

Wlotzke, U., Baumgartner, R., & Landthaler, M. (1997). [Prosthesis edge nodule and verrucous hyperplasia in leg amputees]. *Z Orthop Ihre Grenzgeb, 135*(3), 233-235.

Wong, C. K. & Edelstein, J. E. (2000). Unna and elastic postoperative dressings: Comparison of their effects on function of adults with amputation and vascular disease. *Arch Phys Med Rehabil, 81*(9), 1191-1198.

Yabanoglu, H., Yagmurdur, M. C., Taskintuna, N., & Karakayali, H. (2012). Early period psychiatric disorders following burn trauma and the importance of surgical factors in the etiology. *Ulus Travma Acil Cerrahi Derg, 18*(5), 436-440.

Yang, N. B., Garza, L. A., Foote, C. E., Kang, S., & Meyerle, J. H. (2012). High prevalence of stump dermatoses 38 years or more after amputation. *Arch Dermatol, 148*(11), 1283-1286.

Zidarov, D., Swaine, B., & Gauthier-Gagnon, C. (2009). Life habits and prosthetic profile of persons with lower-limb amputation during rehabilitation and at 3-month follow-up. *Arch Phys Med Rehabil, 90*(11), 1953-1959.

Ziegler-Graham, K., MacKenzie, E. J., Ephraim, P. L., Travison, T. G., & Brookmeyer, R. (2008). Estimating the prevalence of limb loss in the United States: 2005 to 2050. *Arch Phys Med Rehabil, 89*(3), 422-429. doi: 10.1016/j.apmr.2007.11.005.

2. Attention-Deficit/Hyperactivity Disorder

Heather R. Porter

Attention-Deficit/Hyperactivity Disorder (ADHD) is a neurodevelopmental disorder that interferes with social and academic/occupational functioning or development. According to the *Diagnostic and Statistical Manual of Mental Disorders, 5th Edition*, clients with ADHD have (1) markedly decreased inattention (not due to defiance or comprehension deficits) such as difficulty staying on task and lack of perseverance, organization, and focus, and/or (2) an age-inappropriate level of hyperactivity/impulsivity. Examples of hyperactivity include excessive motor activity and talkativeness. Examples of impulsivity include hasty decisions that could cause harm (APA, 2013). Symptoms must be present before the age of 12 and have lasted for at least six months (APA, 2013). Depending upon the specific symptoms, an ADHD presentation is identified as a predominantly hyperactive/impulsive presentation, a predominantly inattentive presentation, or a combined presentation (inattention and hyperactivity).

Incidence/Prevalence in U.S.

The American Psychiatric Association (APA, 2013) reports that approximately five percent of children and 2.5% of adults have diagnoses of ADHD. However, according to the Centers for Disease Control and Prevention, community samples indicate the prevalence of ADHD is much higher. For example, in 2011 it was estimated that 11% (6.4 million) children age 4-17 had a diagnosis of ADHD (CDC, 2013).

Predominate Age

The average age of ADHD diagnosis is seven years old (CDC, 2013). It is commonly diagnosed once the child reaches school age and problems are noted by teachers. Boys tend to be diagnosed with ADHD more than girls (13.2% vs. 5.6%) (CDC, 2013).

Causes

Currently there is no clearly identified, underlying cause of ADHD. ADHD has a neurobiological basis with heredity having a strong influence in most cases (CDC, 2013). A widely recognized psychopathological model for ADHD theorizes that a deficit in inhibitory control is the underlying symptom. The deficit affects executive functioning, resulting in a broad range of dysfunctional behavior (Wehmeier, Schacht, & Barkley, 2010). In addition to genetics, other factors such as environmental exposures (e.g., high lead concentrations in the blood), brain injury, prenatal exposure to tobacco and alcohol, low birth weight, or difficulties during pregnancy are potential risk factors (CDC, 2013).

Psychosocial factors may also play a role in the development of ADHD. For example, according to Sadock & Sadock (2003) symptoms of ADHD in children with prolonged emotional deprivation (e3 Support and Relationships) have been seen to dissipate once deprivation ends (e.g., by being placed in a loving foster home). Stressful psychological events during childhood can contribute to ADHD-like symptoms, although post-traumatic stress disorder may be a better diagnosis. A child's temperament and the demands of society to adhere to a routine way of behaving and performing might also influence the ADHD diagnosis (Sadock & Sadock, 2003). Research does not support the common myths that ADHD is caused by excessive sugar intake, food additives, excessive viewing of television, poor child management by parents, or social and environmental factors such as poverty or family chaos (CDC, 2013).

Systems Affected

Cognitive testing through single-photon emission computed tomography (SPECT), photon emission tomography (PET), and functional magnetic resonance imaging (fMRI) often reveal decreased cognitive processing ability related to decreased attention span and impulsivity (Bush, 2010). Within multiple ADHD studies, functional abnormalities have been found in cognitive and attention networks including the dorsal anterior midcingulate cortex (daMCC), the dorsolateral prefrontal cortex (DLPFC), the ventrolateral prefrontal cortex (VLPFC), the parietal cortex, the striatum, and the cerebellum (Bush, 2010). Relevant ICF codes are found under b1 Mental Functions, especially b140 Attention Functions, b147 Psychomotor Functions, b160 Thought Functions, and b164 Higher-Level Cognitive Functions.

The daMCC acts within cognitive-reward motor networks to increase the efficiency of decision-making and execution. It is responsible for attention, cognitive processing, target detection, novelty detection, motor control response selection, response inhibition, motivation, error detection, and feedback-based decision making. The DLPFC and VLPFC support vigilance, selective and divided attention, attention shifting, planning, executive control, working memory functions, and behavioral inhibition. The parietal cortex supports attention and spatial processing. The striatum supports executive and motor functions such as attention functions and motivation or reward processing. The cerebellum controls motor, somatosensory, language, verbal working memory, spatial processing, executive functions, and affective processing (Bush, 2010).

Central nervous system involvement can also be observed within activity performance, as a broad spectrum of related impairments is common. These cause activity limitations (e.g., inhibition, visual-motor impairment) and participation restrictions (e.g., difficulty engaging in schoolwork, leisure, and interpersonal relationships). Use d1 Learning and Applying Knowledge codes.

Emotional health may additionally be affected with increased incidences of depression and interpersonal problems that may be a direct result of an organic problem or an indirect result of people's negative reactions to the client's impaired social skills (see Secondary Problems).

Secondary Problems

Emotional Impairment

It is estimated that, in the U.S., more than one-third of children with ADHD have high levels of emotional difficulties (anger, aggression, frustration, reduced empathy, decreased arousal to stimulation, and emotion dysregulation). They have difficulty moderating or suppressing emotional reactions and show more extreme emotional reactions compared to peers (b126 Temperament and Personality Functions). This makes them appear impulsive; takes an emotional toll on parents and siblings; and leads to poor self-esteem, depression, poor self-perception, a distorted sense of self, and anxiety (Wehmeier, Schacht, & Barkley, 2010).

Co-existing mental health conditions may also contribute to emotional impairment. It is estimated that 65% of individuals with ADHD have a comorbid mental health condition. Between 30% and 90% have oppositional defiant disorder (ODD) or conduct disorder (CD) (Kessler et al., 2006; Harpin, 2005; Bailey, 2013, ADDitude, 2013; Wehmeier et al., 2010). ODD involves an angry/irritable mood, argumentative/defiant behavior, and vindictiveness. CD involves aggression to people and animals, destruction of property, deceitfulness or theft, and serious violations of rules (APA, 2013). See the chapter on ODD and CD for more information about documenting these conditions.

Individuals with ADHD are also at a higher risk for dysthymia, major depressive disorder, and anxiety disorders (Kessler et al., 2006; Harpin, 2005; Bailey, 2013, ADDitude, 2013; Wehmeier et al., 2010). Causes for increased mental health comorbidities might be due to genetics (similar etiology to ADHD) or exposure to repeated social stressors (Wehmeier et al., 2010). For example, in regards to depression, although there are various causes, in the ADHD population academic difficulties, peer relationship difficulties, parent-child relationship difficulties, and interpersonal dysfunction due to inattention symptoms were found to mediate predictions of depression in children with ADHD (Humphreys, et al., 2013). See the chapter on depression for more information about documenting depression with the ICF.

Lastly, secondary emotional impairments, including sadness, frustration, feeling like one doesn't belong, learned helplessness, can arise from the impact of ADHD and comorbid conditions (Wehmeier et al., 2010).

Social Impairment

Often social skills are learned through observation and incidental learning (b126 Temperament and Personality Functions, d155 Acquiring Skills). Because of the nature of their impairment, clients with ADHD have difficulty using this method of learning and consequently have impaired social skills (Rapoport, 2009). Behavioral issues related to ADHD such as inability to delay gratification, jumping up out of a seat at school, emotional lability (easily set off to laugh or cry), perseveration, and unpredictable mood (explosiveness, irritation from minor stimuli) also limit the number and quality of peer social interactions, affecting social skills development.

Rapoport (2009) states that due to the fore-mentioned impairments children with ADHD have difficulty with learning positive social skills for several reasons: (1) ADHD affects their ability to attain knowledge of what comprises a positive social skill. For example, they may not understand the goal of the social interaction or how to perform a specific social skill, such as how to make friends. (2) People in the children's everyday lives fail to provide extra practice and feedback needed for the child to effectively learn social skills. (3) The children's lack of self-control interferes with performing a social-skill behavior. (4) Difficulty with transitions makes positive interactions in social situations challenging. (5) The children may not be aware of their deficits or challenges, or they might be aware of their deficits but have difficulty changing such behaviors because the behaviors are engrained. (6) Children with ADHD misunderstand others' social cues.

The lack of age-appropriate social skills typically causes problems fitting in with peers. Studies have shown that children who have a problem fitting in with their peers are at a higher risk for "anxiety, behavioral and mood disorders, substance abuse, and delinquency as teenagers" (National Resource Center on AD/HD, 2004). Likewise, parents of children with ADHD report that their children have three times more peer problems (21.1% vs. 7.3%) and ten times more difficulties that interfere with friendships (20.6% vs. two percent) compared to peers who do not have ADHD. Up to 70% of children with ADHD have no close friends by third grade, due to behav-

ioral issues and they are more likely to become involved in deviant peer groups if social rejection continues (Wehmeier, Schacht, & Barkley, 2010). Document social skills impairments using codes under d7 Interpersonal Interactions and Relationships and difficulties acquiring skills with d155 Acquiring Skills.

Dislike for School

The acquisition, retention, and display of knowledge are all hampered by ADHD and other secondary disorders, such as a learning disability or communication disorder. The negative reactions of school staff and peers to ADHD behaviors and lowering of self-esteem from academic difficulties can cause children with ADHD to dislike school. This can lead to antisocial behavior and self-defeating, self-punitive behaviors (Sadock & Sadock, 2003). ICF codes d130-d159 Basic Learning and d810-d839 Education can be used to record these deficits.

Impaired Sense of Self

Often clients with ADHD have IQs within the normal range and some even have high IQs (Brown, 2011). They can understand, to some degree, that they are "different" from other children. Often the behaviors associated with the disorder cause others to ostracize or put down individuals with ADHD contributing to impaired self-esteem, self-confidence, and self-image (Harpin, 2005). The environmental concerns can be documented with e425 Individual Attitudes of Acquaintances, Peers, Colleagues, Neighbors, and Community Members.

Physical Activity Deficits

Perceptual motor deficits and general coordination deficits (b147 Psychomotor Functions) can make it difficult for children with ADHD to participate in sports and other high-level physical activities. These deficits also result in increased risk for injuries, hospital admissions, and emergency room visits (CDC, 2013). Consequently, children with ADHD may feel like failures in physical as well as intellectual tasks.

Prognosis

ADHD symptoms diagnosed during elementary school years can continue or change throughout the developmental years. During adolescence, about 50-60% of the diagnosed population continue to experience problematic symptoms including conduct disorder, oppositional defiant disorder, lower academic performance, fewer friends, psychosocial adjustment issues, self-esteem issues, and social skills deficits (Millichap, 2009; Mannuzza & Klein, 2000). About 40% of the diagnosed population experience significant impairment (antisocial personality disorder, arrests, drug abuse) (Mannuzza & Klein, 2000). It is further estimated that 50-70% of the diagnosed population continue to have problems into adulthood (Billingsley-Jackson, 2008; Harpin, 2005).

Of the various impairments associated with ADHD, hyperactivity is usually the first to decline with attention span and impulse control impairments lingering (Millichap, 2009). Individuals usually struggle the most during high school and college because this is when they are challenged the most, both academically and socially, with no opportunity to escape the challenges (Brown, 2011). During adulthood, however, after school obligations have been met, individuals have the opportunity to specialize in areas that are more interesting where they are more likely to experience success (Brown, 2011) and go on to succeed in higher education. Additionally, it is believed that throughout the developmental years, brain function continually improves, resulting in a reduction of ADHD symptoms (Brown, 2011).

Assessment

Typical Scope of Team Assessment

Initial symptoms of ADHD, although recognized most often by parents and teachers, are formally diagnosed by a psychiatrist. The specific criteria for ADHD are defined in the *DSM-5* (APA, 2013). Practice parameters for the assessment of children with ADHD set forth by the American Academy of Child and Adolescent Psychiatry (AACAP) include the following recommendations: (1) Screening for ADHD should be a part of every client's mental health assessment. (2) Evaluation of the preschooler, child, or adolescent for ADHD should consist of clinical interviews with the parent and client, obtaining information about the client's school or day care functioning, evaluation for comorbid psychiatric disorders, and review of the client's medical, social, and family histories. (3) If the client's medical

history is unremarkable, laboratory or neurological testing is not indicated. (4) Psychological and neuropsychological tests are not mandatory for the diagnosis for ADHD, but should be performed if the client's history suggests low general cognitive ability or low achievement in language or mathematics relative to the client's intellectual ability. (5) The clinician must evaluate the client with ADHD for the presence of comorbid psychiatric disorders (Pliszka, 2007).

Common behavior rating scales used in the assessment and monitoring of ADHD include the *Academic Performance Rating Scale; ADHD Rating Scale-IV; Brown ADD Rating Scales for Children, Adolescents, and Adults; Child Behavior Checklist; Conners Parent Rating Scale—Revised; Conners Teacher Rating Scale—Revised; Conners Wells Adolescent Self-Report Scale; Home Situations Questionnaire—Revised; School Situations Questionnaire—Revised; IOWA Conners Rating Scale; Swanson, Nolan, and Pelham (SNAP-IV) and SKAMP Internet site ADHD.NET;* and *Vanderbilt ADHD Diagnostic Parent and Teacher Scales* (Pliszka, 2007). In addition, tools such as the *Therapeutic Recreation Activity Assessment (TRAA)*, the 22 modules in the *Community Integration Program*, the *Comprehensive Evaluation in Recreational Therapy — Psych/Behavioral, Revised (CERT-Psych/R)*, the *Home and Community Social Behavior Scales*, and the *School Social Behavior Scales* can help pinpoint specific functional impairments and restrictions to address in the therapy treatment plan.

Pelham & Fabiano (2008), however, recommend that less time should be spent on time-intensive and expensive clinical assessment interviews. They advocate for evidence-based assessments focused on functional outcomes that include the use of rating scales combined with functional behavior analysis of select target behaviors. These assessments identify antecedent and consequence variables that influence behaviors, which can then be focused upon in treatment. The use of rating scales and functional behavioral analysis in real-life settings aligns well with current recreational therapy assessment methods.

As part of the treatment team, recreational therapists assist in determining the type of ADHD presentation through observing the client's performance in structured tasks that require both capacity (clinic setting) and performance (real life setting). For example, in activities clients with inattentive presentations make careless mistakes (e.g., miss details), have difficulty sustaining attention or get easily distracted, don't follow through with instructions, have difficulty with organization and time management, avoid cognitive challenges, and/or lose things. Clients with hyperactivity/impulsivity presentations have excessive motor activity (trouble sitting still, tapping feet, fidgeting), demonstrate difficulty engaging in quiet play or leisure activities, talk incessantly, inappropriately shout out answers, have difficulty taking turns, inappropriately interrupt others, use other people's things without asking, and/or inappropriately take over situations (APA, 2013).

Areas of Concern for RT Assessment

ADHD symptoms and the ICF implications depend on the client's age. Code educational issues under d810-d839 Education. Other issues that can be assessed by recreational therapy, sorted by age group, are listed below.

Preschool child: Unusually poor intensity of play (d880 Engagement in Play, d9200 Play), excessive motor restlessness (b147 Psychomotor Functions), delayed development (b122 Global Psychosocial Functions), oppositional behavior (b126 Temperament and Personality Functions), and poor social skills (b122 Global Psychosocial Functions, d7 Interpersonal Interactions and Relationships) (Harpin, 2005).

Primary school years: The child may experience academic challenges (any of b1 Mental Functions or d130-d159 Basic Learning), peer rejection (d720 Complex Interpersonal Interactions), low self-esteem, increasing severity of other comorbid conditions, difficulties at home or on outings (d920 Recreation and Leisure), and external locus of control related to ADHD-related problems. The child may also have poor sleep patterns resulting in poor daytime behavior (b134 Sleep Functions). Those who interact with the child may not want to be with the child. Other family members may refuse to care for or baby-sit the child (e415 Individual Attitudes of Extended Family Members). Peers may not invite child to parties or out to play (d720 Complex Interpersonal Interactions). Strained family relationships may cause additional social or financial difficulties that result in feelings of sadness or exhibition of oppositional and aggressive behavior by the child (d760 Family Relationships). Parents can be especially affected, including lack of self-care due to provision of constant supervision (d5 Self-Care); disrupted parent-child relationships (d7600 Parent-Child Relationships); reduced parenting efficacy (d7600 Parent-Child Relationships); and increased parental stress, particularly in mothers. Children who display deviant behaviors are associated with increased parental alcohol consumption (d240 Handling Stress and Other Psychological Demands). Siblings may also be negatively affected with physical violence, verbal aggression, manipulation, and increased caregiving responsibilities for the sibling with ADHD, since they may feel the need to watch over and protect the child. They may feel anxious, worried, or sad given the totality of the situation (d7602 Sibling Relationships) (Harpin, 2005).

Adolescence: There is a possible reduction in hyperactivity; however, inattention, impulsiveness, and inner restlessness often remain (b130 Energy and Drive Functions, b140 Attention Functions, b147 Psychomotor Functions). Other findings may include a distorted sense of self (b180 Experience of Self and Time Functions), disruption of the normal development of self, development of aggressive/antisocial behavior (b126 Temperament and Personality Functions), parent-teen conflict (d7600 Parent-Child Relationships), severe lack of friendships (d720 Complex Interpersonal Interactions), and increased risk for problem behaviors. Potential problem behaviors, which can be scored with Activities and Participation codes, include substance abuse, academic failure, intentional injury, attempted suicide, repetition of grade, dropping out of school, school detention or expulsion, teenage pregnancy, criminal behavior and incarceration, sexually transmitted diseases, dismissal from a job, and driving fast and not paying attention resulting in traffic violations, tickets, and accidents) (Harpin, 2005).

Adult life: Clients are more likely to be dismissed from employment and have difficulty finding a job where they experience success. There may be work-related problems such as interpersonal conflicts, lateness, absenteeism, excessive errors, and inability to accomplish their workload (d845 Acquiring,

Keeping, and Terminating a Job). There may also be personal relationship difficulties (d7 Interpersonal Interactions and Relationships), increased risk of substance abuse, particularly by those who do not take medication for ADHD (d570 Looking After One's Health). They may have difficulty parenting, especially if their child has ADHD, leading to cyclical difficulties (d7600 Parent-Child Relationships) (Harpin, 2005).

Other common findings that are not age-specific include:

Ability to focus on meaningful tasks: Despite having difficulty with focusing attention, individuals with ADHD are often able to focus without difficulty on tasks that hold personal interest and meaning (e.g., playing an instrument, baking) (Brown, 2011). When a person desires to achieve something "good" or avoid something "bad" (a motivational behavior that holds intrinsic meaning), dopamine is released in the body that encourages action, encouraging and motivating the desired or needed behavior. Score this area by choosing a participation code that reflects the particular meaningful activity — e.g., d9203 Crafts (Salamone, 2012).

Participation restrictions: Due to cognitive, motor, and social deficits associated with ADHD, participation restrictions will be seen in everyday activities, including recreation, leisure, play, and community activities. Score this area by choosing a participation code that reflects the particular activity where participation restrictions are experienced — e.g., d9201 Sports (Litner & Ostiguy, 2000).

Leisure engagement (d920 Recreation and Leisure): Participation in games and crafts can be difficult due to a lack of fine motor skills (Parker, 1988). Poor visual-motor integration, sequencing, and problem-solving skills can make competitive sports activities frustrating (Parker 1998). Poor memory impacts remembering instructions (Parker, 1988; Reeve 1993). Use ICF codes in b140-b189 Specific Mental Functions to score these deficits. Those with inattentive presentations have difficulty adapting to change, have a tendency to socially withdraw, and may be ignored by peers, resulting in a dislike for team or group-oriented activities (Brown, 1997). Those with hyperactive/impulsive presentations have difficulty understanding interpersonal dynamics and reading social cues, resulting in being singled out for causing problems, which in turn

causes feelings of anger and acts of aggression causing rejection by peers (Reeve, 1994). These could be documented using codes in b110-b139 Global Mental Functions. Variability in play, leisure, and recreation performance causes others to view the individual as lazy and unmotivated (Goldstein & Goldstein, 1990). Due to leisure engagement difficulties, the client may have an unhealthy leisure balance and tend to gravitate towards more solitary activities that don't challenge deficit areas.

Observation of strengths: A review of the literature by Litner & Ostiguy (2000) found that individuals with ADHD, despite having many challenges, also present with unique strengths including resiliency, ingenuity, creativity, spontaneity, boundless energy, sensitivity to others, inquisitiveness, imagination, resourcefulness, observational skills, and empathy. They say "[t]he challenge is to offer recreation programs designed to harness and build on the many strengths of the children and youth" (Litner & Ostiguy, 2000, p. NL).

Quality of life: ADHD is associated with decreased social and emotional well-being, impacting quality of life (Wehmeier, Schacht, & Barkley, 2010).

ICF Core Set

An ICF Core Set for ADHD has not yet been published. Visit the ICF Research Branch website at http://www.icf-research-branch.org/icf-core-sets-projects-sp-1641024398/other-health-conditions/icf-core-set-for-cp-for-cy/494-icf-core-set-for-attention-deficit-hyperactivity-disorder-adhd for a description of how the ICF Core Set for ADHD is currently being developed.

Treatment Direction

Whole Team Approach

Practice parameters for the treatment of children with ADHD set forth by AACAP include the following recommendations: (1) A well-thought-out and comprehensive treatment plan should be developed for the client with ADHD. (2) The initial psychopharmacological treatment of ADHD should be a trial with an agent approved by the Food and Drug Administration (FDA) for the treatment of ADHD. (3) If none of the agents result in satisfactory treatment of the client with ADHD, the clinician should undertake a careful review of the diagnosis and then consider behavior therapy and/or the use of medications not approved by the FDA for the treatment of ADHD. (4) During the psychopharmacological intervention for ADHD, the client should be monitored for side effects that emerge because of treatment. (5) If the client with ADHD has a robust response to psychopharmacological treatment and subsequently shows normal functioning, then using just psychopharmacological treatment for the ADHD may be sufficient. If the client with ADHD has a less than optimal response to medication, has a comorbid disorder, or experiences stressors in family life, then psychosocial treatment in conjunction with medication treatment if often beneficial. (6) Clients should be assessed periodically to determine whether there is continued need for treatment or if symptoms remain present and cause impairment. (7) Clients treated with medication for ADHD should have their height and weight monitored throughout treatment because stimulant treatments are associated with stunted growth and doses need to be adjusted for changes in weight (Pliszka, 2007).

Pelham & Fabiano (2008), however, after conducting a comprehensive literature analysis on psychosocial interventions for ADHD, do not agree with AACAP recommendations of medication being the first line of treatment and argue that in a "relative risk-benefit analysis...behavioral treatments should be employed as the first line intervention and that medication should be added as an adjunct when indicated" (p. 208). They further note that due to the chronic nature of ADHD:

> it is inappropriate to think that a brief, time-limited treatment regimen, whether it be behavioral, pharmacological, or combined, will be a sufficient and effective intervention for a child with ADHD. For most children with ADHD and their families, chronic, intensive, pervasive, palatable treatment that promotes engagement and adherence to the selected regime for protracted periods of time will be required. (p. 209)

Unfortunately, only about 60% of youth with ADHD report having received services related to their disorder (National Institutes of Mental Health, 2011) and current treatment focuses mainly on core daytime symptoms that occur during the school day

(Harpin, 2005). Harpin (2005) strongly recommends that more treatment is focused outside of the school day (early mornings, after school, weekends) which are "frequently unaffected by current treatment regimes [and] can negatively impact child and family functioning and fail to optimize self-esteem and long term mental health development" (p. i6).

Additionally, given the early onset of ADHD, it is important to treat the disorder as early as possible with a broad range of interventions including counseling, parent/teacher/sibling education and training, behavior therapy, pharmacotherapy, methods of behavior management and modification, special education services, summer treatment programs, and contingency management methods (Wehmeier et al., 2010). It is also noted by Wehmeier et al. (2010) that interventions for ADHD are most helpful when they assist with the performance of a particular behavior at the place and time of performance in the natural environment. Consequently, it is important to provide assistance with the time, timing, and timeliness of behavior. To be effective in altering the prognosis, treatment must be maintained over extended time (months to years), with interventions occurring periodically in the long term.

Recreational Therapy Approach

Recreational therapists work with clients with ADHD in many different settings including community recreation programs, schools, and rehab settings with ADHD as a secondary diagnosis. Interventions include those that increase functioning in particular environments, with special attention given to the development of social skills, a healthy sense of self, and a balanced leisure lifestyle.

The value of play and leisure (d880 Engagement in Play, d920 Recreation and Leisure) for this population cannot be understated. It can "make a crucial difference in the self-esteem and self-worth of youth with ADHD,...provide an opportunity for youth with ADHD to 'fit in' and provide a context for enhancing strengths that offer increased opportunities for recognition,...[and help to develop] important skills to succeed in life" (Litner & Ostiguy, 2000, p. NL). The inherent characteristics of leisure activities, coupled with the internal motivation to participate, driven by personal meaning and interest, aid in the development of critical life skills: Cooking and music teach measuring, timing, sequencing, and creative judgment. Martial arts teach discipline, attention, coordination, self-concept, and motor planning. Board games teach learning rules, sequential judgment, and receiving feedback on mistakes. Building objects and crafts teach fine motor development, visual judgment, sequencing, planning skills, concentration, fine motor coordination, and work habits (Litner & Ostiguy, 2000).

Leisure additionally provides individuals with ADHD opportunities to develop social networks (d7 Interpersonal Interactions and Relationships), improve mental functions through leisure skills and interests (b1 Mental Functions), escape pressures and rules of academic and school life, and engage in activities that have more flexibility and variety (d240 Handling Stress and Other Psychological Demands). Leisure also may develop and strengthen confidence through success in leisure activities (b126 Temperament and Personality Functions), which in turn motivates continued participation and skill building (b130 Energy and Drive Functions, d155 Acquiring Skills). Participants develop skills, positive behaviors, and interpersonal awareness in a pleasant and natural way, experience opportunities for choice and control (d177 Making Decisions), as well as an outlet for excess energy or feelings of aggression (b147 Psychomotor Functions, b130 Energy and Drive Functions, b152 Emotional Functions). Developing competence in managing leisure time leads to self-empowerment (b126 Temperament and Personality Functions) (Litner & Ostiguy, 2000).

Recreational Therapy Interventions

A task force sponsored by the American Psychological Association conducted a comprehensive review of the literature to identify the best evidence-based psychosocial practices for the treatment of ADHD (Pelham & Fabiano, 2008). The review concluded that the following psychosocial practices met the criteria to be well-established and effective interventions for the treatment of ADHD:

Behavioral Parent Training (BPT): This typically consists of an eight- to twelve-week formal training program for parents of children with ADHD. Through discussion, coaching, and role-play it teaches parents how to alter, influence, and change their child's behavior through behavior modification, including how to identify and manipulate antecedents and consequences of behavior, how to target and

monitor problem behaviors, how to reward positive behavior through tangible and intangible rewards, and how to decrease undesired behavior through planned ignoring, time out, and other non-physical discipline techniques. Those implementing the program should read the referenced article for program details (Chronis et al., 2004). Creative, alternative methods for delivering BPT are also being piloted and explored (Chronis et al., 2004). One study mentioned by Chronis et al. (2004) is an eight-week program called Coaching Our Acting-Out Children: Heightening Essential Skills (COACHES) aimed at increasing involvement of fathers of children with ADHD, as many fathers do not attend BPT. In the first hour, fathers are taught how to employ basic parenting strategies (e.g., time out, positive praise) while their children practice soccer drills. During the second hour, a soccer game is played. During the game, the fathers stand on the sidelines and "coach" their own child throughout the game using the behavioral strategies learned earlier. The clinician stands with the fathers on the sidelines and provides feedback to the fathers throughout the game. A randomized controlled trial comparing traditional BPT to COACHES is underway and results have not yet been published. See Chronis et al. (2004) for more ideas on enhancing BPT. Therapists can demonstrate the gains from these techniques by documenting changes in d760 Family Relationships.

Behavioral Classroom Management (BCM): BCM describes contingency management procedures (e.g., point systems, time outs, reward programs) used by teachers in the classroom. These procedures are gradually faded and replaced with a Daily Report Card (DRC). Findings also indicated that prudent negative consequences are superior to contingent praise alone; brief time outs work better than longer ones; and response cost programs are more effective than reward programs (Pelham & Fabiano, 2008). Recreational therapists who work in school systems using BCM can use these techniques in recreational therapy sessions to provide consistency. Success can be measured with d1 Learning and Applying Knowledge and d2 General Tasks and Demands, as well as other ICF codes.

Behavioral Peer Interventions (BPI): The review by Pelham & Fabiano (2008) found that traditional office-base social skills training (SST) produces minimal effects, and that more intensive BPIs, such as those offered through summer intensive programs, are needed to impact peer relations (d7 Interpersonal Interactions and Relationships). Summer intensive BPI programs focus on behavioral interventions for peer problems in recreational settings. Interventions are typically daylong programs for five to eight weeks delivering anywhere from 200 to 400 hours of treatment compared to the typical 10 to 20 hours of treatment in traditional social skills training (SST) programs. The summer intensive programs usually consist of brief segments of SST followed by coached group play in recreational activities (d920 Recreation and Leisure) concurrent with contingency management systems (e.g., point system, time-out). The program typically focuses on teaching sports skills and team membership skills. BPI allows for objective observations and frequency counts of social behaviors over a long period of time, in addition to adult ratings of social skills as outcome measures. These long-term measures are something that short-term, clinic-based SST programs cannot accurately provide. This is one of the primary strengths of a BPI program. Within the BPI program, BPT is typically provided concurrently and home-based contingencies are often employed as well. Most notable in the review was that BPI often produces "acute effects comparable to those produced by medication…The odds ratio for BPI alone is four to five times greater than that reported for medication alone…[and children are] 6 to 19 times more likely to meet their daily behavioral goals, including goals focused on peer interactions" (p. 197). On the downside, the review also noted that BPI is more costly then BPT and BCM, more difficult to implement in community settings, and is the least available of all the evidence-based practices for ADHD. This highlights the unique and much needed role of recreational therapy. Outside of running summer intensive BPI programs, the review stated that "[i]t is possible that something approximating the intensive summer BPIs could be conducted in after-school programs or on Saturdays in clinic settings where there is access to recreational resources, but this approach has not yet been tested" (p. 209).

Despite the identification of the above interventions as being well-established and effective interventions, further research is needed to answer critical questions such as the identification of the necessary and effective aspects and components of behavioral interventions, the sequence in which stimulants and behavioral interventions should be initiated, ways to generalize treatment effects, and methods of providing behavioral treatments cost effectively (Pelham & Fabiano, 2008).

Within the recreational therapy literature, other effective interventions may be found.

An anger management program aimed at facilitating appropriate expression of anger in children with ADHD was found to reduce externalization of anger and increase anger control as reported by parents (b152 Emotional Functions, d7 Interpersonal Interactions and Relationships) (Marcus & Mattiko, 2007). The study consisted of 38 children (ages six-twelve) who were in a 13-week double-blind, placebo-controlled medication trial at the National Institutes of Health. During this trial, the children participated in the recreational therapy anger management program five times a week for two hours a day through the 13-week study. The anger management program consisted of seven steps: (1) group brainstorming of possible expressions of anger, (2) judging each idea as either positive or negative, (3) each child choosing three positive ideas from the list to use as strategies for dealing with angry feelings, (4) each child reciting their anger strategies, (5) practicing implementation of strategies during RT sessions and integrating the behaviors into home and school environments (feedback provided by parents), (6) processing behaviors as a group and role-playing to act out alternative strategies, and (7) reinforcing activities to practice dealing with anger and frustration (e.g., board games). Steps 1 through 3 took place in the initial one to one and a half hours of the program. Step 4 was done a minimum of five times a week at the end of each session. Steps 5 and 6 were done one to two hours a week. Step 7 was done two to three hours a week.

In addition to social skills and behavior, recreational therapists address the multitude of cognitive, psychological, and motor ADHD-related deficits. As supported in the previously reviewed literature, recreational therapists utilize play, recreation, leisure, and community activities of interest to the client to encourage focus on skill development and the release of dopamine to further enhance motivation and focus for continued participation. Real life settings are also utilized whenever possible to improve skill transfer and to enhance the development of realistic life skills, such as coping with unexpected outcomes and responding to contextual factors that are not easily replicated in structured settings. Recreational therapy sessions, whether individual or group based, are crafted to meet the needs and desires of the individuals and families. In addition, plans are developed and put into place for post-discharge participation to increase the likelihood of skill maintenance, psychological-emotional well-being, and quality of life. Changes can be noted in b1 Mental Functions and several of the Activities and Participation chapters including d1 Learning and Applying Knowledge, d2 General Tasks and Demands, and d7 Interpersonal Interactions and Relationships.

For recreational therapists working in community recreation services for children with ADHD, the following suggestions by Litner & Ostiguy (2000) should be considered to maximize outcomes: (1) Provide structure and consistency. Have clear expectations, clear understanding of acceptable and unacceptable behavior and resultant consequences, predictable routine, consistent and clear instructions, and clearly established rules and target behaviors. (2) Plan the activities so the participants can succeed. Make changes to the environment to facilitate success through adaptations and modifications. Design activities that focus on skill development. Plan participation components such as pre-selecting teams and rotating individuals during activities. Use organizational tools such as checklists to help children stay on task and transition. Put materials into individual bags to improve organization. (3) Create a positive environment. Limit environmental stimuli that could increase distraction, create enriching experiences to foster motivation, use techniques to encourage continued motivation such as direct questions or individual responsibilities, provide a welcoming and safe/supportive environment, and provide incentives for participation. (4) Increase motivation to participate. Use meaningful activities that are relevant to interests, provide opportunities for social interaction with peers in varying contexts, showcase individual strengths, and use humor and novelty to build enthusiasm and energy. Modify the environment for better focus by adding music and changing tone of voice, emotional vibe, and color. Review materials and instructions before beginning the task, demonstrate new materials and skills to help with organization of thoughts and decrease likelihood

of difficulties, and use experiential learning. (5) Build self-esteem. Foster a sense of identity, belonging, and purpose; encourage independence; reinforce social and behavior limits while promoting trust, self-respect, and responsibility; and teach problem-solving strategies and interpersonal skills that promote good self-esteem. (6) Select appropriate programs and services. Consider the size of the program, skills required to participate, staff knowledge about ADHD, complexity of rules, activity structure, opportunities for hands-on learning and cooperative play, etc.

From an ICF point of view, create a therapeutic environment and document changes in the deficits noted during the assessment process.

Resources

ADHD Aware
www.adhdaware.org
Run by and for people with ADHD with the purpose of empowering children, adults, and families affected by ADHD, educating those who interact with people with ADHD, and enlightening all people as to the courage and competence of the ADHD community.

Attention Deficit Disorder Association
www.add.org
Provides information, resources, and networking opportunities to help adults with ADHD lead better lives.

Children and Adults with Attention-Deficit/Hyperactivity Disorder (CHADD)
www.chadd.org
Provides education, advocacy, and support for individuals with ADHD. Publishes materials to keep members and professionals current on research advances, medications, and treatments affecting individuals with ADHD. There is a free electronic newsletter, *Attention* magazine.

Technical Assistance Center on Social-Emotional Intervention for Young Children
www.challengingbehavior.org
Identifies, disseminates, and promotes the implementation of evidence-based practices in order to improve the social, emotional, and behavioral functioning of young children with or at risk for delays or disabilities.

References

ADDitude. (2013). Oppositional defiant disorder. Retrieved from http://www.additudemag.com/adhd-web/article/4646.html.

American Psychiatric Association. (2013). *Diagnostic and statistical manual of mental disorders, fifth edition.* Washington, DC: American Psychiatric Publishing.

Bailey, E. (2013). ADHD and conduct disorder. Retrieved from http://www.healthcentral.com/adhd/related-conditions-196325-5.html.

Billingsley-Jackson, K. A. (2008). Adult attention deficit/hyperactivity disorder: Personality characteristics in DSM-IV-TR diagnosed and symptomatic samples. ProQuest, ISBN 054974777X.

Brown, T. E. (2011). The mysteries of ADD and high IQ. Retrieved from http://www.psychologytoday.com/blog/the-mysteries-add/201108/the-mysteries-add-and-high-iq.

Brown, T. E. (1997). The faces of "inattention" ADD beyond hyperactivity. Proceedings of Ninth Annual CHADD Conference (183185). New York.

Brown, T. E. (2001). The mysteries of ADD and high IQ. *Psychology Today.* Retrieved from http://www.psychologytoday.com/blog/the-mysteries-add/201108/the-mysteries-add-and-high-iq.

Bush, G. (2010). Attention-deficit/hyperactivity disorder and attention networks. *Neuropsychopharmacology, 35*(1), 278-300.

Centers for Disease Control and Prevention. (2013). Attention-deficit/hyperactivity disorder: Data and statistics. Retrieved from http://www.cdc.gov/ncbddd/adhd/data.html.

Chronis, A. M., Chacko, A., Fabiano, G. A., Wymbs, B. T., & Pelham, W. E. (2004). Enhancements to the behavioral parent training program for families with ADHD: Review and future directions. *Clinical Child and Family Psychology Review, 7*(1), 1-27.

Goldstein, S. & Goldstein, M. (1990). *Managing attention disorders in children: A guide for practitioners.* New York: John Wiley and Sons.

Harpin, V. A. (2005). The effect of ADHD on the life of an individual, their family, and community from preschool to adult life. *Archives of Disease in Childhood, 90*(Suppl 1), i2-i7.

Humphreys, K. L., Katz, S. J., Lee, S. S., Hammen, C., Brennan, P. A., & Najman, J. M. (2013). The association of ADHD and depression: Mediation by peer problems and parent-child difficulties in two complementary samples. *Journal of Abnormal Psychology, 122*(3), 854-867.

Kessler, R. C., Adler, L., Barkley, R., Biederman, J., Conners, C. K., Demler, O., Faraone, S. V., Greenhill, L. L., Howes, M. J., Secnik, K., Spencer, T., Bedirhan-Ustun, T., Walters, E. E., & Zaslavsky, A. M. (2006). The prevalence and correlates of adult ADHD in the United States: Results from the National Comorbidity Survey Replication. *American Journal of Psychiatry, 163*(4), 716-723.

Litner, B. & Ostiguy, L. (2000). Understanding attention deficit hyperactivity disorder: Strategies and consideration for inclusion of youth in leisure services. *Journal of Leisurability, 27*(2), 11-18.

Mannuzza, S. & Klein, R. G. (2000). Long-term prognosis in attention-deficit/hyperactivity disorder. *Child and Adolescent Psychiatric Clinics of North America, 9*(3), 711-26.

Marcus, D. & Mattiko, M. (2007). An anger management program for children with attention deficit hyperactivity disorder. *Therapeutic Recreation Journal, 41*(1), 16-28.

Millichap, J. G. (2009). *Attention deficit hyperactivity disorder handbook: A physician's guide to ADHD.* New York: Springer Publishing.

National Institutes of Mental Health. (2011). Majority of youth with mental disorders may not be receiving sufficient services. Retrieved from http://www.nimh.nih.gov/news/science-news/2011/majority-of-youth-with-mental-disorders-may-not-be-receiving-sufficient-services.shtml.

National Resource Center on AD/HD. (2004). About AD/HD: Causes and pathophysiology. www.help4adhd.org/en/about/causes.

Parker, H. (1998). Introduction to ADHD: Practical strategies for parents. Proceeding of the 10th Annual CHADD Conference, New York, NY, 138-139.

Parker, H. (1988). *The attention deficits disorder workshop for parents, teachers, and kids.* Plantation, FL: Impact Publications.

Pelham, W. E. & Fabiano, G. A. (2008). Evidence-based psychosocial treatment for attention-deficit/hyperactivity disorder. *Journal of Clinical Child and Adolescent Psychology, 37*(1), 184-214.

Pliszka, S. (2007). Practice parameter for the assessment and treatment of children and adolescents with attention-deficit/hyperactivity disorder. *American Academy of Child and Adolescent Psychiatry, 47*(6), 894-921.

Rapoport, E. M. (2009). *ADHD and social skills: A step-by-step guide for teachers and parents.* Lanham, MD: R&L Education.

Reeve, R. (1993). The academic impact of ADD. *Attention, 1*(1), 8-12.

Sadock, B. & Sadock, V. (2003). *Synopsis of psychiatry, 9th edition.* Philadelphia: Lippincott, Williams & Wilkins.

Salamone, J. D. (2012). The mysterious motivational functions of mesolimbic dopamine. *Neuron, 76*(3), 470.

Wehmeier, P. M., Schacht, A., & Barkley, R. (2010). Social and emotional impairment in children and adolescents with ADHD and the impact on quality of life. *Journal of Adolescent Health, 46*(3), 209-217.

3. Autism Spectrum Disorder

Jo Ann Coco-Ripp and Rachel L. Smith

Autism Spectrum Disorder (ASD) is a new *DSM-5* diagnosis that reflects a scientific consensus that four previously separate disorders are actually a single condition with different levels of symptom severity in two core domains. ASD now encompasses the previous *DSM-IV* Autistic Disorder (autism), Asperger's Disorder, Childhood Disintegrative Disorder, and Pervasive Developmental Disorder Not Otherwise Specified (APA, 2013). Specific diagnostic criteria for ASD can be found in the *DSM-5* (APA, 2013) and include: (1) deficits in social communication and social interaction, including social-emotional reciprocity; nonverbal communication behaviors; and developing, maintaining, and understanding relationships; and (2) restricted, repetitive patterns of behavior, interests, or activities, including stereotyped or repetitive motor movements, use of objects, or speech; insistence on sameness, inflexible adherence to routines, or ritualized patterns of behavior; highly restricted or fixated interests of abnormal intensity and/or focus; or hyper/hypo reactivity to sensory input. Symptoms are present during early development and cause significant functional impairment. The *DSM-5* further divides ASD into three severity levels depending upon the level of support required: Level 1 requires support, Level 2 requires substantial support, and Level 3 requires very substantial support (APA, 2013)

ASD is a neurodevelopmental disorder that is diagnosed on behavioral and developmental characteristics rather than medical, anatomic, or specific genetic markers (Firth, 2008). There is no single behavior that is always seen in ASD, nor is there a single behavior that can disqualify an individual from being diagnosed with ASD (Schreibman, 2005). Rather, it is the collection of social, communication, and behavioral impairments that create the disorder, or, more aptly, that individual's ASD (Firth, 2008; Schreibman, 2005). There is a wide spectrum of functionality in ASD, with the highest functioning individuals scoring far above average on intelligence testing and the lowest on the spectrum scoring far below. This chapter speaks generally about ASD as a spectrum. For more information on the specific conditions and levels of functioning, see the resources listed at the end of the chapter.

Incidence/Prevalence in U.S.

ASD is the fastest growing developmental disability in the United States with one out of every 110 children being diagnosed somewhere on the autism spectrum (Center for Disease Control and Prevention, 2011). There is a four to one male to female ratio, meaning that one in 70 boys and one in 315 girls are diagnosed with ASD in the United States (Lord & Bishop, 2010). This translates into approximately 730,000 Americans aged 0-21 falling somewhere on the spectrum, and between one and one and a half million Americans of all ages with ASD (Firth, 2008; Autism Society of America [ASA], 2010). A full one percent of the population aged three to seven has ASD (ASA, 2010). In the last 20 years (1990-2010) there has been a 172% increase of cases of ASD (Lord & Bishop, 2010), and current estimates say that there is a 10-17% increase in ASD annually (ASA, 2010). Researchers are unclear whether higher rates reflect an expansion of the diagnostic criteria, increased awareness, differences in study methodology, or a true increase in frequency of ASD (APA, 2013).

Predominant Age

Age of onset in ASD is hard to identify. Many children with ASD are diagnosed at 18-36 months (APA, 2000). However, it is not uncommon for higher functioning children to not be diagnosed until they enter elementary school (five to eight years old) when the severity of their social impairment becomes more apparent (Firth, 2008). In fact, some cases of ASD are not diagnosed until adolescence or adulthood. More, some parents notice that their child is developing abnormally in infancy and others recognize a pattern of typical development that then slows or regresses. What is important to note is that ASD is a neurodevelopmental disorder, and an early disruption of typical neurodevelopment is present even if it not caught until later in life.

Causes

The etiology of ASD is unknown. In the past ten years there have been great strides made towards understanding the disorder. However, what is becoming clear is that there is a long way to go before the underlying cause, or more likely causes, of autism are known (Volkmar & Wiesner, 2009). There are three broad areas of research into the etiology of autism that have shown promise in explaining the disorder: genetics, neurological structure and development, and environmental factors.

Genetics: In 1977, Folstein and Rutter found that monozygotic (identical) twins were more likely to share autism than were dizygotic (fraternal) twins. More, incidence rates of autistic disorder among siblings of autism increases from a one in 1000 to a one in 80 (sometimes documented as one in 50) chance of having ASD (Volkmar & Wiesner, 2009). However, the specific genes involved have not been located to date. In fact, researchers are not sure how many genes play into the disorder. Estimates range from four to more than 20. It appears that different manifestations of ASD have different genetic factors. Much research is being done in this area, and there is great hope that the specific genes will be identified within the next 10 or so years.

Neurological structure and development: The first reason most researchers believe that there is a neurological component to autism is that children with autism are more likely to develop epilepsy than are typically developing children (Volkmar & Wiesner, 2009). As the technology for studying the brain has advanced, researchers have found that about half of children with autism have abnormal electroencephalograms (EEG). While there is no autism-specific pattern of abnormality, the high number of children with unusual EEGs speaks to there being an underlying, probably structural, brain

difference between typically developing individuals and individuals with ASD. More recently, researchers have found that individuals with ASD have smaller and fewer Purkinje cells than typically developing individuals, most noticeably in the cerebellum (Firth, 2008). There is also evidence that the cells of individuals with ASD tend to be less densely packed in the limbic systems (Firth, 2008). Finally, the frontal cortex of individuals with ASD tends to be made of smaller and more isolated cells than in typically developing brains (Firth, 2008). Much like genetics, there is great hope for making significant strides in understanding the neurology of ASD over the next 10 years.

Environmental factors: Theories that environmental factors, such as pesticide use or immunizations, contribute to autism are the most controversial in terms of the disorder's etiology. Most researchers agree that there is little evidence for a direct environmental cause of autism. However, there are countless anecdotal accounts of parents using bio-medical treatments that rid the child's body of toxins and cure the child of autism. This does not work for everyone, but the experiences of the individuals it has worked for cannot be disputed. That being said, it should be noted that the more severe the autism, the less likely it is that the bio-medical treatments will work. Therefore it can, and probably should, be argued that while environmental factors can lead to a better or worse prognosis, they are not the cause of the disorder.

Many current studies are being undertaken to explore the causes of ASD. The Study to Explore Early Development (SEED) is a multi-year study funded by the CDC (2011). SEED is the largest U.S. study looking at factors that may put children at risk for ASD or other developmental disabilities. Learning more about the risk factors can assist with finding causes for ASD.

Systems Affected

ASD affects social interactions and the ability of the person to accept and adapt to changes in the environment. Specific diagnostic criteria for ASD, as delineated by the *DSM-5* (APA, 2013), include five diagnostic criteria and three severity levels. A summary of the levels and criteria are provided below, followed by a description of the severity levels.

There are five specific diagnostic criteria. The first looks at persistent deficits in social communication and social interaction in three categories: social-emotional reciprocity (d7 Interpersonal Interactions and Relationships); nonverbal communication behaviors used in social interactions (d315 Communicating with — Receiving — Nonverbal Messages, d335 Producing Nonverbal Messages); and developing, maintaining, and understanding relationships (d710 Basic Interpersonal Interactions, d720 Complex Interpersonal Interactions). The second criteria looks at restricted, repetitive patterns of behavior, interests, or activities with the presence of at least two of the following four observation categories: stereotyped or repetitive motor movements, use of objects, or speech; insistence on sameness, inflexible adherence to routines, or ritualized patterns of behavior; highly restricted, fixated interests of abnormal intensity or focus; or hyper- or hypo-reactivity to sensory input (b1 Mental Functions, especially b140 Attention Functions, b152 Emotional Functions, b160 Thought Functions, and b167 Mental Functions of Language, d131 Learning Through Actions with Objects, d133 Acquiring Language). The third criterion is that symptoms are present during early development. The fourth is that the symptoms cause significant functional impairment. The fifth criteria requires ruling out other possible explanations for the symptoms.

It should be noted that individuals previously diagnosed using the *DSM-IV-TR* (APA, 2000) categories of autistic disorder, Asperger's disorder, or pervasive developmental disorder not otherwise specified will now be given the diagnosis of ASD. Individuals who have marked deficits in social communication but do not meet other symptom criteria should be considered for the diagnosis of social communication disorder.

The *DSM-5* divides ASD into three severity levels depending on the level of support required (APA, 2013):

Level 1, requires support: Deficits in social communication cause noticeable impairments in initiating and maintaining social interactions. The inflexible behaviors interfere with functioning in one or more situations.

Level 2, requires substantial support: The marked deficits in social communication skills are apparent even when support systems are in place. The restricted, repetitive behaviors are significant enough that they are obvious to a casual observer and cause distress when change is required.

Level 3, requires very substantial support: Severe deficits in social communication result in very limited initiation of interactions and minimal response to others. The restricted, repetitive behaviors are extremely inflexible and the inability to change focus markedly interferes with functioning in all activities.

Secondary Problems

Common secondary conditions in ASD include epilepsy (seizure disorder), sleep disorders, hyperactivity, anxiety, and depression (Volkmar & Wiesner, 2009). However, the most concerning and problematic secondary conditions in ASD are sensory processing dysfunctions, cognitive impairment, and self-injurious behaviors. These are discussed in detail below.

Sensory processing dysfunctions: Most, if not all, individuals with ASD have sensory processing difficulties. There are three primary types of sensory problems in ASD: sensory over-responsivity, sensory under-responsivity, and sensory seeking (Volkmar & Wiesner, 2009).

- Sensory over-responsivity is caused by the brain not being able to inhibit sensations effectively (Kranowitz, 2005). Individuals tend to have "melt-downs" regularly, because they cannot control how their brain responds to stimuli (b152 Emotional Functions, b156 Perceptual Functions).
- Sensory under-responsivity occurs when individuals with ASD react less intensely to sensory information than normally developing individuals (b2 Sensory Functions and Pain). Here it seems to take much more neural activity to reach a responsive threshold (Kranowitz, 2005). For example, many parents report that their child with autism seems to feel no pain when s/he falls or great pain is required before their child will respond (b280 Sensation of Pain).
- Sensory seeking individuals need more intense sensory input than typically developing children. These individuals often exhibit high levels of self-stimulation (b156 Perceptual Functions, b160 Thought Functions) and tend to bump,

press, spin, and jump more than other children (Kranowitz, 2005).

As a final word on sensory processing in ASD, it should be noted that many individuals with ASD tend to have a mixed sensory processing disorder. They might be unable to stand loud noises, but seek physical sensory stimulation constantly (Kranowitz, 2005). This greatly affects the way they adapt and understand the world around them, and it is key to understand an individual's sensory profile before developing any kind of programming, especially recreation programming. Understanding what sensations an individual loves and hates can help create an environment where the individual thrives. On the other hand, not knowing how the individual processes sensory information can lead to an individual having a melt-down and possibly never getting to participate in that day's activity.

Cognitive impairment: Approximately 50% of individuals with ASD have below average intelligence, with the other 50% exhibiting average to above average intelligence. However, it is not just cognitive deficits or surpluses that mark the cognitive characteristics of autism. It has been shown that most individuals with ASD think completely differently than typically developing individuals (Volkmar & Wiesner, 2009). This is best explained by Temple Grandin when she describes the way children with autism think as being similar to Google images (Grandin, 2010). Individuals with ASD think visually, rather than linguistically (b160 Thought Functions). This means that cognition is very literal and concrete. It has also been noted that children with autism tend to process information more slowly than typically developing children (Volkmar & Wiesner, 2009). This is often attributed to their strength in visual processing. It seems to take longer to find the correct picture associated with the word in question and apply it within a new or different setting (b167 Mental Functions of Language) (Volkmar & Wiesner, 2009). And, some individuals with ASD are unable to generalize across situations (b164 Higher-Level Cognitive Functions), so that a skill mastered in one environment cannot be completed in another because the way the individual understands the behavior is contingent on the specific environment it was learned in (Volkmar & Wiesner, 2009).

Self-injurious behavior: About 10% of individuals with ASD exhibit self-injurious behavior (SIB)

(Schreibman, 2005; Volkmar & Wiesner, 2009). SIB is any behavior that is self-inflicted and causes physical injury to the individual (b126 Temperament and Personality Functions, b152 Emotional Functions, d240 Handling Stress and Other Psychological Demands) (Neisworth & Wolfe, 2005). Common SIBs include biting hands and arms, scratching or hitting face, head banging, pinching, and eye gouging (Neisworth & Wolfe, 2005). Less common are abusive behaviors towards others. Both of these behaviors have been shown to improve with positive behavioral interventions.

Prognosis

No single known cure currently exists for ASD; however, most children greatly improve with both treatment and age (NIMH, 2011). There is no single best treatment package for all children with ASD. One point that most professionals agree on is that early intervention is important; another is that most individuals with ASD respond well to highly structured, specialized programs (NIMH, 2011). A majority of individuals with ASD will need support and services throughout their lifetime (Volkmar & Wiesner, 2009). However, with the appropriate support and services, most individuals with ASD will find employment, form relationships, and continue to learn and to develop throughout their lives (NIMH, 2011).

According to the *DSM-5* (APA, 2013) the best established prognostic factors for individual outcomes with ASD are presence or absence of associated intellectual disability and language impairment and additional mental health problems. For example, functional language by age five years is a good prognostic sign while additional mental health problems lead to a poorer prognosis. Epilepsy, as a comorbid diagnosis, is associated with greater intellectual disability and lower verbal ability. Functional consequences of ASD for young children are impacted by rate or effectiveness of learning, especially in settings where social interaction with peers is part of the process. Extreme difficulties in planning, organizing, and coping with change may negatively impact academic achievement, even for students with above-average intelligence. For adults there may be consequences for health caused by reduced help seeking due to isolation and communication difficulties. Strategies to offset these functional limitations can be managed for positive outcomes of independent living and gainful employment.

Assessment

Typical Scope of Team Assessment

Assessment usually involves input from parents or family and across several contexts such as home, school (for older child), and community. Observation, interview, and standardized measurement tools are used. These may include the *Autism Diagnosis Interview—Revised* (ADI-R) and the *Autism Diagnostic Observation Schedule* (ADOS-G) (National Institute of Mental Health, 2011). The ADI-R is a structured interview that contains over 100 items and is conducted with a caregiver. It consists of four main factors — the child's communication, social interaction, repetitive behaviors, and age-of-onset. The ADOS-G is an observational measure used to uncover socio-communicative behaviors that are often delayed, abnormal, or absent in children with ASD. Still another instrument often used by professionals is the *Childhood Autism Rating Scale*. It aids in evaluating the child's body movements, adaptation to change, listening response, verbal communication, and relationship to people. It is suitable for use with children over two years of age. The examiner observes the child and also obtains relevant information from the parents. The child's behavior is rated on a scale based on deviation from the typical behavior of children of the same age (National Institute of Mental Health, 2011). Each case is highly individualized; nevertheless, most approaches focus on the areas of behavior (d2 General Tasks and Demands, d7 Interpersonal Interactions and Relationships), communication (d3 Communication), and socialization (d7 Interpersonal Interactions and Relationships, d9 Community, Social, and Civic Life).

In a case study approach, Kennedy et al. (2000) found that assessment of causes for stereotypical behavior is not as important as individual analysis of approaches to successfully manage the behaviors. Research suggests that physical exercise provides some reduction of stereotypic behaviors in children with ASD (Petrus et al., 2008). Thus, within the scope of evaluation, analysis of physical or movement-related behavior is suggested (d4 Mobility).

Areas of Concern for RT Assessment

Within recreational therapy, a variety of additional assessment approaches are used. These often depend on program settings. In one inpatient program for children, as reported by Rothwell, Piatt, and Mattingly (2008), the *School Social Behavior Scales* (SSBS) assessment is used for evaluation of social skills (d740 Formal Relationships, d750 Informal Social Relationships). The SSBS is comprised of two scales: Social Competence and Antisocial Behavior. These two concepts, social competence and antisocial behavior, are not dichotomous, but are related. Although these concepts are linked (i.e., poor social competency means it is more likely the child will engage in antisocial behaviors), the nature of the relationship is unknown, thus, they are measured in two different scales. The Social Competency scale includes 32 positively worded questions divided into three subscales (interpersonal skills, self-management skills, and academic skills). Interpersonal skills consists of 14 items that measure social skills needed for establishing positive relationships with and gaining acceptance among peers. Self-management includes 10 items that measure social skills related to self-restraint, cooperation, and compliance to school rules and expectations. Academic skills consists of eight items that measure competent performance of and engagement in academic tasks. The Antisocial Behavior Scale includes 33 items divided into three subscales (hostile-irritable, antisocial-aggressive, disruptive-demanding). Hostile-irritable consists of 14 items that describe behaviors considered to be self-centered, irritating, and annoying and likely to lead to rejection by peers. Antisocial-aggressive consists of 10 behavioral descriptors that relate to violation of school rules and harm or threats to others. Disruptive-demanding includes nine items that reflect ongoing school activities where the client places inappropriate demands on others, such as continually seeking teacher's attention.

In the school setting, the therapist often uses results from tests already completed to plan for a treatment approach that is complementary with others yet unique in the interventions used for specific annual goals for the student.

Findings from assessments used in community settings vary widely depending on the organization's mission. Often, a therapist working in a community setting will have access to education or clinical records and can supplement this information with a specific assessment for the setting. For example, if a child is involved in aquatic therapy through a municipal park program, the therapist may complete additional tests to ascertain skills and behaviors related directly to the intervention being considered.

The complete assessment process will provide information on the core outcomes: social skills, communication, and behavior (Warren et al., 2012). Most often findings from observations are based on multiple settings and indicate the amount of deviation from typical development. For example, the comparison for a very young child in the area of communication might be shown by the differences outlined below (Clark, Gulati, & Johnston, 2008).

- Typically developing child: Uses gestures, pointing and showing to communicate; begins to use single words; may imitate or echo utterances of others for a short time; draws attention to self or interesting objects; and requests information, such as asking WH questions (who, what, when, where, why, how).
- Child with ASD: Rarely uses pointing; often uses contact gestures; may use persistent echolalia; rarely draws attention to objects or seeks information; and does not use eye gaze in focusing on objects of attention.

Thus, the RT assessment results related to communication could say, "Client demonstrated communication deficits in these areas: using gestures and pointing to indicate wants and needs; echoing utterances of others in the playroom, at meals, with family, and during story time in excess of typically developing patterns for age four; and during weekly observation touched adult on elbow or arm about five times per request for up to six episodes a day." ICF scores for b140 Attention Functions, b1142 Orientation to Person, b167 Mental Functions of Language, d335 Producing Nonverbal Messages, d350 Conversation, and other relevant codes would also be provided. For other ages, the findings usually continue to be reported as deviations from developmental norms.

Other typical results related to communication show that imitation is rare in language development. Children with ASD are more interested in environmental sounds and noises than in interacting with others (b340 Alternative Vocalization Functions).

Development of language and social skills in children with autism does not often follow a pattern (Mayo Clinic, 2011). There is a wide variability exhibited in results for children of the same age.

Results related directly to social skills show limited turn taking or ability to grasp the concept of sharing (White, Keonig, & Scahill, 2006). Other social skill findings show that initiating interaction with another is minimal or atypical. For example, the child will repeat a request many times or use a contact gesture such as tapping on another person's arm repetitively in spite of receiving a response. These can be scored with d710 Basic Interpersonal Interactions.

A typically developing child may exhibit enjoyment in an activity, but observation of a child with autism shows very little expression of joy or positive emotion (b126 Temperament and Personality Functions). Other actions demonstrated by a child with autism are narrow range of interests in play, activity, or toys. For example, the child may play with the same toy for a long period of time (b140 Attention Functions), and sometimes in an atypical way (d9200 Play). So instead of playing with a toy car as a vehicle, the child may toss the car up and down as if it were a ball. This "play" behavior may extend for long periods of time.

As a consequence of the communication deficits, atypical behavior patterns, and limited social skills, children with autism have great difficulty interacting with peers in typical play activities (White, Keonig, & Scahill, 2006). For example, in situations where the communication includes elements of humor, sarcasm, or metaphors, the child with autism may show limited or no response to the intended messages or have great difficulty interpreting the nonliteral format (d315 Communicating with — Receiving — Nonverbal Messages) (National Autism Center, 2011; White, Keonig, & Scahill, 2006). Playing alone is a common assessment observation. Lack of imaginative or imitating behavior at the level of the typically developing child is also a finding that shows up as a problem area on assessments (d710 Basic Interpersonal Interactions, d9200 Play). As a result of the social skill difficulties and communication problems, a child with autism often has trouble developing friendships (d720 Complex Interpersonal Interactions).

Results from screening and assessment related to the three core primary areas of social skills, communication, and behavior can be summarized by review of the charts from initial and ongoing diagnosis based on the DSM criteria (APA, 2000; Mayo Clinic, 2011) as well as additional items for these three areas in standardized RT assessments. In addition, typical RT assessment findings will provide further information related to setting-specific needs, such as a primary program or modality. For example, an agency that provides aquatic therapy may have results that cover that area or an organization which offers animal-assisted therapy will have findings directly connected to that program. It is recommended that RT findings extend results of social skills, communication, and behavior to link to RT programs being offered or planned.

ICF Core Set

An ICF Core Set for ASD is currently under development. Go to http://www.icf-research-branch.org/icf-core-sets-projects-sp-1641024398/other-health-conditions/icf-core-set-for-autism-spectrum for more information.

Treatment Direction

Whole Team Approach

There is no one best approach or single best treatment path for a child with ASD. One point upon which most professionals do agree is that early intervention is critical; another is that most individuals with ASD respond well to highly structured, specialized programs. Applied behavior analysis (formerly known as behavior modification) has become widely accepted as an effective treatment. Many years of research have demonstrated the efficacy of applied behavioral methods in reducing inappropriate behavior and in increasing communication, learning, and appropriate social behavior. The goal of behavioral management is to reinforce desirable behaviors and reduce undesirable ones (National Institute of Mental Health, 2011). Mayo Clinic (2011) suggests individualized and structured approaches work best for all age levels. A cooperative group effort among professionals should seek treatment directed to increasing social (d7 Interpersonal Interactions and Relationships) and communication skills (d3 Communication) and decreasing unacceptable behaviors (d710 Basic Interpersonal Interactions, d720 Complex Interpersonal Interactions) for the child with ASD. Even though the child will not outgrow ASD, nor can it be cured, most make great progress and learn to function well with these approaches.

In 2009, the National Autism Center completed a comprehensive, multi-year effort called the National Standards Project. Its goal was to identify the level of research support available for interventions for children and adolescents with ASD. The findings include 11 established treatments that have been thoroughly researched and have sufficient evidence to confidently support a high level of effectiveness based on evidence presented. The 11 established treatments are (National Autism Center, 2009, p. 39)

Antecedent package: These interventions typically involve events that precede the occurrence of the target behavior to be increased or decreased; examples of actions include time delays, stimulus variation, or environmental enrichment. This is suitable for many deficits.

Behavioral package: These interventions are designed to reduce problem behavior and teach functional alternative behaviors or skills through the application of basic principles of behavior change; examples of actions include token economy strategies and task analyses. This is also suitable for many deficits.

Comprehensive behavioral treatment for young children: These treatment programs are also referenced as applied behavioral analysis programs or behavioral inclusive program and early intensive behavioral intervention; these interventions are comprehensive, intense, used across all settings and behaviors (home, school, play, etc.), and for children under age eight.

Joint attention intervention: The focus is on teaching a child to respond to the nonverbal social bids of others (d315 Communicating with — Receiving — Nonverbal Messages) or to initiate joint attention interactions (d710 Basic Interpersonal Interactions). Examples include pointing to objects, showing items or activities to another person, and following eye gaze.

Modeling: An adult or peer provides a demonstration of the target behavior either live or video-taped (d710 Basic Interpersonal Interactions). This could be used in conjunction with other techniques or as an intervention strategy on its own.

Naturalistic teaching strategies: These interventions may include providing a stimulating environment, encouraging conversation, milieu teaching, providing choices and direct/natural reinforcers, and rewarding reasonable attempts. These improve e3 Support and Relationships to reduce observed deficits.

Peer training package: This strategy focuses on teaching children (peers or siblings) without disabilities strategies for facilitating play and social interactions with children on the autism spectrum. Typical programs may be best buddies or circle of friends. These use e320 Friends to improve observed deficits in d710 Basic Interpersonal Interactions and d750 Informal Social Relationships.

Pivotal response treatment: These training strategies focus on pivotal behavior areas such as self-initiation (d210 Undertaking a Single Task, d220 Undertaking Multiple Tasks) or social communication (d350 Conversation). The intervention involves parents and is conducted across multiple setting.

Schedules: These interventions use lists to complete activities, such as steps in a task or sequences in a skill (d210 Undertaking a Single Task, d220 Undertaking Multiple Tasks). The mode of communication can be verbal, written, visual, or other ways that meet the individual's needs.

Self-management: These interventions involve promoting independence by training individuals to regulate their own behavior by recording the occurrence/non-occurrence of the target behavior and using self-selected motivational strategies for achievement (d230 Carrying Out Daily Routine). Having the clients set their own goals is a suggested strategy to include in these interventions.

Story-based intervention package: These interventions are based on a narrative, descriptive, written, or oral perspective telling of a task, skill, or action to be accomplished in a story format. There are many story-based programs available, but the format can be applied by the recreational therapist in any area for a variety of needs. Pictures, text, audio, video, and combined delivery of the story can be used.

A full document on the findings from the study and the treatments is available by visiting the National Standards Project area on the NAC website (National Autism Center, 2011).

Recreational Therapy Approach

Approaches for RT depend on the individual with ASD and the setting. Often the treatment is part of the school's Individualized Education Plan (IEP) for the student. If a specific goal is on the IEP, then plans are made to achieve it over the academic year. Plans may include target dates for incremental achievement. Universities, human service agencies, and public recreation providers frequently collaborate with schools to provide therapy for children with autism. Waller and Wozencroft (2010) describe a long-term affiliation with RT students at the University of Tennessee and local school districts. Some of the outcomes sought by the school are improving social skills and enhancing positive behavior (d7 Interpersonal Interactions and Relationships). The children's needs for routine and consistency are met with techniques of intentional re-direction, frequent reminders, and visual cues through the therapeutic activities used in this partnership (d2 General Tasks and Demands).

In any setting the therapist must also follow current, existing applied behavior analysis plans for the child even if it is not a direct treatment in RT. Behavior plans may include tokens or levels and the therapist must be familiar with the details of the plan.

Specific attention on play, recreation, and leisure frequently mean some components of the treatment plan will be carried out by the RT based on context or content. For example, a child in a residential treatment program who needs to learn to tolerate groups (d9205 Socializing) may have weekly community outings that are part of the program provided by RT.

Recreational Therapy Interventions

Much of the published evidence-based information relates to children but not directly to RT interventions. Solish, Perry, and Minnes (2010) found that children with ASD participate in fewer activities than their typical peers (d920 Recreation and Leisure). They also found that friendship with peers was minimal (d750 Informal Social Relationships) and engagement in activities was primarily with adults (e.g., d920 Recreation and Leisure). This research would suggest that interventions might be more effective supporting peer friendship development (d720 Complex Interpersonal Interactions) in the interventions focused on communication (d3 Communication) and social skills (d710 Basic Interpersonal Interactions). It might also encourage increasing engagement and involvement of children with ASD in activities with peers rather than parents or other adults.

An intervention based on the use of LEGO blocks has shown promise in increasing peer socialization skills (d710 Basic Interpersonal Interactions, d720 Complex Interpersonal Interactions) (Owen et al., 2008). The idea behind LEGO therapy is to motivate children to work together by building in pairs or groups of three (d8803 Shared Cooperative Play). A therapist guides the children in specific tasks, guiding them in following social rules as they build. Although this intervention has not been reported to be used by recreational therapy, it appears to be a promising one to explore as an effective approach.

Another study relates to young adults with ASD. García-Villamisar and Dattilo (2010) conducted a yearlong leisure intervention with young adults with ASD. The intended outcomes were stress reduction and an increase in factors related to quality of life. The interventions included engagement in exercise, playing games and doing crafts, attending events, and participating in other recreation activities. From baseline to the end of the intervention 12 months later there was a significant decrease in overall scores of stress levels (d240 Handling Stress and Other Psychological Demands) for participants. There was also a significant increase in the four factors of quality of life that were measured (satisfaction, independence, competence, and social interaction), as well as the total score for quality of life. Relevant ICF codes include b125 Dispositions and Intra-Personal Functions, b126 Temperament and Personality Functions, b130 Energy and Drive Functions, d710 Basic Interpersonal Interactions, and d720 Complex Interpersonal Interactions. It is interesting to note that anxiety and depression may become a problem that develops for persons with ASD as they approach adulthood.

Many interventions are focused on social skills, behavior, and communication. These interventions often encompass recreation, leisure, and play activities. Quality evidence-based research needs to be published for specific RT interventions or the collaborative aspects of RT in comprehensive programs.

Functional Skills and Education, Training, and Counseling

Functional skills typically addressed for children and adults with ASD are communication, social skills, and acceptable behavior. Education and training typically focuses on improving social skills and communication, as well as decreasing maladaptive behavior, if needed. Among best practices, a growing body of empirical work highlights ideas for improvement in these areas. Social skills groups and video modeling have accumulated necessary evidence to be classified as evidence-based practices (Reichow & Volkmar, 2010). From data collected through the Autism Treatment Network, a group of 15 autism centers, *Health-Related Quality of Life* (HRQoL) was found to be significantly lower for children with ASD than those of typically developing counterparts (Kuhlthau et al., 2010). Furthermore, when compared to normative data from children with chronic conditions, analysis revealed that children with ASD demonstrated worse HRQoL for total, psychosocial, emotional, and social functioning, but did not demonstrate differing scores for physical and school functioning. HRQoL was not consistently related to ASD diagnosis or intellectual ability. However, it was consistently related to internalizing and externalizing problems as well as repetitive behaviors, social responsiveness, and adaptive behaviors. Associations among HRQoL and behavioral characteristics suggest that treatments aimed at improvements in these behaviors may improve HRQoL. Therefore, the greatest improvements will be seen when focus is placed on improving behavior (d720 Complex Interpersonal Interactions) and social skills (d710 Basic Interpersonal Interactions).

Community Integration

Children and adults with ASD are provided many opportunities for treatment in community recreation settings. Opportunities range from segregated programs to inclusion in ongoing recreation activities with support. Recent findings from a search for best practices in inclusive service delivery (ISD) across the U.S. indicated the use of inclusion support staff as a prevalent practice to address the need for direct support for persons with ASD participating in recreation (Miller, Schleien, & Bowens, 2010). Data gathered from inclusion facilitators and administrators from 15 public recreation agencies identified as successful with ISD yielded significant details regarding the use of this staffing practice. Inclusion support staff were essential in assisting participants with disabilities in regard to acquisition of leisure and social skills (d155 Acquiring Skills); participating fully with adaptations, physical assistance, and prompting (d920 Recreation and Leisure); and successful social interactions with peers (b122 Global Psychosocial Functions, d750 Informal Social Relationships). Miller, Schleien, and Bowens (2010) also found the process to be extremely individualized, meaning the inclusion staff need to be highly skilled and able to develop plans for the individual with whom they are working. Staff also need to be very knowledgeable about the diagnostic characteristic of the person, in this case about ASD.

Parents (d760 Family Relationships), immediate family (e310 Immediate Family, and Caregivers (e340 Personal Care Providers and Personal Assistants) need support as well as training or education to provide the most appropriate care for their child with ASD. Education may focus on community resources and the value of play in diverse environments. Recreation skill development may include a focus on communication, behavior, or social skills, as well, with a parent or caregiver acting as the individual coach. This role of coach or behavior specialist in a recreation setting may need to be part of training for parents in a family-centered group or individual sessions. Helping family or caregivers learn behavioral support for a child can be done without the child with ASD in role-play or simulation formats to increase confidence in carrying out the techniques in real life situations.

Health Promotion

Many organizations and agencies exist for promoting healthy development for persons with ASD. Some groups provide support for parents, family members, and caregivers. Autism Speaks and the Global Autism Collaboration are examples of two such groups. Information on a wide array of topics, such as nutrition or local events, can be found. The resources section lists some of the more well-known.

Children with ASD essentially need the same healthcare as other children following such typical good health guidelines as eating nutritious food, including physical activity and exercise in daily routines, drinking water, getting sufficient sleep, and others (d570 Looking After One's Health). In addition, parents or caregivers of children with ASD might need to find healthcare providers who are familiar and comfortable in providing care for persons with ASD. Furthermore, a behavioral change or behavioral issue may be because the person with ASD has a medical problem s/he cannot describe. For instance, head banging could be related to a disability, or it could be due to a headache or toothache. For this reason, it is important to find out if there is a physical problem before making changes in a person's treatment or therapy. Due to communication issues related to the ASD diagnosis, careful attention to healthy behavior and following good health guidelines is important for a healthy lifestyle.

Miscellaneous

Some disorders share common characteristics with ASD and some may occur simultaneously (be comorbid) with ASD. The most frequently occurring are anxiety and depression, attention-deficit/hyperactivity disorder, obsessive-compulsive disorder, psychotic disorders, bipolar disorder, and oppositional defiant disorder. It is highly recommended that therapists working with an individual with ASD become familiar with characteristics of these disorders so referrals for further screening, diagnosis, and treatment can be provided.

Resources

Autism Speaks

www.autismspeaks.org/

Autism Speaks provides general information about ASD, as well as funds and disseminates cutting edge research into understanding, treating, and hopefully one day curing ASD. It also provides excellent resources that allow for individuals to get involved in the autism community and help support families and individuals who live with ASD every day.

Autism Society

www.autism-society.org

The Autism Society webpage offers many resources and great information about ASD. It also serves as an excellent way to locate local branches of the autism society in your area. Finally, the Autism Society webpage has excellent information on getting treatment, and where to find help locally.

Autism guide for parents

www.nimh.nih.gov/health/publications/a-parents-guide-to-autism-spectrum-disorder/complete-index.shtml

Provides an excellent comprehensive overview of ASD for parents and caregivers.

Autism (journal)

aut.sagepub.com/

Autism is a major, peer-reviewed, bi-monthly, international journal, providing research of direct and practical relevance to help improve the quality of life for individuals with autism or autism-related disorders. It is interdisciplinary in nature, focusing on evaluative research in all areas, including intervention, diagnosis, training, case study analyses of therapy, education, neuroscience, psychological processes, evaluation of particular therapies, quality of life issues, family issues and family services, medical and genetic issues, and epidemiological research.

Autism Treatment

www.neurologychannel.com/autism/treatment.shtml

A great place to start when trying to understand how ASD is treated. Provides an overview of the major treatment options, and has a great handout of questions for parents to ask doctors.

Autism practitioner manual for education settings

www.nationalautismcenter.org/learning/practitioner.php

This website provides a free educator's manual entitled, *Evidence-Based Practice and Autism in the Schools: Educator Manual.*

Global Autism Collaboration

www.GlobalAutismCollaboration.com

The mission of the Global Autism Collaboration is to network and collaborate with autism organizations worldwide to generate necessary legal and social change to deal with the global autism health crisis.

American Academy of Pediatrics

www.healthychildren.org

The mission of the American Academy of Pediatrics is to attain optimal physical, mental, and social health and well-being for all infants, children, adolescents, and young adults. Many links and resources for professionals.

Vanderbilt Evidence-Based Practice Center

www.effectivehealthcare.ahrq.gov/ehc/products/106/656/CER26_Autism_Report_04-14-2011.pdf

The Vanderbilt Evidence-Based Practice Center systematically reviewed evidence on therapies for children ages two to 12 with autism spectrum disorder (ASD). The focus was on treatment outcomes, modifiers of treatment effectiveness, evidence for generalization of outcomes to other contexts, and evidence to support treatment decisions in children ages zero to two years at risk for an ASD diagnosis. This document is a compilation of information from reliable sources on studies for many areas of treatment and multiple types of outcomes. It is very helpful to find tables and summaries of so much information on ASD therapies in one place.

References

American Psychiatric Association. (2013). *Diagnostic and statistical manual of mental disorders, fifth edition.* Washington, DC: American Psychiatric Association.

American Psychiatric Association. (2000). *Diagnostic and statistical manual of mental disorders, fourth edition, text revision.* Washington, DC: American Psychiatric Association.

Autism Society of America. (2010). Facts and statistics. Retrieved from http://www.autism-society.org/about-autism/facts-and-statistics.html.

Centers for Disease Control and Prevention. (2011). Autism spectrum disorders. Retrieved from http://www.cdc.gov/ncbddd/autism/index.html.

Clark, T., Gulati, S., & Johnston, J. (2008). Diagnosis and assessment of autism spectrum disorder. Children's Hospital Boston ©. Retrieved from http://www.childrenshospital.org/clinicalservices/Site2143/Documents/Autism%20+%20Deaf%20FINAL%20%28Copy%20Proctected%29.pdf.

Firth, U. (2008). *Autism: A very short introduction.* New York: Oxford University Press.

Folstein, S. & Rutter, R. (1977). Infantile autism: A genetic study of 21 twin pairs. *The Journal of Child Psychology and Psychiatry, 18*(4), 297-321.

García-Villamisar, D. A. & Dattilo, J. (2010). Effects of a leisure programme on quality of life and stress of individuals with ASD. *Journal of Intellectual Disabilities Research, 54*(7), 611-619.

Grandin, T. (2010). *Thinking in Pictures: My Life with Autism.* New York: Knopf Doubleday.

Kennedy, C. H., Meyer, K. A., Knowles, T., & Shukla, S. (2000). Analyzing the multiple functions of stereotypical behavior for students with autism: Implications for assessment and treatment. *Journal of Applied Behavior Analysis, 33*(4), 559-571.

Kranowitz, C. S. (2005). *The out-of-sync child: Recognizing and coping with sensory processing disorder,* 2nd edition. New York: Penguin Group.

Kuhlthau, K., Orlich, F., Hall, T. A., Sikora, D., Kovacs, E. A., Delahaye, J., & Clemons, T. E. (2010). Health-related quality of life in children with autism spectrum disorders: Results from the autism treatment network. *Journal of Autism and Developmental Disorders, 40*(6), 721-729.

Lord, C. & Bishop, S. L. (2010) Autism spectrum disorders: Diagnosis, prevalence, and service for children and families. *Sharing Child and Youth Development Knowledge. 24*(2), 1-27.

Mayo Clinic. (2011). Autism. Retrieved from http://www.mayoclinic.com/health/autism/DS00348.

Miller, K. D., Schleien, S. J., & Bowens, F. (2010). Support staff as an essential component of inclusive recreation services. *Therapeutic Recreation Journal, 44*(1), 35-49.

National Autism Center. (2009). Evidence-based practice and autism in the schools: A guide to providing appropriate interventions to students with autism spectrum disorders. Retrieved from http://www.nationalautismcenter.org/learning/ed_manual.php.

National Autism Center. (2011). National Standards Report. Retrieved from http://www.nationalautismcenter.org/nsp/.

National Institute of Mental Health. (2011). Autism spectrum disorders (pervasive developmental disorders). Retrieved from http://www.nimh.nih.gov/health/topics/autism-spectrum-disorders-pervasive-developmental-disorders/index.shtml#.

Neisworth, J. T. & Wolfe, P. S. (2005). *The autism encyclopedia.* Baltimore: Paul H. Brookes.

Owens, G., Granader, Y., Humphrey, A., & Baron-Cohen, S. (2008). LEGO Therapy and the Social Use of Language Programme: An evaluation of two social skills interventions for children with high functioning autism and Asperger syndrome. *Journal of Developmental Disorders, 38*, 1944-1957.

Petrus, C., Adamson, S. R., Block, L., Einarson, S. J., Sharifnejad, M., & Harris, S. R. (2008) Effects of exercise interventions on stereotypic behaviours in children with autism spectrum disorder. *Physiotherapy Canada, 60*(2), 134-145.

Reichow, B. & Volkmar, F. R. (2010). Social skills interventions for individuals with autism: Evaluation for evidence-based practices within a best evidence synthesis framework. *Journal of Autism and Developmental Disorders, 40*(2), 149-166.

Rothwell, E., Piatt, J., & Mattingly, K. (2006). Social competence: Evaluation of an outpatient recreation therapy treatment program for children with behavioral disorders. *Therapeutic Recreation Journal, 40*(4), 241-254.

Schreibman, L. (2005). *The science and fiction of autism.* Cambridge: Harvard University Press.

Siegel, B. (2003). *Helping children with autism learn.* New York: Oxford University Press.

Solish, A., Perry, A., & Minnes, P. (2010). Participation of children with and without disabilities in social, recreational and leisure activities. *Journal of Applied Research in Intellectual Disabilities, 23*, 226-236.

Volkmar, F. R. & Wiesner, L. A. (2009). *A practical guide to autism.* Hoboken: John Wiley & Sons, Inc.

Waller, S. N. & Wozencroft, A. J. (2010). Public school-university partnership model project TRiPS: A school-based learning opportunity for therapeutic recreation students. *Therapeutic Recreation Journal, 44*(3), 223-233.

Warren, Z., Veenstra-VanderWeele, J., Stone, W., Bruzek, J. L., Nahmias, A. S., Foss-Feig, J. H., Jerome, R. N., Krishnaswami, S., Sathe, N. A., Glasser, A. M., Surawicz, T., McPheeters, M. L. (2012). Therapies for children with autism spectrum disorders. Comparative effectiveness, Review No. 26. (Prepared by the Vanderbilt Evidence-based Practice Center under Contract No. 290-2007-10065-I.) AHRQ Publication No. 11-EHC029-EF. Rockville, MD: Agency for Healthcare Research and Quality. April 2011. Available at: www.effectivehealthcare.ahrq.gov/reports/final.cfm.

White, S. W., Keonig, K., & Scahill, L. (2007). Social skills development in children with autism spectrum disorders: A review of the intervention research. *Journal of Autism Developmental Disorders, 37*, 1858-1868. doi: 10.1007/s10803-006-0320-x.

4. Back Disorders and Back Pain

Heather R. Porter

There are various back disorders and conditions that cause acute or chronic back pain. Acute pain begins suddenly, lasts less than six months, and typically disappears once the underlying condition is resolved. Chronic pain remains active for six months or more, and the underlying causes may or may not be able to be resolved (Cleveland Clinic Foundation, 2009).

Incidence/Prevalence in U.S.

Anywhere from 30-50% of the U.S. population reports back pain within a three to twelve month window (Clinical Key Elsevier, 2012; Centers for Disease Control, 2012).

Predominant Age

Although back disorders and back pain can occur at any age, peak prevalence is between 45 and 59 years of age, with the first episode occurring between the ages of 20 and 40 years old (Clinical Key Elsevier, 2012). It is the most common reason for work disability in clients 40 years old and younger (Clinical Key Elsevier, 2012).

Causes

Common causes of back pain include degenerative causes (e.g., osteoarthritis, degenerative disk disease, spondylolisthesis), muscular causes (e.g., myofascial pain, paraspinal muscle strain), mechanical causes (e.g., prolapsed intervertebral disk), referred pain (e.g., endometriosis, hip joint pain, abdominal aortic aneurysm), vertebral fractures (e.g., osteoporosis), cancer (e.g., bony metastases, multiple myeloma), infection (e.g., vertebral osteomyelitis, spinal tuberculosis, diskitis, epidural abscess), vascular conditions (e.g., epidural hematoma), rheumatological conditions (e.g., rheumatoid arthritis, ankylosing spondylitis, psoriatic arthritis,

reactive arthritis), lesions causing spinal cord or cauda equina compression, heavy manual labor, obesity, and psychosocial factors such as job dissatisfaction or depression (Clinical Key Elsevier, 2012).

Individuals who have a low socioeconomic status and engage in jobs requiring heavy physical labor, static posture, bending and twisting, lifting, repetitive work, and vibration are also more likely to experience back disorders and back pain (Clinical Key Elsevier, 2012). Frequency of back pain also appears to correlate with perceived lack of social support at work, limited control at work, having an excessive workload, low job satisfaction, perceived inadequacy of income, and performance of unskilled or manual tasks (Moore, 2010).

Systems Affected

Back disorders and back pain primarily affect the musculoskeletal system. The basic symptoms are recorded using b28013 Pain in Back and other aspects of b280 Sensation of Pain. Other ICF codes include s120 Spinal Cord and Related Structures, s760 Structure of Trunk, and s770 Additional Musculoskeletal Structures Related to Movement.

Pain, especially chronic pain, can impact psychological, emotional, social, and cognitive health, as described in the Secondary Problem section.

Secondary Problems

A review of the literature by Moore (2010) identified several psychosocial issues related to chronic low back pain:

Life changes: Chronic low back pain can cause occupational disability (d845 Acquiring, Keeping, and Terminating a Job); financial stress (d850 Remunerative Employment); sleep disruption (b134 Sleep Functions); negative health consequences (b130 Energy and Drive Functions, b152 Emotional Functions); relationship distress (d760 Family Relationships); sexual dysfunction (b640 Sexual Functions); family role changes; and limitations in social, recreational, and household activities (d2 General Tasks and Demands, d4 Mobility, d9 Community, Social, and Civic Life).

Pain avoidance: Clients who fear of pain and avoid movement or activity because of pain-related fear are at risk of disuse, deconditioning, and pain-related disability, resulting in loss of strength and flexibility, obesity, cardiovascular disease, type 2 diabetes, increased pain severity, loss of ability to engage in meaningful activities, depression, and/or emotional distress. Some of the ICF codes include b455 Exercise Tolerance Functions, b7 Neuromusculoskeletal and Movement-Related Functions, b4 Functions of the Cardiovascular, Hematological, Immunological, and Respiratory Systems, b530 Weight Maintenance Functions, and any Activities and Participation codes that are affected. This, in turn, can increase further avoidance behaviors including abnormal postures or movement patterns designed to avoid pain (e.g., limping, guarding, and bracing, b7 Neuromusculoskeletal and Movement-Related Functions). Although such behaviors may reduce feelings of pain and pain-related fear, they can be difficult to renormalize, thus becoming a major obstacle to the process of learning that movement or activity can be performed without negative consequences.

Reinforcement of pain behavior: Behavior that has a positive outcome tends to continue, while behavior that has a negative outcome tends to occur less frequently, as described by operant theory. Contextual factors that can reinforce dysfunctional pain behaviors and cognitions include attention, sympathy, assistance with tasks, financial compensation, avoidance of undesired tasks, ability to engage in meaningful tasks that would not otherwise be possible (e.g., being "out on disability" allows a mother to be a stay at home with her children), and well-meaning healthcare professionals (e.g., recommendations to "take it easy" that reinforce catastrophizing cognitions). Record these using the appropriate Environmental Factors codes.

Depression: Depression is common in chronic low back pain and increases with pain severity, multiple pain problems, and lack of an identified cause of the pain. See the chapter on Major Depressive Disorder for more information about scoring depression symptoms. When depression is a comorbid condition with chronic pain, there is also greater functional impairment, more symptoms without an identified pathology, increased healthcare use, and higher healthcare costs. Individuals who have positive cognitive schemas, healthy coping skills, and social support may experience less emotional distress (and subsequent depression) compared to those who do not. Conversely, those who have negative cognitive schemas (b125 Dispositions and Intra-Personal Functions), unhealthy coping skills (b126 Temperament and Personality Functions), and a lack of social support (e3 Support and Relationships) are more likely to experience chronic low back pain due to lack of resources.

Prognosis

A comprehensive review of the literature by Hayden et al. (2010) found the following related to back pain prognosis:

Among clients who seek primary medical care for back pain, approximately 62% will continue to have pain a year after consultation. Of those who are off from work due to back pain, 16% will continue to be off from work at six months.

For those with acute back pain, 75-90% recover within weeks. However, one-quarter to one-third of those with acute injuries report having back pain again within six to twelve months after consultation. For those with chronic back pain, 60-80% continue to have symptoms at 12-month follow-up, with two-thirds still having pain one to two years after onset. Approximately 60% of individuals with back pain will experience back pain again.

Factors consistently reported in the literature that are associated with poor outcomes include a higher level of functional disability, sciatica, older age, poor general health, increased psychological or psychosocial stress, negative cognitive characteristics, poor relations with colleagues, heavy physical work demands, and presence of compensation. Other factors associated with a poor prognosis include passive coping strategies, somatization, job dissatisfaction, and low educational attainment.

Additionally, Moore (2010) found that individuals who appraise pain as a benign experience are less likely to experience pain and have a faster recovery, compared to those who appraise pain as a severe injury and subsequently become fearful of pain-related movement.

Assessment

Typical Scope of Team Assessment

According to the National Guideline for Low Back Disorders (Hegmann, 2011), the physician conducts an initial assessment focusing on the identification of red flags that could indicate a serious underlying condition. If a condition is suspected, further tests are done to confirm or rule out the possible problems. In the absence of red flags no imaging or further tests are recommended.

The guideline does not provide further guidance related to assessment by other disciplines, but these assessments will usually occur only when red flags have been found. In general, when a client with low back pain is referred to a particular therapy (e.g., recreational therapy, physical therapy, psychology), a full discipline-related assessment is conducted aimed at identifying underlying causes and triggers of pain (b280 Sensation of Pain), functional abilities (b7 Neuromusculoskeletal and Movement-Related Functions), cognitions, such as fear-avoidance behaviors (b126 Temperament and Personality Functions, and contextual issues including available support and resources and personal beliefs scored using Environmental Factors codes. Possible assessment tools include the *Faces Pain Scale, Numeric Rating Scale, Verbal Rating Scale/Graphic Rating Scale, Visual Analog Scale, Brief Pain Inventory, McGill Pain Questionnaire, Katz Index of Activities of Daily Living, Pain Disability Index, Roland-Morris Disability Questionnaire, WOMAC Index, Profile of Chronic Pain: Screen, Chronic Pain Acceptance Questionnaire,* and *Fear-Avoidance Beliefs Questionnaire.*

Areas of Concern for RT Assessment

Recreational therapists who see clients with back problems in an inpatient rehabilitation hospital usually find that the clients have had chronic pain for a long period of time and are there either to rehabilitate from a surgical procedure (e.g., laminectomy) or for general conditioning and pain management.

Clients will typically report a lifestyle of progressive losses associated with chronic pain including loss of activity level, loss of a job, loss of identity from their job, loss of a family role, loss of favorite hobbies or recreational activities, loss of internal locus of control because pain controls everything, loss of relationships, loss of sexuality and intimacy due to pain and psychological stressors, loss of sleep, loss of appetite, loss of positive feelings or depression, and loss of positive self-image including appearance, self-esteem, and confidence. All of these can be scored with the appropriate Activities and Participation codes as listed in the ICF Core Sets for Chronic Pain, Low Back Pain, and Musculoskeletal Conditions. The therapist will find a multitude of dynamics that may need to be addressed including communication skills, self-esteem, sexuality, and leisure issues.

Clients who are unemployed or on workers' compensation often report increased levels of pain since they stopped working. This could be attributed to further deconditioning due to a decreased activity level (b7 Neuromusculoskeletal and Movement-Related Functions) and/or an increased awareness and sensitivity to the pain because other stimuli related to work are no longer available (b280 Sensation of Pain).

Clients with a long-standing history of chronic pain often exhibit signs of learned helplessness and reduced participation or withdrawal from play, recreation, leisure, and community activities (b125 Dispositions and Intra-Personal Functions, b126 Temperament and Personality Functions). Therapists may find that the client has been self-medicating with alcohol or drugs to manage pain levels.

ICF Core Set

ICF Core Sets that might be helpful in identifying relevant ICF codes include Chronic Pain, Low Back Pain, and Musculoskeletal Conditions.

Treatment Direction

Whole Team Approach

In the absence of red flags for serious underlying conditions, the incident is treated with anti-inflammatory medication, adjustments to physical activity levels if needed, and the use of heat or cold to relieve discomfort (b280 Sensation of Pain). The physician reassures the client that low back pain is normal and that ordinary activity should be continued as it leads to the most rapid recovery. Additional education is also provided as needed by the physician to combat any elevated fear-avoidance beliefs (b126 Temperament and Personality Functions).

The National Guideline for Low Back Disorders provides evidence-based information regarding recommended treatments for specific back disorders that are more serious than simple back pain. These include acute low back pain, subacute low back pain, chronic low back pain, radicular pain syndromes, spinal stenosis, spinal fractures, sacroiliitis, spondylolisthesis, and facet degenerative joint disease. Recommendations are also given for prevention of low back disorders and post-operative low back pain (Hegmann, 2011). The treatment recommendations are further broken down into three categories: recommended, no recommendation, not recommended. Refer to the Resources section for information on how to access this document.

For those with chronic low back pain, the National Guidelines for Low Back Disorders recommends the utilization of an interdisciplinary rehabilitation program. A recent review of the literature by Moore (2012) also supports this recommendation, finding that there is strong evidence for the efficacy of interdisciplinary rehabilitation programs for chronic low back pain that include five full days a week of therapy for approximately four weeks. He particularly notes that "reviews have indicated that for non-radicular low back pain, interdisciplinary pain rehabilitation probably has better or at least equal outcomes to more invasive interventions, such as injections or surgery that also carry greater risk of iatrogenic consequences and greater cost" (p. 810).

Recreational Therapy Approach

Recreational therapy employs a holistic and biopsychosocial approach to pain management, with the primary aims of enhancing recovery and quality of life.

Recreational Therapy Interventions

Although not identified as recreational-therapy-specific interventions, the recommended interventions outlined by the National Guideline for Low Back Disorders that fall within the scope of recreational therapy practice (Hegmann, 2011) are provided below:

Interventions Based on Timing

Acute low back pain: Aerobic exercise (b455 Exercise Tolerance Functions), specific stretching exercises (b710 Mobility of Joint Functions), strengthening exercises (b730 Muscle Power Functions), fear avoidance belief training (d240 Handling Stress and Other Psychological Demands), and substance abuse screening (d570 Looking After One's Health).

Subacute low back pain: Aerobic exercise (b455 Exercise Tolerance Functions), specific stretching exercises (b710 Mobility of Joint Functions), strengthening exercises (b730 Muscle Power Functions), trial of aquatic therapy, cognitive behavioral therapy, fear avoidance belief training (d240 Handling Stress and Other Psychological Demands), and ergonomic training (d570 Looking After One's Health).

Chronic low back pain: Aerobic exercise (b455 Exercise Tolerance Functions), specific stretching exercises (b710 Mobility of Joint Functions), strengthening exercises (b730 Muscle Power Functions), trial of aquatic therapy, yoga (for select, highly motivated patients with low back pain lasting more than one year) (e.g., d920 Recreation and Leisure, b710 Mobility of Joint Functions), cognitive behavioral therapy, fear avoidance belief training, psychological evaluation, biofeedback (d240 Handling Stress and Other Psychological Demands), substance abuse screening (d570 Looking After One's Health), ergonomic training (d570 Looking After One's Health), and activity-based approaches to increase the number of healthy activities the person is participating in.

Prevention of low back disorders: Strengthening exercises (b730 Muscle Power Functions), smoking cessation programs and weight loss programs (d570 Looking After One's Health).

Post-operative low back pain: Aerobic exercise (b455 Exercise Tolerance Functions), strengthening exercises (b730 Muscle Power Functions), fear avoidance belief training (d240 Handling Stress and Other Psychological Demands), and substance abuse screening (d570 Looking After One's Health).

Types of Interventions

Psychosocial interventions: In regards to psychosocial interventions for the treatment of chronic low back pain, a review of the literature conducted by

Moore (2010) found that cognitive behavioral therapy (CBT) (b125 Dispositions and Intra-Personal Functions, b126 Temperament and Personality Functions, b130 Energy and Drive Functions, b160 Thought Functions) has strong empirical support, with the particular use of the CBT interventions of cognitive restructuring, exposure therapy, and cognitive behavioral education, all of which are relevant to recreational therapy practice.

Cognitive restructuring: Cognitive restructuring begins with increasing the client's awareness of how thoughts influence behavior and subsequent health. The next step is the identification of assumptions, interpretations, and thoughts and how they influence behavior and subsequent health (e.g., "I'll never get better." "My doctor isn't working hard enough to figure out what is wrong with me." "I'll have more pain if I increase my activity level." "Physical activity is dangerous." "I'll never be able to do the things I enjoy."). Distorted thoughts are then challenged to determine if they are truly rational and supported by evidence. If they are not, the thoughts are replaced with ones that are rational and evidence based (e.g., "It's good for me to remain physically active even if I do experience some pain." "Having pain when I move doesn't mean that I'm causing further injury to myself." "Even though I have back pain I can still do the things I enjoy and be happy."). Improvements should be noted in ICF codes b125 Dispositions and Intra-Personal Functions, b126 Temperament and Personality Functions, b7 Neuromusculoskeletal and Movement-Related Functions, and codes that reflect behavioral changes.

Exposure therapy: "In addition to changing cognitions to bring about more positive emotions and behaviors [as in cognitive behavioral therapy], it is possible to change behavior to produce corresponding adaptive cognitive and emotional changes [through exposure therapy]" (Hegmann, 2011, p. 808). Exposure therapy consists of gradual exposure to a feared stimulus paired with a benign response. The exposure starts out slow and short and gradually increases. Clients don't easily generalize their corrected pain prediction in one task to other tasks, so regular exposure to a wide variety of tasks is recommended. Documentation of changes should be made using codes associated with the stimuli being presented, e.g. b280 Sensation of Pain, b710

Mobility of Joint Functions, and b780 Sensations Related to Muscles and Movement Functions.

Cognitive behavioral education: Cognitive behavioral education programs teach participants about fear-avoidance beliefs and the impact they have on behavior and health, as well as possible self-management strategies to reduce or change such beliefs. This type of intervention has been found to reduce pain, lack of function, and pain-related fear. Changes in beliefs can be scored with b126 Temperament and Personality Functions.

Specific Activities

When individuals have chronic low back pain, or are at risk for developing back pain, participation in specific physical activities and sports warrants particular attention, especially if deficits have been noted in these areas (b455 Exercise Tolerance Functions, d920 Recreation and Leisure, d9201 Sports). For example, a study by Ribaud et al. (2013) sought to understand which leisure-time physical activities and sports can be recommended for clients with chronic low back pain after rehabilitation. They conducted a review of the literature from 1990-2011 related to the efficacy and safety of post-rehabilitation physical activities and sports in chronic low back pain, citing a total of 121 articles. Findings indicate that "moderate but regular physical activity helps to improve fitness and does not increase the risk of acute pain in chronic low back pain patients" (p. 576). Findings for particular sports they reviewed include:

Swimming: Aquatic exercise has demonstrated efficacy, however butterfly stroke should be avoided due to the need for intense effort coupled with hyperlordosis and activation of the erector spinae muscles.

Walking: Walking (slow pace, brisk pace, Nordic walking) is not associated with adverse effects and can therefore be recommended.

Cycling: Cycling can be a beneficial aerobic activity for individuals with lower back pain; however the placement of the client's hands on the handlebars must be even with the client's waist. Handlebars (hand placement) that are below the waist increase kyphosis and resultant back pain.

Tai chi: Appears to offer beneficial effects on chronic low back pain, but further research is needed.

Team sports: Leisure soccer playing can be beneficial in increasing trunk activity and coordination. High-intensity sports that involve physical contact have not been studied and are therefore not recommended at this time.

Tennis: Tennis exposes the player to microtrauma to the spine from repetitive rotational forces applied to the disc, coupled with hyperextension forces. This increases shear forces on the caudal lumbar discs causing back problems. Tennis is not recommended.

Horseback riding: Leisure riding may have beneficial effects. Use of a Western, long-stirrup saddle is recommended for maintenance of lumbar lordosis.

Golf: Golf can be recommended but the player must warm up for at least 10 minutes, not carry the golf bag, and change the golf swing technique to include a shorter back swing to lessen lumbar stress.

Running: Intense running is not recommended, however regular progressive running with proper shoes and insoles can decrease shock transmission to the lumbar spine.

Other Interventions

Other common recreational therapy interventions for the treatment of low back pain include:

Body mechanics and ergonomics (d410 Changing Basic Body Position, d5700 Ensuring One's Physical Comfort): Clients are taught proper body mechanics and ergonomics as they relate to particular play, leisure, recreation, and community activities.

Smoking cessation (d570 Looking After One's Health): Smoking reduces blood flow to the lower spine and causes the spinal discs to degenerate (National Institute of Neurological Disorders and Stroke, 2013). Individuals who smoke have a higher incidence of chronic pain and higher pain intensity scores (Kaye et al., 2012). Over the course of a four-month study of 112 pain clients, clients were told by their physician during each monthly visit that (1) every cigarette has more than 50 poisonous chemicals, (2) smoking cigarettes will shorten your lifespan, (3) your current diagnosis will not improve (e.g., your pain will not lessen) if you continue to smoke (Kaye et al., 2012). They were also offered a multitude of smoking cessation options. At the end of the four months, 93% of the clients reduced the number of cigarettes smoked. Additionally, 68% said they could breathe better, 66% felt better, and 34%

experienced less pain (Kaye et al., 2012). When a person quits smoking, it takes only 72 hours for the mind and body to become nicotine-free and up to 21 days for the number of nicotine-developed brain receptors to drop to levels seen in non-smokers (Polito, 2013). Unfortunately, less than 20% of people who quit for one day are able to quit for six months or more (Messer et al., 2008). Although there are many variables that impede smoking cessation, affective responses to stress and one's own self-efficacy are associated with smoking urges (Niaura et al., 2002). The act of smoking also becomes associated with particular tasks to form habits that are difficult to break. Consequently, recreational therapy that focuses on stress management, relaxation training, coping strategies, and formation of new and healthy habits could be beneficial (d230 Carrying Out Daily Routine).

Endorphin release: Endorphins are neurotransmitters that interact with opiate receptors in the brain to reduce perception of pain. There are over 20 types of endorphins in the human body (Stoppler, 2007). Unlike narcotic pain medication, which is commonly prescribed for back pain, endorphins are not addictive and can have the same effect as morphine and codeine (Stoppler, 2007). In fact, studies have found that the body's endorphins are thousands of times stronger than morphine (Ross, 2009). Narcotic pain medication, although often prescribed for short-term pain relief, can easily turn into long-term use when pain does not subside or addiction ensues. With continued use of narcotic pain medication, the body also builds up a tolerance and higher amounts of narcotic pain medication need to be prescribed to attain the same pain relief (Sprouse-Blum et al., 2010). Consequently, when a client reaches the maximum prescribed amount of narcotic pain medication, and pain becomes excruciating and severely impacts life activities, inpatient rehabilitation is often required to wean the client off of the narcotic pain medication and rally the person's endorphins (d570 Looking After One's Health). Activities that help to increase endorphins include exercise, acupuncture, massages, hot baths and showers, laughter, meditation, guided imagery, and music. Endorphins are also increased by specific foods such as chocolate and hot chili peppers (Hall, 2006).

Stress management and relaxation training (d240 Handling Stress and Other Psychological Demands): Techniques to help cope with chronic back pain include relaxation training to release muscle tension (b735 Muscle Tone Functions); biofeedback to learn how to control body functions; visual imagery, repetition of positive words or phrases, and engaging in activities that distract from painful, negative stimuli (Block, 2007).

Weight reduction and core strengthening (d570 Looking After One's Health): Increased abdominal weight increases stress on the lower back (National Institute of Neurological Disorders and Stroke, 2013). Reducing body weight, particular around the midsection, and strengthening core muscles that support the back muscles can help keep the back in proper alignment, which will reduce further pain (b710 Mobility of Joint Functions).

Psychological and emotional health: Chronic pain can lead to many losses, including job loss, family role loss, and activity loss. These losses can impair self-esteem, self-confidence (b126 Temperament and Personality Functions), and locus of control. Recreational therapists employ interventions that seek to strengthen the client's positive sense of self by choosing activities that induce flow, highlight personal strengths, maximize feelings of success, apply "Looking Glass Self" concepts, change distorted thinking, provide opportunities for control, etc.).

Community integration training: Clients with chronic low back pain often avoid engaging in community activities because they fear the experience of pain in a public place or not being able to find a place to sit and rest. Problem solving for barriers, identifying potential facilitators, and learning how to identify and access resources can be a necessary step to increasing community engagement (d4 Mobility). For those that are severely deconditioned (b740 Muscle Endurance Functions) or have mobility limitations, educating the client about and applying community accessibility and energy conservation techniques (b455 Exercise Tolerance Functions), as well as addressing community mobility skills (d4 Mobility), can be helpful in increasing success in the community (d910 Community Life). Going out into the community to practice these skills is vital to combat distorted thinking, reduce pain-related fears (d240 Handling Stress and

Other Psychological Demands), develop functional skills, improve psychological and emotional health, and enhance quality of life.

Additional education: Clients may require additional education and counseling aimed at specific needs such as sexuality counseling (d770 Intimate Relationships, b640 Sexual Functions), education about the consequences of inactivity (d570 Looking After One's Health), leisure education about the benefits of leisure related to recovery and health and exploration of leisure interests (d570 Looking After One's Health), and/or anger management (b152 Emotional Functions).

Resources

Agency for Healthcare Research and Quality (AHRQ) National Guideline Clearinghouse
www.guideline.gov/content.aspx?id=38438.
Access to the full National Guideline for low back disorders.

American Chronic Pain Association
www.theacpa.org
Facilitates peer support and education for individuals with chronic pain and their families, and raises awareness among the healthcare community, policy makers, and the public at large about issues of living with chronic pain.

Substance Abuse and Mental Health Services Administration
store.samhsa.gov/product/SMA12-4671
A free book titled *A treatment improvement protocol: Managing chronic pain in adults with or in recovery from substance use disorders*.

References

Block, A. R. (2007). Chronic pain coping techniques: Pain management. Retrieved from http://www.spine-health.com/conditions/chronic-pain/chronic-pain-coping-techniques-pain-management.

Centers for Disease Control. (2012). Summary health statistics for U.S. adults: National health interview survey, 2010. Retrieved from http://www.cdc.gov/nchs/data/series/sr_10/sr10_252.pdf.

Cleveland Clinic Foundation. (2009). Acute vs. chronic pain. Retrieved from http://my.clevelandclinic.org/services/Pain_Management/hic_Acute_vs_Chronic_Pain.aspx.

Clinical Key Elsevier. (2012). Back pain. Retrieved from https://www.clinicalkey.com/topics/rheumatology/back-pain.html.

Hall, K. (2006). *A life in balance: Nourishing the four roots of true happiness*. AMACOM.

Hayden, J. A., Dunn, K. M., van der Windt, D. A., & Shaw, W. S. (2010). What is the prognosis of back pain? *Best Practice & Research Clinical Rheumatology, 24*(2), 167-179.

Hegmann, K. T. (2011). *Occupational medicine practice guidelines: Evaluation and management of common health problems and functional recovery in workers, 3rd edition.* Elk Grove Village, IL: American College of Occupational and Environmental Medicine (ACEOM).

Kaye, A. D., Prabhakar, A. P., Fitzmaurice, M. E., & Kaye, R. J. (2012). Smoking cessation in pain patients. *The Ochsner Journal, 12*(1), 17-20.

Messer, K., Trinidad, D. R., Al-Delaimy, W. K., & Pierce, J. P. (2008). Smoking cessation rates in the United States: A comparison of young adult and older smokers. *American Journal of Public Health, 98*(2), 317-322.

Moore, J. E. (2010). Chronic low back pain and psychosocial issues. *Physical Medicine and Rehabilitation Clinics of North America, 21*(4), 801-815.

National Institute of Neurological Disorders and Stroke. (2013). Low back pain fact sheet. Retrieved from http://www.ninds.nih.gov/disorders/backpain/detail_backpain .htm.

Niaura, R., Shadel, W. G., Britt, D. M., & Abrams, D. B. (2002). Response to social stress, urge to smoke, and smoking cessation. *Addictive Behaviors, 27*(2), 241-250.

Polito, J. R. (2013). Nicotine addiction 101. Retrieved from http://whyquit.com/whyquit/LinksAAddiction.html.

Ribaud, A., Tavares, I., Viollet, E., Julia, M., Herisson, C., & Dupeyron, A. (2013). Which physical activities and sports can be recommended to chronic low back pain patients after rehabilitation? *Annals of Physical and Rehabilitation Medicine, 56*(7-8), 576-594.

Ross, J. (2009). Restoring the natural opioid system with D-Phenylalanine (DPA): A novel therapeutic approach. *Practical Pain Management, 9*(9), 29-31.

Sprouse-Blum, A. S., Smith, G., Sugai, D., & Parsa, F. D. (2010). Understanding endorphins and their importance in pain management. *Hawaii Medical Journal, 69*(3), 70-71.

Stoppler, M. C. (2007). Endorphins: Natural pain and stress fighters. Retrieved from http://www.medicinenet.com/script/main/art.asp?articlekey= 55001.

5. Borderline Personality Disorder

Ruthie Kucharewski and Joy Lauerer

Borderline Personality Disorder (BPD) is a serious psychiatric illness. BPD is most often characterized by pervasive instability in interpersonal relationships, moods, and self-image combined with marked impulsivity. It can best be described as a disorder of mood regulation.

Often times the individual is engaged in unstable, chaotic relationships and makes frantic attempts to avoid real or imagined abandonment. Unable to regulate mood, an individual with BPD may appear dysphoric for a short period of time and a few hours later may be irritable or anxious. Episodes of dysphoria are often disrupted by periods of panic, anger, or despair and the individual rarely finds relief or satisfaction. Episodic mood instability can reflect the individual's reaction to interpersonal stressors and the inability to control the relationship. This mood instability tends to disrupt work and family life and the individual's ability to make long-term plans.

Other behaviors characteristically observed in persons with BPD include a display of impulsivity which can include reckless behaviors such as substance abuse, gambling, engaging in unsafe sex, driving recklessly, or binge eating. Persons diagnosed with borderline personality disorder may exhibit recurring self-injurious behavior, gestures, or threats. Recurrent suicide attempts and self-injurious behaviors often occur when the individual fears rejection or separation or believes that rejection or separation is impending, whether real or imagined. Impulsive aggression is at the core of BPD symptoms and often influences the affective instability (Stuart, 2013). The disorder may cause an individual to feel isolated or lonely due to the inability to maintain and sustain healthy relationships and support systems.

In the past decade, funding for BPD has increased, along with the establishment of several key advocacy groups such as the National Education Alliance for Borderline Personality Disorder (NEA-BPD) and the establishment of the Borderline Personality Disorder Research Foundation (BPDRF). NEA-BPD is an organization that advocates raising awareness about BPD, provides education, and promotes research about BPD. NEA-BPD assisted in having the National Institute of Mental Health (NIMH) and National Alliance of Mental Illness (NAMI) adopt BPD (Gunderson, 2009). All of these organizations advocate, educate, and advance the BPD agenda. As a result of their efforts, in April 2008 the United States House of Representatives unanimously passed HR 1005 which proclaimed the month of May as Borderline Personality Disorder Month. The House Resolution formally legitimized the recognition of a disorder that is responsible for nearly 20% of all clinical psychiatric hospitalizations. The advocacy efforts commanded the public's attention and have raised the level of public awareness of BPD, which will likely support an increase in funding for research efforts and patient access to treatment.

Incidence/Prevalence in U.S.

According to the American Psychiatric Association (2001) prevalence of BPD is roughly two percent of the general population. They also estimate that 20% of the inpatient mental health population and 10% of the mental health outpatient population are diagnosed with BPD. Estimates may vary slightly regarding the general population, but there seems to be agreement that BPD affects two to four percent of the general population. Of the diagnosed, 70-75% are women (Swartz et al., 1990; Nehls, 1999). According to a study by Swartz et al. (1990), the disorder is highly associated with single, young females who are likely of lower economic status and reside in urban areas.

Predominant Age

BPD is most commonly recognized and diagnosed in young adulthood. A diagnosis of BPD in adolescence is generally not recommended. Young adolescent behaviors often mimic borderline personality disorder symptoms and these behaviors are more related to normal adolescent attempts to develop identity and a sense of self. Adolescents may display behaviors that are recognized by clinicians as meeting the criteria for BPD, but the behaviors may be misleading in that the behaviors being exhibited may be linked to substance abuse or identity problems which characterize emotional instability (APA, 2013). BPD is most frequently diagnosed in early adulthood when symptoms appear to peak (Nehls, 1999).

Causes

The exact cause of BPD is unknown; however, numerous theories exist. One theory suggests that a childhood history of neglect, abuse, or separation increases the risk of developing BPD and that environmental stressors may trigger the onset of the disorder in young adulthood (National Institute of Mental Health, 2009). BPD may also have a genetic component. The disorder has been reported to be almost five times more common among first-degree biological relatives than the general populace (APA, 2001). It was also suggested by Swift (2009) that biological irregularities might impair the neural circuits that regulate emotion. And, Miller (2006), who conducted a twin and adoption study, found that personality disorder is 70% inherited. The author was also quick to note, however, that the effect of other factors, such as environmental stressors, should not be ignored. BPD is clearly characterized as having biological abnormalities that potentially interact with psychosocial stressors to result in BPD psychopathology (Ruocco, 2005).

Systems Affected

BPD affects the brain as indicated by detection of abnormalities by magnetic resonance imaging (MRI). Studies have consistently indicated that individuals with BPD typically have smaller volumes of amygdala and hippocampus when compared to control groups without BPD (Ruocco, 2005). Similarly, positron emission tomography (PET) scans have provided additional evidence of abnormalities

of the frontal lobe in persons with BPD (Ruocco, 2005). These observations can be recorded with the ICF code s110 Structure of Brain.

Visual observation of behavior often indicates that emotional health is compromised due to the individual's inability to regulate emotion or mood, identity disturbance, impulsivity, chronic feelings of emptiness, intense anger or difficulty controlling anger, and recurring suicidal behavior. Relevant ICF Body Function codes include b125 Dispositions and Intra-Personal Functions, b126 Temperament and Personality Functions, b130 Energy and Drive Functions, b140 Attention Functions, b152 Emotional Functions, b164 Higher-Level Cognitive Functions, and b180 Experience of Self and Time Functions.

Individuals with BPD often have unstable relationships with family, friends, and co-workers. While they are able to develop significant relationships, their difficulty with mood stability, aggression, and fear of loss may make it challenging for them to engage in and maintain healthy relationships (NIMH, 2013; Substance Abuse and Mental Health Services Administration — SAMHSA, 2010). ICF Activities and Participation codes that cover these relationship issues include d230 Carrying Out Daily Routine, d240 Handling Stress and Other Psychological Demands, d250 Managing One's Own Behavior, d350 Conversation, d355 Discussion, d7 Interpersonal Interactions and Relationships, d9 Community, Social, and Civic Life.

Secondary Problems

Suicide attempts and threats, self-destruction, and self-mutilation are often seen with persons with BPD (James & Taylor, 2008). It's estimated that over 50% of persons with BPD engage in parasuicidal behavior, which includes suicide attempts and gestures of self-harm which are not fatal. Approximately 8-10% commit suicide (James & Taylor, 2008; APA, 2001). Other comorbidities include substance dependence and other psychiatric illnesses such as bipolar disorder, depression, anxiety, schizophrenia, or other personality disorders (APA, 2013; APA 2001). Consequently, the treatment of the individual can become complex, requiring a combination of therapeutic approaches and interventions. Code these issues with b126 Temperament and Personality Functions, b130 Energy and Drive

Functions. See other chapters in this book for ways to code other specific DSM diagnoses.

Individuals with BPD often have high rates of utilization of medical and mental health services due to their chronic debilitating syndrome (Clarkin et al., 2007; Bellino et al., 2010). Psychiatric hospitalizations are often necessary to resolve acute symptoms such as self-mutilation or attention seeking suicide attempts. Long-term, intensive psychotherapy can also be useful, but it is a costly form of treatment (Zanarini, 2009). Persons with BPD account for 20% of psychiatric hospitalizations (NIMH, 2013). They are challenging and emotionally draining on professional care providers, often making them feel uncomfortable or guilty by their demanding demeanor (Gold & Smith, 1991; Harvard Mental Health Letter, 2006). Because persons with BPD often have interpersonal relationship difficulties and lack the ability to appropriately regulate emotions, they sometimes express aggression and violence that alienates a care provider or causes the individual to become involved with the law (Swift, 2009). Code this environmental factor with e450 Individual Attitudes of Health Professionals, if it needs to be considered in treatment.

The inability to define oneself in a positive manner (e.g., "I am a good person.") or have an appropriate self-concept (e.g., "What I think is important.") also presents numerous problems that may cause the individual to devalue him/herself or feel isolated or guilty (Moran, 2011). Without a good self-image, the experience of success in occupation (d845 Acquiring, Keeping, and Terminating a Job) is unlikely due to the constant need for validation and approval (Gunderson, 2006).

Prognosis

BPD is the most serious and most common personality disorder (Bellino, Rinaldi, & Bogetto, 2010). Why is it the "most serious?" Persons with BPD are at a high risk for suicide and self-harm, and the completed suicide rate is 8-10% (Mohr, 2009).

Over time, with effective treatment as described below, individuals with BPD may improve. Gunderson et al. (2011) found that following a decade of treatment approximately 85% of patients achieved remission, but problems with social interactions persisted. Individuals with BPD can experience a significant improvement in mood stability if they become active participants in one or more long-term psychotherapy treatments such as psychodynamic therapy, dialectical behavior therapy, or transference-focused psychotherapy combined with psychopharmacology therapy to decrease specific problems such as irritability, impulsivity, aggressive behavior, and lability (Clarkin et al., 2007; Gunderson, 2009).

BPD often co-occurs with other mood disorders such as post-traumatic stress disorder (PTSD), panic or anxiety disorders, major depressive disorder, or eating disorders, which can complicate prognosis, as well as assessment and diagnosis (APA, 2001). Typically the greatest degree of instability and chaos associated with BPD occurs during early adulthood. As individuals with BPD age, they may experience less instability in social and occupational functioning (Swift, 2009, SAMHSA, 2010). Despite the debilitating aspects of BPD, follow-up studies have found that 10 years after individuals with BPD received help through outpatient mental health clinics almost half of the individual's behavior didn't meet the full diagnostic criteria for BPD (APA, 2013). With this decline in symptoms over a 10-year timeframe, ongoing treatment may lead to a somewhat positive prognosis (SAMHSA, 2010).

Assessment

Typical Scope of Team Assessment

The diagnostic criteria in the DSM-5 (APA, 2013) are utilized as a screening tool to diagnose BPD by considering clinical data such as observation, interviews, self-reports, and family reports.

An individual who presents with five or more of the nine DSM-5 diagnostic criteria would be diagnosed as having BPD (APA, 2013): (1) frantic efforts to avoid real or imagined abandonment; (2) unstable and intense interpersonal relationships alternating between idealization and devaluation; (3) identity disturbance that leads to unstable self-image; (4) impulsivity that is potentially self-damaging; (5) suicidal behavior, gestures, or threats or self-mutilating behavior; (6) affective instability that comes from over-reacting to events; (7) chronic feelings of emptiness; (8) anger problems such as inappropriate anger, intense anger, or difficulty controlling anger; and (9) transient paranoid ideation or dissociative symptoms when stressed. See APA (2013) for more detailed criteria descriptions.

Areas of Concern for RT Assessment

Assessment of the individual typically includes an interview, observation, patient self-report, family member report, and consultation with other treatment team members along with a review of the patient's history and physical information. Common findings include:

Difficulties with affective functionality: Often the patient exhibits emotional instability, which may include volatility, intense episodic depression, anger, panic, unrest, or despair (b125 Dispositions and Intra-Personal Functions, b126 Temperament and Personality Functions, b130 Energy and Drive Functions). This wide range of emotions may be caused or reflect the individual's response to stresses, particularly interpersonal ones (Gunderson, 2009).

Need for safety precautions to ensure the safety of the individual and/or others: Collaboration and communication with other members of the treatment team is essential in the treatment of persons with BPD. Modifications to the treatment plan and therapeutic environment may be needed, such as developing specific risk management policies for terminating treatment, boundary definition, and ensuring that the physical environment is safe and secure to minimize the risk of suicide, self-mutilation, etc. (e150 Design, Construction, and Building Products and Technology of Buildings for Public Use, e340 Personal Care Providers and Personal Assistants, e450 Individual Attitudes of Health Professionals, e580 Health Services, Systems, and Policies) (APA, 2001).

Difficulty controlling anger: Anger (b130 Energy and Drive Functions, b152 Emotional Functions) often occurs in the patient when there is a disruption in the patient's relationships or the patient is feeling or sensing abandonment (APA, 2001).

Impulsivity: May occur if the patient feels misunderstood or unjustly accused of something (b130 Energy and Drive Functions, d570 Looking After One's Health) (APA, 2001).

Affective instability: The patient displays irritability, anxiety, and may exhibit episodic dysphoria that may last a few hours (b152 Emotional Functions) (APA, 2001).

Problematic social functioning: The patient fails to conform or has difficulty conforming to social norms (d240 Handling Stress and Other Psychological Demands, d7 Interpersonal Interactions and Relationships) (APA, 2013).

Interpersonal relationship difficulty: The patient experiences difficulty establishing or maintaining meaningful relationships due to a real or imagined fear of abandonment (d7 Interpersonal Interactions and Relationships) (APA, 2013).

Recurring suicide attempts or ideation: The patient may have inflicted self-harm or had several failed suicide attempts. More than 70% of individuals with BPD have attempted suicide at least once (b130 Energy and Drive Functions, b152 Emotional Functions) (SAMHSA, 2010).

Losing self in relationships: The patient tends to have intense relationships and has unrealistic expectations of others including demanding they spend all of their time together (b180 Experience of Self and Time Functions) (APA, 2013).

Manipulation: The patient may try to control the relationship and often attempts to control the expectations of the other person in the relationship (d7 Interpersonal Interactions and Relationships) (APA, 2013).

Splitting: The patient may see people or situations as "good or bad" or "black or white" (d7 Interpersonal Interactions and Relationships) (APA, 2001). The patient will try to split the treatment team so that the current set of "good" people are working against the current set of "bad" people, making treatment much less effective for the patient.

Depression: The patient often experiences depression as a comorbid disorder. It frequently follows fear of abandonment, failed relationships, etc. Approximately 41-83% of individuals with BPD have experienced major depression (APA, 2001). See the chapter on Major Depressive Disorder for more information on scoring this comorbidity.

ICF Core Set

An ICF Core Set for Borderline Personality Disorder has not been developed.

Treatment Direction

Whole Team Approach

A psychiatrist or psychiatric nurse practitioner is often the leader of the treatment team. The team commonly consists of nurses, mental health technicians, social workers, recreational therapists, and occupational therapists. Treatment often consists of a combination of modalities, pairing medication and psychosocial interventions. Treatments, as indicated in the *Practice Guideline for the Treatment of Patients with Borderline Personality Disorder*, consist of recommendations that are coded on a scale which indicates varying degrees of clinical confidence (APA, 2001).

Developed in 2001 by psychiatrists, the *Practice Guideline for the Treatment of Patients with Borderline Personality Disorder* (APA, 2001) offers treatment recommendations, but does not ensure successful outcomes for all individuals with BPD. The APA guideline is a practical guide for the management of BPD for persons over 18 years of age. The practice guideline is divided into three parts: Part A contains treatment recommendations and recommendations to develop and implement a treatment plan; Part B provides evidence in support of the treatment recommendations; and Part C identifies future research needs.

Psychodynamic psychotherapy: Psychodynamic psychotherapy is a therapy that employs three major perspectives: ego psychology, object relations, and self-psychology. This therapy provides the patient with a supportive/explorative intervention to investigate unconscious behavior patterns and to aid the patient in delaying impulsive reactionary behaviors (b125 Dispositions and Intra-Personal Functions, b126 Temperament and Personality Functions, b130 Energy and Drive Functions, b164 Higher-Level Cognitive Functions, b180 Experience of Self and Time Functions).

Dialectical behavioral therapy (DBT): DBT involves pairing two opposing concepts such as rational thinking with emotional thinking with the objective of achieving interpersonal effectiveness. DBT is a combination of individual and group therapy which is aimed at educating and teaching the person with BPD self-soothing techniques to help manage mood swings, regulate intense emotional situations, and to provide an opportunity for self-awareness (b125 Dispositions and Intra-Personal Functions, b126 Temperament and Personality Functions, b130 Energy and Drive Functions, d7 Interpersonal Interactions and Relationships).

Cognitive behavioral therapy (CBT): CBT involves focusing attention on a set of dysfunctional, automatic thoughts or imagined beliefs and learning and practicing new non-maladaptive behaviors (b125 Dispositions and Intra-Personal Functions, b126 Temperament and Personality Functions, b130 Energy and Drive Functions). The patient is required to scrutinize core beliefs and the behaviors associated with them. CBT is a more structured therapy than psychodynamic therapy and more emotionally balanced. CBT and DBT are often led by the therapist and require the patient to work on specific things between therapy sessions.

Group therapy: Group therapy provides an opportunity for the individual to be in a supportive environment with other individuals (d7 Interpersonal Interactions and Relationships). Groups are often led by a professional or they may have a specific membership such as other individuals with common problems or the same diagnosis. Some self-help groups may also be considered and many individuals with BPD tend to find them less threatening and more acceptable to belong to.

Family therapy: Family Therapy is prescribed to assist the individual in improving prior chaotic or dysfunctional relationships, while also serving as a modality to educate and increase family members' understanding of BPD (d760 Family Relationships).

Pharmacology: Pharmacological approaches are varied and include the use of antidepressants, mood stabilizers, and antipsychotic agents. Any of the assessed ICF deficiencies may be targeted with pharmacology.

Recreational Therapy Approach

The approach utilized by recreational therapy will depend on the person's age and the mission of the agency. In general, RT utilizes a functional improvement approach based predominantly on education and practice of newly acquired skills to counteract environmental stressors and to assist in promoting and facilitating positive social interactions (Carter & Van Andel, 2011).

If the recreational therapist is aware of the possibility of some of problematic behaviors, the RT can provide meaningful therapeutic experiences to assist the patient in achieving treatment goals and help develop treatment goals with the patient so the patient can experience success.

Working with persons with BPD can be challenging and physically exhausting at times. Individuals with BPD have interpersonal relationship difficulties and dysfunctional emotional regulation and can be confrontational with care providers. The RT should have clear interpersonal boundaries and provide structure and direction to assist the patient (e355 Health Professionals, e450 Individual Attitudes of Health Professionals, e580 Health Services, Systems, and Policies). RTs can develop boundaries through the use of contracts, which can also be part of the treatment plan. Clear and consistent boundaries can strengthen the therapeutic relationship by indicating consistency of care and commitment from the care provider. The contract can also serve as a partnership between the patient and the care provider, which can help to increase patient trust and alleviate any fear of abandonment.

Recreational Therapy Interventions

BPD is complex in that it is the illness that produces the behavior, not the person, and symptoms are treated to manage the behaviors (Moran, 2011). The *DSM-5* (2013) has identified specific diagnostic criteria to diagnose BPD. Many individuals with BPD will exhibit a combination of those criteria and will be treated somewhat similarly, but with attention being given to individual differences. It is universally accepted among healthcare providers that psychosocial interventions remain the primary treatment for individuals with BPD (SAMHSA, 2010; Gunderson, 2009; James & Taylor, 2008; APA, 2001). In SAMHSA's 2010 "Report to Congress on BPD" two evidence-based psychotherapeutic interventions (DBT and family therapy) were identified as successful interventions when supplemented with medication. SAMHSA (2010) also acknowledges that while much research has been done over the past 20 years, there is still a need for more research to support best practices in the field and it has developed programs to promote evidence-based practices in service delivery for persons with BPD.

Since RTs are integral members of the treatment team and are instrumental in providing services to persons with mental health disorders, they should choose the appropriate interventions, keeping in mind that treatment modalities that utilize psychosocial interventions will most likely be fairly successful in improving functional abilities. RTs can and should also be involved in research to help determine the efficacy of interventions and to improve treatment outcomes (Kinney & Kinney, 2001). Additionally, whenever possible, RTs should utilize research studies as a basis for practice (Lee & McCormick, 2002).

Functional Skills

In many psychiatric settings there is a need to improve a patient's functional skills, which frequently requires a clinical or therapeutic intervention to assist the patient in developing new coping behaviors for dealing with life crises (d240 Handling Stress and Other Psychological Demands) (Kinney & Kinney, 2001). The RT develops interventions to decrease or diminish negative patient behaviors and to help the patient acquire new skills to achieve treatment goals. Improvement of such skills might include: self-concept (b114 Orientation Functions), confidence (b126 Temperament and Personality Functions), social interaction and interpersonal skills (d7 Interpersonal Interactions and Relationships), anger management and impulsive behavior management (b130 Energy and Drive Functions), recognition of suicidal ideation and splitting (b164 Higher-Level Cognitive Functions), etc.

Individuals with BPD require interventions that provide the opportunity to learn and practice appropriate social behaviors (d7 Interpersonal Interactions and Relationships) so that they exhibit socially acceptable behaviors to develop and maintain healthy relationships. The RT would likely provide individual and group therapy sessions to educate and facilitate social skills, coping skills, and stress and anger management groups to assist the patient in becoming proficient in managing his/her own behavior for a better lifestyle (b125 Dispositions and Intra-Personal Functions, b126 Temperament and Personality Functions, b130 Energy and Drive Functions, b180 Experience of Self and Time Functions) (Carter & Van Andel, 2010). Treatment interventions may be done individually or in small groups. This typically depends on patient goals and objectives and agency resources (Kinney & Kinney, 2001).

Education, Training, and Counseling

Patient education is most likely to occur in a heterogeneous ambulatory group in conjunction with individual and group treatment (Yalom & Leszcz, 2005). Session duration should be determined by the individual's ability to focus on the task and remain involved in the task. Because therapists can sometimes be hailed as saviors and friends one minute and be denounced the next minute, it is important to make sure that the patient is aware of acceptable and appropriate behaviors and consequences for undesirable behavior (d7 Interpersonal Interactions and Relationships). This would typically be discussed by the RT prior to the beginning of the session (Harvard Mental Health Letter, 2006; Kinney & Kinney, 2001). It is also important to provide this information to the patient so that the roles and responsibilities are clearly understood and so that the therapist can set appropriate personal and interpersonal boundaries to provide structure to aid the patient (Swift, 2005).

Opportunities to practice newly learned behaviors and timely feedback about behavior and progress should also be provided. As necessary, counseling sessions should be scheduled with the patient to address any treatment issues that might be too threatening or embarrassing to address in a therapeutic group setting (Yalom & Leszcz, 2005). It is essential for the RT to recognize that one patient with BPD can be markedly different from another patient.

Because observation of behavior is largely subjective, it may be difficult for the RT to measure deficits in interpersonal relationships when working with individuals with BPD. It may be necessary to rely on formal, standardized assessment tools associated with RT or personality disorders. These include objective scales, such as the *Comprehensive Evaluation in Recreational Therapy: Psych/Behavioral, Revised* (CERT Psych/R) or the *Leisure Assessment Inventory* (LAI) (burlingame & Blaschko, 2010). Identifying the appropriate assessment tool is essential to assist the RT in placing the patient in the right intervention and to measure outcomes (Stumbo, 2002).

Community Integration

When appropriate behaviors are demonstrated, community integration training is provided to allow the individual to practice newly acquired skills in a real-life social setting (d7 Interpersonal Interactions and Relationships). Immersion into the community should be paced appropriately so that the individual can regulate and demonstrate the appropriate emotions (b152 Emotional Functions). The RT should conduct community site visit evaluations to ensure the safety of the patients by determining the

appropriateness of the community facility, physical accessibility, opportunities available for inclusive programming, etc. (e150 Design, Construction, and Building Products and Technology of Buildings for Public Use, e340 Personal Care Providers and Personal Assistants, e450 Individual Attitudes of Health Professionals, e580 Health Services, Systems, and Policies) (Long, 2008).

A community integration program (CIP) can help alleviate a patient's discomfort by providing an opportunity with the support of an RT who is aware of the patient's anxieties and needs and who can adapt the trip to assist the patient in achieving positive outcomes (Armstrong & Lauzen, 1994). In 1994, Armstrong and Lauzen implemented a CIP with clients which included an initial screening and assessment to develop a treatment plan in conjunction with the client. The treatment plan contains six specific modules which cover community experiences to assist the patient in successfully integrating into the community. These include community environment, cultural activities, community activity, transportation, physical activity, and independent activity. In Armstrong and Lauzen's book, *Community Integration Program*, they described a CIP at Harborview Medical Center in Seattle, Washington, and provided a table of research studies, which confirmed the efficacy of similar community integration programs. While the table does not contain specific studies involving individuals with BPD, at least one of the studies can likely be duplicated with individuals with BPD. Specifically, Bullock and Howe (1991) found that subjects who participated in their study showed improvement in behavioral functioning, adjustment to disability, autonomy, and quality of life. Very little research has been done on the effectiveness of CIPs; this would be an area worthy of further research (Long, 2008).

Also worth noting is that the initial development of Armstrong and Lauzen's Harborview Medical Center CIP was for persons with spinal cord injury, but for the book they adapted modules for use by patients with traumatic brain injury, stroke, and psychiatric disorders.

Health Promotion

According to Mohr (2009), all members of the treatment team should encourage clients to maximize health-seeking behaviors to achieve overall wellness (d570 Looking After One's Health). Individuals with BPD are encouraged to adopt and maintain healthy self-care, adequate nutrition, appropriate amounts of sleep, regular dental care, weight control, good hygiene, and healthy sexual habits. RTs should promote health strategies for clients with disabilities; clients should be encouraged to engage in wellness activities by scheduling regular preventative tests and medical exams to detect visual, hearing, and dental concerns so that they can learn to live well despite their disabling condition (Shank & Coyle, 2002).

Research studies have demonstrated that by improving the quality of life through leisure experiences and decreasing the incidence of secondary conditions associated with disabilities, individuals have the potential to develop a trait known as "hardiness," which allows a person to cope more effectively in stressful situations (d240 Handling Stress and Other Psychological Demands) (Shank & Coyle, 2002). Individuals with BPD would benefit greatly from participation in health promotion programs aimed at improving coping skills.

RTs also have the ability to offer disease prevention programs which focus on avoiding illness by encouraging clients to take responsibility for their health. Examples of such programs include walking and fitness (b455 Exercise Tolerance Functions), social clubs (d910 Community Life), and nutrition education combined with a healthy cooking intervention (d570 Looking After One's Health). Quality of life is often shaped by interactions, experiences, and opportunities that exist in an individual's physical and social environment. It is also very subjective and personal. Quality of life is not the absence of disease nor is it a cure for disabling conditions. It positively contributes to life satisfaction, which can reduce disabling symptoms (Shank & Coyle, 2002; McCormick, 1999). Persons with chronic mental health issues could benefit from treatment programs that address health and wellness to improve their quality of life (Shank & Coyle, 2002).

Resources

American Psychiatric Association (APA)
www.psych.org
Founded in 1844, it is the largest psychiatric organization representing over 38,000 psychiatrists. The organization ensures humane care and effective treatment for persons with mental disorders, devel-

opmental disabilities, and substance-related disorders.

National Institute of Mental Health (NIMH)
nimh.nih.gov
NIMH was established to further the understanding and treatment of mental illnesses through research to assist in the prevention, recovery, and cure of mental illness.

Substance Abuse and Mental Health Services Administration (SAMHSA)
samhsa.gov
A federal government agency that was established by Congress in 1992 to effectively target substance abuse and mental health services to the people most in need.

References

American Psychiatric Association. (2013). *Diagnostic and statistical manual of mental disorders (5th ed.).* Washington, DC: American Psychiatric Association.

American Psychiatric Association. (2001). *Practice guideline for the treatment of patients with borderline personality disorder.* Washington, DC: American Psychiatric Association.

Armstrong, M. & Lauzen, S. (1994). *Community integration program* (2nd ed.). Ravensdale, WA: Idyll Arbor, Inc.

Bellino, S., Rinaldi, C., & Bogetto, F. (2010). Adaptation of interpersonal psychotherapy to borderline personality disorder: A comparison of combined therapy and single pharmacotherapy. *The Canadian Journal of Psychiatry, 56*(2), 74-80.

Bullock, C. C. & Howe, C. Z. (1991). A model therapeutic recreation program for the reintegration of persons with disabilities into the community. *Therapeutic Recreation Journal, 25,* 7-17.

burlingame, j. & Blaschko, T. (2010). *Assessment tools for recreational therapy and related fields* (4th ed.). Enumclaw, WA: Idyll Arbor, Inc.

Carter, M. J. & Van Andel, G. (2011). *Therapeutic recreation: A practical approach* (4th ed.). Long Grove, IL: Waveland Press.

Clarkin, J., Levy, K., Lenzenweger, M., & Kernberg, O. (2007). Evaluating three treatments for borderline personality disorder: A multiwave study. *American Journal of Psychiatry, 164,* 922-928.

Gold, M. & Smith, P. (1991).Therapeutic recreation service and borderline personality disorder. *Therapeutic Recreation Journal, 3,* 61-64.

Gunderson, J. G. (2006). A BPD brief: An introduction to borderline personality disorder. The Borderline Personality Disorder Resource Center, 1-13.

Gunderson, J. G. (2009). Borderline personality disorder: Ontogeny of a diagnosis. *American Journal of Psychiatry, 165*(5), 530-539.

Gunderson, J. G., Stout, R. L., McGlashan, T., Shea, T., Morey, L., Grilo, C., Zanarini, M., & Skodol, A. (2011). Ten-year course of borderline personality disorder: Psychopathology and function from the collaborative longitudinal personality disorders study. *Archives of General Psychiatry, 68*(8), 827-837. doi: 10.1001/archgenpsychiatry.2011:37.

Harvard Mental Health Letter. (2006). Borderline personality disorder: Treatment. Harvard University, July, 3-6. Cambridge, MA.

James, L. & Taylor, J. (2008). Associations between symptoms of borderline personality disorder, externalizing disorders and suicide-related behaviors. *Journal of Psychopathology of Behavior Assessment, 30,* 1-9.

Kinney, J. S. & Kinney, W. B. (2001). Psychiatry and mental health. In Austin, D. R. & Crawford, M. E. (Eds.). *Therapeutic recreation: An introduction* (3rd ed.). Needham Heights, MA: Allyn & Bacon.

Lee, Y. & McCormick, B. (2002). Toward evidence-based therapeutic recreation practice. In D. R. Austin, J. Dattilo, & B. P. McCormick (Eds.), *Conceptual foundations for therapeutic recreation* (pp. 165-183). State College, PA: Venture Publishing.

Long, T. (2008). Therapeutic recreation and mental health. In T. Robertson and T. Long (Eds.). *Foundations of therapeutic recreation: Perceptions, philosophies, and practices for the 21st century. (pp. 145-163).* Champaign, IL: Human Kinetics.

McCormick, B. (1999). Contributions of social support and recreation companionship to the life satisfaction of people with persistent mental illness. *Therapeutic Recreation Journal, 33*(4), 304-319.

Miller, M. (2006). Borderline personality disorder: Origins and symptoms. *Harvard Mental Health Letter, 22,* 1-3.

Mohr, W. (2009). *Psychiatric mental health nursing: Evidence-based concepts, skills and practices (7th ed.).* Philadelphia, PA. Lippincott Williams & Wilkins.

Moran, M. (2011). Long journey led to advances in understanding, treating BPD. *Psychiatric News, 46*(6), 16.

National Institute of Mental Health. (2013). Borderline personality disorder. Retrieved on from http://www.nimh.nih.gov/health/topics/borderline-personality-disorder/index.shtml.

Nehls, N. (1999). Borderline personality disorder: The voice of patients. *Research in Nursing & Health, 22,* 285-29.

Ruocco, C. (2005). Re-evaluating the distinction between axis I and axis II disorders: The case of borderline personality disorder. *Journal of Clinical Psychology, 61*(12), 1509-1523.

Shank, J. & Coyle, C. (2002). *Therapeutic recreation in health promotion and rehabilitation.* State College, PA: Venture Publishing.

Stuart, G. (2013). Social responses and personality disorders. In G. Stuart (Ed.), *Principles and practices of psychiatric nursing* (10 ed., p. 410). St. Louis, MO: Elsevier Mosby.

Stumbo, N. (2002). *Client assessment in therapeutic recreation services.* State College, PA: Venture Publishing.

Substance Abuse and Mental Health Services Administration. (2010). Report to Congress on borderline personality disorder. Retrieved on May 26, 2011 from http://store.samhsa.gov/product/SMA11-4644.

Swartz, M., Blazer, D., George, L., & Winfield, I. (1990). Estimating the prevalence of borderline personality disorder in the community. *Journal of Personality Disorders, 4*(3), 257-72.

Swift, E. (2009). Borderline personality disorder: Etiology, presentation and therapeutic relationship. *Mental Health Practice, 13*(3), 22-25.

Yalom, I. D. & Leszcz, M. (2005). *The theory and practice of group psychotherapy* (5th ed.). New York: Basic Books.

Zanarini, M. C. (2009). Clinical overview: Psychotherapy of borderline personality disorder. *Acta Psychiatrica Scandinavica, 120,* 373-377.

6. Burns

Heather R. Porter

A burn is damage to body tissue that is caused by chemicals, electricity, heat, or radiation (Centers for Disease Control [CDC], 2013). Burns are described, or graded, by a combination of severity and percentage of body injured. The severity of burns is described by "degrees" (CDC, 2013; Perdue et al., 2011):

First-degree burns: Involves the top layer of skin (epidermis). Signs include redness, pain from touch, and mild skin swelling. No evidence of blisters or skin separation. When rubbed with a gloved finger, the burn tissue does not separate from the underlying dermis (referred to as a negative Nikolsky's sign). One example of a first-degree burn is a mild sunburn.

Second-degree burns (also referred to as partial-thickness burns): Involves the top two layers of skin, both the epidermis and part of the dermis. Signs include deep reddening of the skin, pain, blisters, and glossy appearance from leaking fluid.

Third-degree burns: Penetrates the entire thickness of the skin and permanently destroys tissues. It extends through the dermis, destroying all epidermal and dermal elements. Signs include loss of skin layers, dry and leathery skin. Skin may appear charred or have patches that appear white, brown, or black. It is often painless, although pain may be caused by patches of first- and second-degree burns which often surround third-degree burns.

Fourth-degree burns: Burns that extend deep into soft tissue, muscle, or bone, leading to deep burn necrosis.

Burns are also described by the total body surface area (TBSA) or body surface area (BSA) using the Berkow Formula (Perdue et al. 2011). The Berkow Formula assigns percentages to each body area depending on the client's age. The age ranges used are under one year, one to four years, five to nine years, 10 to 14 years, 15 years, and adult. The percentages vary by age because body proportions change with age. The percentages of burn areas are then tallied to determine the TBSA. For an adult, the head is 7%, neck 2%, anterior trunk 13%, posterior trunk 13%, right buttock 2.5%, left buttock 2.5%, genintalia 1%, right upper arm 4%, left upper arm 4%, right lower arm 3%, left lower arm 3%, right hand 2.5%, left hand 2.5%, right thigh 9.5%, left thigh 9.5%, right leg from the knee down 7%, left leg from the knee down 7%, right foot 3.5%, and left foot 3.5% (Perdue et al., 2011).

Incidence/Prevalence in U.S.

Every year, 1.1 million burn injuries require medical attention. Approximately 50,000 of these require rehospitalization, 20,000 are major burns involving at least 25% of the total body surface, and 4,500 people die (CDC, 2013).

Over 300 children ages 0-19 are treated in emergency rooms for burn-related injuries every day, with two deaths resulting from burns (CDC, 2012). Approximately one third of clients admitted to a burn center are children (Purdue et al., 2011).

Up to 10,000 people die every year from burn-related infections (CDC, 2013).

On the average in the United States in 2004, someone died in a fire nearly every 135 minutes, and someone was injured every 30 minutes (CDC, 2013).

Burns are the third most frequent cause of childhood injury resulting in death, after motor vehicle accidents and drowning (Toon et al., 2011).

Predominant Age

Groups at increased risk of fire-related injuries and deaths include: children four years and younger, adults 65 years and older, African-Americans and Native Americans, the poorest Americans, people living in rural areas, and people living in manufactured homes or substandard housing (CDC NCIPC, 2004).

Causes

Four causes cover most of the burns seen: (1) scald burns and cooking-related tasks, which primarily affect children and are related to hot beverages, soup, microwaved food; (2) tap water burns, which are usually seen in children and older adults; (3) inappropriate use of highly flammable liquids such as gasoline or lighter fluid, most often involving adults; and (4) electrical and chemical burns, primarily seen in adults (Perdue et al., 2011).

Sources of burn injuries include smoking, intoxication, suicide attempts, and assaults (Perdue et al., 2011).

Approximately five to 15 percent of individuals who sustain a burn also sustain a traumatic injury. Examples include motor vehicle accidents, explosions, and falls from jumping from a fire (Perdue et al., 2011).

Six to 20 percent of all abuse cases are burn injuries and severe burns are reported in about 10% of all childhood abuse cases (Toon et al., 2011)

Systems Affected

Even though a burn may appear to affect only the tissue damaged, a significant burn affects almost all areas of health. (See Secondary Problems.)

Secondary Problems

A variety of secondary complications can be seen in the burn population due to the extensive impact on multiple domains of health and life. A review of the literature by Wiechman (2011) found:

Psychological or emotional distress (d240 Handling Stress and Other Psychological Demands): Substantial distress is most noticeable within the first two years after the initial burn injury, resulting in such problems as sleep disturbances, body image concerns, sexual problems, mood disorders, and anxiety disorders, all potentially contributing to decreased quality of life. Acute stress disorder is estimated to be present in about 11-32% of the burn population. Post-traumatic stress disorder (PTSD) is present in about 23-33% of the burn population three to six months post injury and 15-45% at one year post injury. Without treatment, PTSD doesn't appear to subside over time. Other symptoms related to

psychological or emotional distress may include nightmares, intrusive thoughts, hypervigilance, and avoidance. See the chapter on PTSD for more information about related ICF coding.

Depression (b152 Emotional Functions): Symptoms of depression in the burn population vary widely from two to 22 percent during the first year post injury and three to 54 percent after the first year of injury.

Pain (b280 Sensation of Pain): Burn pain can fluctuate over time. There are also many factors that contribute to pain, making it difficult to predict. Some of the factors include physiological responses to pain medication, psychosocial variables (e.g., pain tolerance, anxiety, depression), and premorbid behavior issues. The size and location of the burn are not reliable pain predictors. To assist in describing pain, it is generally classified into five types: background pain (noticed when at rest, low to moderate intensity, long duration), procedural pain (noticed when undergoing wound care, intense, brief), breakthrough pain (noticed unexpected at rest or during procedures, pain spikes), postoperative pain (following operations, predictable, temporary), and chronic pain (continuing after all wounds are healed or lasting more than six months, may be due to nerve damage). Chronic pain occurs in about 30% of clients and commonly interferes with work, sleep, and daily activities. Large body surface areas affected by the burn and skin grafting correlate positively with chronic pain.

Locus of control (b160 Thought Functions, b164 Higher-Level Cognitive Functions, d740 Formal Relationships): Clients typically experience reduction or loss of internal locus of control due to multiple treatments, exhaustion of coping resources, high pain levels, being in an unfamiliar environment, dependency on others, lack of input on schedules and routines, and uncertainty about their future related to appearance, wound status, work, survival, etc.

Sleep (b134 Sleep Functions): Quality and quantity of sleep can be affected by the hospital environment, treatments, metabolic imbalance, being woken up during the night to take vital signs, itching (pruritus) when wound begins to heal, pain, anxiety, depression, and medications.

Pruritus (itching) (b840 Sensation Related to the Skin): Pruritus occurs in the early stages of wound healing, peaks at six months post burn, and declines after the first year following the injury in both healed and grafted skin. It is a result of inflammation, dryness, damage to the skin, and nerve damage and regeneration.

Body image dissatisfaction (b180 Experience of Self and Time Functions): Changes in appearance due to scarring, contractures, changes in skin pigmentation, or amputation can impact self-esteem and body image. Individuals who are at particular risk of body image dissatisfaction include those that have visible scars, depression, and poor coping skills. Females and those who premorbidly placed a high level of importance on their appearance are more likely to have body image dissatisfaction.

Fatigue (related to muscle weakness) (b455 Exercise Tolerance Functions, b730 Muscle Power Functions): deLateur & Shore (2011) conducted a literature review on fatigue in the burn population and noted the following. Fatigue, due to catabolism (muscle wasting) and hypermetabolism (increased metabolic activity leading to extreme weight loss), is common in both adults and children with burn injuries, significantly impacting return to school, work, and community life (d9 Community, Social, and Civic Life). Without special intervention, strength and aerobic capacity return at a slow and gradual rate over about two years, although full strength and aerobic capacity may never be attained.

Prognosis

Mortality rates can be crudely estimated by using the Prognostic Burn Index also called the Baux Index. This is calculated by adding the person's age and the total body surface area burned. For inhalation injuries another 17 is added. Currently, in the best units, about half the patients survive when the score is 130-140 (Oliver, 2013).

Treatment is complicated by burn size and depth, body part, client's age, preexisting disease, and presence of other trauma, such as smoke inhalation during a fire (Perdue et al., 2011).

Client motivation, pre-burn psychological morbidity, family support, and socio-economic background influence outcomes (Falder et al., 2009).

Children under the age of two and adults older than 50 are at a higher risk for complications and death (Perdue et al., 2011).

Individuals who are ill or have a disability are at a greater risk for having a burn injury due to mobility and/or sensory impairment issues. Others at greater risk are those who smoke while on oxygen — often seen with chronic obstructive pulmonary disease (Perdue et al., 2011).

Individuals with substance abuse disorders, diabetes, chronic obstructive pulmonary disease, and other medical comorbidities have a lower survival rate, longer lengths of stays, and poorer overall outcomes (Wiechman, 2011).

Individuals with severe burns requiring hospitalization often have preexisting chaos and dysfunction in their lives (e.g., depression, personality disorders, substance abuse). Mental health symptoms can be exacerbated during hospitalization due to continuation of dysfunctional coping mechanisms. This may result in increased lengths of stay and more serious psychopathological conditions upon discharge (Wiechman, 2011).

Individuals who had an anxiety or depressive disorder before they sustained a burn injury are at greater risk for developing post-traumatic stress disorder (Wiechman, 2011). High pain levels during inpatient rehabilitation are associated with long-term distress (Wiechman, 2011).

Individuals with visible burns to their face or hands, report more emotional distress compared to those who have less visible burns (Wiechman, 2011).

Approximately 60-80% of adults return to work by one year after burn injury (Esselman, 2011). Barriers include physical abilities, working conditions, wound issues, concerns about appearance and working with others, being afraid to leave home, being afraid of the workplace, depressed mood, pain, neurological problems, impaired mobility, psychiatric issues, lack of an individualized rehab plan, and lack of psychological support. Facilitators include ability to set goals during the rehab process, persistence, willpower, ability to take action, family support, and a strong social network (Esselman, 2011).

Children who sustain a burn injury, on average, return to school in eight to ten days. Approximately one third have an in-person school reentry visit by a member of the burn team or have a phone call or educational materials, such as a video, sent to the school to assist with reintegration (Esselman, 2011). However, a single visit to the school is not sufficient to be called community integration training, nor effective enough to resolve the complex issues surrounding school reintegration (Blakeney,

Partridge, & Rumsey, 2007). See the Resources to access a free e-book on school transitioning.

The CDC (2013) reports recovery based on the severity of the burn as follows: First-degree burns and all but the most severe of second-degree burns will heal in one to three weeks without medical intervention. Without medical intervention some of the second-degree burns will heal leaving a skin surface that is normal to slightly pitted and with inconsistent pigmentation of the skin. Severe second-degree burns and less severe, small-area third degree burns may benefit from elective skin grafts and generally take more than three weeks to heal. Pitted, flat, and shiny skin with uneven pigmentation and scar tissue should be expected. Most third-degree and fourth-degree burns will not heal well without medical intervention.

Assessment

Typical Scope of Team Assessment

Falder and colleagues (2009) recommended that the multidisciplinary burn assessment include seven core domains: (1) skin (s810 Structure of Areas of Skin, looking at protection, repair, and sensation), (2) neuromuscular function (b730 Muscle Power Functions, b740 Muscle Endurance Functions, and s7 Structures Related to Movement, looking at joint mobility, muscle strength, low limb function, hand and upper limb function, and cardiovascular fitness), (3) sensory function and pain (b280 Sensation of Pain, looking at pain intensity and itch), (4) psychological function (b125 Dispositions and Intra-Personal Functions, b126 Temperament and Personality Functions, and b180 Experience of Self and Time Functions, including the possibility of post-traumatic stress disorder and depression), (5) physical role function (d4 Mobility and d8 Major Life Areas, to assess functional independence and ability to return to work), (6) community participation (d9 Community, Social, and Civic Life, especially social reintegration), and (7) perceived quality of life (d240 Handling Stress and Other Psychological Demands and other deficits that might reduce the quality of life, such as b280 Sensation of Pain). Falder et al. (2009) further recommend the following assessment methods: goniometry and composite finger flexion for joint mobility; dynamometers, free weights, and manual muscle testing for strength; single and tandem leg stance, tandem walk, and *Timed Up and Go (TUG)* for lower limb function; The *QuickDASH* (Disability of the Arm, Shoulder, and Hand) for upper extremity function; the *Shuttle Run* (modified incremental shuttle walk test) for cardiovascular fitness; the *Brief Pain Inventory (BPI)* and the *Abbreviated Burn Specific Pain Anxiety Scale* for pain; the *Questionnaire for Pruritus Assessment* for itch; structured interviews, the *Clinician Administered PTSD Scale (CAPS)*, the *Structured Clinical Interview for DSM (SCID)*, *Impact of Events Scale (IES)*, *Davidson Trauma Scale (DTS)*, *Beck Depression Inventory (BDI)*, the *Hospital Anxiety and Depression Inventory II (HADS)* for psychological function; the *Canadian Occupational Performance Measure (COPM)*, the *Modified Barthel Index (MBI)*, and the *Functional Independence Measure (FIM)* for physical role function; the *Community Integration Questionnaire* and the *Craig Handicap Assessment and Reporting Technique (CHART)* for community participation; and the *SF-36*, the *Sickness Impact Profile (SIP)*, and the *Burn Specific Health Scale (BSHS)* for perceived quality of life. In addition to these assessments, Wiechman (2011) recommends use of the *Post-Traumatic Stress Disorder Symptom Checklist — Civilian Version (PCL-C)* to screen for PTSD and nine-item *Patient Health Questionnaire* to screen for depression.

Areas of Concern for RT Assessment

In addition to the issues reviewed in Secondary Problems, the recreational therapist can anticipate a wide array of issues related to play, leisure, recreation, and community engagement. For example, engagement in preferred play, leisure, recreation, and community activities may now have new or added physical, social, or psychological challenges. These may require activity-specific skill development and adaptation, education and counseling, and integration training. Unhealthy leisure patterns may emerge, including social withdrawal and lack of participation, impacting recovery and health. Some ICF codes that may be affected include d4 Mobility, d5 Self-Care, d7 Interpersonal Interactions and Relationships, d8 Major Life Areas, and d9 Community, Social, and Civic Life.

ICF Core Set

An ICF Core Set for Burns has not yet been developed.

Treatment Direction

Whole Team Approach

The first step is the acute management of the burns. The CDC (2013) and Perdue et al. (2013) recommend:

First-degree burn: Apply cool water compresses for the first day. Take over-the-counter oral pain medication to alleviate pain and decrease inflammation. Remoisturize the skin through topical agents (e.g., aloe vera, Eucerin, Aveeno, Lubriderm). Cover the burn with a sterile, non-adhesive bandage or clean cloth. Most first-degree burns heal without further treatment. However, if burns cover a large area of the body or if the person is an infant or older adult, medical attention should be sought.

Second-degree burn: Immerse in fresh, cool water or apply cool compresses for 10-15 minutes. Dry with a clean cloth and cover with sterile gauze. Do not break blisters. Elevate burned arms or legs. Take steps to prevent shock by laying the person flat, elevating the feet about 12 inches, covering the person with a coat or blanket. However, do not put the person in this position if a head, neck, or back injury is suspected or if it makes the person uncomfortable. Seek immediate medical advice. Spontaneous healing typically occurs within seven to 28 days. For deeper partial thickness burns, excision and skin grafting might be needed.

Third-degree burn: Cover the burn lightly with sterile gauze or clean cloth. Don't use material that could leave lint on the burn. Take steps to prevent shock by laying the person flat, elevating the feet about 12 inches, covering the person with a coat or blanket. However, do not put the person in this position if a head, neck, or back injury is suspected or if it makes the person uncomfortable. Elevate the burned area higher than the person's head when possible. Keep the person warm and comfortable. Watch for signs of shock. Do not place a pillow under the person's head if the person is lying down and there is an airway burn because this can close the airway. Seek immediate medical attention. Third-degree burns require skin grafting and topical antimicrobials for wound closure. Prior to grafting, eschar (dead tissue) needs to be debrided.

Fourth-degree burn: Seek medical attention immediately. Often requires a surgical skin flap closure or extremity amputation.

Once in the medical system, a multidisciplinary approach is recommended because the variety of life functions impacted by a burn injury influence long-term adjustment (Falder et al., 2009). The majority of clients with severe burns will be treated in a burn unit, a specific area in the hospital that has the specialized staff and equipment necessary to treat severe burns.

Burn care usually consists of three phases (Supple, 2013). Throughout all phases the treatment team is concerned with preventing infection and reducing functional loss typically caused by scar tissue. These treatments primarily address the ICF Body Structures codes.

Emergent phase: The first phase lasts from one to three days. During this time the treatment revolves around stabilization, transport, balancing the client's fluid needs, and evaluating other injuries and comorbid conditions.

Acute phase: The second phase constitutes the majority of the time the client is in the hospital and focuses on infection control, wound care, pain control, nutritional support, surgical intervention, therapy, and psychosocial support.

Rehabilitative phase: The third phase goes from complete wound closure through the active scar maturation process and usually lasts one to two years. However, rehabilitation may be a life-long process due to reconstructive procedures, contracture releases, and overcoming community integration issues (d4 Mobility, d7 Interpersonal Interactions and Relationships, d8 Major Life Areas, and d9 Community, Social, and Civic Life).

There are three major elements of rehabilitation for burns (other than surgery) that are critical for the therapist to understand. They are debridement procedures, splinting, and pressure garments.

Debridement is the removal of contaminated or foreign material from the burn site. The burn (and, often the entire person) is cleaned a minimum of twice daily to remove caked antimicrobials (antibacterial creams and lotions), to keep the injured area clean, to remove any dead tissue, and to remove bacteria. There are three methods used to remove contaminated or foreign material: mechanical — scrubbing the burn site until it is clean, surgical — cutting away the excess material, and enzymatic — using enzymes to dissolve the dead tissue and unwanted foreign material (Supple, 2013). While all of these methods may be used, most clients who are hospitalized are "tubbed" in a whirlpool to soften and loosen the unwanted material prior to physically scrubbing the area. This is a very painful process that happens twice a day. Clients are usually given morphine or similar pain medication. However, the nerves are so raw in the area that the pain medication is usually inadequate to reduce pain to a tolerable level.

Splinting is used in all three phases of burn care to address concerns documented with the ICF Body Structures codes and d4 Mobility. It is used in the emergent phase for edema control and pressure relief, in the acute phase for tissue elongation and graft protection, and in the rehabilitation phase for tissue elongation (Dewey, Richard, & Parry, 2011). Scarring of the burn site is often significant. Scar tissue has limited stretching ability. If the burn was deep enough, the client also lost some muscle tissue, ligaments, and tendons. Splinting may be used to help immobilize a burn site while newly grafted material adheres to the body. It is critical from an early stage to increase and maintain range of motion through the healing and scar tissue development process. Splinting helps reduce the severity of contractures, prevent deformity, and maximize the flexibility of scar tissue (Dewey et al., 2011). Splinting is a major component of most treatment for burns on extremities, helping maintain desired ligament and skin length and decreasing the incidence of contractures.

There are three phasing of splinting: primary splints, post-graft splints, and follow-up splints (DiGregorio, 1984; Dewey, 2013). Primary static splints (splints without moving parts) are used during the acute and pre-graft phase to prevent loss of range of motion. These splints are worn at all times except when staff or the client is working on range of motion exercises, skin care, or self-care. Post-graft splints are crafted before the grafting surgery and then worn for five to fourteen days after surgery to allow healing of the grafted area. Follow-up splints are worn for up to two years after the burn while the tissues in the burn site mature. Whenever possible, the splint wearing time is restricted to sleeping and it is eventually discontinued when the clients is able to maintain range of motion without constantly wearing the splint. Follow-up splints may be static or dynamic.

Pressure garments are tight elastic clothing specially designed to restrict blood flow to developing scar tissue and to inhibit the growth of raised scar tissue (Hoeman, 2008). After significant burns, normal tissue is replaced with scar tissue. Restricting the growth of scar tissue helps promote long-term range of motion and limits disfigurement. Clients will wear pressure garments over the burned portion of the body twenty-three hours a day, taking them off only for hygiene and skin care (Hoeman, 2008). Clients should have at least two specially fitted sets of pressure garments, allowing the garments to be washed when they are soiled.

Recreational Therapy Approach

Recreational therapists work with the team approach outlined above. Their specific role is to identify and provide opportunities for enjoyable activities to help with pain management (b280 Sensation of Pain), engage the client in appropriate physical activities to minimize scar formation and increase physical function (d4 Mobility), teach the client relaxation techniques to help with pain management, and address issues and skills related to community integration (d4 Mobility, d7 Interpersonal Interactions and Relationships, d8 Major Life Areas, and d9 Community, Social, and Civic Life), including issues related to adjustment. Clients often get the feeling that every member of the medical staff causes them pain. The recreational therapist may be the exception.

Recreational Therapy Interventions

Community integration: The need for community integration training related to school, work, and community life is noted throughout burn rehabilitation literature due to the impact of burns on multiple domains of functioning. Blakeney and colleagues (2007) note the following issues for community integration: Burn survivors say everyday social interactions, such as, shopping, being in public places, and taking public transportation, are challenging due to the staring and curiosity of others. Self-image and self-worth are damaged and self-consciousness and anxiety are increased. Survivors feel sad and angry about how they look, as they are unaccustomed to their new physical appearance. Survivors don't want to put their family members in uncomfortable situations in the community. Survivors "find little assistance from burn care professionals in their struggle to live their lives with burn scar disfigurement beyond discharge from their acute hospitalizations" (p. 598) and they desire further assistance in learning how to deal with community situations (e580 Health Services, Systems, and Policies). Family members of burn survivors report related distress. A review of the literature by Blakeney et al. (2007) identified powerful statistics to support the need for community integration: 30-50% of adult burn survivors complain of chronic and pervasive social strain (difficulty coping with the behavior of other or their own behavior in social situations), 20-30% of adult burn survivors demonstrate moderate to severe psychological and/or social difficulties, 50% of child burn survivors lack adaptive strategies for social reintegration and have diminished social competence. The authors conclude that research on community integration training is much needed in the burn population and identify five priority research areas. See Blakeney et al. (2011) for details. Use ICF codes b125 Dispositions and Intra-Personal Functions, b126 Temperament and Personality Functions, b130 Energy and Drive Functions, and b180 Experience of Self and Time Functions to describe treatment for emotional aspects for survivors. Teaching physical abilities required to move about in the community addresses issues documented with d4 Mobility. Working on interpersonal concerns addresses ICF codes d7 Interpersonal Interactions and Relationships, d8 Major Life Areas, and d9 Community, Social, and Civic Life.

Progressive exercise (b455 Exercise Tolerance Functions): According to a review of the literature by deLateur and Shore (2011), individuals who sustain a severe burn injury need to engage in a gradually progressive exercise program, based on interests and available resources, for at least 12 weeks after rehabilitation to increase muscle strength (b730 Muscle Power Functions) and aerobic capacity (b455 Exercise Tolerance Functions). The goal is to create a program that can be continued long term. The authors recommend that therapists ask a client to track the number of minutes engaged in the chosen

form of exercise for 10 days. At the end of 10 days, the client averages the number of minutes exercised, including any zero-minute days (e.g., walked 100 minutes over the course of 10 days, 100 minutes divided by 10 days = 10 minutes on average per day), and then subtract 10% to determine the daily recommended quota (e.g., 10 minutes on average per day, minus 10% = nine minutes per day). Each week, one extra minute should be added until 30 minutes a day is reached. It is important to note that "if no more activity than performance of activities of daily living is the norm, the individual will gradually lose both muscle mass and aerobic endurance, eventually ending up back in the 'frail' category" (p. 349). Although not stated in the review, recreational therapists should assist the client in finding forms of physical activity that hold personal meaning for the client and induce a sense of flow to promote motivation and sustained performance (b130 Energy and Drive Functions).

Pain management (b280 Sensation of Pain): Nonpharmacological pain management interventions that can be utilized by recreational therapists include distraction techniques to avoid painful stimuli, virtual reality to decrease attention to painful stimuli, relaxation imagery or guided imagery to create a full sensory image in the client's mind, deep breathing, progressive muscle relaxation, a quota system (Therapy procedures are performed to the tolerance set by the client. Once tolerance is reached, the client is rewarded with a break. Then the procedure begins again.), positive reinforcement, cognitive restructuring (changing negative and distorting thoughts, such as "I can't do this." to more positive self-talk such as "I can cope with this."), and forced choice (The client is given two options, one of which must be chosen, allowing the client to have more choice and control over the painful task.) (Wiechman, 2011). When choosing a coping strategy, therapists should be aware of the client's preferences and past coping styles, rather than force a particular coping strategy. For example, clients who prefer an "avoidant" coping style where they prefer not to know what is going on and give up control to the clinician, tend to gravitate towards distraction techniques to avoid painful stimuli. Those who prefer an "approach" coping style where they want to know what is going on, tend to become frustrated with distraction techniques (Wiechman, 2011). Giving the clients techniques that match their preferences is part of remedying deficits in b130 Energy and Drive Functions.

Sleep issues (b134 Sleep Functions): Quality and quantity of sleep, as reviewed in Secondary Problems, can impact therapy performance, pain control, adjustment, and wound healing. According to Wiechman (2011), several interventions can be helpful. These include sleep hygiene (providing the best routine for sleep), stimulus control (bed is used only for sleeping), sleep restriction (staying in bed only when asleep), cognitive behavioral therapy (changing dysfunctional thoughts that disrupt sleep), relaxation therapy, and light therapy to address disruption of circadian rhythms. Although not stated in the article, these can be appropriately integrated into recreational therapy through instruction about techniques and when addressing activity patterns.

Body image and self-esteem (b125 Dispositions and Intra-Personal Functions, b126 Temperament and Personality Functions, b180 Experience of Self and Time Functions): The utilization of cognitive behavioral strategies and adaptive coping strategies, along with social skills training can help enhance self-esteem (b126 Temperament and Personality Functions) and improve social competence (d7 Interpersonal Interactions and Relationships) (Wiechman, 2011). The "Changing Faces" program in Britain and "BEST" program in the U.S. focus on image enhancement and social skills. (See Resources for more information.)

Summer burn camps: Summer burn camps provide opportunities to engage in activities and social interactions designed to enhance self-esteem (b126 Temperament and Personality Functions), skills (d155 Acquiring Skills), and relationships (d7 Interpersonal Interactions and Relationships) in a safe and accommodating environment (Rimmer et al., 2007). Camp activities, such as archery, arts and crafts, horseback riding, rappelling, life skills, team building, are designed to foster success that builds self-confidence, sense of mastery, and a positive sense of self (Rimmer et al, 2007). Although literature on summer burn camps is scarce, there is evidence supporting its value. For example, Rimmer et al. (2007) conducted a study of children who attended a one-week burn camp. They found that camp enhanced the children's self-esteem, the self-esteem continued to improve over the next year, and the self-esteem remained relatively stable by the end

of the second year. The authors recommend that "parents and burn centers should strongly consider including attendance at burn camp in the rehabilitation strategies of burn surviving children, whenever possible" (p. 339).

Other interventions that may be helpful that are not found in burn-specific literature include:

Medical play: Medical play and preparation helps children and adolescents work through the anger, misunderstandings, and fear associated with burns (e.g., b126 Temperament and Personality Functions, d240 Handling Stress and Other Psychological Demands).

Leisure: Leisure opportunities (d920 Recreation and Leisure) should be provided in the hospital setting for coping, maintenance of self-identity, and skill enhancement. Leisure education and counseling explain leisure's importance for recovery and health (d570 Looking After One's Health).

Peer counseling: Peer counseling visits and identification of support groups (e3 Support and Relationships) provide additional community resources for the patient.

Prevention: Only 60% of Americans have a fire escape plan and only 25% have practiced it (CDC, 2013). Smoke alarms reduce the risk of dying in a fire by 50% (CDC, 2013).

Resources

Berkow Formula
www.uwmedicine.org/harborview/Documents/Burn-Stabilization-Protocol.pdf
UW Medicine, Harborview Medical Center. Go to the web page to access the Berkow Formula.

BEST Program
www.phoenix-society.org/programs/bestimageenchancement/
Developed by the Phoenix Society for Burn Survivors, the BEST program was developed to help individuals with disfigurements reintegrate back into the community. It includes three steps: STEPS (Self-talk, Tone of voice, Eye contact, Posture, Smile) which assists with projecting social comfort and confidence, RYR (Rehearse Your Response) which is used to manage questions, and The Staring Tool which is used to respond to stares.

Changing Faces
www.changingfaces.org.uk

A charity for people and families who are living with conditions, marks, or scars that affect their appearance. Gives practical and emotional support to adults, children, and their families. Provides training, support, and advice to professionals in health and education. Aims to change public attitudes towards people with an unusual appearance through campaigns, lobbying, and pushing for equal rights. Provides extensive resources for individuals, families, and healthcare providers.

www.changingfaces.org.uk/Resources-and-Guides
Changing Faces has also developed the REACH OUT Weekend Program. It is written for professionals to enable them to offer an intensive three- to four-day event for groups of young people with significant disfigurements to their face, hands, and/or bodies from burn injuries or similar visibly disfiguring conditions. It includes a CD-ROM training manual with an introduction for program directors, the REACH OUT DVD, one copy of Living with a Disfigurement, and three self-help guides for children and young people: Looking Different Feeling Good, What Happened to You?, and Do Looks Count? A variety of other publications and programs are also available in the Resource Guide on the website.

Model Systems Knowledge Translation Center (MSKTC) for Burns
www.msktc.org/burn
The MSKTC works closely with researchers in the four Burn Injury Model Systems to develop resources for people living with burn injuries and their supporters. These evidence-based materials are available in a variety of platforms such as printable PDF documents, videos, and slideshows.

Phoenix Society for Burn Survivors
www.phoenix-society.org
The leading national non-profit organization dedicated to empowering anyone affected by a burn injury through peer support, education, and advocacy. Membership is free and there are a multitude of resources, including a 212-page e-book titled *The Journey Back: Resources to Assist School Reentry after Burn Injury or Traumatic Loss, Revised Version II.*

References

Blakeney, P., Partridge, J., & Rumsey, N. (2007). Community integration. *Journal of Burn Care Research, 28*(4), 598-601.

Centers for Disease Control. (2012). Burn safety: The reality. Retrieved from http://www.cdc.gov/Safechild/Burns/.

Centers for Disease Control. (2013). Mass casualties: Burns. Retrieved from http://emergency.cdc.gov/masscasualties/burns.asp.

Centers for Disease Control National Center for Injury Prevention and Control. (2004). Fire deaths and injuries. Retrieved from www.cdc.gov/ncipc/factsheets/fire.htm.

deLateur, B. J. & Shore, W. S. (2011). Exercise following burn injury. *Physical Medicine and Rehabilitation Clinics of North America, 22*(2), 347-350.

Dewey, W. S., Richard, R. L., & Parry, I. S. (2011). Positioning, splinting, and contracture management. *Physical Medicine and Rehabilitation Clinics of North America, 22*(2), 229-247.

DiGregorio, V. (1984). *Rehabilitation of the burn patient*. New York: Churchill Livingston.

Esselman, P. C. (2011). Community integration outcome after burn injury. *Physical Medicine and Rehabilitation Clinics of North America, 22*(2), 351-356.

Esselman, P. C., Ptackek, J. T., Kowalske, K., Cromes, G. F., deLateur, B. J., & Engrav, L. H. (2001). Community integration after burn injuries. *Journal of Burn Care and Rehabilitation, 22*(3), 221-227.

Falder, S., Browne, A., Edgar, D., Staples, E., Fong, J., Rea, S., & Wood, F. (2009). Core outcomes for adult burn survivors: A clinical overview. *Burns, 35*, 618-641.

Hoeman, S. P. (2008). *Rehabilitation nursing: Prevention, intervention, and outcomes*. Elsevier Health Sciences.

Oliver, R. (2013). Burn resuscitation and early management. Retrieved from http://emedicine.medscape.com/article/1277360-overview.

Perdue, G. F., Arnoldo, B. D., & Hunt, J. L. (2011). Acute assessment and management of burn injuries. *Physical Medicine and Rehabilitation Clinics of North America, 22*(2), 201-212.

Rimmer, R. B., Fornaciari, G. M., Foster, K. N., Bay, C. R., Wadsworth, M. M., Wood, M., & Caruso, D. (2007). Impact of a pediatric residential burn camp experience for burn survivors' perceptions of self and attitudes regarding the camp community. *Journal of Burn Care & Research, 28*(2), 334-341.

Supple, K. G. (2013). Burn injury care. Retrieved from http://nursing.advanceweb.com/article/burn-injury-care-2.aspx?CP=2.

Toon, M. H., Maybauer, D. M., Arceneaux, L. L., Fraser, J. F., Meyer, W., Runge, A., & Maybauer, M. O. (2011). Children with burn injuries — assessment of trauma, neglect, violence and abuse. *Journal of Injury and Violence Research, 3*(2), 98-110.

Wiechman, S. A. (2011). Psychosocial recovery, pain, and itch after burn injuries. *Physical Medicine and Rehabilitation Clinics of North America, 22*(2), 327-345.

7. Cancer

Heather R. Porter

Cancer is the generic name given to a group of more than 100 diseases where abnormal cells divide and grow out of control (American Cancer Society [ACS], 2012). As cancer advances, the cancer cells can invade other parts of the body (metastasize), spreading to nearby tissue or moving through the blood or lymphatic system (ACS, 2012). The location where the cancer originates dictates the name of the cancer (ACS, 2012). For example, cancer that begins in the breast, even if it metastasizes to the liver, is called breast cancer, not liver cancer. General signs and symptoms of cancer include unexplained weight loss, fever, fatigue, pain, and skin changes, Specific forms of cancer have other or additional signs and symptoms. For example, a change in bowel habits might be a sign of colon cancer and lumps in the breast might be a sign of breast cancer (ACS, 2012).

Incidence/Prevalence in U.S.

Approximately 13 million people in the U.S. currently have cancer and half of all men and one-third of all women in the U.S. will develop cancer during their lifetimes (ACS, 2012). In 2010 the most prevalent cancers were breast cancer (about 2.8 million) and prostate cancer (about 2.6 million). These were followed by melanoma (about 922,000), endometrial cancer and uterine sarcoma (about 600,000), urinary bladder cancer (about 564,000), thyroid cancer (about 535,000), and non-Hodgkin's lymphoma (about 509,000) (ACS, 2012). Approximately 379,000 children had cancer in 2010, of which 50% were males and 50% were females (ACS, 2012). Childhood cancer affects approximately 17.5% of the population ages 0-19, with leukemia and brain or nervous system cancers being most prevalent (Centers for Disease Control and Prevention [CDC], 2010). In 2010, approximately 11% of individuals living in assisted living or other residential care had cancer and approximately 43% of those in hospice care had a primary diagnosis of cancer (CDC, 2013).

Predominate Age

Anyone, at any age, can have cancer. Certain cancers, however, are more prevalent at certain ages (NCI, 2013b). For example, in those under the age of 20, brain and nervous system cancers occur much more frequently than bladder cancer (NCI, 2013b). The median age for being diagnosed with cancer, when all cancer site data is included, is 66 years old (NCI, 2013b).

Causes

Cancer can be caused by lifestyle choices (e.g., smoking, alcohol, high body weight, poor eating habits, poor activity levels, too much exposure to ultraviolet rays and sunlight), environmental factors (e.g., radiation, chemicals), and/or genetics. One out of every 20 cases of cancer is directly linked to inherited genes (ACS, 2012).

Systems Affected

The specific body systems involved, and the extent to which they are involved, will vary depending on the type of cancer. Cancers that are life threatening will also affect the whole physical structure, cognitive processes, and psychological, emotional, and spiritual health.

Secondary Problems

Side effects from cancer treatment vary widely due to a multitude of factors including the treatment chosen, the client's age and health, and the individual's response to the specific treatment. The three most invasive treatments are surgery, chemotherapy, and radiation. Surgery complications include pain, a partially collapsed lung, blood clots, fatigue, muscle atrophy, anesthesia effects, confusion or delirium, and infection (WebMD, 2013). Chemotherapy effects include nausea, vomiting, loss of appetite, hair loss, mouth sores, and low blood cell counts that increase risk for infection, bleeding, bruising, and anemia. Radiation effects include skin irritation and fatigue (ACS, 2012). Individuals with advanced cancer often experience a greater number of physical, emotional, and spiritual symptoms (Campbell & Campbell, 2012). These include pain, dyspnea, constipation, fatigue, poor sleep, anxiety, depression, and grief.

Prognosis

Information from the U.S. National Cancer Institute's Surveillance Epidemiology and End Results (SEER) database from 2008-2010 was used to predict the risk of developing and the risk of dying from particular cancers (ACS, 2012b). In males, the overall risk of dying from cancer is 22.9%, with the largest number of deaths coming from lung or bronchus cancer (6.6%), prostate cancer (2.7%), and colon and rectal cancer (2.1%). In women, the overall risk of dying from cancer is 19.3%; with the largest number of deaths due to lung or bronchus cancer (5.0%), breast cancer (2.7%), and colon and rectal cancer (1.9%) (ACS, 2012b). In 2013, it is expected that over 580,000 people will die of cancer (ACS, 2012b). Data analyzed from 2003-2009 indicate that, on average, 65.8% of people are still living five years after having a cancer diagnosis (NCI, 2013a).

Assessment

Typical Scope of Team Assessment

If cancer is suspected, tests, such as x-rays, blood tests, and biopsies, are ordered to determine if cancer is indeed present. Once cancer is diagnosed, it is "staged." Cancer staging is an assessment used by treatment teams that helps determine the appropriate treatment protocols for the client. It helps determine the client's prognosis and helps compare treatment results across different facilities. Most types of cancers have specific stages based on the number of cancer cells and the degree to which the cancer has spread to other parts of the body.

In the United States the National Cancer Institute manages the Surveillance, Epidemiology, and End Results Program (SEER) to help identify the most promising treatment protocols. Clinical data is submitted to SEER using a Summary Staging Scale that has five levels (National Cancer Institute [NCI], 2013a):

In situ: early cancer that is present only in the layer of cells in which it began.

Localized: cancer that is limited to the organ in which it began, without evidence of spread.

Regional: cancer that has spread beyond the original (primary) site to nearby lymph nodes or organs and tissues.

Distant: cancer that has spread from the primary site to distant organs or distant lymph nodes.

Unknown: describes cases for which there is not enough information to indicate a stage.

The SEER Staging Scale helps compare data for all types of cancers. The most commonly used, clinically based staging system for cancers that form tumors is the TNM (tumor size, if the cancer has spread to the lymph nodes, and if the cancer has metastasized or spread to other parts of the body). Not all cancers have TNM designations. The TNM Staging System is provided below (NCI, 2013a):

Primary Tumor (T)

TX: Primary tumor cannot be evaluated.

T0: No evidence of primary tumor.

Tis: Carcinoma is situ (CIS). Abnormal cells are present but have not spread to neighboring tissue. Although CIS is not cancer, it may become cancer and is sometimes called preinvasive cancer.

T1, T2, T3, T4: Size and/or extent of the primary tumor.

Regional Lymph Nodes (N)

NX: Regional lymph nodes cannot be evaluated.

N0: No regional lymph node involvement.

N1, N2, N3: Degree of regional lymph node involvement based on number and location of lymph nodes.

Distant Metastasis (M)

MX: Distant metastasis cannot be evaluated.

M0: No distant metastasis.

M1: Distant metastasis is present.

To illustrate the use of the TNM system, consider a client who has T3 N2 M0 breast cancer. This means that the tumor is large (T3) and has spread outside the breast to nearby lymph nodes (N2), but has not spread to other parts of the body (M0). For many cancers, TNM combinations correspond with one of five cancer stages, as reflected below (NCI, 2013a):

Stage 0: Carcinoma in situ.

Stage I, II, and III: Higher numbers indicate more extensive disease, as seen by larger tumor size and spread of the cancer beyond the organ in which it first developed to nearby lymph nodes and/or tissues or organs adjacent to the location of the primary tumor.

Stage IV: The cancer has spread to distant tissues or organs.

If the ICF is used for reporting the physical aspects of cancer, the Body Structure codes would be cited, along with specific functional problems, such as b435 Immunological System Functions.

Areas of Concern for RT Assessment

Being diagnosed with cancer is often a life-altering event. While the majority of clients diagnosed with cancer will survive, a diagnosis of cancer often causes clients to stop and re-evaluate their lives. The treatment phase of cancer often leaves the client very ill, with limited energy and limited appetite (b130 Energy and Drive Functions, b280 Sensation of Pain, d230 Carrying Out Daily Routine). Cancer treatment is also time-consuming, whether it is given in outpatient or inpatient settings. Major normal activities need to be significantly reduced to accommodate the number of hours associated with treatment, the lack of energy, and the lack of overall health (b134 Sleep Functions, d230 Carrying Out Daily Routine, d4 Mobility, d6 Domestic Life, d7 Interpersonal Interactions and Relationships, d8 Major Life Areas, d9 Community, Social, and Civic Life). Given all of these major changes, the potential for death due to the cancer, and the stress put on relationships important to the client, a secondary diagnosis of depression may also be of concern (b130 Energy and Drive Functions, b152 Emotional Functions). Not all cancers have pain associated with the cancer, but some have severe pain (b280 Sensation of Pain). Pain and the treatment for pain (including the use of narcotics) also negatively impact the client's ability to function. Specific cancers will affect specific body functions, such as lung cancer affecting b440 Respiration Functions. These additional functional limitations and related deficits in Activities and Participation should also be described.

ICF Core Set

Many ICF Core Sets identify relevant ICF codes. Some of the Core Sets that can be consulted are Breast Cancer, Chronic Pain, and Head and Neck Cancer.

Treatment Direction

Whole Team Approach

Treatment of cancer will vary depending on a variety of variables including the type of cancer, stage of cancer, client's age and medical history, and location of the cancer. Common treatments include surgery, chemotherapy, radiation, hormone therapy, stem cell transplants, bone marrow transplants, and immunotherapy (ACS, 2012).

Recreational Therapy Approach

The recreational therapy approach will vary depending primarily on the setting (e.g., intensive care, outpatient, summer camp for kids that have cancer), the cancer stage (advanced, remission), treatment side effects, level of support, prognosis, and client wishes.

Recreational Therapy Interventions

Exercise: Mishra and colleagues (2012) conducted a systematic review of the literature of randomized controlled trials (RCTs) on the effect of exercise in individuals undergoing active cancer treatment, looking at outcomes and health-related quality of life (HRQoL). A total of 56 RCTs were found with a total of 4826 participants. Exercise interventions varied and included walking, cycling, strength training, resistance training, yoga, and qigong. Findings suggest that exercise interventions resulted in improvements in HRQoL, physical functioning, role function, and social functioning from baselines to 12-week and six-month follow-ups (d6 Domestic Life, d7 Interpersonal Interactions and Relationships, d8 Major Life Areas, d9 Community, Social, and Civic Life). In the subcategory of breast cancer, exercise interventions led to a significant reduction in anxiety (b152 Emotional Functions). For other cancers they found significant reductions in depression, fatigue, and sleep disturbances, and improvements in HRQoL, emotional wellbeing, physical functioning, and role function (b130 Energy and Drive Functions, b134 Sleep

Functions, b455 Exercise Tolerance Functions, b730 Muscle Power Functions, d4 Mobility, d920 Recreation and Leisure). Findings also indicated that moderate to vigorous exercise had greater effects compared to mild exercise. The authors note that the findings need to be interpreted cautiously due to the high risk of bias in the studies. Although not stated by the authors, exercise abilities and limitations across clients with cancer will vary widely. Therefore, prior to engaging in any form of leisure time physical activity, the therapist must get clearance from the treating physician along with specific precautions and parameters.

Cognitive behavioral interventions: A systematic review of the literature was conducted from 1990-2002 on psychosocial interventions for individuals with advanced cancer (Uitterhoeve et al., 2004). Findings indicated that behavioral therapy for individuals with advanced cancer is frequently utilized as a single or combined intervention to help clients learn how to relax skeletal muscles, divert attention from pain and stressful thoughts, change distorted thinking and beliefs, enhance their sense of control, and reinforce adaptive behavior (b126 Temperament and Personality Functions, b152 Emotional Functions, d240 Handling Stress and Other Psychological Demands, b280 Sensation of Pain). The authors noted that the majority of the studies measured anxiety and depression, followed by physical functioning and quality of life. The studies generally lacked much-needed measures on social, spiritual, and existential aspects of quality of life. In another review of the literature of psychosocial interventions for individuals with advanced cancer, Campbell and Campbell (2012) described cognitive behavioral interventions to identify and modify negative thoughts, beliefs, and expectations; relieve physical symptoms; reduce emotional distress; and enhance social support and self-efficacy (b126 Temperament and Personality Functions, b152 Emotional Functions, d240 Handling Stress and Other Psychological Demands, b280 Sensation of Pain). They further noted that the specific interventions of cognitive restructuring, problem solving, guided imagery, and psychoeducational interventions related to the diagnosis were used (d2 General Tasks and Demands). Also found were meaning-making interventions and specific behavioral interventions designed to increase the use of healthy adaptive

behaviors and decrease unhealthy maladaptive behaviors. In the Campbell and Campbell (2012) review, findings indicated that the interventions were effective in people who have early stage cancer. Findings related to the efficacy of these interventions for individuals who have advanced stage cancer are limited and require further research.

Pain management: Gaertner and Schiessl's (2013) review of the literature on pain management interventions (b280 Sensation of Pain) for individuals with cancer found that pharmacological and non-pharmacological interventions can be helpful. Skills training to, for example, reduce catastrophizing and change distorted thoughts and education, such as relaxation training, were efficacious. The authors found that "the experience of loss, fundamental loneliness, and existential pain substantially add to the experience of cancer pain which has lead to the development of the concept of 'total pain'" (p. 328).

Life review: Ando and colleagues (2010) conducted a randomized controlled trial of 68 individuals with terminal cancer to study the effect of the *Short-Term Life Review* (STLR) interview on spiritual well-being, anxiety, depression, suffering, and elements of good death (b126 Temperament and Personality Functions). The control group received two sessions of general support and the experimental group received two STLR sessions, each lasting 30 to 60 minutes. The STLR sessions consisted of discussions about eight questions (person-centered manner, nonjudgmental, supportive) and developing a simple album reflecting the individual's narrative. The album was developed during the first session and consisted of positive and negative keywords expressed during the interviews. Photos and drawings that related to the words were cut from books and magazines and pasted into the album to make it beautiful and memory provoking. In the second session, the client and therapist reviewed and finalized the album together with the goal of encouraging the individual to feel continuity of the self from past to present, to accept life completion, and to be satisfied with his/her life. At the end of the second session, the album was given to the individual to keep. Although not measured, it was thought that the presentation of the album might help the individuals feel as if their lives were much more impressive and valuable. Findings indicated that the STLR alleviated anxiety and depression, improved spiritual well-being, increased sense of meaning, reduced psycho-existential suffering, led to a peaceful mind, increased feelings of life completion, and allowed for a good death (b126 Temperament and Personality Functions).

Art: A systematic review of the literature related to art therapy and cancer from inception to December 2008 was conducted by Wood, Molassiotis, and Payne (2011). A total of 14 studies were found. Symptoms investigated included emotional, physical, social, and global functioning, as well as existential and spiritual concerns. A variety of measures were used including questionnaires, in-depth interviews, patients' artwork, therapists' narratives, and stress markers in saliva samples. The narrative synthesis found that while art therapy was used as a psycho-therapeutic approach at all stages of cancer, it was most frequently used with women who had breast cancer. Art therapy is utilized to manage treatment-related symptoms and facilitate psychological adjustments to loss, change, and cancer survival (b126 Temperament and Personality Functions). The authors concluded that research in this area is still in its infancy. Although recreational therapists are not art therapists, the modality of art is utilized by recreational therapists to facilitate functioning, psychological and emotional health, and quality of life. More research in this area is needed.

Yoga: A systematic review of the literature was conducted from inception to April 2008 on the outcomes of yoga for individuals with cancer (Smith & Pukall, 2009). A total of six RCTs, two non-controlled studies, and one program evaluation were found. Positive results were identified that included improvements in sleep, b134 Sleep Functions; quality of life, b125 Dispositions and Intra-Personal Functions; stress levels, d240 Handling Stress and Other Psychological Demands; mood; and social well-being, b126 Temperament and Personality Functions. Variability across studies and methodological limitations prevented yoga from being identified as a specific intervention for the treatment of cancer symptoms. It's usefulness as an exercise regime has been shown, as discussed in the Exercise intervention above. More research is needed.

Spirituality: In a review of the literature by Campbell and Campbell (2012), spiritual needs (d930 Religion and Spirituality) of individuals with advanced cancer are common, including the need for

hope; gratitude; receiving love; forgiveness; creating meaning and purpose; connection with family, friends, spiritual community, or deity from their faith; a belief in the concept of something bigger than one-self; and spiritual/religious practices. The reviewers further noted that spiritual symptoms include expressions of existential distress; loss of meaning; the need for forgiveness; and isolation from family, friends, community, and religious images. ICF codes addressed include d7 Interpersonal Interactions and Relationships and d9 Community, Social, and Civic Life.

Music interventions: A systemic review of the literature from 1970 to 2012 was conducted by Archie, Bruera, and Cohen (2013) to identify the benefits of music-based interventions (MBI) in palliative cancer care. Findings indicated that MBI may have a positive impact on pain (b280 Sensation of Pain), anxiety (b126 Temperament and Personality Functions), and quality of life.

Rehabilitation-specific interventions: A review of the literature from Egan and colleagues (2013) sought to identify rehabilitation interventions post-cancer treatment aimed at ameliorating functional impairments. Evidence, although limited, identified physical functioning (b7 Neuromusculoskeletal and Movement-Related Functions, d4 Mobility), fatigue (b455 Exercise Tolerance Functions), pain (b280 Sensation of Pain), sexual functioning (b640 Sexual Functions), cognitive functioning (b1 Mental Functions, d1 Learning and Applying Knowledge), depression (b126 Temperament and Personality Functions), employment (d840-d859 Work and Employment), nutrition (d570 Looking After One's Health), and participation (any related d code) as possible areas for intervention, including psychoeducation interventions.

Other interventions: Other recreational therapy interventions that are not reflected in literature include: activity balance (d920 Recreation and Leisure) to help the client to identify and plan activity engagement that addresses physical, emotional, interpersonal, and cognitive needs or desires within the abilities and limitations of the client (d570 Looking After One's Health); activity modification based on abilities and limitations to maximize participation and outcomes (e140 Products and Technology for Culture, Recreation, and Sport); time management to help the client prioritize activities based on abilities, support, health, and meaning (d230 Carrying Out Daily Routine); energy conservation training to minimize fatigue and enhance engagement in meaningful activities (b455 Exercise Tolerance Functions); and medical play to reduce fear related to cancer treatments (d880 Engagement in Play).

Resources

American Cancer Society (ACS)

www.cancer.org

The ACS is the nationwide, community-based, volunteer health organization dedicated to eliminating cancer as a major health problem by preventing cancer, saving lives, and diminishing suffering from cancer through research, education, advocacy, and service.

www.cancer.org/cancer/cancerbasics/other-sources-of-cancer-information

An ACS web page with over 100 sources of cancer information.

National Cancer Institute at the National Institutes of Health

www.cancer.gov

Coordinates the National Cancer Program, which conducts and supports research, training, health information dissemination, and other programs with respect to the cause, diagnosis, prevention, and treatment of cancer, rehabilitation from cancer, and the continuing care of cancer patients and the families of cancer patients.

References

American Cancer Society. (2012). Cancer basics. Retrieved from http://www.cancer.org/cancer/cancerbasics/index.

Ando, M., Morita, T., Akechi, T., & Okamoto, T. (2010). Efficacy of short-term life-review interviews on the spiritual well-being of terminally ill cancer patients. *Journal of Pain and Symptom Management, 39*(6), 993-1002.

Archie, P., Bruera, E., & Cohen, L. (2013). Music-based interventions in palliative cancer care: A review of quantitative studies and neurobiological literature. *Support Cancer Care, 21*, 2609-2624.

Campbell, C. L. & Campbell, L. C. (2012). A systematic review of cognitive behavioral interventions in advanced cancer. *Patient Education and Counseling, 89*(1), 15-24.

Centers for Disease Control and Prevention. (2010). 2010 childhood cancer by primary site. Retrieved from http://apps.nccd.cdc.gov/uscs/childhoodcancerbyprimarysite.aspx.

Centers for Disease Control and Prevention. (2013). FastStats: Cancer. Retrieved from http://www.cdc.gov/nchs/fastats/cancer.htm.

Egan, M. Y., McEwen, S., Sikora, L., Chasen, M., Fitch, M., & Eldred. S. (2013). Rehabilitation following cancer treatment. *Disability and Rehabilitation, 35*, 2245-2258.

Gaertner, J. & Schiessl, C. (2013). Cancer pain management: What's new? *Current Pain and Headache Report, 17*, 328.

Mishra, S. I., Scherer, R., Snyder, C., Geigle, P. M., Berlanstein, D., & Topaloglu, O. (2012). Exercise interventions on health-related quality of life for people with cancer during active treatment. *The Cochrane Database of Systematic Reviews, 8*.

National Cancer Institute. (2013a). Cancer staging. Retrieved from http://www.cancer.gov/cancertopics/factsheet/detection/staging.

National Cancer Institute. (2013b). SEER stat fact sheets: All cancer sites. Retrieved from http://seer.cancer.gov/statfacts/.

Smith, K. B. & Pukall, C. F. (2009). An evidence-based review of yoga as a complementary intervention for patients with cancer. *Psycho-Oncology, 18*, 465-475.

Uitterhoeve, R. J., Vernooy, M., Litjens, M., Potting, K., Bensing, J., DeMulder, P., & van Achterberg, T. (2004). Psychosocial interventions for patients with advanced cancer: A systematic review of the literature. *British Journal of Cancer, 91*, 1050-1062.

WebMD. (2013). 8 common surgery complications. http://www.webmd.com/healthy-aging/features/common-surgery-complications.

Wood, J. M, Molassiotis, A., & Payne, S. (2011). What research evidence is there for the use of art therapy in the management of symptoms in adults with cancer? A systematic review. *Psycho-Oncology, 20*, 135-145.

8. Cerebral Palsy

Dawn R. DeVries

Cerebral palsy, commonly referred to as CP, describes a group of symptoms and neurological disorders that appear in early childhood and infancy (Mayo, 2010; NINDS, 2009; Reaching for the Stars, 2013). Cerebral means that it has to do with the brain, and palsy refers to muscle problems or weakness (National Dissemination Center for Children with Disabilities (NICHCY), 2010; Reaching for the Stars, 2013; CDC, 2012b; NINDS, 2012). These neurological problems are the result of non-progressive damage to areas of the brain that control movement and coordination, such as the cerebellum and basal ganglia (Griffin, Fitch, & Griffin, 2002; NICHCY, 2010; NINDS, 2012; Odding, Roebroeck, & Stam, 2006; Reaching for the Stars, 2013). Damage to these areas also affects muscle tone, endurance, strength, and speech (Griffin et al., 2002; Odding et al., 2006). The effects of CP vary in each person depending on the severity of the damage to the brain. Some may have cognitive impairments and minimal physical problems, while others may have a clear physical disability but not a cognitive one (AAP, 2013; CDC, 2012b; Mayo, 2010; NICHCY, 2010; Reaching for the Stars, 2013). There are four types of CP (CDC, 2012a; CDC, 2012b; March of Dimes, 2007; NICHCY, 2010; NINDS, 2009, 2012; Reaching for the Stars, 2013; Torpy, 2010):

Spastic CP: 70-80% of all people with CP; muscles are stiff and can be permanently contracted; muscles are tight and tone is increased; further classified by which limbs are affected.

Athetoid or dyskinetic CP (also referred to as choreoathetoid or dystonic CP): 10-20% of all people with CP; slow, uncontrolled movements usually in extremities and face; low muscle tone; frequently dysarthria (difficulty coordinating the muscles needed for speech); intelligence is rarely affected in this type of CP.

Ataxic CP: 5-10% of all people with CP; balance and depth perception most affected; poor coordination; unsteady wide-based gait.

Mixed: Combination of any of the above types; may have combination of high and low tone or stiffness and involuntary movements.

Types are further classified based on the physical area affected:

Diplegia: only legs are impacted.

Hemiplegia: only half of the body is impacted, usually one side of the body in both extremities.

Quadriplegia: both upper and lower extremities are impacted; may also include facial and trunk muscles.

General symptoms of cerebral palsy (Mayo, 2010; McRae et al., 2009; NINDS, 2009, 2012; NICHCY, 2010; Reaching for the Stars, 2013) include:

- Ataxia (poor muscle coordination)
- Poor muscle control
- Spasticity or tight muscles
- Atypical gait (scissoring particularly with spastic CP)
- Drooling
- Swallowing and/or eating difficulties
- Speech impairments in clarity and articulation
- Difficulty with fine motor tasks
- Toe walking
- Atypical muscle tone (too high or too low)
- Involuntary movements or tremors

Incidence/Prevalence in U.S.

CP is one of (if not) the most common motor disability affecting children (CDC, 2012b; Davis et al., 2009; Geytenbeek, 2011; Groff, Lundberg, & Zabriskie, 2009; Ketelaar et al., 2008; Longo, Badia & Orgaz, 2013; Vargus-Adams & Martin, 2011; von der Luft et al., 2008). It is estimated that approximately 800,000 children and adults in the United States display signs and symptoms of CP (March of Dimes, 2007; NINDS, 2012) and that 17,000,000 people worldwide live with CP (Reach for the Stars, 2013). Approximately 10,000 infants are diagnosed with CP annually, along with an additional 1,200-1,500 preschool-age children (NINDS, 2012; Reaching for the Stars, 2013). CP is found in one out of every 303 eight-year-olds in the U.S. (CDC, 2012c; Kirby et al., 2011). Its prevalence is lower in Hispanic children than in black or white children (Boyle et al., 2011; CDC, 2012a).

The incidence and prevalence of CP has changed little in recent years. Even with improvements in medical care for pregnant women and during delivery, the incidence of CP has remained the same (Griffin et al., 2002; NINDS, 2012), not just in the United States but also around the world (Griffin et al., 2002; Odding et al., 2006; Winter et al., 2002). Data from around the world (Australia, Europe, Sweden, and Scotland) also indicates similar incidences of CP in babies of low birth weight or premature birth (CDC, 2012a).

Predominant Age

CP is difficult to diagnose before birth or during early development due to variations that occur in milestone achievement (NINDS, 2012; Reaching for the Stars, 2013). Consequently, CP is typically diagnosed in the early developmental years, most frequently by 18 months but sometimes taking up to three years (March of Dimes, 2007; NINDS, 2009, 2012; Reaching for the Stars, 2013). Developmental delays, such as the inability to grasp, sit up, or crawl, are the primary observed indication of CP. Other signs include changes in muscle tone from low (hypotonia) to high (hypertonia), abnormal posture, and retained early childhood reflexes (March of Dimes, 2007; Reaching for the Stars, 2013). Physicians diagnose CP by focusing on motor skills to evaluate delays while ruling out other disorders that cause movement problems. Individuals diagnosed with CP live with the neurological disorder for the duration of their lives (CDC, 2012b; Reaching for the Stars, 2013).

Causes

Approximately 70-80% of CP cases occur prenatally (CDC, n.d.; March of Dimes, 2007; Reaching for the Stars, 2013), and are caused by genetic conditions, infection, maternal bleeding or seizures, abnormal brain development, lack of oxygen, stroke, and intrauterine growth restriction (CDC, 2012a, 2012b; Griffin et al., 2002; Mayo 2010; NINDS, 2012; Reaching for the Stars, 2013). New research is also showing a link between cerebral palsy and abnormalities with the placenta (NINDS, 2012). Less than 10% occur during labor and delivery (Goh & Flynn, 2010). Causes that occur during birth include breech position, infections, lack of oxygen, stroke, multiple births, and jaundice (Griffin et al., 2002; Odding et al., 2006; Reaching for the Stars, 2013; March of Dimes, 2007; Mayo 2010; CDC, 2012a; NINDS, 2012). The remaining cases occur within the first years of life due to head injury, viral or bacterial infections affecting the central nervous system (such as meningitis), seizures, motor vehicle accidents, and child abuse (CDC, 2011; CDC, 2012a; Griffin et al., 2002; Reaching for the Stars, 2013; Mayo, 2010). Children born prematurely (earlier than 37 weeks) or with a low birth weight (3.5 pounds or less) are at greatest risk for CP (CDC, 2011; Odding et al., 2006; March of Dimes, 2007, Reaching for the Stars, 2013; CDC, 2012a; AAP, 2013; NINDS, 2012).

Systems Affected

The systems affected will vary depending on the severity of CP and the location of the brain injury (Mayo, 2010; March of Dimes, 2007; NINDS, 2009; Reaching for the Stars, 2013; NINDS, 2012; NICHCY, 2010; CDC, 2012b; McRae et al., 2009; Groff et al., 2009; Geytenbeek, 2011).

Nervous system: decreased muscle control; involuntary movement and/or spasticity; seizures; sensory processing and hyper-responsiveness or hypo-responsiveness to stimuli; cognitive impairment or delay; hearing impairment; vision impairment; speech impairment; sensation or perception abnormalities. Relevant ICF codes for these Body Functions deficits include b147 Psychomotor Functions, b210 Seeing Functions, b230 Hearing Functions, b235 Vestibular Functions, b260 Proprioceptive Function, b265 Touch Function, b3 Voice and Speech Functions, and b7 Neuromusculoskeletal and Movement-Related Functions.

Skeletal system: joint pain or discomfort; hyperextensive joints (b7 Neuromusculoskeletal and Movement-Related Functions).

Muscular system: hypotonic or hypertonic tone; spasticity; poor control; poor, low, or delayed coordination; hyperextension of extremities; fine motor impairments; gross motor impairments; impaired balance; may use assistive device (walker, crutches, wheelchair) for mobility; potential for contractures due to inability to move extremities independently (b7 Neuromusculoskeletal and Movement-Related Functions, d4 Mobility).

Digestive system: swallowing problems; may have feeding tube (b510 Ingestion Functions).

Respiratory system: breath support; may need ventilator or respirator depending on muscle involvement and tone; decreased endurance; breathing difficulty related to posture (b440 Respiration Functions, b445 Respiratory Muscle Functions, b455 Exercise Tolerance Functions).

Urinary system: problems with bowel and bladder continence due to muscle control (b525 Defecation Functions, b620 Urination Functions).

Secondary Problems

The Metropolitan Atlanta Developmental Disabilities Surveillance Program (a CDC research site) showed that 59% of eight-year-olds with CP had another developmental disability (CDC, 2012a). Many sources (Fowler et al., 2007; March of Dimes, 2007; Odding et al., 2006; NICHCY, 2010; Reaching for the Stars, 2013; UCP, 2013; Mayo, 2010; AAP, 2013; NINDS, 2012; Straub & Obrzut, 2009) list additional disabilities commonly occurring with CP. These disabilities include:

- *Intellectual disability*: Intellectual disability is the most common secondary disability in CP. Statistics indicated that 40-67% of children with CP will have intellectual disabilities (CDC, 2012a; NINDS, 2012). See the Intellectual Disability chapter for ICF codes.
- *Epilepsy or seizures*: Approximately 35-50% of individuals with CP have epilepsy or seizures (CDC, 2012a; NINDS, 2012; Gaskin & Morris, 2008). See the Epilepsy chapter for ICF codes.
- *Both intellectual disability and seizure disorder*: Occurs in about 25% of the CP population (CDC, 2012a). Additionally, 20-40% of those with cerebral palsy and intellectual disability will also have epilepsy (NINDS, 2012).
- *Behavioral problems*: Approximately 25% of children with CP have behavior problems in-

cluding attention-deficit/hyperactivity disorder, dependency, oppositional defiance disorder, and general hyperactivity (Odding et al., 2006) See chapters in this book that cover each of these conditions for information on ICF codes.

- *Learning disabilities*: Approximately 40% of children with CP have learning disabilities (Straub & Obrzut, 2009). See the Intellectual Disability chapter for ICF codes.
- *Sensory impairments*: Anywhere from 15-62% of children with CP have vision impairments and about six percent have a hearing impairment (CDC, 2012a). In adults with CP, 25-39% have vision problems, and 8-18% have hearing difficulties (NINDS, 2012). Approximately 75% of children with CP will develop strabismus (commonly referred to as lazy eye) (AAP, 2013). Code these with b210 Seeing Functions and b230 Hearing Functions.
- *Feeding difficulties and/or malnutrition*: This includes choking, long feeding time, need for gastric tube, underweight, sucking problems, swallowing, and silent aspiration. Approximately 57% of children with CP have sucking problems during the first year of life, and 38% have swallowing difficulties; 80% have been fed via a tube at some point in their lives; and 50% are either overweight or underweight (Odding et al., 2006; Mayo, 2010). Code with b510 Ingestion Functions, b530 Weight Maintenance Functions, and b560 Growth Maintenance Functions.
- *Lung problems*: About 33% experience a pulmonary infection in a six-month period (b450 Additional Respiratory Functions).
- *Chronic pain*: Pain, particularly back, foot, ankle, knee, and shoulder pain, and headaches, occur in approximately 28% of adults with CP (b280 Sensation of Pain) (Odding et al., 2006).
- *Autism*: Occurs in approximately nine percent of the CP population (CDC, 2012a). See the Autism chapter for ICF codes.

In addition to the above, individuals with CP can have a variety of other secondary complications related to neurological damage or physical limitations including:

- Inadequate or low levels of physical fitness (b455 Exercise Tolerance Functions) (Fowler et al., 2007; Siebert et al., 2010).

- Balance issues (b235 Vestibular Functions, d4 Mobility) (Siebert et al., 2010; Mayo, 2010; Reach for the Stars, 2013).
- Fatigue and cardiovascular disease (b455 Exercise Tolerance Functions) (Fowler et al., 2007; NINDS, 2012; Mayo, 2010). In one study, 31% of adults with spastic CP reported severe fatigue of physical origin that may have been related to low fitness levels (Nieuwenhuijsen, van der Slot, et al., 2011). The researchers indicated that this may be related to physical activity level and/or physical fitness, or a combination of the two, as well as behavioral factors.
- Musculoskeletal problems such as weakness, contractures, arthritis, kyphosis, osteoporosis, scoliosis, osteopenia (low bone density), and decreased range of motion (Bartlett & Palisano, 2002; Benda, McGibbon, & Grant, 2003; Fowler et al., 2007; Odding et al., 2006; Reaching for the Stars, 2013; Mayo, 2010; AAP, 2013; NINDS, 2012). Code with b7 Neuromusculoskeletal and Movement-Related Functions.
- Difficulty processing stimulation including over- or under-response to auditory, tactile, and visual stimuli; impacting ability to manipulate objects (b7 Neuromusculoskeletal and Movement-Related Functions, d4 Mobility) (Clayton et al., 2003; NICHCY, 2010; NINDS, 2012; Mayo, 2010; March of Dimes, 2007; Reach for the Stars, 2013).
- Incontinence (about 23%) (b620 Urination Functions) (Odding et al., 2006).
- Speech difficulties, with the most common being dysarthria (b3 Voice and Speech Functions) (Odding et al., 2006; Geytenbeek, 2011).
- Drooling due to swallowing disorder (effects 10-58% of children with CP) (b510 Ingestion Functions) (Erasmus et al., 2012).
- Breathing difficulties due to impaired postural control (b445 Respiratory Muscle Functions) (Reaching for the Stars, 2013).
- Skin breakdown (b820 Repair Functions of the Skin) (Reaching for the Stars, 2013; AAP, 2013).
- Contractures (b735 Muscle Tone Functions) (Mayo, 2010; Gaskin & Morris, 2008).
- Problems with spatial awareness due to decreased sense of position of a part of their body (b260 Proprioceptive Function) (AAP, 2013; Reach for the Stars, 2013).

- Depression or distress (Mayo, 2010; UCP, 2013a). See the chapter on Depression for relevant ICF codes.

Prognosis

CP is permanent and incurable. Once diagnosed, individuals live the remainder of their lives with this disability. Most individuals have a typical life span (NICHCY, 2010; NINDS, 2012), but life expectancy of an individual with CP can vary depending on the severity of the person's disability (Hutton & Pharoah, 2006; Strauss et al., 2008). There are many complex factors that impact the life expectancy of an individual with CP, including seizure diagnosis, motor skills, and cognitive abilities (Hutton & Pharoah, 2006). The earlier treatment begins for an individual with CP, the more likely they will enjoy "near-normal adult lives," whether that is through minimizing the effects of CP or adapting life to their abilities (NINDS, 2012).

Assessment

Typical Scope of Team Assessment

Medical doctors and allied health professionals complete developmental monitoring and screening to evaluate the child's motor functioning and neurological development. This team works "to develop a plan to help the child reach his or her full potential" (CDC, 2012b). A child with CP may have a developmental pediatrician, a pediatric neurologist, an ophthalmologist for vision problems, an orthodontist for braces, a physiatrist for physical medicine and rehabilitation issues, a gastroenterologist for feeding difficulties, an otolaryngologist or otologist for hearing issues, a geneticist, and an orthopedic surgeon (Reaching for the Stars, 2013; Mayo, 2010; March of Dimes, 2007; NINDS, 2012).

For many children, the first team assessment occurs prior to the age of three, when a child receives early intervention services (NICHCY, 2010; CDC, 2012b). Occupational, physical, and speech therapists, along with a social worker and/or special educator, complete the assessment to develop the Individual Family Service Plan (IFSP) (NICHCY, 2010, AAP, 2013; CDC, 2012b). It will address the child's needs as well as the services to be provided to help the family and child. The goal is to begin therapy and improve the child's functioning and chance of success.

The IFSP evolves into the Individualized Education Plan (IEP) when the child enters the school system. This is usually at age three under the Individuals with Disabilities Education Act [IDEA] (NICHCY, 2010; CDC, 2012b). As with the IFSP, the IEP identifies needs and services that will help the child function in the school setting and may include OT, PT, SLP, special education instruction, and/or assistive technology (NICHCY, 2010). Recreational therapy may be provided through the school system as a related service (NCPAD, 2006).

Areas of Concern for RT Assessment

The recreational therapist conducts a comprehensive assessment, including medical chart review, client and/or family interviews, standardized assessments, and functional observation. Standardized assessments that may be used by a recreational therapist include:

Gross Motor Function Measure: A reliable tool for measuring changes in gross motor function (Davis et al., 2011; Ko & Kim, 2013; Mac Keith Press, 2002).

KIDSCREEN: An instrument that is aimed at health-related quality of life (HRQoL) and measures "physical well-being, psychological well-being, moods and emotions, self-perception, autonomy, parent relations and home life, social support and peers, school environment, social acceptance, and financial resources" (Davis et al., 2011, p. 113; KIDSCREEN Group, 2011).

Cerebral Palsy Quality of Life Questionnaire for Children (CP QoL-Child): A reliable and valid tool to evaluate interventions aimed at improving quality of life in pediatrics (Davis et al., 2011; University of Melbourne Australia, 2013; Waters et al., 2007).

Physical Activity and Disability Survey (PADS): This is a tool to measure physical activity in people with disabilities and chronic neurological problems, such as CP (Gaskin & Morris, 2008; Kayes et al., 2009; Rimmer, Riley, & Rubin, 2001).

School Social Behavior Scales (SSBS) and *Home and Community Social Behavior Scales (HCSBS)*: The SSBS is a tool completed by the therapist, while the HCSBS is a tool completed by the family. The purpose of these tools is "to measure the social competence and antisocial behavior patterns of

youth" (burlingame & Blaschko, 2010, p. 460). This would be used for the pediatric population (5-18 years) related to social skills, self-management, and social behaviors.

Social Attributes Checklist — Assessing Young Children's Social Competence: This is another tool used to evaluate pre-school through elementary school age children's social behavior and social competence over a period of three to four weeks (burlingame & Blaschko, 2010).

Therapeutic Recreation Activity Assessment (TRAA): The TRAA uses tasks and activities to look at functional skills, personal strengths and weaknesses, as well as an individual's perception of their social and activity skills (burlingame & Blaschko, 2010). It has been evaluated for use with individuals with functional losses from causes such as traumatic brain injuries, developmental disabilities, and psychiatric impairments. CP would fit into the developmental disabilities category in using this tool.

State Technical Institute's Leisure Assessment Process (STILAP): This assessment tool measures participation patterns in adolescents with physical disabilities (burlingame & Blaschko, 2010). It looks at current and future interests, as well as the balance of the client's leisure experience.

Children's Assessment of Participation and Enjoyment (CAPE): This tool explores leisure and recreational activities children six years and older engage in during a four-month period (Longo et al., 2013; Majnemer et al., 2011; Palisano et al., 2011).

Preferences for Activities of Children: This companion to the CAPE looks at the preferred activities of children (Palisano et al., 2011).

Some common areas of assessment include:

Physical: Strength, endurance, mobility, range of motion, flexibility, coordination, balance, movement patterns, fine motor abilities, gross motor skills, bilateral movement, and respiratory abilities (ATRA, 2000; CDC, 2012b; Gaskin & Morris, 2008; Kunstler & Stavola Daly, 2010; Mayo, 2010; NCTRC, 2007; NINDS, 2012; NICHCY, 2010). ICF codes to score these areas include b147 Psychomotor Functions, b235 Vestibular Functions, b260 Proprioceptive Function, b440 Respiration Functions, b445 Respiratory Muscle Functions, b455 Exercise Tolerance Functions, b7 Neuromusculoskeletal and Movement-Related Functions, and d4 Mobility). Research clearly demonstrates that the client's gross motor skills impact participation in recreation and physical activities (Law et al., 2006; Orlin et al., 2010; Shikako-Thomas et al., 2008; Stewart et al., 2012). Additionally, a British study showed that children's activities and participation in recreation are most affected by their level of independence with physical functioning and mobility, rather than speech problems or a seizure disorder (Morris et al., 2006). Groff et al. (2009) states that one way "to improve the physical and psychosocial functioning of individuals with CP... is to offer them opportunities to promote their own good health by developing and maintaining healthy lifestyles" (p. 318).

Cognitive: Long- and short-term memory, attention to task, number and letter identification, problem solving, safety awareness, adaptive behavior, and information processing (AAP, 2013; ATRA, 2000; Mayo, 2010; NCTRC, 2007; Palisano et al., 2011). ICF codes include b140 Attention Functions, b144 Memory Functions, b164 Higher-Level Cognitive Functions, and d1 Learning and Applying Knowledge

Sensory: Vision, hearing, tactile responsiveness, olfactory or taste sensitivities (ATRA, 2000; Mayo, 2010; NCTRC, 2007). ICF codes are in b2 Sensory Functions and Pain.

Social/communication: Receptive language skills, expressive language abilities, augmentative communication, social skills, ability to interact with others, and friendships (ATRA, 2000; Kunstler & Stavola Daly, 2010; Mayo, 2010; NCTRC, 2007; NINDS, 2012; NICHCY, 2010). ICF codes can be found in d3 Communication and d7 Interpersonal Interactions and Relationships. Also consider the people interacting with the client using e3 Support and Relationships and e4 Attitudes. Ulman and Vidoni (2012) reported that social skills improve through games and activities, including peer recognition, respect of others, accepting rules, positive social interaction, and communication. Rothwell, Piatt, and Mattingly (2006) say that, "social interactions during the leisure experience are often more important than the activity itself" (p. 244). Therefore, as part of a leisure evaluation, recreational therapists must also consider a child's social skills and ability to interact with others. At older ages the therapist may need to look at issues like transitioning out of school and into work (d845 Acquiring, Keeping, and Terminating a Job).

Emotional/behavioral: Boundaries, awareness of others, reactions to new situations and people, emotional maturity, self-esteem, self-concept, self-efficacy; societal barriers affecting behaviors; mood issues, such as depression and anxiety, and emotional regulation (ATRA, 2000; Gaskin & Morris, 2008; Groff et al., 2009; Mayo, 2010; NCTRC, 2007; Riley, 2011; von der Luft et al., 2008; Wise, 2002). ICF codes can be found in d240 Handling Stress and Other Psychological Demands, d250 Managing One's Own Behavior, and d7 Interpersonal Interactions and Relationships.

Leisure: Recreation and leisure interests, leisure awareness, adaptive equipment and adaptation needs, family participation and interests, leisure barriers and facilitators, leisure attitudes and values, and leisure needs (ATRA, 2000; Groff et al., 2009; NCTRC, 2007; Orlin et al., 2010). This is an essential area for recreational therapists, particularly because it is "overlooked or given lower priority" by other therapists (Majnemer et al., 2010). Additionally, to increase participation in all leisure and recreation activities, including health promotion activities, recreational therapists utilize activities that are appropriate and of interest to the client to enhance their motivation and desire to participate (Majnemer et al., 2010; Orlin et al., 2010). ICF codes for deficits in the client's leisure are found in d920 Recreation and Leisure. Also consider d4 Mobility as it relates to leisure. Environmental ICF codes are also important during the assessment so that the RT can identify what the client will need to participate successfully in a full and appropriate range of activities. Some of the relevant codes will be found in e1 Products and Technology, e3 Support and Relationships, and e4 Attitudes.

Community skills/inclusion: Assessment should be done on:

- Accessibility of home, community, and recreation environments and removal of barriers: Continued removal of architectural barriers and growth of adapted sports also contribute to the physical health and well-being of children with CP (Fowler et al., 2008). Use e1 Products and Technology and e2 Natural Environment and Human-Made Changes to Environment.
- Inclusion: For school-age children, inclusion in physical education classes, recess, and community programs with peers is important for the

reduction of secondary complications (Fowler et al., 2008), developing social and peer interaction skills (Imms, 2008), and self-esteem development (Dattilo, 2002). Use **e585 Education and Training Services, Systems, and Policies.** Also important is evaluating whether the client has a sense of basic human rights. A deficit in that area can be scored with **d940 Human Rights.**

- Adaptive equipment: Use of adaptive equipment to promote community independence (Mayo, 2010). Use **e1 Products and Technology.**

When the RT assessments are complete, the therapist will have information about the areas required for appropriate treatment. The usual findings for a person with CP include:

Physical: Impaired mobility; use of mobility assistive devices; decreased endurance; extraneous movements; slow task completion (Palisano et al., 2009); fine motor impairments; decreased participation in physical activities such as sports; reduced muscle strength; decreased range of motion; impaired motor control; decreased head, neck, and trunk stability and control; decreased range of motion and/or contractures; and retention of early/primitive reflexes (AAP, 2013; CDC, 2012b; Gaskin & Morris, 2008; March of Dimes, 2010; Mayo, 2010; McRae et al., 2009; Reach for the Stars, 2013). Higher levels of gross motor functioning are associated with higher leisure participation in children with CP (Longo et al., 2013; Palisano et al., 2011).

Cognitive: Varied cognitive ability from impaired to above average. In most cases additional time is needed to process information (NICHCY, 2010). Research has demonstrated that higher intelligence in children with CP is associated with more participation in recreation and leisure (Longo et al., 2013; Palisano et al., 2011).

Sensory: Varied sensory function from impaired to within normal limits. Many however, display hyper- or hyposensitivity to stimuli (NICHCY, 2010).

Social/communication: Varied social and communication function, such as slurred, slow, or difficult to understand speech. Less ability to communicate has been found to be a barrier to leisure participation for children with CP (Palisano et al., 2011). Many have articulation problems (Mayo, 2010; NICHCY, 2010). Many with disabilities experience less social-emotional support (UCP, 2013a).

Emotional/behavioral: Varied emotional and behavioral functioning from impaired to within normal functional limits. May display signs and symptoms of depression, have low social support, and low self-esteem (Gaskin & Morris, 2008; Mayo, 2010). Children with physical disabilities experience more loneliness and more social isolation than peers without disabilities. They have less community involvement and may have fewer friendships because they are perceived as being different (Law et al., 2006; Orlin et al., 2010; Shikako-Thomas et al., 2008).

Leisure: Children with physical disabilities tend to be more passive, engage in less varied activities, and participate in fewer activities of a social or physical nature (Law et al., 2006; Longo et al., 2013; Orlin et al., 2010; Shikako-Thomas et al., 2008). Majnemer et al. (2010) stated that few studies have looked at the leisure preferences of children with disabilities and that having a better understanding of the child's preferences would help promote "child-centered therapeutic approaches" (p. 168). They further stated that "Understanding the incongruities between preferences and actual involvement is important, so that rehabilitation professionals can address barriers that limit participation [for children with CP]" (p. 168). This is a primary focus of recreational therapy. In a study on the ICF, healthcare professionals contributed to a profile of functioning of children with cerebral palsy. When considering children six years old and younger, 37.3% of respondents indicated concerns about recreation and leisure while 26.4% considered it a strength. In children older than six, 43% indicated that limitations in recreation and leisure were a concern versus 22.8% who scored it as a strength (Schiariti et al., 2013).

ICF Core Set

An ICF Core Set for CP has been developed and is expected to be published soon. Go to http://www.icf-research-branch.org/icf-core-sets-projects/other-health-conditions/461-icf-core-sets-for-cerebral-palsy-in-cy.html for more information.

Treatment Direction

Whole Team Approach

Once diagnosed with CP, early intervention services, including recreational therapy, can minimize disability and maximize function (Reaching for the Stars, 2013; CDC, 2012b). The primary goal of treatment is to minimize secondary disability and maximize functioning in daily life to achieve the most independence possible (Reaching for the Stars, 2013; AAP, 2013; NINDS, 2012). "A team of healthcare professionals works with the child and family to identify the child's needs and create an individualized treatment plan to help the child reach his or her maximum potential" (March of Dimes, 2007; CDC, 2012b).

Early intervention services may begin as early as birth or as soon as developmental delays are observed (Reaching for the Stars, 2013; March of Dimes, 2007, CDC, 2012b, AAP, 2013). These services are covered under the Individuals with Disabilities Education Act (IDEA), as well as school-based services. Part C deals specifically with early intervention which covers birth through 36 months; Part B applies to school-aged children, which is defined as those between the ages of three and 21 years (CDC, 2012b; NICHCY, 2010). OT, PT, and SLP are among the services provided under IDEA.

Other medical treatments include medications and assistive devices. Medications can control seizures and reduce spasticity and rigidity (NINDS, 2012, Mayo, 2010; March of Dimes, 2007; Reach for the Stars, 2013). Medications such as Baclofen, Botox, and antiseizure medications may help reduce spasticity or excessive movements (NICHCY, 2010; NINDS, 2012; Mayo, 2010). Additionally, the use of assistive devices, such as orthotics or braces, splints, mobility devices, augmentative communication devices, and computers, can facilitate inclusion in everyday life, enhance quality of life, and improve functioning (NICHCY, 2010; NINDS, 2012; Reach for the Stars, 2013).

Recreational Therapy Approach

One of the unique benefits to the recreational therapy approach is the ability to focus on client strengths (ATRA, 2000; Heyne & Anderson, 2012). The purpose of the strengths-based approach is "to help people reach their goals and aspirations related to their well-being and quality of life" (Heyne & Anderson, 2012, p. 111). Recreational therapists can utilize a client's strengths to build upon and improve their overall functioning despite their disability. This is further supported by the fact that healthcare, as seen in the ICF, has shifted its "focus from 'consequences of diseases' to 'functioning' and how it can be improved to achieve a productive and fulfilling life" (Schiariti et al., 2013, p. 1).

As with any client, participation and development of life-long recreation and leisure skills, use of adaptive equipment, community integration, inclusion, and friendship development are important goals and areas for recreational therapists to address with clients who have CP (Majnemer et al., 2010). NINDS (2012) affirms recreational therapy's role working with children with CP: "Parents of children who participate in recreational therapies usually notice an improvement in their child's speech, self-esteem, and emotional well-being."

Additionally, fitness and health promotion are essential for individuals with physical disabilities to promote continued functioning, decrease depression and/or anxiety, improve self-esteem and self-concept, maintain or improve cognitive functioning, prevent secondary disability, improve gross motor skills, and enhance quality of life (Groff et al., 2006; Sable & Gravink, 2005; Gaskin & Morris, 2008; NINDS, 2012). As Gaskin and Morris (2008) point out, "Physical activity has the potential to have a positive influence on these HRQL and psychosocial functioning variables" (p. 147).

Regardless of the type of invention, whether it is functional abilities or leisure, the use of repetitive and controlled tasks is important to facilitate the practice of skills and improve motor learning, particularly the stability of motor patterns in individuals with CP (Valvano, 2004; McRae et al., 2009). Repetitive tasks and activities facilitate motor planning and enhance the individual's ability to learn and complete tasks (Valvano, 2004).

Recreational Therapy Interventions

Functional Skills

Exercise/stretching/fitness: It is important to promote activity and fitness in individuals with CP (d570 Looking After One's Health, d920 Recreation and Leisure). Maintaining muscle strength and endurance (b730 Muscle Power Functions, b455 Exercise Tolerance Functions), cardiovascular and respiratory function (b440 Respiration Functions, b445 Respiratory Muscle Functions), mobility (b235 Vestibular Functions, b260 Proprioceptive Function, d4 Mobility), and joint range of motion and motor skills (b7 Neuromusculoskeletal and Movement-Related Functions) contributes to the person's overall health and functioning, impacting quality of life. "In persons with CP, physical fitness may be even more important to offset the decline in function that might occur with aging and deterioration of CP-related impairments such as reduced range of motion and increased spasticity or pain" (Nieuwenhuijsen et al., 2011, p. 535). Exercise and stretching for individuals with CP can improve all aspects of physical fitness and functioning including cardiovascular functioning, muscle strength, flexibility, body composition, decreased secondary disability, enhanced well-being, range of motion, and hand-eye coordination (Groff et al., 2006; Lopez-Ortiza et al., 2011; NCPAD, 2012; Murphy & Carbone, 2008; Rimmer, n.d.; United Cerebral Palsy, 2012; Wiart et al., 2008; AAP, 2013; UCP, 2013a; UCP, 2013b; Nieuwenhuijsen et al., 2011; Bedini & Thomas, 2012; Rogers et al., 2008; Mobily, 2009).

Aquatic therapy: Benefits of aquatic therapy for individuals with CP include improvements in physical and respiratory functioning, as well as range of motion (Broach & Dattilo, 1996; Getz, Hutzler, & Vermeer, 2006; Chrysagis et al., 2009; Schoolfield, 2008), increased bilateral upper and lower extremity movements and gross motor movements, balance, coordination, range of motion, endurance, strengthening, hand-eye coordination, and development of new leisure skills (Chrysagis et. al, 2009; Peganoff, 1984; Bintzler, 2006; Broach & Dattilo, 1996; Carter, 1998). Warm water reduces muscle tone, relieves pain, and facilitates independent movement (Getz et al., 2006; Bintzler, 2006; Broach & Dattilo, 1996; Mobily, 2009). Psychological benefits include improved mood, self-esteem, and body image, as well as reduced anxiety and depression (Bintzler, 2006; Broach & Dattilo, 1996). It also provides a life-long fitness and leisure activity (Bintzler, 2006; Broach & Dattilo, 1996; Carter, 1998; Schoolfield, 2008). Diagnostic ICF codes that are treated include b125 Dispositions and Intra-Personal Functions, b126 Temperament and Personality Functions,

b235 Vestibular Functions, b260 Proprioceptive Function, b455 Exercise Tolerance Functions, b730 Muscle Power Functions, b735 Muscle Tone Functions, b7 Neuromusculoskeletal and Movement-Related Functions, d4 Mobility, and d920 Recreation and Leisure.

Hippotherapy: Hippotherapy "is the use of a horse as part of an integrated treatment strategy… performed by health professionals" (Hamill, Washington, & White, 2007, p. 24). Benefits for individuals with CP include improved head, neck, and trunk control; posture; gross motor skills; muscle symmetry; self-esteem; endurance; and mobility. Hippotherapy also promotes relaxation and reduction of hypertonia, improves speech, improves motor function, and increases motivation (Benda et al., 2003; Hamill et al., 2007; Shurtleff & Engsberg, 2010; Snider et al., 2007; Sterba et al., 2002). ICF codes that are treated include b125 Dispositions and Intra-Personal Functions, b126 Temperament and Personality Functions, b235 Vestibular Functions, b260 Proprioceptive Function, b3 Voice and Speech Functions, b455 Exercise Tolerance Functions, b730 Muscle Power Functions, b735 Muscle Tone Functions, b7 Neuromusculoskeletal and Movement-Related Functions, d4 Mobility, and d920 Recreation and Leisure.

Therapeutic horseback riding (THBR): THBR is "conducted by non-therapist riding instructors and assistants based upon their training and knowledge of the riders' disabilities and of methods for safely using therapy-trained horses" (Sterba, 2007, p. 68). Davis et al. (2011) added that, "The riding is directed towards improving the rider's ability to receive and process body-wide sensory information from the smooth, rhythmical movements made by the horse" (p. 111). Benefits for individuals with CP include improvements in balance, coordination, upper and lower extremity strength, sitting posture, gross motor skills, gait, riding skills, self-confidence, self-concept, sense of mastery and success, grasp, circulation, relaxation, and emotional and psychological status. Benefits also include reduction in abnormal muscle tone, particularly high tone (Davis et al., 2011; Kunstler & Stavola Daly, 2010; MacKinnon et al., 1995; Moninger, 2008; Sterba, 2007). The Davis et al. (2011) study did not find increases in gross motor function, health or quality of life in children with CP using standardized instruments; however, the study noted that qualitative data was found to indicate that "families perceived the programme to be beneficial to their child's QoL, health, and function" (Davis et al., 2011, p. 117). ICF codes that are treated include b125 Dispositions and Intra-Personal Functions, b126 Temperament and Personality Functions, b235 Vestibular Functions, b260 Proprioceptive Function, b455 Exercise Tolerance Functions, b730 Muscle Power Functions, b735 Muscle Tone Functions, b7 Neuromusculoskeletal and Movement-Related Functions, d4 Mobility, and d920 Recreation and Leisure.

Therapeutic massage (or massage therapy): Massage therapy is considered a part of complementary and alternative medicine and encompasses a variety of techniques to manipulate the muscles and soft tissues in the body (NCCAM, 2010). Massage can be used to improve health, enhance well-being, and reduce pain and anxiety (b280 Sensation of Pain, b152 Emotional Functions) (Brownlee & Dattilo, 2002). There are specific studies to demonstrate the reduction of anxiety (Edwards & Bruce, 2001) and muscle relaxation in individuals with CP (McKechnie et al., 1983). There are contraindications for the use of massage therapy and recreational therapists should be sure to obtain additional training prior to the use of this intervention or consult with a certified massage therapist (Brownlee & Dattilo, 2002).

Education, Training, and Counseling

Recreational therapists provide education and training in the areas of community integration skills and community resources. In a study on the ICF, one of the primary and consistent concerns expressed by youth with CP, their parents, and medical professionals is that of integration into community life (Vargus-Adams & Martin, 2012).

In a school setting, recreational therapists might address developing friendships, improving self-concept and/or self-esteem, transitioning from school to community or workforce, enhancing communication skills, reinforcing daily living skills, developing social skills, utilizing decision-making skills, reinforcing motor skills, facilitating coping skills, and providing opportunities for self-expression (North Carolina Recreational Therapy Association, n.d.).

Adaptive sports (d9201 Sports): Groff et al. (2009) found that eight percent of international athletes with CP competing at the 2005 CP World Championships learned about adaptive sports from a recreational therapist (11% learned from a PT and six percent from an OT).

Community integration skills and resources: Accessibility, advocacy, and removal of barriers are the three main tasks for recreational therapists when promoting community integration.

- *Accessibility*: Accessibility issues in playgrounds, parks, public buildings, community programs, transportation, and activity adaptation affect the leisure participation of children with CP (e.g., e1 Products and Technology, e2 Natural Environment and Human-Made Changes to Environment) (Palisano et al., 2011; Stewart et al., 2012). Weather factors, particularly a lack of snow removal, also interfere with accessibility (e540 Transportation Services, Systems, and Policies, e595 Political Services, Systems, and Policies) (Stewart et al., 2012). By assisting individuals with CP with transition planning and community skills (d4 Mobility), therapists "can support their clients learning how to make informed decisions, by discussing the trade-offs inherent in the choices they are making" (Stewart et al., 2012, p. 176).

- *Advocacy*: Recreational therapists also have an important role to advocate for inclusive environments, accessible facilities, and increased opportunities for participation (e1 Products and Technology and e2 Natural Environment and Human-Made Changes to Environment). Furthermore, social engagement and participation are also important (d9 Community, Social, and Civic Life) (Palisano et al., 2011; Stewart et al., 2012). "Through participation children form friendships, gain knowledge, learn skills, and express creativity" (Palisano et al., 2011, p. 142).

- *Removal of barriers*: Recreational therapists can assist individuals with CP to overcome barriers to participation. Barriers to involvement in leisure include functional and physical impairments, demographic factors, person and family preferences, services and programs available, accessibility of environments, financial costs, time constraints, and the family's ability to adapt (Majnemer et al., 2010; Stewart et al., 2012). Document this work with Environmental Factors ICF codes that reflect specific barriers noted in the client's diagnosis.

Mobile devices as adaptive equipment: Use of the iPad and other new and emerging technologies provides a variety of benefits related to recreational therapy. Apps for communication can assist children who have CP-related speech impairments or are non-verbal to communicate, creating spoken sentences for them (d3 Communication) (Lehman, 2012). Work is also being done to improve the accessibility and use of mobile devices for people with CP and other motor problems in the community. This includes a "scanning interface" that will highlight each letter, button, or link on the screen, one at a time. As the system highlights the desired item, the user simply touches anywhere on the screen to make the selection (Clayton, 2010). The goal is to make communicating using these mobile devices easier, but there are also clear implications for use related to recreational therapy. "A weak diaphragm and poor muscle tone make it difficult to formulate sounds clearly or speak louder. Body movement and coordination also are challenges for children with cerebral palsy" (Lane, 2012). These can be countered by using a mobile communication device. Beyond communication, iPads can be used to work on functional skills such as fine motor skills (d440 Fine Hand Use) (Lane, 2012; Roth, 2013). Additionally, iPads can facilitate leisure involvement through use of a variety of apps and games (d920 Recreation and Leisure). Finally, successful use of the iPad has anecdotally shown improvements in the self-esteem and self-confidence of individuals with CP (b125 Dispositions and Intra-Personal Functions, b126 Temperament and Personality Functions) (Lane, 2012; Roth, 2013).

Leisure and health education: Here the recreational therapist teaches the importance of leisure to prevent secondary disability and enhance quality of life. Improving health and wellness for individuals with CP and reducing overall health disparities and secondary disabilities are important goals (Groff et. al., 2009; Bedini & Thomas, 2012; Mobily, 2009). Document any functional or activity deficit, such as b164 Higher-Level Cognitive Functions, that is improved with this treatment. Educating individuals with CP and their families on nutrition issues and the importance of activity can reduce secondary disabilities such as obesity or diabetes (d570 Looking After One's Health) (Murphy & Carbone, 2008; Rimmer, n.d.; United Cerebral Palsy, 2012).

Relaxation and coping skills: Leisure activity and experiences (including outdoor recreation) aid in developing relaxation skills and dealing with short- or long-term stressors (d240 Handling Stress and Other Psychological Demands) (Hutchinson, Bland, & Kleiber, 2008; Norling & Sibthorp, 2006).

Community Integration and Inclusion

Social skills and inclusion: Inclusion is a significant issue for individuals with CP. Just like individuals without disabilities, "social interaction and relationships to others are consistent features of children with disabilities' perspectives on inclusion and empowerment" (Spencer-Cavaliere & Watkinson, 2010, p. 277). Issues related to inclusion that the recreational therapist must work on with the client include access and being able to enter into play with others, being and feeling like a participant in the activity, and making and having friends (Spencer-Cavaliere & Watkinson, 2010). ICF codes include d7 Interpersonal Interactions and Relationships, d880 Engagement in Play, d920 Recreation and Leisure. Also document work on e3 Support and Relationships.

Participation and inclusion: In adolescence, one of the most common problems is in the area of recreation and leisure, as well as socialization, community integration, and instrumental activities of daily living, such as meal preparation and housework (Nieuwenhuijsen et al., 2009). Benefits of community integration and inclusion include improvements in social skills, friendship, community skills, creative expression, sense of meaning, mobility management, assistive technology, self-esteem, and accessibility (Bedini & Thomas, 2012; Palisano et al., 2009). ICF codes that can be referenced include those in d5 Self-Care, d7 Interpersonal Interactions and Relationships, and d9 Community, Social, and Civic Life.

Advocacy skills: While they are serving as advocates, recreational therapists also have an opportunity to help individuals with CP learn advocacy skills. Palisano et al. (2011) expressed "that the attitude of administrators, instructors, and coaches towards inclusion of a child with a disability is a determinant of successful participation" in recreation and leisure (p. 148). Use d940 Human Rights and e330 People in Positions of Authority.

Health Promotion

Adaptive sports (d9201 Sports): Benefits of participation in adaptive sports for individuals with CP are numerous. Groff, Lundberg, and Zabriskie (2009) found that "the majority of the sample [international athletes competing in the 2005 CP World Championships] either agreed or strongly agreed that adaptive sport positively influenced their overall health (84.9%), quality of life (80.8%), quality of family life (53.4%), and quality of social life (56.1%)" (p. 318). Not only can adaptive sports serve as exercise and a way to improve physical functioning, adaptive sports also have psychosocial benefits including feelings of accomplishment, empowerment, increased self-efficacy, self-confidence, physical confidence, self-esteem, enjoyment of life, sense of well-being, and enhanced mood (Bedini & Thomas, 2012; Groff et al., 2009; Thomas & Bedini, 2011). Respondents in the Bedini and Thomas study (2012), commented that adaptive sports gave them "the chance to feel equal to children without disabilities" (p. 298), as well as to have positive role models. ICF codes that can be treated with adaptive sports include b125 Dispositions and Intra-Personal Functions, b126 Temperament and Personality Functions, b235 Vestibular Functions, b260 Proprioceptive Function, b455 Exercise Tolerance Functions, b7 Neuromusculoskeletal and Movement-Related Functions, d4 Mobility, d7 Interpersonal Interactions and Relationships, d920 Recreation and Leisure, and d940 Human Rights. Benefits provided by particular adaptive sports included:

- Downhill skiing: Improved gross motor skills (lying, rolling, sitting, crawling, standing), and ambulation (running, walking) (Sterba, 2006).
- Basketball: increased strength, energy, and confidence (Bedini & Thomas, 2012).
- Swimming: Improved coordination and muscle strength, enhanced cardiovascular and respiratory functions (Sterba, 2006; Bintzler, 2006; Broach & Dattilo, 1996; Carter, 1998).
- Archery: Improved gross motor coordination, hand-eye coordination, arm/back muscle strength, and balance (Sterba, 2006).
- Dance: Physical, cognitive, and social aspects ranging from coordination, balance, and improved functional ability to follow directions and sequence, interaction with peers, and friendship development (Garcaro, 2011; Lopez-Ortiza et al.,

2011; Sterba, 2006). Youth also experience a sense of identity, pride, and belonging (Kunstler & Stavola Daly, 2010).

- Biking: Strength, endurance when walking, gross motor strength, increased recreational opportunities for family, opportunity for exercise (Siebert et al., 2010; LaPorte, 2010; McRae et al., 2009).
- Yoga: Decreased self-perceptions of anxiety and pain, increased body awareness and strength, specialized breathing techniques to aid attention to task, deep relaxation techniques, decreased muscle tone in children with CP, exercise for low muscle tone areas, stretching and realignment of the spine (a common problem in children with CP), improved range of motion, enhanced coordination (Bonadies, 2004; NCPAD, 2012; Yoga for the Special Child, 2013).

Animal-assisted therapy: Improved communication; increased strength, endurance, psychological/emotional health, social interaction, and energy level; decreased heart rate and blood pressure; reduced anxiety and stress; and motivation for participation in therapy and completion of gross motor tasks (Bibik et al., 2012; Moninger, 2008). ICF codes include b125 Dispositions and Intra-Personal Functions, b126 Temperament and Personality Functions, d4 Mobility, b455 Exercise Tolerance Functions, d7 Interpersonal Interactions and Relationships.

Volunteerism: Recreational therapists can also help clients participate in meaningful volunteer work to enhance their psychological well-being. Benefits include enhanced self-esteem, greater sense of purpose and social connectedness, improved quality of life, community involvement, functional abilities, improved life skills, improved school performance, improved skill in empathy and understanding others, socialization with others, and increased independence (Miller et al., 2005; Murphy & Carbone, 2008; Stewart et al., 2011). ICF codes include b125 Dispositions and Intra-Personal Functions, b126 Temperament and Personality Functions, d7 Interpersonal Interactions and Relationships, and d940 Human Rights.

Therapeutic recreation camping program (d920 Recreation and Leisure): Recreational therapy camping programs have been found to have a positive impact on health-related quality of life among children and adolescents with chronic disabilities, including feeling a sense of community and respect (Bekesi et al., 2011; Dawson & Liddicoat, 2009).

Resources

United Cerebral Palsy
1825 K Street NW, Suite 600
Washington DC 20006
800-872-5827
202-776-0406
www.ucp.org
UCP provides a range of educational, support, and public policy advocacy for individuals with CP. A variety of resources are available to understand the disability and provide resources for daily living, as well as information on state organizations.

Centers for Disease Control and Prevention
www.cdc.gov/ncbddd/dd/ddcp.htm
CDC offers a number of resources and research information on CP, including statistics, demographic information, causes of CP, and life expectancy.

National Institute of Neurological Disorders and Stroke — National Institutes of Health
www.ninds.nih.gov/disorders/cerebral_palsy/cerebral_palsy.htm
NINDS details specifics of CP and its impact on those who have it. NINDS supports research about CP and offers additional resources.

Kids Health
kidshealth.org/parent/medical/brain/cerebral_palsy.html
Kids Health provides an overview and detailed descriptions of CP, and is written in easy-to-understand language for children.

My Child without Limits
www.mychildwithoutlimits.org/
My Child without Limits provides information for families with children up to five years old with disabilities or developmental delays. It also provides a way to connect with other families and resources.

Family Center on Technology and Disability
www.fctd.info
This site provides information on assistive technology, and is funded by the Office of Special Education in the U.S. Department of Education.

National Center on Health, Physical Activity, and Disability
www.ncpad.org
Numerous resources are available about cerebral palsy and other disabilities in relation to physical activities, including information on dance and yoga. There is also a searchable research database.

National Ability Center
www.discovernac.org
The NAC is an organization that is committed to life-long leisure and participation for individuals with disabilities. Located in Park City, Utah, NAC offers a variety of sporting events and resources, including training, clinics, and camps.

Medline
www.nlm.nih.gov/bsd/pmresources.html
A service of the National Institutes of Health with fact sheets and information on cerebral palsy.

Reaching for the Stars
reachingforthestars.org
Reaching for the Stars is a parent-founded foundation focused on preventing, treating, and curing cerebral palsy. A number of resources are available for parents and families along with general information on cerebral palsy.

Pathways Awareness
www.pathwaysawareness.org
800-955-2445
Pathways Awareness is a non-profit organization that creates free resources for both parents and professionals to promote the inclusion of children with disabilities.

March of Dimes Foundation
www.marchofdimes.com
888-MODIMES
March of Dimes is a national non-profit that is focused on helping mothers deliver full-term babies. The organization provides a variety of resources on various disabilities along with statistics and research.

Easter Seals
www.easterseals.com
800-221-6827
Easter Seals is a national non-profit organization that provides therapy and other services, including education, outreach, and advocacy, to individuals with special needs and disabilities.

References

American Academy of Pediatrics. (2013). Health issues: Cerebral palsy. Retrieved from http://www.healthychildren.org/English/health-issues/conditions/developmental-disabilities/ pages/Cerebral-Palsy.aspx.

American Therapeutic Recreation Association. (2000). *ATRA standards of practice*. Alexandria, VA: author.

Bartlett D. J. & Palisano R. J. (2002). Determinants of motor change for children with cerebral palsy: A consensus exercise. *Physical Therapy, 82*, 237-248.

Bedini, L. A. & Thomas, A. (2012). Bridge II Sports: A model of meaningful activity through community-based adapted sports. *Therapeutic Recreation Journal, 46*(4), 284-300.

Bekesi, A., Torok, S., Kokonyei, G., Bokretas, I., Szentes, A., & Telepoczki, G. (2011). Health-related quality of life changes of children and adolescents with chronic disease after participating in a therapeutic recreation camping program. *Health & Quality of Life Outcomes, 9*, 43-52.

Benda, W., McGibbon, N. H., & Grant, K. L. (2003). Improvements in muscle symmetry in children with cerebral palsy after equine-assisted therapy (hippotherapy). *The Journal of Alternative and Complementary Medicine, 9*(6), 817-825.

Bibik, J. M., Cavalier, A. R., Manley, K., & Obrusnikova, I. (2012). Integrating therapy dog teams in physical activity programs for children with autism spectrum disorders: Therapy dog-assisted interventions provide physical, social, and emotional benefits for children with disabilities. *The Journal of Physical Education, Recreation and Dance, 83*(6), 37-41, 47-48.

Bintzler, S. (2006). Research update: Water works wonders. *Parks and Recreation, November*, 36-41.

Bonadies, V. (2004). A yoga therapy program for AIDS related pain and anxiety implications for therapeutic recreation. *Therapeutic Recreation Journal, 38*(2), 148-166.

Boyle, C. A., Boulet, S., Schieve, L. A., Cohen, R. A., Blumberg, S. J., Yeargin-Allsopp, M., Visser, S., & Kogan, M. D. (2011). Prevalence of developmental disabilities in U.S. children, 1997-2008. *Pediatrics, 127*, 1034-1042.

Broach, E. & Dattilo, J. (1996). Aquatic therapy: Making waves in therapeutic recreation. *Parks & Recreation, July*, 38-43.

Brownlee, S. & Dattilo, J. (2002). Therapeutic massage as a therapeutic recreation facilitation technique. *Therapeutic Recreation Journal, 36*(4), 369-381.

burlingame, j. & Blaschko, T. M. (2010). *Assessment tools for recreational therapy and related fields* (4th ed.). Ravensdale, WA: Idyll Arbor, Inc.

Carter, M. (1998). Aquatics: HPERD linkage to health and human services. *Journal of Physical Education, Recreation and Dance, 69*(3), 6-9.

Centers for Disease Control and Prevention. (n.d.). Cerebral palsy among children. Atlanta, GA: author.

Centers for Disease Control and Prevention. (2011). Causes and risk factors of cerebral palsy. Retrieved from http://www.cdc.gov/ncbdd/cp/causes.html.

Centers for Disease Control and Prevention. (2012a). Cerebral palsy. Retrieved from http://www.cdc.gov/ncbddd/cp/index.html.

Centers for Disease Control and Prevention. (2012b). Data and statistics for cerebral palsy. Retrieved from http://www.cdc.gov/ncbddd/cp/data.html.

Centers for Disease Control and Prevention. (2012c). Facts about cerebral palsy. Retrieved from http:/j/www.cdc.gov/ncbddd/cp/facts.html.

Centers for Disease Control and Prevention. (2012d). Tracking and research on cerebral palsy. Retrieved from http://www.cdc.gov/ncbddd/cp/research.html.

Chrysagis, N., Douka, A., Nikopoulos, M., Apostolopoulou, F., & Koutsouki, D. (2009). Effects of an aquatic program on gross motor function of children with spastic cerebral palsy. *Biology of Exercise, 5*(2), p. 13-25.

Clayton, B. (2010). Michigan engineering students develop mobile communications technology for cerebral palsy patients. Retrieved from http://forum.engin.umich.edu/2010/11/mobile-communications-technology-for.html#com.

Clayton, K., Fleming, J. M., & Copley, J. (2003). Behavioral responses to tactile stimuli in children with cerebral palsy. *Physical & Occupational Therapy in Pediatrics, 23*(1), 43-62.

Collingridge, K. (2011). Therapeutic recreation: Getting kids with disabilities outdoors. Retrieved from http://www.parentmap.com/article/therapeutic-outdoor-recreation-for-kids-with-disabilities.

Coyle, C. P., Kinney, W. B., Riley, B., & Shank, J. W. (Eds.). (1991). *Benefits of therapeutic recreation: A consensus view*. Ravensdale, WA: Idyll Arbor, Inc.

Dattilo, J. (2002). *Inclusive leisure services: Responding to the rights of people with disabilities* (2nd ed.). State College, PA: Venture Publishing, Inc.

Davis, E., Davies, B., Wolfe, R., Raadsveld, R., Heine, B., Thomason, P., Dobson, F., & Graham, H. K. (2009). A randomized controlled trial of the impact of therapeutic horse riding on the quality of life, health, and function of children with cerebral palsy. *Developmental Medicine and Child Neurology, 51*(2), 111-119.

Dawson, S. & Liddicoat, K. (2009). "Camp gives me hope": Exploring the therapeutic use of community for adults with cerebral palsy. *Therapeutic Recreation Journal, 43*(4), 9-24.

Edwards, D. & Bruce, G. (2001). For cerebral palsy patients massage makes life better. *Massage Magazine, 92*, 93-110.

Erasmus, C. E., van Hulst, K., Rotteveel, J. J., Willemsen, M. A. A. P., & Jongerius, P. H. (2012). Clinical practice: Swallowing problems in cerebral palsy. *European Journal of Pediatrics, 171*, 409-414.

Fowler, E. G., Kolobe, T. H. A., Damiano, D. L., Thorpe, D. E., Morgan, D. W., Brunstrom, J., & Stevenson, R. D. (2007). Promotion of physical fitness and prevention of secondary conditions for children with cerebral palsy: Section of pediatrics research summit proceedings. *Physical Therapy, 87*(11), 1495-1510.

Garcaro, D. C. (2011). Influence of dance therapy on the functional mobility of children with spastic hemiparetic cerebral palsy. *Motricidad, 7*(3), 3.

Gaskin, C. J. & Morris, T. (2008). Physical activity, health-related quality of life, and psychosocial functioning of adults with cerebral palsy. *Journal of Physical Activity and Health, 5*, 146-157.

Getz, M., Hutzler, Y., & Vermeer, A. (2006). Effects of aquatic interventions in children with neuromotor impairments: A systematic review of the literature. *Clinical Rehabilitation, 20*, 927-936.

Geytenbeek, J. (2011). Prevalence of speech and communication disorders in children with CP. *Developmental Medicine and Child Neurology, 53*(1), 10-11.

Goh, J. & Flynn, M. (2010). *Examination obstetrics and gynaecology*. Elsevier.

Griffin, H. C., Fitch, C. L., & Griffin, L. W. (2002). Causes and interventions in the area of cerebral palsy. *Infants and Young Children, 14*(3), p. 18-23.

Groff, D., Lawrence, E., & Grivna, S. (2006). Effects of a therapeutic recreation intervention using exercise: A case study with a child with cerebral palsy. *Therapeutic Recreation Journal, 40*(4), 269-283.

Groff, D. G., Lundberg, N. R., & Zabriskie, R. B. (2009). Influence of adapted sport on quality of life: Perceptions of athletes with cerebral palsy. *Disability and Rehabilitation*, *31*(4), 318-326.

Hamill, D., Washington, K., & White, O. R. (2007). The effect of hippotherapy on postural control in sitting for children with cerebral palsy. *Physical & Occupational Therapy in Pediatrics*, *27*(4), 23-42.

Heyne, L. A. & Anderson, L. S. (2012). Theories that support strengths-based practice in therapeutic recreation. *Therapeutic Recreation Journal*, *46*(2), 106-128.

Hutchinson, S. L. Bland, A. D., & Kleiber, D. A. (2008). Leisure and stress-coping: Implications for therapeutic recreation practice. *Therapeutic Recreation Journal*, *42*(1), 9-23.

Hutton, J. L. & Pharoah, P. O. D. (2006). Life expectancy in severe cerebral palsy. *Archives of Disease in Childhood*, *91*, 254-258.

Imms, C. (2008). Children with cerebral palsy participate: A review of the literature. *Disability and Rehabilitation*, *30*(24), 1867-1884.

Kayes, N. M., Schluter, P. J., McPherson, K. M., Taylor, D., & Kolt, G. S. (2009). The Physical Activity and Disability Survey — Revised (PADS-R): An evaluation of a measure of physical activity in people with chronic neurological conditions. *Clinical Rehabilitation*, *23*(6), 534-543.

Ketelaar, M., Volman, M. J. M., Gorter, J. W., & Vermeer, A. (2008). Stress in parents of children with cerebral palsy: What sources of stress are we talking about? *Child: Care, Health and Development*, *34*(6), 825-829.

KIDSCREEN Group. (2011). KIDSCREEN: Health related quality of life questionnaire for children and young people and their parents. Retrieved from http://www.kidscreen.org/english/.

Kirby, R. S., Wingate, M. S., Van Naarden Braun, K., Doernberg, N. S., Arneson, C. L, Benedict, R. E. et al. (2011). Prevalence and functioning of children with cerebral palsy in four areas of the United States in 2006: A report from the Autism and Developmental Disabilities Monitoring Network. *Research in Developmental Disabilities*, *32*(2), p. 462-469.

Ko, J. & Kim, M. (2013). Reliability and responsiveness of the gross motor function measure-88 in children with cerebral palsy. *Physical Therapy*, *93*(3), 393-400.

Kunstler, R. & Stavola Daly, F. (2010). *Therapeutic recreation leadership and programming*. Champaign, IL: Human Kinetics.

Lane, T. L. (2012). iPad eases communication for third-grader. Retrieved from http://www.fcps.net/news/features/2011-12/ipad-connection.

LaPorte, C. (2010). Use of therapeutic tricycles to increase activity in an underserved population: Description of an AmTryke demonstration project. *Journal of the National Society of Allied Health*, *Spring/Summer*, 26-33.

Law, M., King, G., King, S., Hurley, P., Rosenbaum, P., Young, N., et al. (2006). Patterns of participation in recreational and leisure activities among children with complex physical disabilities. *Developmental Medicine & Child Neurology*, *48*, 337-342.

Lehman, J. (2012). The best apps for children with cerebral palsy. Retrieved from http://cpfamilynetwork.org/blogs/the-best-apps-for-children-with-cerebral-palsy.

Longo, E., Badia, M., & Orgaz, B. M. (2013). Patterns and predictors of participation in leisure activities outside of school in children and adolescents with cerebral palsy. *Research in Developmental Disabilities*, *34*, 266-275.

Lopez-Ortiza, C., Gladdena, K., Deona, L., Schmidt, J., Girolami, G., & Gaebler-Spira, D. (2011). Dance program for physical rehabilitation and participation in children with cerebral palsy. *Arts & Health*, 1-16.

Mac Keith Press. (2002). Gross motor function measure score sheet. Retrieved from http://motorgrowth.canchild.ca/en/gmfm/resources/gmfmscoresheet.pdf.

MacKinnon, J. R., Noh, S., Lariviere, J., MacPhail, A., Allan, D. E., & Laliberte, D. (1995). A study of therapeutic effects of horseback riding for children with cerebral palsy. *Physical & Occupational Therapy in Pediatrics*, *15*(1), 17-34.

Majnemer, A., Shikako-Thomas, K., Chokron, N., Law, M., Shevell, M. Chilingaryan, G., et al. (2010). Leisure activity preferences for 6- to 12-year-old children with cerebral palsy. *Developmental Medicine and Child Neurology*, *52*(2), 167-173.

March of Dimes. (2007). Cerebral palsy. Retrieved from http://www.marchofdimes.com/professionals/14332_1208.asp.

Mayo Foundation for Medical Education and Research. (2010). Cerebral palsy. Retrieved from http://www.mayoclinic.com/health/cerebral-palsy/DS00302.

McKechnie, A. A., Wilson, F., Watson, N., & Scott, D. (1983). Anxiety states: A preliminary report on the value of connective tissue massage. *Journal of Psychosomatic Research*, *27*(2), 125-129.

McRae, C. G. A., Johnston, T. E., Lauer, R. T., Tokay, A. M., Lee, S. C. K., & Hunt, K. J. (2009). Cycling for children with neuromuscular impairments using electrical stimulation — Development of tricycle-based systems. *Medical Engineering & Physics*, *31*, 650-659.

Miller, K. D., Schleien, S. J., Brooke, P., Frisoli, A. M., & Brooks III, W. T. (2005). Community for all: The therapeutic recreation practitioner's role in inclusive volunteering. *Therapeutic Recreation Journal*, *39*(1), 18-31.

Mobily, K. (2009). Role of exercise and physical activity in therapeutic recreation service. *Therapeutic Recreation Journal*, *43*(2), 9-26.

Moninger, J. (2008). Creature comforts. *Parents*, *83*(9), 166-169.

Morgan, R. (2011). What are the health benefits of leisure and recreation? Retrieved from http://www.livestrong.com/article/438983-what-are-the-health-benefits-of-leisure-recreation/.

Morris, C., Kurinczuk, J. J., Fitzpatrick, R., & Rosenbaum, P. L. (2006). Do the abilities of children with cerebral palsy explain their activities and participation? *Developmental Medicine & Child Neurology*, *48*, 954-961.

Murphy, N. A. & Carbone, P. S. (2008). Promoting the participation of children with disabilities in sports, recreation, and physical activities. Retrieved from http://pediatrics.aappublications.org/content/121/5/1057.full.pdf+html.

National Center for Complementary and Alternative Medicine. (2010). Massage therapy: An introduction. Retrieved from http://nccam.nih.gov/health/massage/massageintroduction.htm?nav=gsa.

National Center on Health, Physical Activity and Disability. (2006). Finding leisure: Therapeutic recreation service. Retrieved from http://www.indiana.edu/~nca/leisureed/find7.html.

National Center on Health, Physical Activity, and Disability. (2012). Yoga for individuals with disabilities. Retrieved from http://www.ncpad.org/295/1834/Yoga~for~Individuals~with~Disabilities.

NCTRC. (2007). Job analysis report. Retrieved from http://www.nctrc.org/documents/NCTRCJAReport07.pdf.

National Dissemination Center for Children with Disabilities (NICHCY). (2010). Cerebral palsy. Retrieved from http://nichcy.org/disability/specific/cp.

National Institute of Neurological Disorders and Stroke. (2009). NINDS cerebral palsy information page. Retrieved from http://www.ninds.nih.gov/disorders/cerebral_palsy/cerebral_palsy.htm.

National Institute of Neurological Disorders and Stroke. (2012). Cerebral palsy: Hope through research. NIH Publication No. 10-159.

Nieuwenhuijsen, C., Donkervoort, M., Nieuwsraten, W., Stam, H. J., Roebroeck, M. E., et al. (2009). Experienced problems of young adults with cerebral palsy: Targets for rehabilitation care. *Archives of Physical Medicine and Rehabilitation, 90*, 1891-1897.

Nieuwenhuijsen, C., van der Slot, W. M. A., Dallmeijer, A. J., Janssens, P. J., Stam, H. J., Roebroeck, M. E., et al. (2011). Physical activity, everyday physical activity, and fatigue in ambulatory adults with bilateral spastic cerebral palsy. *Scandinavian Journal of Medicine and Science in Sports, 21*, 535-542.

Norling, J. C. & Sibthorp, J. (2006). Research update: Mental restoration and recreation. *Parks & Recreation, 41*(3), 30-37.

North Carolina Recreational Therapy Association (NCTRA). (n.d.). Quick list of benefits of including recreation as a related service on an IEP. Retrieved from http://www.nctra.org/Professional/quicklist.html.

Odding, E., Roebroeck, M. E., & Stam, H. J. (2006). The epidemiology of cerebral palsy: Incidence, impairments and risk factors. *Disability and Rehabilitation, 28*(4), p. 183-191.

Orlin, M. O, Palisano, R. J., Chiarello, L. A., Kang, L., Polansky, M., Almasri, N., & Maggs, J. (2010). Participation in home, extracurricular, and community activity among children and young people with cerebral palsy. *Developmental Medicine & Child Neurology, 52*, 160-166.

Palisano, R. J., Chiarello, L. A., Orline, M., Oeffinger, D., Polansky, M., Maggs, J. et al. (2011). Determinants of intensity of participation in leisure and recreational activities by children with cerebral palsy. *Developmental Medicine & Child Neurology, 53*(2), 142-149.

Peganoff, S. A. (1984). The use of aquatics with cerebral palsied adolescents. *The American Journal of Occupational Therapy, 38*(7), 469-473.

Reaching for the Stars. (2013). Cerebral palsy. Retrieved from http://reachingforthestars.org/cerebral-palsy/.

Riley, K. (2011). Effects of a collaborative outpatient therapy program on self-concept of adolescents with depression. *Therapeutic Recreation Journal, 45*(1), 32-46.

Rimmer, J. (n.d.). Cerebral palsy. Retrieved from http://www.ncpad.org/106/813/Cerebral~Palsy.

Rimmer, J. H., Riley, B. B., & Rubin, S. S. (2001). A new measure for assessing the physical activity behaviors of persons with disabilities and chronic health conditions: The Physical Activity Disability Survey. *American Journal of Health Promotion, 16*(1), 34-42.

Rogers, A., Furler, B. L., Brinks, S., & Darrah, J. (2008). A systematic review of the effectiveness of aerobic exercise interventions for children with cerebral palsy: An AACPDM evidence report. Retrieved from http://www.aacpdm.org/resources/outcomes/ReviewAerobicExercise.pdf.

Roth, K. (2013). Adapt with apps (editorial). *Journal of Physical Education, Recreation and Dance, 84*(2), 4-6.

Rothwell, E., Piatt, J., & Mattingly, K. (2006). Social competence: Evaluation of an outpatient recreation therapy program for children with behavioral disorders. *Therapeutic Recreation Journal, 40*(4), 241-254.

Sable, J. & Gravink, J. (2005). The PATH to community health care for people with disabilities: A community-based therapeutic recreation service. *Therapeutic Recreation Journal, 39*(1), 78-87.

Schiariti, V., Masse, L. C., Cieza, A., Klassen, A. F., Sauve, K., Armstrong, R., et al. (2013). Toward the development of the International Classification of Functioning core sets for children with cerebral palsy: A global expert survey. *Journal of Child Neurology, February 21*, 1-10.

Schoolfield, J. (2008). Hydrotherapy can be a key to a happier, healthier and more mobile life. *Aquatic Therapy and Recreation, 38*(12), 50-51.

Shikako-Thomas, K., Majnemer, A., Law, M., & Lach, L. (2008). Determinants of participation in leisure activities in children and youth with cerebral palsy: Systematic review. *Physical & Occupational Therapy in Pediatrics, 28*(2), 155-169.

Shurtleff, T. L. & Engsberg, J. R. (2010). Changes in trunk and head stability in children with cerebral palsy after hippotherapy: A pilot study. *Physical & Occupational Therapy in Pediatrics, 30*(3), 150-163.

Siebert, K. L., DeMuth, S. K., Knutson, L. M., & Fowler, E. G. (2010). Stationary cycling and children with cerebral palsy: Case reports for two participants. *Physical & Occupational Therapy in Pediatrics, 30*(2), 125-138.

Snider, L., Korner-Bitensky, N., Kammann, C., Warner, S., & Saleh, M. (2007). Horseback riding as therapy for children with cerebral palsy: Is there evidence of its effectiveness? *Physical & Occupational Therapy in Pediatrics, 27*(2), 5-22.

Spencer-Cavaliere, N. & Watkinson, E. J. (2010). Inclusion understood from the perspectives of children with disability. *Adapted Physical Education Quarterly, 27*, 275-293.

Sterba, J. A. (2006). Adaptive downhill skiing in children with cerebral palsy: Effect on gross motor function. *Pediatric Physical Therapy, 18*(4), 289-296.

Sterba, J. A. (2007). Does horseback riding therapy or therapist-directed hippotherapy rehabilitate children with cerebral palsy? *Developmental Medicine & Child Neurology, 49*, 68-73.

Sterba, J. A., Rogers, B. T., France, A. P., & Vokes, D. A. (2002). Horseback riding in children with cerebral palsy: Effect on gross motor function. *Developmental Medicine & Child Neurology, 44*, 301-308.

Stewart, D. A., Lawless, J. J., Shimmell, L. J., Palisano, R. J., Freeman, M., Rosenbaum, P. L., et al. (2012). Social participation of adolescents with cerebral palsy: Trade-offs and choices. *Physical & Occupational Therapy in Pediatrics, 32*(2), 167-179.

Straub, K. & Obrzut, J. E. (2009). Effects of cerebral palsy on neuropsychological function. *Journal of Developmental and Physical Disabilities, 21*, 153-167.

Strauss, D., Brooks, J., Rosenbloom, L., & Shavelle, R. (2008). Life expectancy in cerebral palsy: An update. *Developmental Medicine & Child Neurology, 50*, 487-493.

Thomas, A. & Bedini, L. A. (2011). Let me play! Girls with disabilities and physical activity. *Women in Sports and Physical Activity Journal, 20*(1), 104-106.

Torpy, J. M. (2010). JAMA Patient page: Cerebral palsy. *The Journal for the American Medical Association, 304*(9), 1028.

Ulman, J. D. & Vidoni, C. (2012). The fair play game: Promoting social skills in physical education. *Strategies: A Journal for Physical and Sport Educators, 25*(3), 26-30.

United Cerebral Palsy. (2013a). Health and wellness. Retrieved from http://www.ucp.org/resources/health-and-wellness.

United Cerebral Palsy. (2013b). Wellness. Retrieved from http://www.ucp.org/resources/health-and-wellness/wellness.

United Cerebral Palsy. (2012). Physical activity. Retrieved from http://www.ucp.org/resources/health-and-wellness/wellness/physical-activity.

University of Melbourne Australia. (2013). Cerebral palsy quality of life. Retrieved from http://www.cpqol.org.au/.

Valvano, J. (2004). Activity-focused motor interventions for children with neurological conditions. *Physical and Occupational Therapy in Pediatrics, 24*(1/2), 79-107.

Vargus-Adams, J. N. & Martin, L. K. (2011). Domains of importance for parents, medical professionals, and youth with cerebral palsy considering treatment outcomes. *Child: Care, Health and Development, 37*(2), 276-281.

von der Luft, G., DeBoer, B. V., Harman, L. B., Koenig, K. P., & Nixon-Cave, K. (2008). Improving the quality of studies on self concept in children with cerebral palsy. *Journal of Development and Physical Disabilities, 20*, 581-594.

Waters, E., Davis, E., Mackinnon, A., Boyd, R, Graham, H. K., Kai, L. S., Stevenson, R., Bjornson, K., Blair, E., Hoare, P., Ravens-Sieberer, U., & Reddihough, D. (2007). Psychometric properties of the Quality of Life Questionnaire for Children with CP. *Developmental Medicine and Child Neurology, 49*(1), 49-55.

Wiart, L., Darrah, J., & Kembhavi, G. (2008). Stretching with children with cerebral palsy: What do we know and where are we going? *Pediatric Physical Therapy, 20*, 173-178.

Winter, S., Autry, A., Boyle, C., & Yeargin-Allsopp, M. (2002). Trends in the prevalence of cerebral palsy in a population-based study. *Pediatrics, 110*(6), 1220-1225.

Wise, J. B. (2002). Social cognitive theory: A framework for therapeutic recreation practice. *Therapeutic Recreation Journal, 36*(4), 335-351.

Yoga for the Special Child. (2013). Cerebral palsy and yoga. http://www.specialyoga.org/Cerebral_Palsy.html.

9. Cerebrovascular Accident (Stroke)

Marieke Van Puymbroeck, Jared Allsop, and Arlene A. Schmid

A cerebrovascular accident (CVA), also referred to as a stroke, is a disease that affects the arteries in and around the brain. A CVA occurs when a blood vessel that carries oxygen and nutrients to the brain ruptures or is blocked by a clot (American Stroke Association, 2012). When that happens, parts of the brain do not receive the oxygen they require. Due to this lack of oxygen, the brain cells in that part of the brain die. This damage results in neurological impairments (American Stroke Association, 2012). The exact impairments depend on the part of the brain that is damaged. Often medical attention is not sought right away because the symptoms may not seem like a major problem, however, delay in seeking treatment leads to more severe damage since early treatment can restore blood flow to limit the severity of the residual deficits.

The American Stroke Association (2012) has created the acronym F.A.S.T. to remember the sudden signs and symptoms of a CVA.

- **Face Drooping** — If one side of a person's face is numb or droops, the person may be having a stroke (American Stroke Association, 2012). One way to determine if the person has face drooping is to ask the person to smile and make observations about asymmetries.
- **Arm Weakness** — If one arm is numb or weak an individual may be having a stroke (American Stroke Association, 2012). If the person cannot raise both arms without having one of them drift down, the person may be having a stroke.
- **Speech Difficulty** — If the person is having slurred speech or is unable to speak, they may be having a stroke (American Stroke Association, 2012). Ask the person to repeat a simple sentence like "the grass is green."
- **Time to call 911** — If the person is exhibiting any of these signs, call 911 and get the person to the hospital right away (American Stroke Association, 2012).

Additional symptoms of a stroke from the National Stroke Association (2012) include:

- Sudden trouble walking, dizziness, loss of balance or coordination.
- Sudden severe headache with no known cause.
- Sudden nausea, fever, and vomiting distinguished from a viral illness by the speed of onset (minutes or hours versus days).
- Brief loss of consciousness or period of decreased consciousness (fainting, confusion, convulsions, or coma).

If the symptoms resolve within a 24-48 hour period and there are no or very minimal residual effects, the incident is referred to as a transient ischemic attack (TIA), otherwise known as a "mini-stroke" (National Stroke Association, 2012). This is often a warning or precursor to a stroke.

CVAs can be classified by the side of the brain affected, the major cerebral vessel involved, and the reason for the interruption of blood flow (blockage or hemorrhage). There are six major vessels that may be used as descriptors for diagnosis. A list of the arteries and their corresponding effects is as follows (Blesedell, Cohn, & Boyt, 2003):

Internal carotid: contralateral hemiplegia, sensory problems, aphasia (usually left hemisphere), and hemianopia.

Anterior cerebral: contralateral hemiplegia, cognitive deficits, sensory deficits, and aphasia (usually left hemisphere).

Middle cerebral: contralateral hemiplegia (primarily the upper extremity), contralateral hemianopia, sensory deficits, and language deficits.

Posterior cerebral: contralateral hemiplegia, ataxia, and visual deficits including field cuts, cortical blindness, and problems with normal pursuit eye movements.

Basilar: double vision, facial paralysis, visual deficits, and balance or vestibular disturbances.

Cerebellar: vertigo, difficulties in swallowing, ipsilateral ataxia, and changes in sensation.

The side of the brain that is damaged by the CVA affects the symptoms that the client shows:

Left CVA: right hemiplegia, language deficits, slow and cautious behavior style (American Heart Association, 2010).

Right CVA: left hemiplegia, visual deficits, quick and impulsive behavior style (American Heart Association, 2010).

Incidence/Prevalence in U.S.

About 795,000 Americans have a stroke each year with 87% of those cases being an ischemic stroke, 10% an intracerebral hemorrhagic stroke, and three percent a subarachnoid hemorrhage stroke (Roger et al., 2012). An ischemic stroke occurs when a blood vessel that supplies the brain with blood is blocked or obstructed. A hemorrhagic stroke is the result of bleeding in the brain due to a ruptured, weakened blood vessel in the brain. On average, someone in America has a stroke every 40 seconds (American Heart Association Subcommittee, 2008).

Strokes kill more than 135,000 people each year (American Stroke Association, 2012). It is the fourth leading cause of death in the U.S., and it is a leading cause of severe, long-term disability (American Stroke Association, 2012). Even though stroke is more common in men, women have higher rates of stroke deaths than men. There are about seven million Americans who are stroke survivors (National Stroke Association, 2012).

Predominant Age

According to the National Stroke Association (2012), stroke can affect anyone, but there are several risk factors that increase the chances of having a stroke:

- The odds of having a stroke go up with age. Two-thirds of all strokes happen to individuals over age 65 and the stroke risk doubles with each decade past the age of 55.
- African-Americans have a higher stroke risk than other racial groups.

- The risk is higher for people with a family history of stroke.
- Men have a slightly higher stroke risk than women. However, there are more women who have survived a stroke that are over of age of 65 than men because women in the United States live longer.
- Individuals who have diabetes have a higher risk of stroke. This increase in risk may have a connection with circulation problems common in individuals with diabetes.
- Strokes are more common among individuals with low income and a history of drug or alcohol abuse.

Causes

One or more of the following three problems with the vascular system are the primary causes of strokes. First, a stroke may be caused by a blood clot that develops in the brain and blocks blood flow. This is called a thrombosis and is the main cause of ischemic strokes (National Stroke Association, 2012). Second, a blood clot may originate elsewhere in the vascular system and travel to the brain, where it becomes lodged and blocks blood flow. This is called an embolism and is another main cause of ischemic strokes (National Stroke Association, 2012). Third, a blood vessel breaks or ruptures, which causes bleeding in the brain. This is called a hemorrhage and is most often caused by weakened blood vessels and increased blood pressure (National Stroke Association, 2012). Hemorrhages are the causes of intracerebral hemorrhagic strokes and subarachnoid hemorrhage strokes (Roger et al., 2012).

Common stroke risk factors include hypertension, high cholesterol, heart disease, sleep apnea, smoking, alcohol use, heart rhythm disorders, drug use, and body weight above the recommended Body Mass Index (BMI) (American Stroke Association, 2012). Less common but still significant risk factors for women include pregnancy and post-menopause (American Heart Association Subcommittee, 2008). As most stroke risk factors are controllable, most strokes can also be prevented (Heidenreich et al., 2011). By controlling lifestyle components, anyone can significantly reduce the risk of having a stroke. To help decrease the risk of stroke, an individual should eat a healthy diet with low amounts of salt, participate in regular exercise, maintain a healthy weight, avoid tobacco and drugs, limit alcohol consumption, if prescribed prescription medication take it correctly, and stay informed about personal health issues (American Stroke Association, 2012; Heidenreich et al., 2011).

Systems Affected

As a stroke is loss of blood to vital sections of the brain resulting in brain damage (s110 Structure of Brain), a stroke may affect many different cerebral functions. However, a stroke primarily affects an individual's motor, sensory, cognitive, language, and visual functions (American Stroke Association, 2012).

Motor impairments may include hemiplegia, motor planning, muscle power, muscle tone, reflexes, balance, gait, apraxia, and coordination (American Stroke Association, 2012; Kelly-Hayes et al., 1998). Motor impairments are the most common impairment seen after a stroke. They most often are seen in the face, arms, and/or legs (Kelly-Hayes et al., 1998). Relevant ICF codes include b235 Vestibular Functions, b730-b749 Muscle Functions, b750-b789 Movement Functions, and d4 Mobility.

Sensory impairments may include decreased sensory awareness, numbness, tingling, astereognosis, agraphia, and processing problems (American Stroke Association, 2012; Kelly-Hayes et al., 1998). ICF codes to check include b210 Seeing Functions, b240 Sensations Associated with Hearing and Vestibular Functions, and b260 Proprioceptive Function.

Cognitive impairments may include decreases in consciousness functions, calculation abilities, attention, concentration, problem solving, organizing, perception, orientation, time management, planning, judgment, and safety (American Stroke Association, 2012). All of the codes in b1 Mental Functions should be assessed, especially b110 Consciousness Functions, b114 Orientation Functions, b167 Mental Functions of Language. Also relevant are the codes included in d160-d179 Applying Knowledge, d570 Looking After One's Health, and d571 Looking After One's Safety.

Language impairments may include dysphasia in comprehension, reading, and writing, and a decrease in expression and reception of language (aphasia, dysarthria) (American Stroke Association, 2012; Kelly-Hayes et al., 1998). ICF codes include b167 Mental Functions of Language, and codes in d3 Communication.

Visual impairments may include double vision, depth perception problems, and field cuts (b210 Seeing Functions) (National Stroke Association, 2012).

Strokes can also affect emotions, personality, sexual function, as well as bowel and bladder function (American Heart Association Subcommittee, 2009). The extent of the dysfunction depends on the severity and location of brain damage, client's motivation for and participation in rehabilitation, the brain's innate recovery process, and the level of support and encouragement. Review codes b125 Dispositions and Intra-Personal Functions, b126 Temperament and Personality Functions, b130 Energy and Drive Functions, b152 Emotional Functions, b525 Defecation Functions, b620 Urination Functions, b640 Sexual Functions, and d530 Toileting.

The effects of a stroke also depend on the person's age and gender, the type and location of the stroke, and the speed and effectiveness of the medical care. Based upon these variables, an individual can have any number of additional physical, emotional, and/or cognitive effects. Some common post-stroke physical effects include seizures, paralysis, incontinence, spasticity, pain, dysphagia, and fatigue (American Heart Association, 2012). Common post-stroke emotional effects include depression, reflex crying, memory challenges, and one-side neglect (American Heart Association, 2012). The American Heart Association (2012) identifies common post-stroke cognitive effects as dementia, aphasia, apraxia, and diminished short-term and long-term memory.

Secondary Problems

Along with motor, sensory, cognitive, language, and visual limitations, individuals recovering from stroke may also exhibit several secondary problems and limitations. Some of the more common secondary problems and limitations include inactivity, lack of independence and participation, post-stroke depression, and emotional lability.

Many secondary problems associated with recovering from stroke are related to inactivity (Wolfe et al., 2011). Inactivity may result from a lack of mobility, poor coping mechanisms, loss of function, and barriers to recreation and leisure choices (Wolfe et al., 2011). Inactivity can affect an individual's work performance, academic performance, community involvement, and social relationships. ICF codes used to document these deficits include codes in d2 General Tasks and Demands, especially d230 Carrying Out Daily Routine and d240 Handling Stress and Other Psychological Demands, and codes in d4 Mobility, d5 Self-Care, d6 Domestic Life, d7 Interpersonal Interactions and Relationships, d8 Major Life Areas, and d9 Community, Social, and Civic Life.

In addition to post-stroke effects, individuals recovering from stroke may also exhibit a decrease in independence and participation (National Guideline Clearinghouse, 2008). This decrease in independence and participation stems, in part, from a loss of mobility, a loss of ability to perform both activities of daily living (ADLs) and instrumental activities of daily living (IADLs), and an increase in the number and severity of falls (National Guideline Clearinghouse, 2008). ADLs are activities that are associated with the basic self-care functions of life (Bookman et al., 2007). Examples of ADLs include personal hygiene, dressing and undressing, self-feeding, bowel and bladder management, and ambulation. These are coded with d5 Self-Care. IADLs are activities that are not necessary for the basic functions associated with life, but they do allow an individual to live freely in their community (Bookman et al., 2007). Examples of IADLs include taking proper medications, using a telephone, housework, managing money, and shopping for basic groceries or clothing. These are usually coded with d6 Domestic Life.

Associated with these stroke and post-stroke effects comes an increasing burden on the caregivers of individuals recovering from stroke. These caregivers are now required to perform many of the tasks, both ADLs and IADLs, that the individuals recovering from stroke once performed for themselves. Deficits in the availability of caregivers should be coded with e410 Individual Attitudes of Immediate Family Members and the appropriate parts of e3 Support and Relationships. Care for survivors of stroke comes with great financial and emotional costs. In 2008 the indirect and direct cost associated with stroke recovery in the U.S. was just over $34 billion (Roger et al., 2012) and the indirect costs alone are predicted to increase to over $44 billion by 2030 (Heidenreich et al., 2011).

Additionally, around one-third of all individuals recovering from stroke suffer from post-stroke depression (Loubinoux et al., 2012). Post-stroke depression is identified as irritability, trouble sleeping, low self-esteem, fatigue, and withdrawal (Loubinoux et al., 2012). Post-stroke depression can severely hinder an individual's recovery from stroke by reducing motivation to participate in the rehabilitation process. Use ICF codes b125 Dispositions and Intra-Personal Functions, b126 Temperament and Personality Functions, b130 Energy and Drive Functions, and b134 Sleep Functions.

In addition to post-stroke depression, individuals recovering from stroke may also experience emotional lability (Gillespie et al., 2011). Emotional lability is the rapid transition from emotional highs to emotional lows with no apparent provocation. An individual may go from excessive crying to excessive laughing with no discernible explanation. Emotional lability is witnessed in approximately 20% of individuals who have a stroke (Gillespie et al., 2011). Document it with code b152 Emotional Functions.

Prognosis

Since a stroke can affect an individual's motor, sensory, cognitive, language, and visual functions, the results of a stroke vary greatly from individual to individual. The size and location of the stroke also greatly affects an individual's prognosis. According to the National Stroke Association (2012) general recovery guidelines show:

- 10% of individuals recovering from stroke do so almost completely.
- 25% of individuals recovering from stroke do so with minor impairments.
- 40% of individuals recovering from stroke do so with moderate to severe impairments requiring special care.
- 10% of individuals recovering from stroke require care in a long-term care facility.
- 15% die shortly after the stroke.

For individuals recovering from stroke, recovery of affected functions sometimes occurs within six months, but may take a year or more. The exact time frame for optimal recovery of functions following a stroke is debated, ranging from four weeks to twelve weeks (Murphy & Corbett, 2009). However, it is agreed that the sooner an individual enters rehabilitation the better. For some individuals, major life functions will not be recovered, with functional improvements ending as early as five months after a stroke (Bastille & Gill-Body, 2004).

One treatment that has been shown to improve an individual's prognosis following a stroke is tissue plasminogen activator (tPA), which is a medicine that will dissolve the clot. tPA must be administered within three hours of the onset of stroke symptoms for best benefit. The National Institute of Neurological Disorders and Stroke (NINDS) (1995) funded a study that found that eight out of eighteen individuals would not have significant residual disability following stroke if they had tPA administered according to the strict protocol put forth. Six out of eighteen individuals would typically recover without residual disability.

Assessment

In 1998 the American Heart Association undertook a project to construct a global Stroke Outcome Classification system to classify the impairments and disabilities that can occur after an individual has a stroke (Kelly-Hayes et al., 1998). It is a scale that assesses all five major areas of limitation (motor, sensory, cognitive, language, and visual) and provides a summary score of overall stroke functioning, which includes domains affected, impairments, and disabilities (Kelly-Hayes et al., 1998). The Stroke Outcome Classification score is of most use when used in conjunction with standardized assessment instruments. The goal of the American Heart Association's Stroke Outcome Classification project was to provide a reliable measurement that assesses recovery, response to treatments, and long-term impact on individuals recovering from stroke (Kelly-Hayes et al., 1998).

Typical Scope of Team Assessment

Additional stroke assessments vary according to the size, location, and severity of stroke. They measure a wide variety of impairments and issues including mood, fatigue, motor recovery, quality of life, depression, and overall post-stroke functioning. Some standardized assessments widely used with stroke patients include:

The ICF Measure of Participation and ACTivity (IMPACT): The IMPACT is a 32-item measure designed to identify restrictions a person has in the nine categories of activity and participation outlined by the ICF (Post et al., 2008). The scores can be totaled to obtain the score for each of the nine categories, the sub-scale of activity (items 1-19), the sub-scale of participation (items 20-32), or a total score.

Fatigue Severity Scale (FSS): The FSS (Krupp et al., 1989) measures the impact fatigue has on an individual's daily functions. It is a nine-item scale.

Fugl-Meyer Assessment of Motor Recovery after Stroke: The Fugl-Meyer scale (Gladstone, Danells, & Black, 2002) constitutes a 100-point motor domain to measure motor recovery in individuals recovering from stroke. It has high intra-rater reliability, high construct validity, and has been extensively evaluated.

National Institutes of Health Stroke Scale (NIHSS): The NIHSS (Lyden et al., 1994) contains 11 items which help healthcare professionals understand the scope of an individual's impairment from stroke. Each item is rated on range from 0 to 4, with a score of 0 indicating normal function.

Stroke Impact Scale Version 2.0 (SIS-2): The SIS-2 (Duncan et al., 1999) is a self-report measure that assesses eight domains (strength, hand function, ADL/IADL, mobility, communication, emotion, memory, and participation) through 64 different items.

The Short Form Health Survey (SF-36): The SF-36 (Anderson, Laubscher, & Burns, 1996) is a survey that measures quality of life by assessing physical, psychological, and social functions.

Patient Health Questionnaire (PHQ-9): The PHQ-9 is a nine-item validated assessment for depression in the post-stroke population (Kroenke, Spitzer, & Williams, 2001; Williams et al., 2005). The items assess nine symptoms of depression as defined by the DSM. Higher scores indicate more depression symptoms; scores greater than or equal to 10 indicate clinically significant depression.

Additional recreational therapy assessments will greatly add to the healthcare professional's knowledge of the individual's leisure constraints and beliefs. These assessments will allow the recreational therapist to correctly identify the individual's leisure interests, expectations, and limitations (burlingame & Blaschko, 2010). Some widely used recreational-therapy-specific assessments for individuals recovering from stroke include:

Leisure Diagnostic Battery (LDB): The LDB (Witt & Ellis, 1984) is an instrument that measures an individual's perceived freedom and barriers to leisure. It consists of the following five scales: perceived leisure competence, perceived leisure locus of control, leisure needs, playfulness, and depth of leisure involvement.

Comprehensive Evaluation in Recreational Therapy — Physical Disabilities (CERT-PhysDis): The CERT-PhysDis measures functional ability in eight areas over 50 total items (Petajan & White, 2000). It is used to establish the current status of an individual's functional skills as they relate to their leisure choices. The eight areas include gross motor function, fine motor function, locomotion, motor skills, sensory, cognition, behavior, and communication.

Functional Assessment of Characteristics for Therapeutic Recreation — Revised (FACTR-R): The FACTR-R explores the three domains of physical, cognitive, and social functioning through the use of a 33-item assessment (Peterson, Dunn, & Carruthers, 2010). It is used to identify functional skills and behaviors that the individual needs to improve for better functioning.

The rehab team evaluates the individual's abilities and limitations through a variety of these and other assessments relevant to their field of knowledge. In addition, a full inquiry is also conducted on the individual to identify positive and negative support structures, adaptations that need to be made in the individual's home, and additional ways to help promote increased independence and function.

Areas of Concern for RT Assessment

The RT evaluation may reflect any of the following:

Social participation limitations (d9 Community, Social, and Civic Life): The individual's ability to participate in leisure choices, recreation, and community activities may be diminished due to physical and/or cognitive limitations (Schmid et al., 2012a).

Safety concerns (d571 Looking After One's Safety): Due to cognitive limitations the individual may not fully understand safety concerns in connection with participation in complex community activities (Pohjasvaara et al., 2002).

Decreased physical activity (d230 Carrying Out Daily Routine): Due to physical limitations and motor deficiencies the individual may be fatigued when participating in everyday tasks. The person will have to prioritize actions due to lack of mobility, time, and/or energy (Roger et al., 2012).

Functional skill impairments (choose appropriate Body Function or Activities and Participation ICF codes): Due to the post-stroke effects an individual may experience a number of functional skill impairments. These functional skill impairments may include poor balance, decreased vision, hemiparesis, spasticity, pain, fatigue, and dementia (American Heart Association, 2012).

Mood issues (b126 Temperament and Personality Functions): There are many psychosocial challenges associated with stroke. They include depression, emotional lability, anxiety, and cognitive changes (American Heart Association, 2012; Gillespie et al., 2011). Depression is the most common psychiatric disorder, affecting at least one-third of all stroke survivors (Loubinoux et al., 2012).

Fatigue (b455 Exercise Tolerance Functions): Due to physical impairments fatigue is often a limiting factor in the individual's desire to engage in life activities. Between 33% and 77% of stroke survivors identify fatigue as a major barrier to their life activities (Parks et al., 2012).

Decreased cognitive functioning (b1 Mental Functions, d1 Learning and Applying Knowledge): As many as 65% of stroke survivors demonstrate some level of cognitive impairment (Donovan et al., 2008). This decrease in cognition may manifest itself in lack of short-term or long-term memory, aphasia, dysarthria, apraxia, increased mathematical challenges, or auditory overload (American Heart Association, 2012).

Other ICF codes that may be used by the recreational therapist were given in the Systems Affected and Secondary Problems sections.

ICF Core Set

A brief and comprehensive ICF Core Set for Cerebrovascular Accident is available to help guide the therapist in identifying diagnosis-related ICF codes.

Treatment Direction

Whole Team Approach

The whole team approach to stroke rehabilitation is to enhance independence, restore functional skills, adapt for functional losses, and train family or an identified caregiver to assist the client after discharge (Duncan et al., 2005). The treatment team usually focuses on task and skill repetition utilizing familiar activities that may evoke a spontaneous reaction. Examples of familiar activities include singing the alphabet, basic counting and matching activities, picking up a telephone, opening and closing doors, or other simple activities that were a part of the individual's life. These types of activities can help promote neuromotor re-training. Additional approaches that may be taken include:

Constraint-induced movement therapy (CIMT): CIMT works to improve the functioning of upper extremities by constraining the use of the unaffected extremity in order to focus intensive use on the affected extremity (Grotta et al., 2004).

Mental practice and mental imagery: Mental practice and mental imagery is the process of imagining that your body is moving or performing a certain activity while you are physically not performing that action. There is evidence for and against this approach, however many individuals recovering from stroke have found success with its practice (Braun et al., 2006; Butler & Page, 2006; Page, Levine, & Leonard, 2005, 2007).

Mirror visual feedback/mirror therapy (MVF/MT): MVF/MT is a relatively new approach in stroke rehab. MVF/MT involves the use of a large mirror that is correctly positioned so, when individuals recovering from stroke sit in front of the mirror, they see their unaffected arm positioned as their affected arm (Cacchio et al., 2009). This visual illusion seems to promote favorable neurological activity that has an encouraging effect on sensory and motor recovery (Cacchio et al., 2009; Sütbeyaz et al., 2007; Yavuzer et al., 2008).

Recreational Therapy Approach

Recreational therapists follow the whole team approach while addressing secondary complications, participation restrictions, and leisure/recreation adaptations. Recreational therapy's goal is for the individual recovering from stroke to be able to return to living as normal a life as possible, including reducing the risk for an additional stroke, by increasing health promoting activities and re-engaging in enjoyable activities. During inpatient rehabilitation stays, individuals recovering from stroke traditionally stay for two to three weeks and receive six to nine hours of recreational therapy interventions. In outpatient, day treatment, or adapted recreation settings, the length of treatment may be considerably longer. Recreational therapy is also provided in adult day programs, assisted living programs, and skilled nursing facilities. Due to the lack of time during inpatient rehabilitation, the recreational therapist must prioritize and incorporate both restorative and adaptive activities to establish a balanced intervention process. These activities also need to be designed with input from the client and his or her family to meet their situational and emotional needs, as documented during diagnosis, as well as to ensure success and continuity post discharge.

Stroke rehabilitation is based on neurological recovery and can be very complex. The recreational therapist assesses and treats each client while providing stroke risk education (d570 Looking After One's Health), family training (e410 Individual Attitudes of Immediate Family Members), home and leisure adaptations (e.g., e1 Products and Technology, e2 Natural Environment and Human-Made Changes to Environment), community reintegration (d910 Community Life while also addressing related Body Functions and Activities & Participation ICF codes), and the development of life skills to help reduce the future risk of stroke including exercise and stress management (d155 Acquiring Skills, d570 Looking After One's Health). The recreational therapist tailors each of these to the individual, as the intervention will depend on the impairments of the specific client. The therapist will determine what to address first, second, and third based upon the initial assessment and follow-up evaluations. Although no two treatment plans and interventions will be the same, they should all be directed towards the outcome of optimal functioning.

Recreational Therapy Interventions

Recovering from a stroke is a difficult process that is made even more difficult by the complex range of dysfunctions and limitations one may acquire from the stroke. Interventions and modalities that are commonly implemented by recreational therapists for individuals who are recovering from stroke include:

Movement training: This category includes interventions that focus on balance (b235 Vestibular Functions, b755 Involuntary Movement Reaction Functions, d415 Maintaining a Body Position), proprioception (b260 Proprioceptive Function), and gait retraining (b770 Gait Pattern Functions). Yoga is a specific technique that can enhance all of these areas. Studies have found that yoga provides significant benefits for individuals recovering from stroke including increased balance (b235 Vestibular Functions, d415 Maintaining a Body Position), improved mobility (d4 Mobility), increased joint movement (b710 Mobility of Joint Functions), and increased muscle strength (b730 Muscle Power Functions) (Bastille & Gill-Body, 2004; Garrett, Immink, & Hillier, 2011; Lynton, Kligler, & Shiflett, 2007; Schmid et al., 2012b). Others have identified that yoga reduces activity limitations and enhances participation in those who have had a stroke (d9 Community, Social, and Civic Life) (Schmid et al., 2012c; Van Puymbroeck et al., 2012). The benefit of using the Wii video game system in movement training is emerging in the stroke research literature. For example, a pilot study with seven individuals found that functional ability in the upper extremities improved (b7 Neuromusculoskeletal and Movement-Related Functions, d4 Mobility), as did overall disability score, balance (b235 Vestibular Functions, d415 Maintaining a Body Position), and dexterity (d440 Fine Hand Use) following one hour on the Wii on 10 consecutive days (Mouawad et al., 2011).

Physical activity/exercise: Resistance training has been shown to improve muscle strength, power (b730 Muscle Power Functions), and endurance (b740 Muscle Endurance Functions) in affected and unaffected extremities of stroke survivors (Flansbjer et al., 2008; Lee et al., 2010). In addition, exercise therapy for individuals recovering from stroke has been suggested to be beneficial in terms of increasing strength (b730 Muscle Power Functions), fitness (d570 Looking After One's Health, b455 Exercise Tolerance Functions), ADLs (d5 Self-Care, d230 Carrying Out Daily Routine), and improvements in walking (d450 Walking) (Veerbeek et al., 2011). As lack of strength and decreased muscle endurance are both limitations for individuals recovering from

stroke, interventions that focus on strengthening muscles should be utilized. Additionally, aquatic therapy programs have also been shown to be beneficial at increasing muscle strength and balance in individuals recovering from stroke (Noh et al., 2008). Furthermore, exercise in a variety of forms has been shown to be an effective tool in increasing mobility (Flansbjer et al., 2008; Lee et al., 2010; Veerbeek et al., 2011; Wevers et al., 2009). Finally, aerobic exercise that considers the ability level and comorbid conditions of the individual has been shown to improve walking speed (b137 Psychomotor Functions, d450 Walking), endurance (b455 Exercise Tolerance Functions), mood (b126 Temperament and Personality Functions), cognition (b163 Basic Cognitive Functions, b164 Higher-Level Cognitive Functions), and reduce risk for additional stroke (Lindsay, Gubitz, & Bayley, 2010; Teasell, Foley, & Salter, 2007).

Music: Research has shown that music, music-based activities, and speech can all positively affect mood (b126 Temperament and Personality Functions) and increase cognition (b163 Basic Cognitive Functions, b164 Higher-Level Cognitive Functions) in individuals recovering from stroke (Forsblom et al., 2009; Särkämö et al., 2010; Särkämö et al., 2008; van Wijck et al., 2012). Furthermore, a study that used musical instruments (a MIDI-piano or electronic drum pads) 15 times over three weeks, in addition to standard rehabilitation, improved speed, precision, and smoothness of movements (b137 Psychomotor Functions, d4 Mobility) compared to individuals who received standard rehabilitation only (Schneider et al., 2007). Consequently, RT-based interventions should consider the use of music for improving mood and targeted, intentional goal attainment.

Social interactions and engagement: Due to the functional limitations that are associated with stroke, social relationships (d710-d729 General Interpersonal Interactions, d750 Informal Social Relationships) may be ignored to preserve time and energy for more basic functions. However, these social relationships are important to the overall health of the individual, and research has indicated that stroke survivors who received emotional support made substantial improvements, even for those with low functional ability to start (Glass & Maddox, 1992). The recreational therapist can help the individual identify interests, past social groups, and friendships.

The therapist can then work on training and interventions that assist the individual in learning the skills required to facilitate social situations (d710-d729 General Interpersonal Interactions).

Recreation participation: Another important aspect of improving social participation is helping individuals post-stroke engage in enjoyable activities (d920 Recreation and Leisure). A study revealed that leisure rehabilitation was more effective than occupational therapy or a control group in scores for leisure rehabilitation (Drummond & Walker, 1995). Recreational therapists can tailor adaptive recreation activities to the needs of the individual recovering from stroke, to encourage full participation in enjoyable activities. Therapists can also help patients identify community resources for active participation post-rehabilitation.

Resources

American Stroke Association
7272 Greenville Ave.
Dallas, TX 75231
888-4-STROKE
www.strokeassociation.org
The American Stroke Association provides great information on new research, new medications, new procedures, and additional resources. They also provide support groups, newsletters, various help topics, current research, information on preventing and recovering from a stroke, and more. They also offer the Stroke Connection magazine and a section of the website for health professionals.

National Stroke Association
9707 E. Easter Lane, Suite B
Centennial, CO 80112
800-STROKES (800-787-6537) or 303-649-9299
www.stroke.org
The National Stroke Association offers information on risk reduction, the Stroke Smart magazine, and personal stories of stroke. The website also offers a resource center full of information about stroke, as well as the latest research on stroke and stroke recovery.

National Institute of Neurological Disorders and Stroke (NINDS)
P.O. Box 5801
Bethesda, MD 20824
Voice: 800-352-9424 or 301-496-5751

TTY: dial 711
www.ninds.nih.gov
NINDS funds a lot of stroke-related research. On the website, one can find out about stroke-related clinical trials that are currently enrolling subjects, as well as recently breaking stroke news.

References

American Heart Association. (2010). Heart disease and stroke statistics: Our guide to current statistics and the supplement to our heart and stroke facts. 2008 Update at-a-glance. Retrieved from American Heart Association.

American Heart Association. (2012). Effects of stroke. From http://www.strokeassociation.org/STROKEORG/About-Stroke/EffectsofStroke/Effects-of-Stroke_UCM_308534_SubHomePage.jsp.

American Heart Association Subcommittee. (2008). AHA statistical update. *Circulation, 117*, e25-e146.

American Heart Association Subcommittee. (2009). Evidence table. *Circulation, 119*(3), 480-486.

American Stroke Association. (2012). Stroke warning signs. From http://www.strokeassociation.org/STROKEORG/Warning-Signs/Stroke-Warning-Signs_UCM_308528_SubHomePage.jsp.

Anderson, C., Laubscher, S., & Burns, R. (1996). Validation of the Short Form 36 (SF-36) health survey questionnaire among stroke patients. *Stroke, 27*(10), 1812-1816.

Bastille, J. V. & Gill-Body, K. M. (2004). A yoga-based exercise program for people with chronic poststroke hemiparesis. *Physical Therapy, 84*(1), 33-48.

burlingame, j. & Blaschko, T. (2010). *Assessment tools for recreational therapy and related fields* (4th ed.). Enumclaw, WA: Idyll Arbor.

Blesedell, E., Cohn, E. S., & Boyt, B. A. (2003). *Willard & Spackman's occupational therapy*. New York: Lippincott.

Bookman, A., Harrington, M., Pass, L., & Reisner, E. (2007). *Family caregiver handbook*. Cambridge, MA: Massachusetts Institute of Technology.

Braun, S. M., Beurskens, A. J., Borm, P. J., Schack, T., & Wade, D. T. (2006). The effects of mental practice in stroke rehabilitation: A systematic review. *Archives of Physical Medicine and Rehabilitation, 87*(6), 842-852.

Butler, A. J. & Page, S. J. (2006). Mental practice with motor imagery: Evidence for motor recovery and cortical reorganization after stroke. *Archives of Physical Medicine and Rehabilitation, 87*(12), 2-11.

Cacchio, A., De Blasis, E., De Blasis, V., Santilli, V., & Spacca, G. (2009). Mirror therapy in compleregional pain syndrome type 1 of the upper limb in stroke patients. *Neurorehabilitation and Neural Repair, 23*(8), 792-799.

Donovan, N. J., Kendall, D. L., Heaton, S. C., Kwon, S., Velozo, C. A., & Duncan, P. W. (2008). Conceptualizing functional cognition in stroke. *Neurorehabilitation and Neural Repair, 22*(2), 122-135.

Drummond, A. & Walker, M. (1995). A randomized controlled trial of leisure rehabilitation after stroke. *Clinical Rehabilitation, 9*(4), 283-290.

Duncan, P. W., Wallace, D., Lai, S. M., Johnson, D., Embretson, S., & Laster, L. J. (1999). The Stroke Impact Scale Version 2.0 evaluation of reliability, validity, and sensitivity to change. *Stroke, 30*(10), 2131-2140.

Duncan, P. W., Zorowitz, R., Bates, B., Choi, J. Y., Glasberg, J. J., Graham, G. D., … Reker, D. (2005). Management of adult stroke rehabilitation care: A clinical practice guideline. *Stroke, 36*(9), e100-e143.

Flansbjer, U. B., Miller, M., Downham, D., & Lexell, J. (2008). Progressive resistance training after stroke: Effects on muscle strength, muscle tone, gait performance and perceived participation. *Journal of Rehabilitation Medicine, 40*(1), 42-48.

Forsblom, A., Laitinen, S., Särkämö, T., & Tervaniemi, M. (2009). Therapeutic role of music listening in stroke rehabilitation. *Annals of the New York Academy of Sciences, 1169*(1), 426-430.

Garrett, R., Immink, M. A., & Hillier, S. (2011). Becoming connected: The lived experience of yoga participation after stroke. *Disability and Rehabilitation, 33*(25-26), 2404-2415.

Gillespie, D. C., Joice, S., Lawrence, M., & Whittick, J. (2011). Interventions for post-stroke disturbances of mood and emotional behaviour: Recommendations from SIGN 118. *International Journal of Therapy and Rehabilitation, 18*(3), 166-176.

Gladstone, D. J., Danells, C. J., & Black, S. E. (2002). The Fugl-Meyer assessment of motor recovery after stroke: A critical review of its measurement properties. *Neurorehabilitation and Neural Repair, 16*(3), 232-240.

Glass, T. A. & Maddox, G. L. (1992). The quality and quantity of social support: Stroke recovery as psycho-social transition. *Soc Sci Med, 34*(11), 1249-1261.

Grotta, J. C., Noser, E. A., Ro, T., Boake, C., Levin, H., Aronowski, J., & Schallert, T. (2004). Constraint-induced movement therapy. *Stroke, 35*(11 suppl 1), 2699-2701.

Heidenreich, P. A., Trogdon, J. G., Khavjou, O. A., Butler, J., Dracup, K., Ezekowitz, M. D., ... Khera, A. (2011). Forecasting the future of cardiovascular disease in the United States: A policy statement from the American Heart Association. *Circulation, 123*(8), 933-944.

Kelly-Hayes, P. M., Robertson, J. T., Broderick, J. P., Duncan, P. W., Hershey, L. A., Roth, E. J., ... Trombly, C. A. (1998). The American Heart Association stroke outcome classification. *Stroke, 29*(6), 1274-1280.

Kroenke, K., Spitzer, R. L., & Williams, J. B. (2001). The PHQ-9: Validity of a brief depression severity measure. *J Gen Intern Med, 16*(9), 606-613.

Krupp, L. B., LaRocca, N. G., Muir-Nash, J., & Steinberg, A. D. (1989). The Fatigue Severity Scale. Application to patients with multiple sclerosis and systemic lupus erythematosus. *Archives of Neurology, 46*(10), 1121-1123.

Lee, M. J., Kilbreath, S. L., Singh, M. F., Zeman, B., & Davis, G. M. (2010). Effect of progressive resistance training on muscle performance after chronic stroke. *Medicine and Science in Sports and Exercise, 42*(1), 23-34.

Lindsay, M., Gubitz, G., & Bayley, M. (2010). On behalf of the Canadian Stroke Strategy Best Practices and Standards Writing Group. *Canadian Best Practice Recommendations for Stroke Care (Update 2010). Ottawa, Ontario Canada: Canadian Stroke Network.*

Loubinoux, I., Kronenberg, G., Endres, M., Schumann-Bard, P., Freret, T., Filipkowski, R. K., ... Popa-Wagner, A. (2012). Post-stroke depression: Mechanisms, translation and therapy. *Journal of Cellular and Molecular Medicine, 16*(9), 1961-1969.

Lyden, P., Brott, T., Tilley, B., Welch, K., Mascha, E., Levine, S., ... Marler, J. (1994). Improved reliability of the NIH Stroke Scale using video training. NINDS TPA Stroke Study Group. *Stroke, 25*(11), 2220-2226.

Lynton, H., Kligler, B., & Shiflett, S. (2007). Yoga in stroke rehabilitation: A systematic review and results of a pilot study. *Topics in Stroke Rehabilitation, 14*(4), 1-8.

Mouawad, M. R., Doust, C. G., Max, M. D., & McNulty, P. A. (2011). Wii-based movement therapy to promote improved upper extremity function post-stroke: A pilot study. *Journal of Rehabilitation Medicine, 43*(6), 527-533.

Murphy, T. H. & Corbett, D. (2009). Plasticity during stroke recovery: From synapse to behaviour. *Nature Reviews Neuroscience, 10*(12), 861-872.

National Guideline Clearinghouse. (2008). Occupational therapy practice guidelines for adults with stroke. From http://guidelines.gov/content.aspx?id=15290.

National Institute of Neurological Disorders and Stroke PA Stroke Study Group. (1995). Tissue plasminogen activator for acute ischemic stroke. *New England Journal of Medicine, 333*(24), 1581-1587. doi: 10.1056/NEJM199512143332401.

National Stroke Association. (2012). What is stroke? From http://www.stroke.org/site/PageServer?pagename=stroke.

Noh, D. K., Lim, J. Y., Shin, H. I., & Paik, N. J. (2008). The effect of aquatic therapy on postural balance and muscle strength in stroke survivors — a randomized controlled pilot trial. *Clinical Rehabilitation, 22*(10-11), 966-976.

Page, S. J., Levine, P., & Leonard, A. (2007). Mental practice in chronic stroke: Results of a randomized, placebo-controlled trial. *Stroke, 38*(4), 1293-1297.

Page, S. J., Levine, P., & Leonard, A. C. (2005). Effects of mental practice on affected limb use and function in chronic stroke. *Archives of Physical Medicine and Rehabilitation, 86*(3), 399-402.

Parks, N. E., Eskes, G. A., Gubitz, G. J., Reidy, Y., Christian, C., & Phillips, S. J. (2012). Fatigue Impact Scale demonstrates greater fatigue in younger stroke survivors. *The Canadian Journal of Neurological Sciences, 39*(5), 619-625.

Petajan, J. H. & White, A. T. (2000). Motor-evoked potentials in response to fatiguing grip exercise in multiple sclerosis patients. *Clinical Neurophysiology 111*(12), 2188-2195.

Peterson, C. A., Dunn, J., & Carruthers, C. (Eds.). (2010). *Functional assessment of characteristics for therapeutic recreation, revised.* Ravensdale, WA: Idyll Arbor.

Pohjasvaara, T., Leskelä, M., Vataja, R., Kalska, H., Ylikoski, R., Hietanen, M., ... Erkinjuntti, T. (2002). Post-stroke depression, executive dysfunction and functional outcome. *European Journal of Neurology, 9*(3), 269-275. doi: 10.1046/j.1468-1331.2002.00396.x.

Post, M. W., de Witte, L. P., Reichrath, E., Verdonschot, M. M., Wijlhuizen, G. J., & Perenboom, R. J. (2008). Development and validation of IMPACT-S, an ICF-based questionnaire to measure activities and participation. *J Rehabil Med, 40*(8), 620-627. doi: 10.2340/16501977-0223.

Roger, V. L., Go, A. S., Lloyd-Jones, D. M., Benjamin, E. J., Berry, J. D., Borden, W. B., ... Fox, C. S. (2012). Heart disease and stroke statistics — 2012 update: A report from the American Heart Association. *Circulation, 125*(1), e2-e220.

Särkämö, T., Pihko, E., Laitinen, S., Forsblom, A., Soinila, S., Mikkonen, M., ... Laine, M. (2010). Music and speech listening enhance the recovery of early sensory processing after stroke. *Journal of Cognitive Neuroscience, 22*(12), 2716-2727.

Särkämö, T., Tervaniemi, M., Laitinen, S., Forsblom, A., Soinila, S., Mikkonen, M., ... Laine, M. (2008). Music listening enhances cognitive recovery and mood after middle cerebral artery stroke. *Brain, 131*(3), 866-876.

Schmid, A. A., Van Puymbroeck, M., Altenburger, P. A., Dierks, T. A., Miller, K. K., Damush, T. M., & Williams, L. S. (2012a). Balance and balance self-efficacy are associated with activity and participation after stroke: A cross-sectional study in people with chronic stroke. *Archives of Physical Medicine and Rehabilitation, 93*(6), 1101-1107. doi: 10.1016/j.apmr.2012.01.020.

Schmid, A. A., Van Puymbroeck, M., Altenburger, P. A., Schalk, N. L., Dierks, T. A., Miller, K. K., ... Williams, L. S. (2012b). Poststroke balance improves with yoga: A pilot study. *Stroke, 43*(9), 2402-2407.

Schmid, A. A., Van Puymbroeck, M., Miller, K. D., & Schalk, N. (2012c). Group yoga intervention leads to improved balance and balance self-efficacy after stroke. *BMC Complementary and Alternative Medicine, 12*(Suppl 1), 222.

Schneider, S., Schonle, P., Altenmuller, E., & Munte, T. (2007). Using musical instruments to improve motor skill recovery following a stroke. *Journal of Neurology, 254*(10), 1339-1346.

Sütbeyaz, S., Yavuzer, G., Sezer, N., & Koseoglu, B. F. (2007). Mirror therapy enhances lower-extremity motor recovery and motor functioning after stroke: A randomized controlled trial. *Archives of Physical Medicine and Rehabilitation, 88*(5), 555-559.

Teasell, R., Foley, N., & Salter, K. (2007). EBRSR: Evidence-based review of stroke rehabilitation. London (ON): EBRSR.

Van Puymbroeck, M., Schmid, A. A., Miller, K. D., & Schalk, N. (2012). Improved activity, participation, and quality of life for individuals with chronic stroke following an 8-week yoga intervention. *BMC Complementary and Alternative Medicine, 12*(Suppl 1), 039.

van Wijck, F., Knox, D., Dodds, C., Cassidy, G., Alexander, G., & MacDonald, R. (2012). Making music after stroke: Using musical activities to enhance arm function. *Annals of the New York Academy of Sciences, 1252*(1), 305-311.

Veerbeek, J. M., Koolstra, M., Ket, J. C. F., van Wegen, E. E. H., & Kwakkel, G. (2011). Effects of augmented exercise therapy on outcome of gait and gait-related activities in the first 6 months after stroke: A meta-analysis. *Stroke, 42*(11), 3311-3315.

Wevers, L., van de Port, I., Vermue, M., Mead, G., & Kwakkel, G. (2009). Effects of task-oriented circuit class training on walking competency after stroke: A systematic review. *Stroke, 40*(7), 2450-2459.

Williams, L. S., Brizendine, E. J., Plue, L., Bakas, T., Tu, W., Hendrie, H., & Kroenke, K. (2005). Performance of the PHQ-9 as a screening tool for depression after stroke. *Stroke, 36*(3), 635-638.

Witt, P. & Ellis, G. (1984). The Leisure Diagnostic Battery: Measuring perceived freedom in leisure. *Loisir et Société, 7*(1), 109-124.

Wolfe, C. D. A., Crichton, S. L., Heuschmann, P. U., McKevitt, C. J., Toschke, A. M., Grieve, A. P., & Rudd, A. G. (2011). Estimates of outcomes up to ten years after stroke: Analysis from the prospective South London Stroke Register. *PLoS medicine, 8*(5), e1001033.

Yavuzer, G., Selles, R., Sezer, N., Sütbeyaz, S., Bussmann, J. B., Köseoğlu, F., & Stam, H. J. (2008). Mirror therapy improves hand function in subacute stroke: A randomized controlled trial. *Archives of Physical Medicine and Rehabilitation, 89*(3), 393-398.

10. Chronic Obstructive Pulmonary Disease

Heather R. Porter

Chronic obstructive pulmonary disease (COPD) is a condition that makes it difficult to breathe. To understand this group of diseases it is important to have a good working model of lung functions. Think of a lung as an upside down tree. When a breath is taken in by the mouth or nose it travels down the trachea (the tree trunk) and branches into large tubes (heavy branches called "bronchi") and small tubes (thin branches called "bronchioles"). At the end of the small tubes are alveoli, something like the leaves on a tree. These are small air sacs with very thin walls. In these walls are capillaries. When air is taken into the alveoli the capillaries in the air sac walls capture the oxygen and carry it into the bloodstream. The airways (trachea, bronchi, and bronchioles), the lung tissue itself, and the alveoli are elastic. The lung expands when a breath is taken in and contracts/collapses when air is exhaled.

There are two types of COPD that interfere with the normal functioning of the lung by obstructing or interfering with part of the breathing system (National Heart, Lung, and Blood Institute [NHLBI], 2014):

Chronic bronchitis: Chronic bronchitis is chronic inflammation of the bronchial tubes with an increase in mucus and mucus secreting cells. The mucus obstructs the bronchioles, making it difficult to breathe in and out. The person coughs to try to clear the mucus and becomes short of breath with exertion. Chronic bronchitis is associated with prolonged exposure to bronchial irritants. Smoking is the most common cause of chronic bronchitis.

Emphysema: In emphysema, the walls of the alveoli begin to break down and the lung loses its elasticity. So instead of having many small alveoli, only a few large air sacs remain. To picture this, think about two bubbles touching each other. Each bubble has its own outer surface, just like the alveoli. In alveolar wall breakdown, the wall that keeps the two bubbles separate breaks down and makes one large bubble. In the lung, less alveoli and bigger air sacs cause a problem. There is less surface area for the exchange of oxygen and carbon dioxide. When combined with the loss of lung elasticity, air can become trapped in the large alveoli leading to poor air exchange and shortness of breath. Chronic bronchitis is often the cause of emphysema.

Incidence/Prevalence in U.S.

COPD is the third leading cause of death in the United States (American Lung Association [ALA], 2013). In 2011, about 12.7 million Americans reported having COPD. Since 24 million people reported having impaired lung function, COPD may be underdiagnosed (ALA, 2013). In 2011, 10.1 million people reported having chronic bronchitis and 4.7 million reported having emphysema (ALA, 2013).

Predominant Age

Chronic bronchitis and emphysema are most common in middle to older age (45-65+) (ALA, 2013). Chronic bronchitis occurs in women twice as often as men. Emphysema occurs almost equally in men and women (ALA, 2013).

Causes

The primary cause of COPD is smoking, which accounts for approximately 85-90% of COPD cases (ALA, 2013). This includes all smoked tobacco products (cigarettes, pipe, cigars). Only a small number of people develop COPD from other air allergens, such as prolonged exposure to fumes, chemicals, or secondhand smoke (ALA, 2013). In rare cases, COPD can be caused by alpha 1 antitrypsin deficiency, which is a gene-related disorder in which low levels of alpha 1 antitrypsin lead to deterioration of the lung (ALA, 2013). People who have this deficiency and smoke are instructed to stop smoking, since smoking causes the disease to progress more rapidly.

Systems Affected

COPD primarily affects the lungs, although other systems may be affected. ICF codes used to document systems affected by COPD include b440 Respiration Functions, b450 Additional Respiratory Functions, and s430 Structure of Respiratory System.

Secondary Problems

A survey by the American Lung Association in 2000 indicated that COPD limits work ability (51%) (d840-d859 Work and Employment), physical ability (70%) (b7 Neuromusculoskeletal and Movement-Related Functions, d4 Mobility), household chores (56%) (d6 Domestic Life), social activities (53%) (d9 Community, Social, and Civic Life), sleeping (50%) (b134 Sleep Functions), and family activities (46%) (d9 Community, Social, and Civic Life) (ALA, 2013). Individuals with COPD are also more susceptible to respiratory infections, pulmonary hypertension (high blood pressure in the arteries that bring blood to the lungs), heart problems (such as cardiovascular disease and myocardial infarction), lung cancer, and depression (Mayo Clinic, 2014). Document these using codes b126 Temperament and Personality Functions, b410 Heart Functions, b415 Blood Vessel Functions, b420 Blood Pressure Functions, and b435 Immunological System Functions.

People with COPD may additionally have poor nutrition (d570 Looking After One's Health), poor muscle strength (b730 Muscle Power Functions) and endurance (b455 Exercise Tolerance Functions), skeletal disease such as decreased bone density (s7 Structures Related to Movement), psychosocial issues including anxiety, learned helplessness, loss of internal locus of control (b126 Temperament and Personality Functions), and sensory problems (b156 Perceptual Functions) (Lan, Nici, & Wallack, 2011). Many of these problems are due to frequent hospitalizations, decreased activity level, deconditioning, medications, lack of sufficient oxygen, and poor adjustment and coping strategies.

Prognosis

Damage to the lungs from COPD cannot be reversed, however the progression of the disease can be slowed with smoking cessation (ALA, 2010). The prognosis (years of life, quality of life, functional abilities) depends upon the severity of the disease.

Assessment

Typical Scope of Team Assessment

The physician takes a medical history, listens to the client's lungs, and performs a breathing test to confirm the diagnosis of COPD. A common breathing test is the spirometry test. The client blows into a tube that measures the amount of air the lungs can hold and how fast the client can exhale. Results of the test help the physician to determine the severity of the disease. Levels are usually reported as at risk, mild, moderate, or severe. Other tests may include a chest x-ray and an arterial blood gas test to determine how much oxygen is in the blood. The treatment team evaluates the client's current level of functioning in all domains and develops a treatment plan that predominantly reflects exercise training and education.

Areas of Concern for RT Assessment

The recreational therapist will commonly find that the client's lifestyle has become increasingly isolative and homebound. Recreational activities are usually limited, with the majority of the client's time being spent watching television, napping, reading, or engaging in other activities that require little or no physical exertion. It is not uncommon for people with moderate to severe COPD to remain in the home for weeks or months at a time. There is often high anxiety surrounding any activity that requires physical exertion and feelings of depression are commonly reported from lack of social contact and having to cope with a chronic disease that greatly limits the client's ability to participate in activities that s/he once enjoyed. Some clients can become quite bitter and angry about their situation, contributing to distancing from friends and family. A history of falls and complaints about loss of balance are common due to weakened muscles, loss of flexibility, poor endurance, and other aspects of deconditioning. Clients are typically unaware of the connection between exercise and pulmonary health or dismiss suggestions to exercise with comments like, "The doctor just doesn't understand that I can't do that." Learned helpless and external locus of control are also common findings.

In addition to the codes listed in the Systems Affected and Secondary Systems, the recreational therapist should document problems found in codes b110 Consciousness Functions, b114 Orientation Functions, b130 Energy and Drive Functions, b134 Sleep Functions, b140 Attention Functions, b260 Proprioceptive Function, b410 Heart Functions, b430 Hematological System Functions, b450 Additional Respiratory Functions, b510 Ingestion Functions, b810 Protective Functions of the Skin, b820 Repair Functions of the Skin, d177 Making Decisions, d240 Handling Stress and Other Psychological Demands, d410 Changing Basic Body Position, d415 Maintaining a Body Position, d420 Transferring Oneself, d450 Walking, d460 Moving Around in Different Locations, d465 Moving Around Using Equipment, d540 Dressing, d910 Community Life, and d920 Recreation and Leisure.

ICF Core Set

Two ICF Core Sets that might be helpful in identifying relevant ICF codes are Cardiopulmonary Conditions and Obstructive Pulmonary Diseases.

Treatment Direction

Whole Team Approach

Since COPD is a progressive disease, the goal is to slow down the progression of the disease, preserve quality of life, relieve symptoms, reduce frequency and severity of exacerbations, and improve overall health and ability to exercise (ALA, 2010). This may include the following multi-disciplinary interventions (Jacob, 2012; NHLBI, 2010; Lan, Nici, & Wallack, 2011):

Medications and oxygen therapy: Inhaled steroids or bronchodilators may be prescribed to open up the airways to make it easier to breathe. Oxygen therapy may be provided as needed or throughout the day. Lack of adequate oxygen can damage organs, decrease alertness, induce feelings of fatigue, and cause shortness of breath. ICF codes treated include b110 Consciousness Functions, b114 Orientation Functions, b130 Energy and Drive Functions, b140 Attention Functions, b410 Heart Functions, b430 Hematological System Functions, and b450 Additional Respiratory Functions.

Exercise training: Exercise training is a cornerstone of pulmonary rehabilitation. Exercise training consists of endurance (b455 Exercise Tolerance Functions), strength (b730 Muscle Power Functions), and flexibility training (b710 Mobility of Joint Functions) to improve functioning related to deconditioning. Endurance training is predominantly addressed through walking and use of a stationary bicycle to enhance abilities to complete daily activities such as caring for oneself (d5 Self-Care, d6 Domestic Life). Strength training may include lifting weights, unsupported arm exercises, and TheraBands. Upper body training improves the flexibility of the respiratory muscles and muscle coordination resulting in improved oxygen efficiency. Flexibility training is addressed through range of motion and stretching exercises.

Education and psychosocial support: Clients are taught about (1) COPD and their role in managing it with the hope that it will increase compliance with recommendations; (2) energy conservation and work simplification techniques; (3) their medications actions, side effects, proper dosage, and proper use; (4) oxygen therapy (what it is, how to connect and disconnect oxygen, how to use a nasal cannula, safety issues, transport issues); (5) a living will, including whether they would like to write a living will; (6) importance of getting vaccines, particularly flu and pneumococcal vaccines to decrease risks of developing illnesses; (7) the need to quit smoking to slow down the progression of the disease along with strategies and products to assist with smoking cessation; (8) the need to stay away from pollutants and allergens that can affect lung function; (9) benefits of exercise; (10) stress management and relaxation techniques; (11) coping techniques; and (12) how to access resources. Each of these modules should be tied to a particular deficit noted in the assessment process.

Breathing techniques: Clients are taught and encouraged to use breathing techniques to help when feeling short of breath, addressing issues documented with b440 Respiration Functions, b445 Respiratory Muscle Functions, b450 Additional Respiratory Functions, and b455 Exercise Tolerance Functions.

- *Pursed-lip breathing (PLB)*: Pursed lip breathing is used when the client feels short of breath from activity, stress, or anxiety. Short and rapid breathing patterns are common in people who have COPD. PLB makes the client focus on a slower breathing pattern. When the lips are pursed while exhaling, pressure within the airway increases, which helps to keep the airway open. When inhaling with the lips pursed, the major portion of the work is transferred from the diaphragm to the ribcage muscles. Resting the diaphragm also helps to reduce shortness of breath. Technique: The client is instructed to purse his/her lips (as if to whistle or blow out a candle) and slowly exhale for four to six seconds.

- *Leaning forward posture*: Leaning forward posture is helpful to reduce shortness of breath because it reduces respiratory effort. A client who is short of breath should sit down and lean forward (e.g., rest arms on a tabletop) and then perform PLB to open up the airway.

Nutritional counseling: People with COPD often do not have an adequate dietary intake. They also burn more calories with minimal activities because of increased resting energy expenditure, have difficulty obtaining food from the market because they don't have enough energy to accomplish shopping activities, and may lack a healthy adaptation for this problem. Poor nutritional intake also affects the client's energy, which makes it even harder to obtain food. The treatment team educates clients with COPD about the importance of maintaining a proper weight and receiving adequate nutrition to maintain strength (d570 Looking After One's Health, and covering problems noted in b455 Exercise Tolerance Functions, d620 Acquisition of Goods and Services, and d630 Preparing Meals). This is also coupled with problem solving and resource awareness to help with carryover. On the opposite side of the spectrum, obesity can also affect respiratory function. Extra body weight puts a greater strain on the respiratory system, especially for activities that require the client to stand or walk. Clients who are overweight are encouraged to decrease body fat. Issues that surround the person's ability to obtain healthy food (e.g., eating home delivery fast food is easier that going to the supermarket) need to be addressed and counseling sessions with a nutritionist are recommended to develop healthy meal plans.

Self-image changes: The incorporation of exercise into the client's daily routine after discharge can be very difficult for clients on many different levels. It is a new way of thinking and behaving. People who are seen in inpatient rehabilitation for COPD typically have moderate to severe COPD and have mostly adapted to the COPD by giving up activities that cause shortness of breath, specifically activities that require physical exertion. This results in staying at home more; having fewer social contacts; deconditioning from lack of exercise; experiencing feelings of depression, anxiety, and/or isolation; lack of outside stimulation with possible disorientation; and difficulties in obtaining supplies from the community. Energy is typically reserved and spent only on necessary self-care activities, such as bathing, dressing, and simple meal preparation. Breaking this long-term cycle of behavior can be difficult and adopting a different view of pulmonary care through exercise may not be easily accepted. Although clients experience the pulmonary benefits of exercise firsthand while at the rehabilitation center and may verbalize their intention to follow an exercise program after discharge, carryover is often poor. To increase the likelihood of exercise carryover, problem solving, resource awareness, education, and development of a positive self-image must be included in the rehabilitation program. Codes that can be addressed with this part of treatment include b130 Energy and Drive Functions, b134 Sleep Functions, b455 Exercise Tolerance Functions, d177 Making Decisions, d240 Handling Stress and Other Psychological Demands, d910 Community Life, and d920 Recreation and Leisure.

Adaptive equipment: The prescription of adaptive equipment can help decrease the amount of energy used for specific tasks. This may include a mobility aid such as a cane, walker, or wheelchair; a self-care piece of equipment such as a dressing stick or a reacher; or a recreational aid such as lightweight gardening tools (d4 Mobility, e140 Products and Technology for Culture, Recreation, and Sport).

Psychosocial and behavioral intervention: This includes individual or group therapy that focuses on stress management and relaxation training, techniques for managing anxiety and panic to help reduce shortness of breath, techniques for managing feelings of depression, and discussions about healthy coping techniques (b126 Temperament and Personality

Functions, d240 Handling Stress and Other Psychological Demands). Ongoing support groups can be helpful for people with COPD and their families.

Recreational Therapy Approach

The recreational therapist addresses many of the topics described in the team approach. The difference is that the recreational therapist puts a much stronger focus on integration of these skills into the client's real-life environment, particularly related to engagement in recreation, leisure, and community activities that promote health and quality of life. Tying the changes to the client's interests increases the chances that the client will follow through with the suggested changes (b130 Energy and Drive Functions).

Recreational Therapy Interventions

Recreational therapists employ many of the interventions previously described, as they relate to leisure, recreation, and community engagement. This includes engagement in physical activity and knowledge of its benefits, energy conservation and work simplification, oxygen management during recreation and community activities, smoking cessation through developing new and healthy coping mechanisms and healthy "distractions" to break the habit, staying away from allergens and pollutants inherent in particular leisure and community activities, stress management and relaxation training, general coping techniques to combat anxiety and depression, accessing resources related to leisure and community engagement, breathing techniques, self-image, and adaptive equipment recommendations. Relevant ICF codes were included in the detailed descriptions of these interventions.

Additional RT interventions focus on using recreation as a modality to reduce the deficits noted in the diagnosis. Document how these interactions reduce deficits in d7 Interpersonal Interactions and Relationships, d8 Major Life Areas, and d9 Community, Social, and Civic Life. Also document how they increase the client's compliance with other interventions being carried out by the treatment team. Noting how social interactions and recreation and leisure activities improve compliance with specific treatment goals demonstrates their value in the overall treatment process. Possible interventions include:

Exploration of leisure interests, attitudes, and values: Given the progressive nature of the disease, individuals commonly give up leisure activities due to COPD symptoms and complications. In an effort to increase physical activity, social support, and psychological well-being, re-engagement in enjoyable leisure activities is needed. Individuals might have difficulty identifying leisure interests and require leisure interest exploration. Individuals might also have preconceived attitudes about leisure (e.g., "Working in the garden is something I like to do, but it isn't something I have to do, so there is no need for me to do it anymore.") and lack knowledge about the value of recreation, leisure, and community activities related to COPD management and health.

Activity pattern development: Assisting the client in developing a well-balanced activity pattern for post-discharge participation can be helpful in combating the tendency to fall back into a sedentary lifestyle. An activity pattern consists of a menu of activities, which are then plugged into a weekly schedule. When working on the activity pattern, the discussion topics include balancing choices, the timing of activities as it relates to other activities and functioning, and outside resources. The client must learn to allow opportunities for rest breaks, complete physically demanding activities at a time when the client has the most energy, and effectively take advantages of outside resources, such as a daughter who is usually available on Saturday mornings to go shopping.

Leisure resource awareness: Clients might require education about home and community leisure resources related to activity engagement, such as items available in the home for leisure engagement, scholarship funds available to pay for membership at the local Y, transportation services, and places to go in the community to engage in leisure activities. Identified resources are often written down and given to the client for future reference.

Enhancement of social support: Since individuals with COPD tend to be isolative, their social support network diminishes, along the related benefits, such as having others to confide in, having help with problem solving, testifying to the value of one's life, and feeling a sense of love and belonging. Opportunities to develop and enhance social support should be routinely explored through clubs, organizations, Skype, email, leisure activities where one can meet others who have similar interests, and other activities.

Community integration training: The therapist goes into the community with the client to apply techniques in the clients real-life environment, problem solve for unforeseen barriers, and bolster self-efficacy related to independent engagement.

Resources

Agency for Healthcare Research and Quality, National Guideline Clearinghouse

www.guideline.gov

For COPD guidelines see

www.guideline.gov/content.aspx?id=23801

National Heart, Lung, and Blood Institute

www.nhlbi.nih.gov

Stimulates basic discoveries about the causes of disease, enables the translation of basic discoveries into clinical practice, fosters training and mentoring of emerging scientists and physicians, and communicates research advances to the public.

References

American Lung Association. (2013). Chronic obstructive pulmonary disease: Fact sheet. Retrieved from http://www.lung.org/lung-disease/copd/resources/facts-figures/COPD-Fact-Sheet.html.

American Lung Association. (2010). State of lung disease in diverse communities. Retrieved from http://www.lung.org/assets/documents/publications/solddc-chapters/copd.pdf.

Jacob, E. (2012). *Medifocus guidebook on chronic obstructive pulmonary disease*. Medifocus.

Lan, C. K., Nici, L., & Wallack, R. Z. (2011). Pulmonary rehabilitation. In Hanania, N. A. & Sharafkhaneh, A. (Eds.). *COPD: A guide to diagnosis and clinical management* (pp 167-190). New York: Humana Press.

Mayo Clinic. (2014). COPD complications. Retrieved from http://www.mayoclinic.org/diseases-conditions/seo/basics/complications/CON-20032017.

National Heart, Lung, and Blood Institute. (2014). What is COPD? Retrieved from http://www.nhlbi.nih.gov/health/health-topics/topics/copd/.

National Heart, Lung, and Blood Institute. (2010). What is pulmonary rehabilitation? Retrieved from http://www.nhlbi.nih.gov/health/health-topics/topics/pulrch/.

11. Diabetes Mellitus

Heather R. Porter

Diabetes mellitus (DM) is a complex disease that occurs when insulin production is too low (or lacking entirely) or when the body is unable to effectively use the insulin it produces because of defects in the insulin receptors. The result is that the body does not metabolize carbohydrates, protein, or fat correctly, leading to severe complications and death if it is not treated.

The body, in its normal state, manufactures insulin to transport sugar in the form of glucose into cells. The cells use the sugar for energy. In diabetes, the body does not properly produce or use insulin. Therefore, glucose builds up in the blood causing a variety of health problems. Many cases of DM go undetected because the symptoms mimic symptoms of other problems. The symptoms include excessive thirst, extreme hunger, frequent urination, unusual weight loss, increased fatigue, irritability, and blurry vision. It is often seeking medical attention for another health problem, such as a circulation problem or a wound that won't heal, that results in the diagnosis of DM.

There are four primary classifications of diabetes (Centers for Disease Control and Prevention [CDC], 2011).

Type 1 diabetes (T1D): Insulin dependent diabetes mellitus (IDDM) and juvenile-onset diabetes are now called T1D. T1D develops when the body's immune system destroys the pancreatic beta cells that make insulin. It primarily occurs in children and young adults. Risk factors for T1D include autoimmune, genetic, and environmental factors.

Type 2 diabetes (T2D): Non-insulin dependent diabetes mellitus (NIDDM) and adult-onset diabetes are now T2D. It is the most common form of diabetes accounting for 90-95% of diabetes cases. The body does not produce enough insulin or the cells cannot use the insulin properly so there is a build-up of glucose in the bloodstream. If glucose levels are not reduced, damage can occur to many body systems including the eyes, kidneys, nerves, and heart. T2D is associated with older age, obesity, family history of diabetes, prior history of gestational diabetes, impaired glucose tolerance, physical inactivity, and race/ethnicity. Clients who have T2D can usually control their blood glucose by following a special diabetic diet, participating in a regular exercise program, achieving and maintaining ideal body weight, and taking oral medication. Insulin may also be needed.

Gestational diabetes (GD): During pregnancy some women develop GD, a form of glucose intolerance. GD occurs more frequently among African-Americans, Hispanic/Latin Americans, and Native Americans. It is also more common among obese women and women with a family history of diabetes. During pregnancy, GD requires treatment to normalize maternal blood glucose levels to avoid complications in the infant.

Pre-diabetes: Pre-diabetes is a condition that occurs when a person's blood glucose levels are higher than normal but not high enough for a diagnosis of T2D.

Incidence/Prevalence in U.S.

According to the Centers for Disease Control and Prevention (2011), diabetes is the seventh leading cause of death in the U.S. It currently affects 25.8 million Americans or 8.3% of the population. About 18.8 million have been diagnosed and seven million have not been diagnosed. It is one of the leading causes of blindness, kidney failure, and lower extremity amputations. If current trends continue, one out of three adults will have diabetes by 2050. Recent information about the 43% drop in childhood obesity among all two- to five-year-olds suggest that the trends may be changing (Tavernise, 2014).

More than 13,000 young people are diagnosed with T1D every year (CDC, 2013). It is difficult to distinguish between T1D and T2D in children using currently available medical tests (CDC, 2013). It is also difficult to diagnose children and adolescents with T2D because it can go undiagnosed due to lack of (or mild) symptoms (CDC, 2013). Consequently, trying to estimate prevalence in this population is challenging (CDC, 2013).

GD ranges from two to ten percent of pregnancies; and women who had GD have a 35-60% chance of developing diabetes in the next 10-20 years (National Diabetes Information Clearinghouse [NDIC], 2011).

It is estimated that about 79 million U.S. adults 20 years of age and older have prediabetes.

Predominant Age

In 2010, approximately 11.8% of American men and 10.8% of American women 20 years of age or older had diabetes (NDIC, 2013). Approximately 25% of U.S. older adults (65+) had diabetes (NDIC, 2013).

In 2010, approximately 215,000 American youth younger than 20 years of age had T1D or T2D (NDIC, 2013). The rate of T2D has been steadily growing in this population (NDIC, 2013; CDC, 2013).

When compared to non-Hispanic white adults, the risk of being diagnosed with diabetes is approximately 18% higher among Asian Americans, 66% higher among Hispanics/Latinos, and 77% higher among non-Hispanic blacks (NDIC, 2013).

Causes

T1D: T1D is caused by an autoimmune disease, predominantly hereditary, that attacks and destroys beta cells in the pancreas. Environmental factors such as viruses, infections, and foods are thought to trigger the autoimmune reaction (NDIC, 2011).

T2D: T2D is triggered by a combination of genetic, personal, and environmental factors. Heredity seems to play a role. African Americans, Alaska Natives, American Indians, Pacific Islanders of American descent, and Hispanics/Latinos have a higher risk. Having a parent or sibling with T2D also increases risk. Personal factors that increase risk include obesity, being middle-aged, physical inactivity, high blood pressure, bad cholesterol

levels; polycystic ovary syndrome, prediabetes, acanthosis nigricans (a dark rash around the neck or armpits), and history of cardiovascular disease (NDIC, 2011). In women the risk is increased when they give birth to a baby over nine pounds or have a history of GD. Lack of physical activity results in insulin resistance where muscle, fat, and liver cells stop responding properly to insulin, forcing the pancreas to compensate by producing extra insulin. Some of the responses include abnormal glucose production by the liver, which continues to produce high levels of glucose after a meal when glucose levels and insulin are high, problems with cell signaling that affect the regulation of insulin and glucose, and beta cell dysfunction that causes abnormal insulin release (NDIC, 2011; NDIC, 2013). Metabolic syndrome is another risk factor. The cluster of symptoms for metabolic syndrome include elevated fasting blood glucose levels of 100 mg/dl or higher; waist circumference of 40 inches or more for men and 35 inches or more for women; high blood pressure of 130 mmHg or higher systolic blood pressure and 85 mmHg or higher diastolic blood pressure; and low levels of good cholesterol with HDL below 40 mg/dl for men and below 50 mg/dl for women. The waist measurement matters even if the person's Body Mass Index is in the healthy/normal range (NDIC, 2012). Obesity, low level of physical activity, and exposure to diabetes in uterus are believed to be major contributors to the increase in T2D among children and adolescents (CDC, 2013)

GD: GD is caused by hormonal changes and metabolic demands associated with pregnancy, along with genetic, environmental, and personal factors (NDIC, 2011).

Systems Affected

Diabetes affects the endocrine system. In the ICF it is documented with code b540 General Metabolic Functions. Other bodily systems can be subsequently affected through the disease process, as described in the Secondary Problems section. Despite pharmacological and lifestyle interventions, diabetes is not always easily controlled. Although controlling diabetes decreases the risk of developing problems from the disease, it does not guarantee that the disease will not affect other systems.

Secondary Problems

Secondary metabolic problems depend on the severity of the disease. All of the problems dealing with blood sugar and blood ketones are documented with b540 General Metabolic Functions, b545 Water, Mineral, and Electrolyte Balance Functions, and b610 Urinary Excretory Functions. Possible problems include:

Hypoglycemia: This is when blood sugar becomes too low. Symptoms include shakiness, dizziness, sweating, hunger, headache, pale skin color, sudden moodiness or behavior changes, clumsy or jerky movements, seizure, difficulty paying attention, confusion, and tingling sensations around the mouth. If hypoglycemia occurs, blood sugar can be raised by ingesting 15 grams of simple carbohydrates, such as glucose tablets, one-half cup of fruit juice, two tablespoons of raisins, one tablespoon of sugar or honey, eight ounces of nonfat or 1% milk, or several pieces of hard candy. Clients are taught to carry glucose testing supplies (glucometer and test strips) and a form of sugar at all times to manage hypoglycemia. Clients are encouraged to check their glucose level as soon as they feel low glucose coming on. After blood glucose is tested and treatment is started, glucose should be rechecked at 15-20 minutes to see if the level went back up. If glucose is still low and symptoms persist, treat it again with more sugar and wait another 15-20 minutes to check the blood glucose again. If blood glucose levels do not rise, the client could pass out. If this occurs, immediate treatment is required, such as an injection of glucagon or emergency treatment in a hospital. The client is educated on how to self-inject glucagon and told to train others (family, friends, coworkers) on how to inject it if s/he passes out. If glucagon is not available, the client will need to be taken to the closest emergency room for treatment of low blood glucose (ADA, 2013b).

Hyperglycemia: This is when blood glucose becomes too high. This could be caused by injection of too little insulin or when the body is not using insulin effectively. The signs and symptoms of hyperglycemia include high levels of sugar in the urine, frequent urination, and increased thirst. Exercising can often lower blood glucose, however if blood glucose is above 240 mg/dl, the urine must be checked for ketones with a urine stick. If ketones are present, exercise is contraindicated because it will increase the ketone level and can further raise the blood glucose level. Any time blood glucose levels stay high, the client will need to seek further treatment (ADA, 2013a).

Ketoacidosis: This is a serious condition where excess ketones and acidosis develop because of faulty carbohydrate metabolism. When carbohydrates can't be used for fuel, the body metabolizes proteins instead. The waste products include so many ketones that the body can't get rid of all of them in the urine. It mostly occurs in clients who have T1D and can rarely occur in clients with T2D. Ketoacidosis usually develops slowly, but when vomiting occurs, the condition can develop within a few hours. The first symptoms of ketoacidosis are thirst or a very dry mouth, frequent urination, high blood glucose levels that are detected using a glucometer, and high levels of ketones in the urine that are detected by a urine stick. Next, other symptoms occur, such as constantly feeling tired, dry or flushed skin, nausea, vomiting, abdominal pain, difficulty breathing, a fruity odor on the breath, a hard time paying attention, or confusion. Ketoacidosis is life threatening and requires immediate treatment (ADA, 2014b).

Hyperosmolar hyperglycemic nonketotic syndrome (HHNS): HHNS can take days or weeks to develop. It occurs in both T1D and T2D, although it is most common in T2D. It is usually brought on by an illness or infection. In HHNS, the blood glucose levels rise and the body tries to get rid of the excess glucose through the urine. At first, the body makes lots of urine and later the amount of urine becomes less and very dark. The client may become very thirsty from so much loss of fluid. Even if the client is not thirsty, s/he is to drink lots of liquids because of the chance of becoming dehydrated. Severe dehydration will lead to seizures, coma, and eventually death. Warning signs of HHNS include a blood glucose level over 600 mg/dl, dry and parched mouth, extreme thirst (although this may gradually disappear), warm and dry skin that does not sweat, high fever of over 101°F, sleepiness or confusion, loss of vision, hallucinations, and weakness on one side of the body (ADA, 2013c).

Other problems will be found. They should be documented using ICF codes that describe the deficits observed. The problems include (NDIC, 2011; ADA, 2014b):

Hypertension: Approximately two-thirds of adults with diabetes have high blood pressure (b420 Blood Pressure Functions).

Heart disease and stroke: Heart disease is the leading cause of diabetes-related deaths. Adults with diabetes are twice as likely to have heart disease or stroke (b410 Heart Functions, b415 Blood Vessel Functions). See the chapters on Cerebrovascular Accident and Heart Disease for more information.

Blindness: Approximately one-third of individuals 40 years of age or older with diabetes have diabetic retinopathy (b210 Seeing Functions).

Kidney disease: Diabetes is the leading cause of kidney failure, accounting for about 45% of all new kidney failure cases (b545 Water, Mineral, and Electrolyte Balance Functions, b610 Urinary Excretory Functions).

Nervous system disease: Approximately 60-70% of adults with diabetes have mild to severe nervous system damage including impaired sensation or pain in hands or feet, slowed digestion, carpal tunnel syndrome, and erectile dysfunction. About 30% of adults with diabetes have impaired sensation in the feet, which is a contributing factor to lower extremity amputations. ICF codes that need to be considered include b265 Touch Function, b270 Sensory Functions Related to Temperature and Other Stimuli, and b280 Sensation of Pain.

Amputations: More than 60% of non-traumatic lower extremity amputations are due to diabetes. See the chapter on Amputations for ICF codes to use.

Dental disease: Almost one-third of people with diabetes have severe periodontal diseases with loss of attachment of the gums to the teeth measuring five millimeters or more. ICF codes include d5201 Caring for Teeth and s320 Structure of Mouth.

Complications of pregnancy: Poorly controlled diabetes before conception and during the first trimester of pregnancy can cause major birth defects in five to ten percent of pregnancies and spontaneous abortions in 15-20% of pregnancies. Poorly controlled diabetes during the second and third trimesters of pregnancy can result in excessively large babies, posing a risk to the mother and the child.

Other complications: Because diabetes reduces functioning of the energy production systems, people with diabetes often have lower energy levels and less tolerance for exercise. These can be documented with codes b130 Energy and Drive Functions, b455 Exercise Tolerance Functions, and b530 Weight Maintenance Functions. Lifestyle choices are part of the reason people have T2D. Treatable areas can be documented with ICF codes d240 Handling Stress and Other Psychological Demands, d450 Walking, or other exercise codes. Because diabetes requires additional care in maintaining health, deficits may also be noted in d520 Caring for Body Parts and d570 Looking After One's Health. Uncontrolled diabetes often leads to biochemical imbalances that can cause acute, life-threatening events, such as diabetic ketoacidosis and hyperosmolar (nonketotic) coma (b110 Consciousness Functions). People with diabetes are more susceptible to many other illnesses and, once they acquire these illnesses, often have worse prognoses than people without diabetes.

Prognosis

T1D: Clients who have T1D will need to take insulin via an insulin pump or injections for their entire life, as well as engage in healthy eating, physical activity, and regular glucose testing (NDIC, 2013). There are no known methods to prevent or cure T1D.

T2D: The prognosis for people who have T2D will vary depending on the level of glucose control that client is able to maintain. In some cases, if the client loses enough weight, individuals with T2D are able to reduce or eliminate medication (NDIC, 2013).

GD: After giving birth, GD generally resolves; however, after pregnancy, five to 10% of women with GD have T2D (NDIC, 2013).

Pre-diabetes: Clients with pre-diabetes can prevent the development of T2D through diet and exercise. Thirty minutes a day, five times a week, of moderate physical activity and a seven percent reduction in body weight produces about a 58% reduction in diabetes, as the glucose levels return to normal ranges (American Diabetes Association [ADA], 2014a).

Assessment

Typical Scope of Team Assessment

There are three tests that determine if a client has pre-diabetes or diabetes in non-pregnant women (ADA, 2014a; NDIC, 2012). One is the fasting blood glucose test (FBG), also called the fasting plasma glucose test (FPG). A fasting blood glucose level between 100 and 125 mg/dl signals pre-diabetes and greater than 126 mg/dl confirms diabetes. The second test is the oral glucose tolerance test (OGTT). The client has to fast and then drink a glucose-rich beverage. Two hours after drinking the beverage, a blood glucose level is taken. A level between 140 and 199 mg/dl signals pre-diabetes and a level greater than 200 mg/dl confirms diabetes. The last test is the A1c test, also called the hemoglobin A1c, HbA1c, or glycohemoglobic test. It is a blood test that provides information about the client's average blood glucose levels over the past three months. An A1c level of 5.7% to 6.4% indicates prediabetes, while 6.5% or greater indicates diabetes. It is important to note that glucose levels from these tests can vary. Results can differ among tests and from one test to the next. One test may indicate diabetes, while another test does not or last month's levels indicated diabetes, but this month's levels indicated prediabetes (NDIC, 2012). Each of the three tests also measures glucose differently. Results can also vary due to laboratory testing variables. Consequently, continued monitoring is important to look for patterns of increased glucose levels to confirm the diagnosis.

In addition to testing, questions are asked to ascertain whether or not the client exhibits symptoms of diabetes including increased urination, increased thirst, unexplained weight loss, fatigue, blurred vision, increased hunger, and sores that don't heal (NDIC, 2012).

In women who are pregnant, diabetes is tested between 24 and 28 weeks of pregnancy using a three-hour fasting glucose challenge (a 100-gram glucose drink). Before drinking the glucose, a fasting blood draw is taken. Blood is also drawn once each hour during the test. A diagnosis of GD is given if one or more of the glucose levels are high. The standards are fasting levels of 95 or above; levels one hour after the drink of 180 or above; levels two hours after the drink of 155 or above; or levels three hours after drink of 140 or above (NDIC, 2012).

The primary metabolic effects of diabetes are documented in the ICF using b540 General Metabolic Functions. Other complications are documented as described in Secondary Problems.

Clients are admitted to a rehabilitation facility when disabling complications from diabetes occur. The healthcare team assesses the past and present management of the disease to plan future treatment and analyzes the client's lifestyle to identify areas for intervention.

Areas of Concern for RT Assessment

If the client is seen in a rehabilitation facility with a secondary diagnosis of diabetes and a primary diagnosis of a complication of diabetes, such as stroke, heart disease, or amputation, it can be suspected that blood glucose levels have not been effectively managed via medication, insulin, and/or lifestyle changes. Since diabetes can affect many body systems, and the severity of diabetes can vary depending upon how well glucose levels were controlled, specific findings will vary by client. Recreational therapists can expect to find deficits in a variety of personal and environmental factors that may need interventions, such as smoking, lack of physical activity, and missing social supports. Code these using d570 Looking After One's Health, b455 Exercise Tolerance Functions, d910 Community Life, and d920 Recreation and Leisure.

ICF Core Set

ICF Core Sets that might be helpful in identifying relevant ICF codes, depending upon the client's diabetes-related complications include Chronic Ischemic Heart Disease, Diabetes Mellitus, and Obesity.

Treatment Direction

Whole Team Approach

Once a client is diagnosed with diabetes, the team seeks to control the client's glucose levels through pharmacology and lifestyle changes. Data from 2007-2009 indicate that the majority of adults with diabetes were treated with oral medication only (58%), followed by no medication (16%), insulin and oral medication (14%), and insulin only (12%) (NDIC, 2011). ICF codes b540 General Metabolic Functions, b545 Water, Mineral, and Electrolyte Balance Functions, and b610 Urinary Excretory Functions can be referenced for this treatment.

The client is educated about lifestyle changes to manage glucose levels and prevent secondary complications. The treatment team or diabetes self-management education programs, as described by Mensing (2004) can provide the education. This education is vitally important, as it has been found that people who do not receive diabetes education show a fourfold increased risk of a major complication (Nicolucci et al., 1996). Treatment to reduce deficits in self-care can be coded with d520 Caring for Body Parts and d570 Looking After One's Health.

Some of the specific educational components include (ADA, 2014a; NDIC, 2013):

Proper nutrition: Adhering to a diabetic diet will help with glucose control and reduce central body fat to help cells respond better to insulin (b530 Weight Maintenance Functions).

Regular physical activity: Thirty minutes a day of moderate physical activity can: build and maintain muscle mass that burns calories and increases glucose uptake, lower blood glucose levels, improve the body's response to insulin, reduce or even eliminate the need for diabetes medication by lowering blood glucose levels, lower cholesterol and reduce blood pressure, improve circulation, and reduce the risk for heart disease and stroke. Weight loss and exercise are the most important modifiable lifestyle behaviors in managing diabetes (Horton, 1998). Regular physical activity has also been associated with positive changes in self-efficacy, self-esteem, and psychological stress (Castaneda, 2000). ICF codes include b130 Energy and Drive Functions, b455 Exercise Tolerance Functions, b530 Weight Maintenance Functions, d240 Handling Stress and Other Psychological Demands, d450 Walking, or other exercise codes, d520 Caring for Body Parts and d570 Looking After One's Health.

Cardiovascular disease: The risk of cardiovascular disease can be lowered with diet, weight loss, exercise, and smoking cessation. Improved control of cholesterol and lipids can reduce cardiovascular complications by 20-50% (b410 Heart Functions, b415 Blood Vessel Functions).

Smoking: Smoking compromises the cardiovascular system and increases the risk for diabetic complications such as amputation and myocardial infarction. Smoking may even have a role in the development of T2D (d570 Looking After One's Health).

Preventive care practices for eyes, feet, and kidneys: Laser therapy for diabetic eye disease can reduce severe vision loss by 50-60%. About 65% of adults with diabetes have improved vision with prescription eyeglasses (b210 Seeing Functions). Comprehensive foot care programs can reduce am-

putation risk by 45-85% (d520 Caring for Body Parts). Lowering blood pressure can reduce decline in kidney function by 30-70% (b545 Water, Mineral, and Electrolyte Balance Functions, b610 Urinary Excretory Functions).

Glucose Level Awareness

Clients are taught to be aware of the symptoms of too much or too little glucose in the blood. Depending on the client's level of competence, the client and/or his/her caretakers are taught how to check for blood glucose levels and ketones (b540 General Metabolic Functions, b545 Water, Mineral, and Electrolyte Balance Functions, d570 Looking After One's Health).

Glucose levels are measured using a glucometer (also called a glucose meter). A disposable glucose-reading strip is placed into the glucometer. The finger is then pricked using a lancet (a tiny needle inserted into a spring-loaded lancing device). The finger is squeezed to produce a small droplet of blood. The blood droplet is then placed on the reading strip. Within a matter of a few seconds, the glucometer will display the glucose reading. The physician will tell the client how frequently to check glucose levels, as this can vary, usually from one to four times a day. Additional glucose level tests should also be done when abnormal symptoms are experienced. Glucose readings are written down in a log to identify patterns and monitor glucose control. The log is reviewed at medical appointments to determine if adjustments in testing or medications are needed.

Ketones are tested using a urine stick. The client simply holds the urine stick underneath the urine stream when using the bathroom or collects the urine in a cup and dips the stick into the urine. Ketones are tested when glucose is greater than 300 mg/dL; when the client is sick; or when the client is nauseous or vomiting, tired, thirsty, in a fog, or having abdominal pain, difficulty breathing, dry mouth, or "fruity" smelling breath.

The client is instructed to always have a source of sugar available for hypoglycemia, to get treatment for hyperglycemia, and get immediate treatment for ketoacidosis.

Track ABCs of Diabetes

A (A1c Target and Blood Glucose Targets): A1c should be below seven percent, blood glucose levels before meals should be 90-130 mg/dl and one to two hours after the start of the meal should be less than 180 mg/dl. Reducing A1c blood test results by one point can reduce the risk of microvascular complications by 40% (b415 Blood Vessel Functions).

B (Blood Pressure Target): Blood pressure should be below 140/80 mmHg. Blood pressure control can reduce cardiovascular disease by approximately 33-50%, and can reduce microvascular disease by approximately 33%. In general, for every 10-mmHg reduction in systolic blood pressure, the risk for any complication related to diabetes is reduced by 12%. Reducing diastolic blood pressure from 90 mmHg to 80 mmHg reduces the risk of major cardiovascular events by 50% (b415 Blood Vessel Functions, b420 Blood Pressure Functions).

C (Cholesterol Targets): LDL (bad) cholesterol should be under 100 mg/dl, HDL (good) cholesterol should be above 40 mg/dl for men and above 50 mg/dl for women, and triglycerides should be under 150 mg/dl. Improved control of cholesterol levels can reduce cardiovascular complications by 20-50% (b415 Blood Vessel Functions). Clients should include at least 14 grams of fiber daily for every 1,000 calories consumed, decrease saturated and trans fat, and consume no more than 300 milligrams a day of cholesterol.

Recreational Therapy Approach

Therapists focus on education about diabetes and its complications and how they will affect the client's level of independence, functioning, and quality of life. Education in the clinic, however, is not enough. Therapists also teach clients how to manage diabetes in real-life settings through integration training. This helps to increase feelings of self-efficacy and leads to better outcomes (Jack, 2003).

Recreational therapists also look for lifestyle changes that the client can make to improve his/her prognosis, such as helping a client find better exercise and eating patterns. The therapists can also work on raising the level of self-efficacy of the client so that the client has the ability and desire to follow through on a healthier lifestyle.

Recreational therapists who work with clients who have diabetes must also know how to test for ketones, blood glucose levels, and take vital signs if needed during treatment sessions, including community integration training sessions.

Recreational Therapy Interventions

Interventions will vary depending on the severity of the disease and secondary problems and conditions. Interventions that relate to the general management of diabetes include:

Education and counseling: The therapist teaches the client about diabetes as it relates to involvement in activity (e.g., monitoring glucose levels in a community setting) and how to minimize the risks of complications from the disease through lifestyle changes in the areas of nutrition, exercise, smoking cessation, blood pressure control, and weight control. Education and counseling also include problem solving for overcoming barriers related to lifestyle changes, leisure education and counseling for leisure values, attitudes and beliefs that impact behavior, activity-specific education and counseling on how to conserve energy in the community, and activity adaptations and modifications to maximize participation. Many of the above can be coded as b455 Exercise Tolerance Functions, d240 Handling Stress and Other Psychological Demands, d520 Caring for Body Parts, and d570 Looking After One's Health.

Skill development: The therapist assists the client in developing skills related to the education and counseling provided including physical activity skills, such as aerobic capacity; relaxation training, such as deep breathing and progressive muscle relaxation; and checking glucose levels in a community setting. Choose the appropriate ICF code related to the specific skill (e.g., b455 Exercise Tolerance Functions, d240 Handling Stress and Other Psychological Demands, d520 Caring for Body Parts, and d570 Looking After One's Health) or choose a general skill development code, such as d155 Acquiring Skills.

Leisure time physical activity (LTPA): Engagement in LTPA deserves special attention. Skeletal muscles are responsible for burning 70-85% of the glucose in the bloodstream (Cartee, 1994), so an exercise program that decreases body fat and increases muscle mass is ideal (Castaneda, 2000). For people with diabetic retinopathy and/or neuropathy, sustained isometric muscle contractions increase the risk for retinal detachment and vitreous hemorrhage, so they should be avoided. Light weights and high repetitions with exercises that are adapted for the client's abilities and limitations are usually appropriate. Clearance by the client's physician is required prior to engaging in physical activity. Foot injuries should be avoided with proper footwear, adequate fluids are required, and glucose levels will need to be monitored any time the exercise routine is modified. Physical activities that the client can continue to engage in after discharge promotes continued engagement. A study of 26 adults with T2D utilizing the Leisure Meanings Gained and Outcomes Scale reported increased minutes of LTPA when participants experienced a sense of connection or belonging with individuals and groups. The positive feelings included attributes of belonging, such as feeling loved, a sense of connection or belonging within the self, a sense of building one's identity, a sense of control and power over one's self and things, a sense of competence/mastery, the experience of positive emotions of escalation, the experience of positive emotions of well-being, a sense of hope and optimism, and a feeling of continuing personal growth and development (Porter, Shank, & Iwasaki, 2012). The authors stated that, "Systemically structured leisure counseling, provided by a recreational therapist early in the disease process, aimed at identifying, exploring, and enhancing the experience of such personal meanings in LTPA may prove helpful in diabetes management" (p. 202). Previous studies with various populations have demonstrated that the feeling of enjoyment is associated with more minutes of LTPA (DiLorenzo et al., 1998; Johnson & Heller, 1998; Lindgren & Fridlung, 1999; Tsai, 2005; Dishman et al., 2005; Williams et al., 2006). The Porter et al. (2012) study "expands upon this finding and identifies underlying personal meaning as a modifiable variable for affecting the experience of positive emotion and subsequent LTPA engagement" (p. 212). The study also found that the longer participants engaged in their LTPA routines, the more they experienced a sense of internal balance, a sense of control and power over self and things, opportunities to reflect control and power to others, and human growth and development in new and different directions, "indicating that personal meanings can be further enhanced through long-term LTPA engagement" (p. 212). Potential opportunities for recreational therapists recommended by the authors include (1) designing transdisciplinary interventions aimed at the identification, exploration, and enhancement of personal meaning in physical activity for clients with T2D, framed within the Leisure Well-Being Model based on positive psychology; (2) delivering presentations at multidisciplinary conferences on diabetes prevention, management, and education to share information about research such as that reported in the study and associated leisure-related interventions; and (3) designing and disseminating self-management strategies and resources that reflect meaning-centered leisure engagement. Choose the specific ICF codes that most closely align with the desired outcome (e.g., d570 Looking After One's Health, b455 Exercise Tolerance Functions, d920 Recreation and Leisure).

Miscellaneous

Special Note about Insulin

Insulin can be stored at room temperature for about a month before it expires, however it can last much longer if stored in the refrigerator (ADA, 2014c). It cannot be placed in extreme heat like the glove compartment of a car or exposed to freezing temperatures (ADA, 2014c). Therefore, clients who need to take insulin into the community must be educated on its correct storage.

Resources

National Certification Board for Diabetes Educators
www.ncbde.org
Provides national certification for diabetes educators.

American Diabetes Association
www.diabetes.org
An organization that seeks to prevent and cure diabetes and to improve the lives of all people affected by diabetes.

References

American Diabetes Association. (2014a). Diagnosis diabetes and learning about prediabetes. Retrieved from http://www.diabetes.org/diabetes-basics/diagnosis/.
American Diabetes Association. (2014b). Complications. Retrieved from http://www.diabetes.org/living-with-diabetes/complications/.
American Diabetes Association. (2014c). Insulin. Retrieved from http://www.diabetes.org/living-with-diabetes/treatment-and-care/medication/insulin/.
American Diabetes Association. (2013a). Hyperglycemia. Retrieved from http://www.diabetes.org/living-with-diabetes/treatment-and-care/blood-glucose-control/hyperglycemia.html.
American Diabetes Association. (2013b). Hypoglycemia. Retrieved from http://www.diabetes.org/living-with-

diabetes/treatment-and-care/blood-glucose-control/hypoglycemia-low-blood.html.

American Diabetes Association. (2013c). Hyperosmolar Hyperglycemic Nonketotic Syndrome (HHNS). Retrieved from http://www.diabetes.org/living-with-diabetes/complications/hyperosmolar-hyperglycemic.html.

Cartee, J. D. (1994). Influence of age on skeletal muscle glucose transport and glycogen metabolism. *Med Sci Sports Exercise, 26*, 577-585.

Castaneda, C. (2000). Type 2 diabetes mellitus and exercise. *Nutrition in Clinical Care, 3*(6), 349-358.

Centers for Disease Control and Prevention. (2011). Diabetes: Success and opportunities for population-based prevention and control. Retrieved from http://www.cdc.gov/chronicdisease/resources/publications/AAG/ddt.htm.

Centers for Disease Control and Prevention. (2013). Children and diabetes: More information. Retrieved from http://www.cdc.gov/diabetes/projects/cda2.htm.

DiLorenzo, T. M., Stucky-Ropp, R. C., Vander Wal, J. S., & Gotham, H. J. (1998). Determinants of children's physical activity. *Preventive Medicine, 27*, 470-477.

Dishman, R. K., Motl, R. W., Saunders, R., Felton, G. Ward, D. S., Dowda, M., & Pate, R. R. (2005). Enjoyment mediates effects of a school-based physical-activity intervention. *Medical Science of Sports Exercise, 37*(3), 478-487.

Horton, E. (1998). Exercise and diabetes mellitus. *Med Clin North America, 72*, 1301-1321.

Jack, L. (2003). Diabetes self-management education research: An international review of intervention methods, theories, community partnerships, and outcomes. *Dis Manage Health Outcomes, 11*(7), 415-428.

Johnson, N. & Heller, R. (1998). Prediction of patient non-adherence with home-based exercise for cardiac rehabilitation: The role of perceived barriers and perceived benefits. *Preventive Medicine, 27*, 56-64.

Lindgren, E. & Fridlung, B. (1999). Influencing exercise adherence in physically non-active young women:

Suggestion for a model. *Women in Sport & Physical Activity Journal, 8*(2), 17-44.

Mensing, C. (2004). National standards for diabetes self-management education. *Diabetes Care, 27*, Sup 1.

National Diabetes Information Clearinghouse. (2013). National diabetes statistics, 2011. Retrieved from http://diabetes.niddk.nih.gov/dm/pubs/statistics/#fast.

National Diabetes Information Clearinghouse. (2011). Causes of diabetes. Retrieved from http://diabetes.niddk.nih.gov/dm/pubs/causes/.

National Diabetes Information Clearinghouse. (2012). Diagnosis of diabetes and prediabetes. Retrieved from http://diabetes.niddk.nih.gov/dm/pubs/diagnosis/.

National Diabetes Information Clearinghouse. (2013). Diabetes overview. Retrieved from http://www.diabetes.niddk.nih.gov/dm/pubs/overview/index.aspx.

Nicolucci, A., Cavaliere, D., Scorpiglione, N., Carinci, F., Capani, F., Tognoni, G., & Benedetti, M. M. (1996). A comprehensive assessment of the avoidability of long-term complications of diabetes. *Diabetes Care, 19*, 927-933.

Porter, H. R., Shank, J., Iwasaki, Y. (2012). Promoting a collaborative approach with recreational therapy to improve physical activity engagement in type 2 diabetes. *Therapeutic Recreation Journal, XLVI*(3), 202-217.

Tavernise S. (2014). Obesity rate for young children plummets 43% in a decade. *New York Times.* 2/25/14. Retrieved from http://www.nytimes.com/2014/02/26/health/obesity-rate-for-young-children-plummets-43-in-a-decade.html.

Tsai, E. (2005). A cross-cultural study of the influence of perceived positive outcomes on participation in regular active recreation: Hong Kong and Australian university students. *Leisure Sciences, 27*, 385-404.

Williams, D. M., Papandonatos, G. D., Napolitano, M. A., Lewis, B. A., Whiteley, J. A., & Marcus, B. H. (2006). Perceived enjoyment moderates the efficacy of an individually tailored physical activity intervention. *Journal of Sport and Exercise Psychology, 28*(3), 300-309.

12. Epilepsy

Susan E. Lynch

Epilepsy is a medical condition that affects brain neurons and causes abnormal signals. These abnormal signals may be caused by an imbalance of neurotransmitters or defects in the connections between neurons in the brain. When the abnormal signals cause a brief, strong surge of electrical activity that affects a portion or all of the brain, it is called a seizure. Seizures can last from a few seconds to a few minutes. Having a seizure does not necessarily mean that a person has epilepsy. Only when a person has had two or more unprovoked seizures is s/he diagnosed with epilepsy (National Institute of Neurological Disorders and Stroke [NINDS], 2013).

Seizures

The Centers for Disease Control and Prevention (2013) classify seizures into two major categories — *focal seizures* and *generalized seizures*. Not all seizures can be easily defined as either focal or generalized. Some people have seizures that begin as focal seizures but then spread to the entire brain. The NINDS (2013) list typical forms of focal and generalized seizures as documented below.

Focal seizures: Also called partial seizures, these begin in a localized area of the brain. They are frequently labeled by the area of the brain in which they originate.

- Simple focal seizure: Individuals remain conscious but experience unusual feelings or sensations. They can experience sudden and unexplainable emotions. They may also have unrealistic heightening of their senses.
- Complex focal seizure: Individuals experience an altered consciousness, in which they may experience a dreamlike experience that lasts a few seconds. They may display strange, repetitious behaviors called automatisms such as blinks, twitches, or mouth movements, or may experi-

ence auras (unusual sensations that warn of an impending seizure).

Generalized seizures: Generalized seizures are a result of abnormal neuronal activity that occurs in more than one area of the brain. These seizures may cause loss of consciousness, falls, or muscle spasms.

- Absence seizures: A momentary loss of consciousness of just a few seconds usually with no other symptoms. The muscles seem to jerk or twitch, and at times individuals seem to just stare into space. This may lead to the individual being unaware that they are having a seizure, only knowing that they have lost time. These seizures are sometimes referred to as petit mal seizures.
- Tonic seizures: These seizures cause stiffening of the back, leg, and arm muscles.
- Clonic seizures: Seizures of this type cause repetitive, rhythmic jerks that involve both sides of the body at the same time.
- Myoclonic seizures: Jerks or twitches of the upper body, arms, or legs are typical of these seizures.
- Atonic seizures: Seizures in this category cause a loss of normal muscle tone, which often results in a fall.
- Tonic-clonic seizures: A typical symptom of these seizures includes stiffening of the body and repeated jerks of the arms and/or legs as well as loss of consciousness. These are sometimes referred to as grand mal seizures.

Status epilepticus is a potentially life-threatening condition in which a person either has an abnormally prolonged seizure or does not fully regain consciousness between seizures. A prolonged seizure is one lasting longer than five minutes (Sirven, & Waterhouse, 2003). For reasons that are poorly understood, people with epilepsy have an increased risk of dying suddenly for no apparent reason (Donner, Smith, & Snead, 2001).

Different Kinds of Epilepsy

Just as there are many different kinds of seizures, there are many different kinds of epilepsy syndromes. These syndromes are disorders characterized by a specific set of symptoms that include epilepsy. Some of these syndromes appear to be hereditary, and for others the cause is unknown (NINDS, 2013). The Epilepsy Foundation of America (2012c) cites examples of epilepsy which include:

Absence epilepsy: Repeated seizures that cause momentary lapses of consciousness and usually have no lasting effect on intelligence or other brain functions.

Frontal lobe epilepsy: Seizures begin in the frontal lobe. Signs of this type of epilepsy can include muscle weakness or significant social effects that involve brief episodes of screaming or inappropriate sexual behavior. These seizures usually last less than a minute, are less likely to be followed by confusion or fatigue, and often occur in a series.

Temporal lobe epilepsy (TLE): This form of epilepsy can affect memory and learning due to damage to the hippocampus. It is the most common epilepsy syndrome occurring in childhood with focal seizures often associated with auras.

Neocortical epilepsy: Characterized by seizures that originate from the external surface layer of the brain. These seizures can cause strange sensations, visual hallucinations, emotional changes, and/or muscle spasms.

Lennox-Gastaut syndrome: Most children with this syndrome experience some degree of impaired intellectual functioning, along with developmental delays and behavioral issues.

Rasmussen's encephalitis: A rare, progressive type of epilepsy in which half of the brain shows continual inflammation. It is characterized by frequent seizures, loss of motor skills and speech, hemiparesis, dementia, and mental deterioration.

Incidence/Prevalence in U.S.

Epidemiologists base their estimates on peer-reviewed studies of medical records at specific institutions or in defined local communities. According to the CDC (2013), more than two million people in the United States (about one in one hundred) have experienced an unprovoked seizure or been diagnosed with epilepsy. More than 200,000 people are diagnosed with epilepsy every year (CDC, 2013). Incidence is highest in the first year of life, decreases in adolescence, and rises again dramatically after the age of 65 and is higher among racial minorities than among Caucasians. Incidence is greater in socially disadvantaged populations, males are slightly more likely to develop epilepsy, and in 70% of new cases there is no apparent reason. Traumatic head injuries can lead to epilepsy, so an increased incidence is expected among the veterans of the wars in Afghanistan and Iraq who have sustained head injuries (Epilepsy Foundation of America, 2012c).

Predominant Age

According to the Epilepsy Foundation of America (2012c), incidence is highest under the age of two and over 65. The basic, underlying risk of developing epilepsy is about one percent. It is estimated that epilepsy can be expected to develop in individuals in certain high-risk populations such as: 25.8% of children with intellectual disabilities, 13% of children with cerebral palsy, 50% of children with a diagnosis of intellectual disabilities and cerebral palsy, 10% of individuals with Alzheimer disease, 22% of persons who had a cerebrovascular accident (stroke), 8.7% of children of mothers with epilepsy, 2.4% of children of fathers with epilepsy, and 33% of people who have had a single, unprovoked seizure.

Causes

Epilepsy can be caused by medical conditions that affects the normal pattern of neuron activity, however it is important to note that in 70% of epileptic cases no direct cause can be identified (Epilepsy Foundation of America, 2012c). If a specific diagnosis of cause cannot be made, then the epilepsy will be described according to seizure type. For example, seizures are called symptomatic if they can be linked to identifiable diseases or brain abnormalities. Seizures are called cryptogenic when no cause can be found. A seizure that can be linked to a genetic cause is called an idiopathic or primary seizure. Causes of seizures (and sometimes epilepsy) are further divided into acute and remote causes. An acute cause classification depends on whether there is active brain disease and a remote cause is determined by whether the brain abnormality is the result of an injury caused by a previous event.

The most common causes discovered by research (NINDS, 2013) include:

Brain damage: In many cases, epilepsy develops as a result of brain damage from disorders that alter the brain such as traumatic brain injury, alcoholism, brain tumors, hydrocephalus, and Alzheimer's disease. Epilepsy can also develop if the brain is deprived of oxygen. Sometimes the brain's attempts to repair itself after a brain injury or stroke may inadvertently generate abnormal nerve connections that lead to epilepsy.

Infectious disease: Infectious diseases such as meningitis, AIDS, and viral encephalitis can lead to epilepsy. Epilepsy can also result from a parasitic infection of the brain called neurocysticercosis.

Intolerance to wheat gluten: Epilepsy also can result from intolerance to wheat gluten (celiac disease).

Brain development abnormalities: Metabolic disorders, cerebral palsy, Landau-Kleffner syndrome, autism, maternal infections, and poor nutrition can cause abnormalities during brain development, which may lead to disturbed neuron activity and epilepsy.

Genetic abnormalities: Abnormalities in genes that control development may have a partial role in contributing to epilepsy, perhaps by increasing a person's susceptibility to seizures that are triggered by an environmental factor.

Systems Affected

Epilepsy affects the central nervous system. A temporary disturbance of motor, sensory, or mental function may occur depending on the area of the brain affected by seizure activity (NINDS, 2013).

Secondary Problems

Secondary problems from epilepsy can be due to the effect of electrical discharges in or near the limbic system, secondary medication effects, psychological reactions to epilepsy, social factors, comorbid conditions, and/or sleep disorders (Ettinger & Kanner, 2006; Whatley, DiIorio, & Yeager, 2010). Secondary problems include depression, anxiety, migraine headaches, insomnia, and verbal or visual memory loss.

Prognosis

Most people with epilepsy lead normal lives. The impact of epileptic seizures on functional abilities and life activities varies depending on the frequency and severity of the epileptic seizures (American Academy of Neurology, 2013). Some individuals may go months or years between seizures, and others may have daily epileptic events (NINDS, 2013). Children with particular forms of epilepsy that resist treatment, such as Lennox-Gastaut syndrome, have a shorter life expectancy and an increased risk of cognitive impairment (NIH, Office of Rare Disease Research, n.d.).

Assessment

Typical Scope of Team Assessment

When a person has two or more seizures, the diagnosis of epilepsy is considered. To be formally diagnosed with epilepsy, a multi-step process is followed (NINDS, 2013):

1. A detailed medical history is taken, including symptoms and duration of the seizures.
2. A thorough neurological exam with EEG monitoring is done to detect abnormalities in the brain's electrical activity. Video and EEG monitoring are often used together to determine the nature of the seizures. Brain scans are done as appropriate. These include computed tomography (CT), positron emission tomography (PET), magnetic resonance imaging (MRI), single photon emission tomography (SPECT), magnetoencephalogram (MEG), magnetic resonance spectroscopy (MRS), and/or near-infrared spectroscopy (NIS). CT and MRI scans reveal the structure of the brain, which can identify brain tumors and cysts. PET is used to monitor the brain's activity and detect abnormalities in its functioning. SPECT is sometimes used to locate seizure foci in the brain. In some cases, the MEG (an experimental type of brain scan) is used to detect magnetic signals generated by neurons deep in the brain. Another experimental brain scan is a magnetic resonance spectroscopy (MRS) that can detect abnormalities in the brain's biochemical processes. Near-infrared spectroscopy (NIS) is a technique that can detect oxygen levels in brain tissue.

3. Blood samples are taken to determine if a person has a metabolic or genetic disorder associated with the seizures. It is also used to check for underlying problems such as infections, lead poisoning, anemia, and diabetes.

4. Developmental, neurological, and behavioral tests are often used to determine how epilepsy is affecting the person.

5. Identification of the type of seizure is made by the type of behavior and brain activity.

6. The team determines whether the seizure disorder falls within a recognized syndrome.

Documentation of the results can be made with ICF codes related to mental functions (b110 Consciousness Functions, b140 Attention Functions) and structure of the brain (s110 Structure of Brain). Secondary effects are reported with the appropriate codes. Most will be from codes in b1 Mental Functions and d1 Learning and Applying Knowledge.

Areas of Concern for RT Assessment

The anticipated findings will vary depending on the severity, the type of epilepsy, the effect of the seizures, and side effects of the medication (NINDS, 2013). Possible findings include:

- Decreased involvement or withdrawal from activities due to misunderstanding of epilepsy (b130 Energy and Drive Functions, d230 Carrying Out Daily Routine, d240 Handling Stress and Other Psychological Demands, d7 Interpersonal Interactions and Relationships, d9 Community, Social, and Civic Life) (Ettinger, Reed, & Cramer, 2004).

- Depression (b126 Temperament and Personality Functions) (Lee, Lee, & No, 2010).

- Over-concern about safety and over-protection limiting choices and options which could lead to learned helplessness, liability concerns, and fear (b125 Dispositions and Intra-Personal Functions, d250 Managing One's Own Behavior, d8 Major Life Areas, d9 Community, Social, and Civic Life) (Jacoby, 2002).

- Development of behavioral and emotional issues based on embarrassment; frustration; or bullying, teasing, and avoidance in school and other social settings (b125 Dispositions and Intra-Personal Functions, d570 Looking After One's Health, d7 Interpersonal Interactions and Relationships, d9 Community, Social, and Civic Life, e3 Support and Relationships) (Whiting, 2007; Mittan, 2010; Plioplys, Dunn, & Caplan, 2007).

- Memory issues: Damage to the left side of the brain causes difficulty with verbal memory, such as remembering conversations and written material, while damage to the right side can affect visual memory, such as scenes or directions. Memory loss can also be caused by side effects of medications (Hermann et al., 2010). Code with b144 Memory Functions.

- Photosensitivity: Epileptic seizures can be brought on by flickering light sources such as computer screens or fluorescent lights (e240 Light) (Shigihara & Tanaka, 2010; Epilepsy Foundation of America, 2012b).

- Learning, cognitive, and school difficulties for children due to stigma, as well as seizure type (d130-d159 Basic Learning, d160-d179 Applying Knowledge, d7 Interpersonal Interactions and Relationships, e3 Support and Relationships) (Whiting, 2007; Plioplys, Dunn, & Caplan, 2007).

Risk of seizures may restrict involvement in life activities such as driving (d475 Driving) and recreational activities (d9 Community, Social, and Civic Life). Some states refuse driver's licenses to people with epilepsy. The issue whether persons with epilepsy can safely participate in contact sports such as football, hockey, and boxing is controversial (Dubow & Kelly, 2003). The risk of drowning or serious injury in water sports such as swimming, scuba diving, and sailing is greater than that of the general population, though the absolute risk remains small, mostly occurring when unsupervised and without precautions (Lim, 2010). Motor sports should be monitored, because a seizure while driving a vehicle may cause harm to others as well as to the driver (Fountain & May, 2003).

ICF Core Set

An ICF Core Set for Epilepsy has not been developed.

Treatment Direction

Whole Team Approach

Accurate diagnosis of the type of epilepsy is crucial for finding effective treatment. Typical treatment includes a regimen of medication, surgery, implanted devices, diet, and dealing with psychosocial issues (Epilepsy Foundation of America, 2012). Medication, surgery, implanted devices, and dietary changes are performed to address ICF codes b110 Consciousness Functions, b140 Attention Functions, and s110 Structure of Brain. Psychosocial issues generally fall under b126 Temperament and Personality Functions, d7 Interpersonal Interactions and Relationships, and e3 Support and Relationships.

Medication: The most common approach to treating epilepsy is the prescription of antiepileptic drugs (AEDs) (Kwan & Brodie, 2007). More than 20 different antiepileptic drugs are now on the market, all with different benefits and side effects (Kwan & Brodie, 2007). AEDs can be divided into narrow spectrum AEDs, which mostly work for specific types of seizures such as partial, focal, absence, and myoclonic seizures (e.g., Dilantin, Tegretol, Lyrica, Sabril), and broad spectrum AEDs, which have some effectiveness for a wide variety of seizures such as partial, absence, and myoclonic seizures (e.g., Depakote, Lamictal, Topamax, Keppra, Klonopin). Some types of seizures are difficult to treat with any AED. The choice of which drug to prescribe, and at what dosage, depends on many different factors, including the type of seizures a person has, the person's lifestyle and age, and how frequently the seizures occur.

Surgery: When seizures cannot be adequately controlled by medications, the person may be evaluated for surgery. The most common surgical procedure for epilepsy is removal of a *seizure focus*, or small area of the brain where seizures originate. The most common type is a temporal lobectomy, which is performed when epilepsy begins in an area of the temporal lobe (Foldvary-Schaefer & Wyllie, 2007). Small portions of the hippocampus are removed. The hippocampus is a part of the limbic system and is involved in memory processing and controlling emotions.

Implanted device: A device called a vagus nerve stimulator may be surgically implanted. The device delivers short bursts of electrical energy to the brain via the vagus nerve (Epilepsy Foundation of America, 2012a). It is placed under the skin of the chest and attached to the vagus nerve. New exploratory devices include transcranial magnetic stimulation (TMS), a procedure which uses a strong magnet held outside the head to influence brain activity, and implantable devices that deliver drugs to specific parts of the brain (Epilepsy Foundation of America, 2012a).

Diet: The ketogenic diet is a special high-fat, low-carbohydrate diet that helps control seizures in some children with epilepsy who do not respond to antiepileptic medicines. This diet is not recommended for all children and adults because some individuals find it difficult to continue with the diet either because of side effects or because they can't tolerate the food (Epilepsy Foundation of America, 2012c). Therefore, a modified Atkins diet is being studied to determine its effectiveness. The proposed diet includes no fluid or calorie restrictions, strong encouragement of fats, no restrictions on proteins, and carefully monitored carbohydrates.

Psychosocial issues: The team aims to increase a person's confidence in abilities and skills by providing functional interventions. Due to age of onset, frequency of seizures, and intensity of medication regimen, a person may need restoration of psychosocial quality of life (Baker, 2001; Bresnahan, 2004).

Other issues that determine the treatment approach include (NINDS, 2013):

Nature of seizures: Some seizures are minor and do not pose much risk. Other seizures that cause confusion, memory loss, and loss of consciousness present a higher level of risk for injury and require a more complex treatment approach.

Control of seizures: Some individuals become tolerant of AEDs and therefore may need medication adjustment. Treatment changes based on controlled seizures versus seizures that are not controlled. The boundaries are imprecise, because even after years of being seizure-free or controlling seizures, another seizure is always possible.

Activity risk: Different recreational activities can pose different levels of risk. People with seizures usually can participate in low-risk activities, even if their seizures are not well controlled. In regards to high-risk activities, there is no conclusive evidence of prevalence of injury due to a pre-existing condition such as epilepsy. Even so, there are still some physicians who advise against individuals with epilepsy participating in contact sports (Dubow & Kelly, 2003). Usually, the recommendations have been based more on the risk to the athlete or others, if the seizure occurs while participating.

Recreational Therapy Approach

The approach will depend on the person with epilepsy and the setting. The therapist could focus on helping an individual develop insight into acceptance of the disease, learn to advocate for him/herself to dispel stigmas attached to the illness, and develop skills of self-determination through functional interventions. Other directions include assisting with social and community integration, identifying community resources, providing adjustment, co-counseling for anxiety and depression, and placing importance on leisure development.

Recreational Therapy Interventions

Below is a list of possible interventions for individuals who have been diagnosed with epilepsy and/or seizure disorders. There is limited recreational therapy outcome research on interventions used for epilepsy; therefore the information presented is based on research completed by other health care disciplines.

Functional Skills

Physical activity (b125 Dispositions and Intra-Personal Functions, b126 Temperament and Personality Functions, b130 Energy and Drive Functions, d230 Carrying Out Daily Routine, d240 Handling Stress and Other Psychological Demands, d570 Looking After One's Health, d920 Recreation and Leisure): Evidence-based material on possible interventions for persons with epilepsy is limited to sport and physical activity. People with epilepsy and their families are commonly concerned about seizures during exercise, and this fear often results in overprotection, feelings of isolation, and needless restrictions on activity. In fact, it is extremely rare for a person to have a seizure while exercising. Rather than triggering seizures, epilepsy may improve with exercise, and abnormalities on an EEG may decrease during exercise (Dubow & Kelly, 2003; Howard, Radloff, Sevier, 2004). One study examined the relationship between exercise and seizure-frequency

in patients with epilepsy, and found that exercise either leads to fewer seizures or does not change seizure control. Nakken, Bjorholt, and Johannessen (1990) investigated the effect of four weeks of controlled, regular, and intense exercise. Seizures that did occur during the exercise period were not related to the type of activity or intensity of the activity. Apart from the physiological benefits of exercise, improvements in psychosocial functioning and quality of life can be observed. It has been identified in the general population that regular, moderate exercise provides mood benefits, aids in the treatment of depression, and decreases the impact of stressful life events (Hassmen, Koivula, & Uutela, 2000; Wong & Wirrell, 2006). Therefore, it can be assumed that exercise will also improve the psychosocial functioning of the lives of individuals with epilepsy. Furthermore, stress is among the most frequently self-reported precursor of a seizure episode. In view of evidence indicating that sensitivity to stress is reduced after a physical exercise program, physical activity could be used as stress reduction in people with epilepsy (Arida et al., 2010).

Social skills and self-esteem (d7 Interpersonal Interactions and Relationships, b126 Temperament and Personality Functions): During more than 25 years of research, the goals of Social Skills Training (SST) programs have been to promote skill acquisition, maintenance, and generalization as well as to reduce or eliminate problem behaviors that compete with appropriate social skills (Cook et al., 2008; Gresham, 2002). Although there is no empirical study of social skills being conducted on persons with epilepsy, social skill inadequacies can cause peer rejection, social isolation, and academic under-achievement (Spence, 2003). This training assumes that when people improve their social skills or change selected behaviors, they will raise their self-esteem and increase the likelihood that others will respond favorably to them.

Compensatory strategies for memory problems (b144 Memory Functions): Memory deficits are the most frequently measured cognitive impairments in epilepsy patients (Hendriks et al., 2002). Memory can be improved with the use of memory aids, such as prompts with verbal cues, charts to describe steps to complicated tasks, voice recordings of verbal instructions, to-do lists, mnemonic devices, and the use of a journal.

Stress management: People with epilepsy may have seizures when stress is not properly managed (d240 Handling Stress and Other Psychological Demands). Situations that create stress can vary from person to person, but could likely involve heavy workloads, unrealistic timeframes, or interpersonal conflicts. Studies have shown that greater skill in stress management, in other disability populations, is associated with lower levels of anxiety and depression and better overall mental quality of life (Javaheri et al., 2010; Faul, Heather, & Charles, 2010). A stress management program can help people more effectively deal with stress in their lives by analyzing the specific stressors and taking positive actions to minimize their effects. Coding for the purpose of the treatment can be tied to deficits documented in particular social, school, and work areas. Some possible interventions are deep breathing, relaxation, yoga, and exercise.

Education, Training, and Counseling

Leisure education: Discussions about the importance of leisure can assist with decreasing depression, anxiety, and stress experienced by individuals with disability (b125 Dispositions and Intra-Personal Functions, b126 Temperament and Personality Functions, d240 Handling Stress and Other Psychological Demands, d570 Looking After One's Health). Stumbo & Peterson (1998) have noted that individuals with impairments generally experience more barriers to leisure when compared to their peers without disabilities. These barriers can lead to anxiety and stress that individuals with epilepsy experience. Therefore, leisure education can provide individuals with epilepsy the opportunity to learn skill sets that promote community leisure participation (d920 Recreation and Leisure, d910 Community Life), including understanding and reducing barriers (e4 Attitudes, e5 Services, Systems, and Policies), which is an essential component of successful community adjustment (Dattilo & Schleien, 1994).

Education on antiepileptic drugs (AEDs): AEDs are the most common treatment for epilepsy and seizures, but some of the side effects may influence performance (Birrer, Griesemer, & Cataletto, 2002). The side effects include: fatigue and tiredness (b455 Exercise Tolerance Functions); vision problems (b210 Seeing Functions), such as blurred vision;

concentration problems (b140 Attention Functions); impaired coordination (b760 Control of Voluntary Movement Functions); and slower response times (b147 Psychomotor Functions). If these effects are treated, they first need to be noted in the assessment documentation.

Education on exercise: Exercise can alter the levels of AEDs in the blood. AEDs may lead to bone loss associated with osteopenia and osteoporosis. Large studies suggest a doubling of fracture risk in people with epilepsy. Weight-bearing exercise is a preventative intervention for these conditions. Other exercise-related risk factors could include extreme fatigue (b455 Exercise Tolerance Functions), lack of sleep (b134 Sleep Functions), electrolyte loss associated with severe dehydration (b545 Water, Mineral, and Electrolyte Balance Functions), hyperthermia (b550 Thermoregulatory Functions), and hypoglycemia. Noting these effects of exercise would be part of the ongoing assessment of the patient during treatment, as well as a record of treatments being done.

Community Integration

Driving (d475 Driving): People with epilepsy may have driving restrictions. For specific information about a state's regulations involving driving with epilepsy, see

www.epilepsyfoundation.org/living/wellness/transportation/drivinglaws.cfm.

Children and adults with epilepsy are provided many opportunities in community recreation settings (e3 Support and Relationships, e575 General Social Support Services, Systems, and Policies). Opportunities range from segregated programs to inclusion in ongoing recreation activities with support. Recent findings from a search for best practices in inclusive service delivery (ISD) across the U.S. indicated the use of inclusion support staff as a prevalent practice to address the need for direct support for persons participating in recreation (Miller, Schleien, & Bowens, 2010).

Resources

Epilepsy Foundation
www.epilepsyfoundation.org
National charitable organization dedicated to the welfare of people with epilepsy. Works for children and adults affected by seizures through education,

advocacy, services, and research towards a cure. Offers a Legal Defense Program through a fund.

Epilepsy Institute

www.efmny.org

Non-profit organization that provides comprehensive social services and resources for people with epilepsy and their families.

National Institute of Neurological Disorders and Stroke (NINDS)

www.ninds.nih.gov/

NINDS is one of 27 Institutes and Centers that comprise the National Institutes of Health (NIH), within the Department of Health and Human Services (DHHS).

National Organization for Rare Disorders

www.rarediseases.org

Federation of voluntary health organizations dedicated to helping people with rare "orphan" diseases and assisting the organizations that serve them. Committed to the identification, treatment, and cure of rare disorders through programs of education, advocacy, research, and service.

References

American Academy of Neurology. (2013). Epilepsy. Accessed via website http://www.aan.com/.

Arida, R. M., Scorza, F. A., da Silva, S. G., Schachter, S. C., & Cavalheiro, E. A. (2010). The potential role of physical exercise in the treatment of epilepsy. *Epilepsy Behavior, 17*, 432-435.

Baker, G. (2001). Assessment of quality of life in people with epilepsy: Some practical implications. *Epilepsia, 42*(Suppl. 3), 66-69.

Birrer, R. B., Griesemer, B. & Cataletto, M. B. (2002). *Pediatric sports medicine for primary care*. Philadelphia, PA: Lippincott, Williams, & Wilkins.

Bresnahan, D. B. (2004). Psychiatric comorbidity in epilepsy and end stage renal disease. *Wisconsin Medical Journal 103*(6).

Centers for Disease Control. (2013). Epilepsy basics. Accessed via website http://www.cdc.gov/epilepsy/basics/fast.htm/.

Centers for Disease Control. (2003). Living well with epilepsy. Report presented at the National Conference on Public Health and Epilepsy.

Cook, C. R., Gresham, F. M., Kern, L., Barreras, R. B., Thornton, S., & Crews, S. D. (2008). Social skills training for secondary students with emotional and/or behavioral disorders: A review and analysis of the meta-analytic literature. *Journal of Emotional and Behavioral Disorders, 16*, 131-144.

Dattilo, J. & Schleien, S. J. (1994). Understanding leisure services for individuals with mental retardation. *Mental Retardation, 32*(1), 53-59.

Donner, E. J., Smith, C. R., & Snead, O. C. (2001). Sudden unexplained death in children with epilepsy. *Neurology, 57*(3), 430-434.

Dubow J. S. & Kelly J. P. (2003). Epilepsy in sport and recreation. *Sports Medicine, 33*(7), 499-516.

Epilepsy Foundation of America. (2012a). Vagus nerve stimulation. Accessed via website http://www.epilepsyfoundation.org/.

Epilepsy Foundation of America. (2012b) Photosensitivity and epilepsy. Accessed via website http://www.epilepsyfoundation.org/.

Epilepsy Foundation of America. (2012c) Seizures and syndrome. Accessed via website http://www.epilepsyfoundation.org/about/types/.

Ettinger, A. B. & Kanner, A. M. (2006). *Psychiatric issues in epilepsy: A practical guide to diagnosis and treatment.* Philadelphia, PA: Lippincott, Williams, & Wilkins.

Ettinger, A., Reed M., & Cramer J. (2004). Epilepsy impact project group: Depression and comorbidity in community-based patients with epilepsy or asthma. *Neurology, 63*, 1008-14.

Faul, L.A., Heather, S., & Charles, J. (2010). Relationship of stress management skill to psychological distress and quality of life in adults with cancer. *Psycho-Oncology, 19*, 102-109.

Foldvary-Schaefer N. & Wyllie E. (2007). In Goetz C, ed. *Textbook of clinical neurology*. 3rd edition, chap. 52. Philadelphia, PA: Saunders Elsevier.

Fountain, N. B. & May, A. C. (2003). Epilepsy and athletics. *Clinics in Sports Medicine, 22*(3).

Gresham, F. M. (2002). Teaching social skills to high-risk children and youth: Preventive and remedial strategies. In M. R. Shinn, H. M. Walker, & G. Stoner (Eds.), *Interventions for academic and behavior problems II: Preventive and remedial approaches* (pp. 403-43). Bethesda, MD: National Association of School Psychologists.

Hassmen, P., Koivula, N., & Uutela A. (2000). Physical exercise and psychological well-being: A population study in Finland. *Preventative Medicine, 30*(1), 17-25.

Hendriks, M., Aldenkamp, A., Van der Vlugt, H., Alpherts, W., & Vermeulen, J. (2002). Memory complaints in medically refractory epilepsy: Relationship to epilepsy-related factors. *Epilepsy & Behavior, 3*, 165-172.

Hermann, B., Meador, K. J., Gaillard, W. D., Cramer, J. A. (2010). Cognition across the lifespan: Antiepileptic drugs, epilepsy, or both? *Epilepsy & Behavior, 17*, 1-5.

Howard, G. M., Radloff, M., & Sevier, T. L. (2004). Epilepsy and sports participation. *Current Sports Medicine Reports, 3*(1).

Jacoby A. (2002). Stigma, epilepsy and quality of life. *Epilepsy & Behavior, 3*(6S2), 10-20.

Javaheri, R., Neshat-Doost, H. T., Molavi, H., & Zare, M. (2010). Efficacy of cognitive-behavioral stress management therapy on improving the quality of life in females with temporal lobe epilepsy. *Arak Medical University Journal, 13*(2), 32-43.

Kwan P. & Brodie, M. J. (2007). Emerging drugs for epilepsy. *Expert Opinion on Emergency Drugs, 3,* 407-22.

Lee, S. A., Lee, S. M., & No, Y. J. (2010). Factors contributing to depression in patients with epilepsy. *Epilepsia, 51*(7), 1305-1308.

Lim, S. L. (2010). Sports and safety in epilepsy. *Neurology Asia, 15*(supplement 1), 25-27.

Miller, K. D., Schleien, S. J., & Bowens, F. (2010). Support staff as an essential component of inclusive recreation services. *Therapeutic Recreation Journal, 44*(1), 35-49.

Mittan, R. J. (2010). Epilepsy and learning disabilities: Part 1 — diagnosing and solving school learning disabilities in epilepsy. *Exceptional Parent, 40*(8), 33-35.

Nakken, K. O., Bjorholt, P. G., & Johannessen, S. I. (1990). Effect of physical training on aerobic capacity, seizure occurrence and contact sports. *Epilepsia, 31*, 88-94.

National Institutes of Health Office of Rare Disease Research. (n.d.). Lafora Disease. Accessed via website http://rarediseases.info.nih.gov/GARD/Condition/8214/Lafora_disease.aspx.

National Institute of Neurological Disorders and Stroke (NINDS). (2013). Seizures and epilepsy: Hope through research. Accessed via website http://www.ninds.nih.gov/.

National Seizure Disorders Foundation. (2011). Seizure disorder effects: How you can help. Access via website http://nationalseizuredisordersfoundation.org/category.

Plioplys, S., Dunn, D. W., & Caplan, R. (2007). 10-year research update review: Psychiatric problems in children with epilepsy. *Journal of the American Academy of Child and Adolescent Psychiatry, 46*(11), 1389-1402.

Shigihara, Y. & Tanaka, M. (2010). Relationship between fatigue and photosensitivity. *Behavioral Medicine, 36*, 109-112.

Sirven, J. I. & Waterhouse, E. (2003). Management of status epilepticus. *American Family Physician, 68*(3), 469-76.

Spence, S. H. (2003) Social skills training with children and young people: Theory, evidence and practice. *Child and Adolescent Mental Health, 8*(2), 84-96.

Stumbo, N. J. & Peterson, C. A. (1998). The leisure ability model. *Therapeutic Recreation Journal, 32*(2), 82-96.

Whatley, A. D., DiIorio, C. K., & Yeager, K. (2010). Examining the relationships of depressive symptoms, stigma, social support and regimen-specific support on quality of life in adult patients with epilepsy. *Health Education Research, 25*(4), 575-584.

Whiting, C. (2007). The school experiences of children with epilepsy. Unpublished master's thesis, Brock University, St. Catharines, Ontario, Canada.

Wong, J. & Wirrell, E. (2006) Physical activity in children/teens with epilepsy compared with that in their siblings without epilepsy. *Epilepsia, 47*(3), 631-639.

13. Feeding and Eating Disorders

Heather R. Porter and Laurie Jake

In the *Diagnostic and Statistical Manual of Mental Disorders, 5th edition* (*DSM-5*), there are eight types of feeding and eating disorders: (1) anorexia nervosa, (2) bulimia nervosa, (3) binge-eating disorder, (4) pica, (5) rumination disorder, (6) avoidant/restrictive food intake disorder, (7) other specified feeding or eating disorders, and (8) unspecified feeding or eating disorders (American Psychiatric Association [APA], 2013). Each is defined below. For this chapter the focus will be on anorexia nervosa, bulimia nervosa, and binge-eating disorder, as these are the most common diagnoses in healthcare settings (APA, 2013; AED, 2014):

Anorexia nervosa (AN): Primary symptoms of this disorder include refusal to maintain body weight at or above a minimally normal weight for height, body type, age, and activity level; intense fear of weight gain or being fat; feeling fat or overweight despite dramatic weight loss; extreme concern with body weight and shape; and loss of menstrual periods in girls and women post-puberty. Warning signs include sudden weight loss, extreme dieting, food rituals such as taking very small bites or eating foods in a certain order, hair loss, dry skin or hair, brittle nails, and growth of fine, downy hair on the face and body.

Bulimia nervosa (BN): Primary symptoms include recurrent episodes of eating large quantities of food in short periods of time, often secretly, without regard to feelings of hunger or fullness, and to the point of feeling out of control while eating; following these binges with some form of purging or compensatory behavior to make up for the excessive calories taken in, which might include self-induced vomiting, laxative or diuretic abuse, fasting, and/or obsessive or compulsive exercise; and extreme concern with body weight and shape. Warning signs include disappearance of large amounts of food, frequent trips to the bathroom after meals, calluses on knuckles from using fingers to induce vomiting, and swelling of the face.

Binge-eating disorder (BED): Binge-eating disorder has primary symptoms similar to bulimia nervosa, including frequent episodes of eating large quantities of food in short periods of time, often secretly, without regard to feelings of hunger or fullness; frequently feeling out of control during binges; eating large quantities of food rapidly without really tasting the food; eating alone; and feelings of shame, disgust, or guilt after a binge, *but* there are no purging or compensatory behaviors. Warning signs include sudden weight gain and disappearance of large amounts of food.

Pica: The persistent eating of nonfood or nonnutritive substances that is developmentally inappropriate and is not supported by any particular cultural or social practice.

Rumination disorder (RD): The frequent and repeated regurgitation of food, such as bringing swallowed food back up into the mouth and then re-chewing, re-swallowing, or spitting out the food. The disorder is not due to a medical condition or within the course of other eating disorders.

Avoidant/restrictive food intake disorder (ARFID): Avoidance or restriction of food intake resulting in failure to meet nutritional and energy needs resulting in significant weight loss, significant nutritional deficiency, dependence on enteral feeding or oral nutritional supplements, or marked interference with psychosocial functioning. The disorder is not due to lack of food availability, cultural practice, or a medical condition, and does not occur with anorexia nervosa or bulimia nervosa.

Other specified feeding or eating disorder: Includes other feeding or eating disorders that do not meet the full criteria of the previously reviewed disorders. Examples include: (1) atypical anorexia nervosa, which includes all the criteria except that weight is within or above the normal range, (2) bulimia nervosa of low frequency and/or limited duration, (3) binge-eating disorder of low frequency and/or limited duration, and (4) purging disorder, which is recurrent purging to influence weight or shape in absence of binge eating.

Unspecified feeding or eating disorder: This includes disorders of feeding and eating that do not meet the criteria for any specific eating disorder or there is insufficient information to make a more specific diagnosis These still require treatment because they cause distress or limit functioning.

Although it is not a formal diagnosis in the *DSM-5*, a growing problem in the eating disorder realm is diabulimia, a dual diagnosis of diabetes and an eating disorder (National Eating Disorders Association [NEDA], 2012). In this disorder, individuals who have diabetes refuse to take or significantly reduce their insulin, which causes the body to "purge" calories through glycosuria (loss of glucose through the urine) (NEDA, 2012). It is estimated that this behavior occurs in 14% of young women with Type 1 diabetes, and 50% of women who have Type 2 diabetes and an eating disorder (Shaw & Favazza, 2010). Health risks of this behavior include high glucose levels, glucose in the urine, exhaustion, thirst, inability to think clearly, severe dehydration, muscle loss, diabetic ketoacidosis, high cholesterol, bacterial skin infections, yeast infections, menstrual disruption, staph infections, retinopathy, neuropathy, peripheral arterial disease, atherosclerosis, steatohepatitis, stroke, coma, and death (NEDA, 2012). Most alarming is the rate of mortality among this population. The mortality rate is 35% and severe health consequences, including blindness and kidney failure, can occur within several years (Eating Disorder Hope [EDH], 2013b). Possible signs of diabulimia include an A1C level of 9.0 or higher on a continuous basis, unexplained weight loss, persistent thirst and frequent urination, preoccupation with body image, blood sugar levels that do not match A1C results, depression, mood swings, fatigue, secrecy about blood sugars/insulin injections/eating, repeated bladder and yeast infections, low sodium and potassium, increased appetite especially for sugary foods, and cancelled doctor's appointments (NEDA, 2012).

Although feeding and eating disorders are often placed in the category of addictions, they are a unique form of mental illness that includes components of disordered thinking, addictive behaviors, and physical complications. Unlike other addictive behaviors, one cannot simply abstain from eating, which creates unique challenges for treatment and recovery.

Incidence/Prevalence in U.S.

Eating disorders affect up to 24 million Americans (National Association of Anorexia Nervosa and Associated Disorders [ANAD], 2014).

Within the last decade, eating disorders in those under the age of 12 rose by 119% (Eating Disorders Coalition [EDC], 2008) and account for approximately four percent of all childhood hospital admissions (EDC, 2008).

It is estimated that 95% of all dieters will regain lost weight within five years and that 35% of "normal dieters" will progress to pathological dieting, of which 20-25% will progress to partial or full-syndrome eating disorders (ANAD, 2014).

It's estimated that the prevalence of eating disorders among athletes is 13% (and 20% in elite athletes), with the highest risk for females in aesthetic sports, such as gymnastics, ballet, and figure skating (ANAD, 2014). Athletes have similar psychological profiles to those with AN, putting them at increased risk for an eating disorder: perfectionism, high self-expectation, competitiveness, hyperactivity, repetitive exercise routines, compulsiveness, drive, tendency toward depression, body image disturbance, pre-occupation with dieting and weight (ANAD, 2014). Female athletes are most at risk for developing an eating disorder due to high expectations about body composition and performance; however they are believed to be underdiagnosed in this population due to denial. Others see them as doing what they need to do in order to succeed, rather than viewing the unhealthy behavior as a problem (EDH, 2012a).

AN is the third most common chronic illness among adolescents (EDC, 2008; ANAD, 2014). About nine out of 1,000 people have AN during the course of their life. Men are less likely to have AN compared to women with estimates that range anywhere from 3:12 to 10:11 (AED, 2014). However, men are less inclined to seek treatment, and screening for AN in the male population by healthcare practitioners may be overlooked, contributing to a false prevalence statistic (AED, 2014). AN has been seen in boys as young as eight years old (EDH, 2012).

BN is seen in about 1-1.5% of the female population during the course of their life (AED, 2014). Like AN, men are less likely to have BN compared to women with estimates ranging from 1:3 to 1:10 (AED, 2014). However, men are less inclined to seek treatment, and screening for BN in the male population by healthcare practitioners may be overlooked, contributing to a false prevalence statistic (AED, 2014).

It is estimated that 10-15% of people with AN or BN are male (ANAD, 2014). Among gay men, it is estimated that 14% have BN and 20% have AN (ANAD, 2014).

BED affects 35 out of 1,000 people during the course of their life (AED, 2014). Approximately 40% of those with BED are males (EDH, 2012).

Predominant Age

About 95% of those who have an eating disorder are between the ages of 12 and 25.8 (ANAD, 2014).

Both AN and BN typically begin during early-to-mid adolescence (AED, 2014).

BED typically begins during adolescence, but most people present for treatment in middle adulthood (AED, 2014).

The development, re-appearance, or escalation of an eating disorder in middle adulthood is thought to be triggered by drastic or unexpected life transitions including divorce or separation, aging body, empty nest, parent's death, and unexpected illness (EDH, 2013).

Approximately 25% of college-aged women engage in bingeing and purging as a weight-management technique (ANAD, 2014).

About one-half of teenage girls and one-third of teenage boys use unhealthy weight control behaviors including skipping meals, fasting, smoking cigarettes, vomiting, and taking laxatives (ANAD, 2014).

Causes

Eating disorders are complex and are influenced by a wide variety of genetic and environmental factors. Although no defined cause has been established, factors include (ANAD, 2014; NEDA, 2014; AED, 2014; Bailer & Kaye, 2010; EDC, 2008):

Genetics: Eating disorders tend to run in families; therefore it is believed that genetics play a role.

In some literature, it is estimated that 50-80% of eating disorders are caused by genetics.

Biological issues: There's some evidence that serotonin, a naturally occurring brain chemical, may influence eating behaviors. The behaviors of restricting food intake, bingeing, and purging have been shown to alter brain structure, metabolism, and neurochemistry in ways that make it difficult for individuals to discontinue the behaviors. Also, once individuals begin to starve themselves, binge eat, or purge, those behaviors in and of themselves can alter brain chemistry and exacerbate the eating disorder.

Psychological or interpersonal issues: Eating disorders may develop or be triggered as a result of searching for control, coping with stress or trauma, personality factors, family issues, low self-esteem, feelings of inadequacy or lack of control in life, depression, anxiety, anger, stress, loneliness, troubled personal relationships, difficulty expressing emotions and feelings, a history of being teased or ridiculed based on size or weight, or a history of physical or sexual abuse. People with eating disorders may have pre-existing psychological and emotional problems that contribute to the disorder, including low self-esteem, perfectionism, impulsive behavior, and troubled relationships. Studies have shown that there are a high number of people suffering with eating disorders who have been subjected to some form of emotional, physical, or sexual abuse. Many of these individuals have found that their eating disorders help to protect them, repress or block out the memories, or numb their feelings. Disordered eating may also arise due to an inability to mourn and/or cope with death, loss, or abandonment. The person may subsequently attempt to numb his/her feelings through restriction, bingeing, and purging. There is a great deal of debate about the role of family in the causes of an eating disorder. Particular styles of family behavior may increase risk for psychopathology in general, including eating disorders. Eating disorders also have substantial co-morbidity with other mental health disorders including depression, anxiety, obsessive-compulsive disorder, post-traumatic stress disorder, and personality disorders.

Social/societal issues: Today's culture often promotes and reinforces a desire for thinness. Peer pressure and what people see in the media may fuel this desire to be thin, particularly among young girls. With unrealistic pressures to obtain the "perfect" body, the constant influx of images of perfection, and narrow definitions of beauty, the media and societal expectations definitely influence self-esteem and self-worth. From a very early age, girls learn that in order to be accepted, they must emulate these unhealthy media messages. Some women internalize society's thinness ideal and when they cannot measure up to the standards set for the female body, they often develop a negative body image. Negative body images can lead some individuals into unhealthy eating patterns and eating disorders. Among several studies, ANAD (2014) found some alarming statistics. The body type portrayed in advertising as the ideal is possessed naturally by only five percent of American females. Forty-seven percent of fifth to twelfth grade girls report wanting to loose weight because of magazine pictures. Sixty-nine percent of fifth to twelfth grade girls report that magazine pictures influence their idea of a perfect body shape. Forty-two percent of first to third grade girls want to be thinner. Eighty-one percent of 10-year-olds are afraid of being fat.

Cultural issues: Cultures that glorify "thinness" or muscularity place a high value on obtaining the "perfect body," have narrow definitions of beauty that include only specific body weights and shapes, emphasize cultural norms that value people on the basis of physical appearance rather than inner qualities and strengths, and display discrimination or prejudice based on size and weight.

Obesity prevention programs: The C. S. Mott Children's Hospital National Poll on Children's Health found that 30% of parents of children aged six to 14 who participated in a school-based childhood obesity prevention program observed behaviors in their children that are commonly seen in eating disorders, including inappropriate dieting, excessive worry about fat in foods, preoccupation with food content and labels, and refusing family meals.

Systems Affected

Individuals with an eating disorder will face a wide range of social, cognitive, emotional, and physical issues. Socially, eating disorders impact family units. Individuals with eating disorders are often withdrawn and socially isolated, since eating disorders are most often practiced in private (d7 Interpersonal Interactions and Relationships). As the illness progresses, individuals with eating

disorders may stop participating in social activities because, for example, they don't want to be forced to eat and need private time to purge (d9 Community, Social, and Civic Life).

Nutritional issues are a significant part of eating disorders with problems including nutritional and caloric intake, eating patterns, eliminated or taboo foods, food rituals, and using food inappropriately to deal with a crisis. ICF codes include d240 Handling Stress and Other Psychological Demands, d250 Managing One's Own Behavior, d550 Eating, d560 Drinking, d570 Looking After One's Health, and d630 Preparing Meals.

Cognitive issues that may arise for an individual with an eating disorder include denial of the illness, severe body image issues, perfectionism, challenges with the need for control, and issues with escape or avoidance thoughts and behaviors. Relevant ICF codes include b125 Dispositions and Intra-Personal Functions, b126 Temperament and Personality Functions, b130 Energy and Drive Functions, b160 Thought Functions, b180 Experience of Self and Time Functions, and d250 Managing One's Own Behavior.

Emotional challenges may include anxiety, depression, decreased self-esteem and self-worth, and inability to express or cope with anger. ICF codes include b125 Dispositions and Intra-Personal Functions, b126 Temperament and Personality Functions, and d240 Handling Stress and Other Psychological Demands.

There are also significant physical issues that are influenced by an eating disorder. Consequently, individuals should always receive a thorough medical evaluation to identify physical issues and complications such as dehydration, low blood pressure, osteoporosis, stomach and digestive complications, arrhythmias (irregular heart beat), and tearing of the esophagus. These can be coded with b410 Heart Functions, b420 Blood Pressure Functions, b510 Ingestion Functions, b515 Digestive Functions, b530 Weight Maintenance Functions, b535 Sensations Associated with the Digestive System, b540 General Metabolic Functions, b545 Water, Mineral, and Electrolyte Balance Functions, and b650 Menstruation Functions. Any structural damage can be noted using s5 Structures Related to the Digestive, Metabolic, and Endocrine Systems and s7 Structures Related to Movement.

Secondary Problems

Eating disorders can cause severe medical issues including cardiac arrhythmia, cardiac arrest, brain damage, osteoporosis, infertility, and death (EDC, 2008).

Almost 50% of people with an eating disorder meet the criteria for depression (ANAD, 2014).

Women who have an eating disorder during pregnancy are at an increased risk for premature labor, low birth weight babies, cardiac irregularities, stillbirth or fetal death, gestational diabetes, miscarriage, preeclampsia, complications during labor, respiratory difficulties, abnormal fetal growth, increased risk of cesarean birth, difficulties breastfeeding, postpartum depression, anxiety or panic attacks, low self-esteem, poor body image, suicidal ideations, withdrawal or social isolation, lack of enjoyment in hobbies or activities, and martial or family conflicts (EDH, 2013a). Code with b152 Emotional Functions, b180 Experience of Self and Time Functions, b660 Procreation Functions, d7 Interpersonal Interactions and Relationships, d9 Community, Social, and Civic Life, and e3 Support and Relationships.

Medical conditions and issues that may co-occur with AN include bone loss, difficulties with temperature regulation, loss of menstrual periods, low heart rate, low blood pressure, anxiety, depression, social isolation, and perfectionism (AED, 2014). Code with b125 Dispositions and Intra-Personal Functions, b126 Temperament and Personality Functions, b130 Energy and Drive Functions, b152 Emotional Functions, b410 Heart Functions, b420 Blood Pressure Functions, b545 Water, Mineral, and Electrolyte Balance Functions, b550 Thermoregulatory Functions, b650 Menstruation Functions, and d7 Interpersonal Interactions and Relationships.

Medical conditions and issues that may co-occur with BN include electrolyte imbalance, esophageal ulcers, tooth decay, anxiety, depression, substance use, and difficulties with impulse control (AED, 2014). Code with b125 Dispositions and Intra-Personal Functions, b126 Temperament and Personality Functions, b130 Energy and Drive Functions, b545 Water, Mineral, and Electrolyte Balance Functions, and s320 Structure of Mouth.

Medical conditions and issues that may co-occur with BED include gastric problems, obesity, obesity-related conditions, anxiety, depression, and substance use (AED, 2014). Code with b152 Emotional Functions, b515 Digestive Functions, and codes discussed in the chapter on Obesity.

Prognosis

In long-term outcome studies, the prognoses for individuals with eating disorders at five to 10 years post treatment are 50% recover, 25% improve with some residual symptoms, and 25% remain ill or die (EDC, 2008). Recovery rates are better in younger individuals who are diagnosed relatively early in the process (AED, 2014).

Eating disorders have the highest mortality rate of any mental illness at 10-20% (ANAD, 2014; EDC, 2008). In females aged 15-24 who have AN, the AN mortality rate is 12 times higher than the rate for all other causes of death (ANAD, 2014). Approximately 20% of people with AN die prematurely from eating disorder complications including suicide and heart problems (ANAD, 2014). Compared to peers without an eating disorder, those with AN are 57 times more likely to die from suicide (EDC, 2008).

Approximately 70% of people with BN recover over time, with better recovery rates in those who have fewer psychiatric issues (AED, 2014). Individuals with BN also have an increased risk of death due to suicide (AED, 2014).

Approximately 70-80% of people with BED recover over time, with better recovery rates in those with fewer interpersonal problems (AED, 2014).

Assessment

Typical Scope of Team Assessment

Prior to developing a treatment plan, a unit psychiatrist, psychologist, or master level therapist conducts an intake interview with the client. An interview commonly includes the administration of the *Eating Attitudes Test* (EAT) (an eating disorder screening tool) and broad medical, psychological, and nutritional assessments to document any significant secondary complications associated with eating disorders (Porter & burlingame, 2006). These areas can be documented with the codes listed in the Systems Affected section.

Medical: Medical tests evaluate body functions such as blood pressure, blood chemistries, urine specific gravity, fluid intake/output, weight, heart function, and bone density. A body mass index

(BMI) is calculated to assess weight, specifically whether a client is underweight, normal, overweight, or obese.

Emotional: An assessment of emotional and cognitive functioning utilizes non-standardized and standardized tools (e.g., *Beck Depression Inventory*, *Body Shape Questionnaire*, and *State-Trait Anxiety Inventory*).

Nutritional: A nutritional assessment evaluates nutritional and caloric intake, eating patterns, eliminated or taboo foods, food preparation (who prepares, how prepared), food rituals, and types of food most likely to be inappropriately used during crisis.

Areas of Concern for RT Assessment

Although there is no specific recreational therapy assessment that has proven valid and reliable specifically for individuals with eating disorders, existing recreational therapy assessment tools may offer important information for effective treatment goals.

In addition to standardized tools, the recreational therapy initial assessment of the client often involves the use of an intake form created by the agency or program. Areas of assessment commonly include leisure function (e.g., current leisure lifestyle, role of leisure related to the eating disorder), leisure skills, social functioning, coping skills, cognition, emotional and psychological issues, especially self-esteem and body image, and leisure attitudes, perceptions, interests, and barriers. The following areas should be included as part of the assessment process:

Healthy leisure choices: Clients with eating disorders often lack the basic skills needed to structure healthy leisure time choices. Social withdrawal, compulsive exercise, and binge/purge behaviors are often engaged in during leisure or unstructured time to the extent that they create a deficit in healthy leisure (d920 Recreation and Leisure).

Intrusive thoughts: Obsessive thoughts about food and body weight, which can occur for hours a day, if not the entire day, can impair everyday functioning, interfere with relationships, and make it difficult to function in social situations (b130 Energy and Drive Functions, b160 Thought Functions, b164 Higher-Level Cognitive Functions, b180 Experience of Self and Time Functions) (Walter & Van Puymbroeck, 2013).

Psychological and emotional issues: These issues include a high need to be in control (b160 Thought Functions, d710 Basic Interpersonal Interactions, d720 Complex Interpersonal Interactions), impaired ability to cope with stress (d240 Handling Stress and Other Psychological Demands), and low self-esteem (b126 Temperament and Personality Functions). Depression may also be present (often accompanied by social isolation) adding to the negative impact on quality of life for clients with eating disorders (b125 Dispositions and Intra-Personal Functions). According to Zerbe (1993), "patients who remain ill over a prolonged period appear to develop a less satisfying lifestyle filled with social and psychological difficulties" (p. 15). Feelings of guilt and shame might also be observed. These feeling often intensify during the course of the illness adding to feelings of not being worthy of enjoyment or pleasure.

Social isolation or impaired social skills: Added to the already difficult issues in maintaining a balanced leisure lifestyle, clients with eating disorders are usually socially isolated, thus limiting their leisure even further. Leisure is also negatively affected by the rigid eating patterns of eating disorder clients. "So many foods become forbidden that regular eating and socializing patterns are disrupted significantly, leaving the individual unable to lead a flexible lifestyle" (Hornyak & Baker, 1989, p. 61). Many social and leisure activities will be avoided because food is involved in the activity. Relevant ICF codes include d710 Basic Interpersonal Interactions, d720 Complex Interpersonal Interactions, d750 Informal Social Relationships, d760 Family Relationships, and d920 Recreation and Leisure.

Leisure attitudes and perceptions: Specific attitudes regarding leisure, such as entitlement to leisure and the value the client places on leisure in their life, often need to be explored with clients, especially women, who have eating disorders. Because clients with eating disorders are primarily women, it is important to distinguish key differences in how women experience leisure. These differences can greatly impact treatment approaches. Women often feel they are not entitled to leisure (Hood, 1997). In women who have eating disorders, this is compounded by their feelings of guilt and shame. Leisure can be guilt producing, rather than a healthy diversion for many clients, and these feelings can prevent women from effectively engaging in healthy leisure pursuits. Women often feel selfish and morally conflicted if they respond to their own needs rather than the needs of those close to them. This is an extremely common way of thinking in women with eating disorders. The result of this pattern of thinking is that many women do not prioritize leisure involvement in their lives unless it serves a specific function in relationship maintenance (d7 Interpersonal Interactions and Relationships, d920 Recreation and Leisure) (Hood, 1997).

Leisure barriers: A number of personal and environmental leisure barriers may prevent individuals with an eating disorder from participating in a healthy leisure lifestyle. Choose appropriate Environmental Factor codes.

Physical complications: Physical complications, such as fatigue and loss of strength, caused by an eating disorder, can leave clients in a very physically distressed state thus impacting healthy leisure participation. Use ICF codes b455 Exercise Tolerance Functions and b730 Muscle Power Functions.

Leisure finances: The financial cost of treatment can leave little discretionary income and clients may feel guilty for using the family's resources for their leisure (d760 Family Relationships, e165 Assets).

Body image disturbance: Body image disturbance, as part of the person's self-image, is often cited as being a central factor in the development and maintenance of an eating disorder (b180 Experience of Self and Time Functions).

Alcohol and drug use: It is very common for bulimic clients to have problems with alcoholism, illicit and prescribed drugs, and non-psychoactive substances, such as laxatives, emetics, diuretics, and diet pills (Woodside, 2008). The reason for this is not fully understood. Code with d570 Looking After One's Health.

ICF Core Set

No ICF core set for Eating Disorders has been published.

Treatment Direction

Although there is a significant lack of evidenced-based practice in the area of recreational therapy for eating disorders, there are accepted practice guidelines that underscore the need for recreational therapy interventions. Practice guidelines set forth by the American Psychiatric Association (APA, 2006) for the treatment of clients with eating disorders, outside of medication treatment, are provided below. Only one in 10 people with an eating disorder receives treatment (EDC, 2008), and only 35% of those who receive treatment receive it at a specialized facility for eating disorders (ANAD, 2014). Treatment can last for months or years, with early, appropriate treatment enhancing recovery prognosis (EDC, 2008).

AN Treatment and Major Outcomes

Nutritional rehabilitation: The first goal is to get the patient back to a minimally healthy weight through nutritional rehabilitation and refeeding programs, vitamin and mineral supplementation, and monitoring of serum potassium and rehydration. This may require treatments including liquid food supplements, nasogastric feedings, and parental feedings. Monitoring and treating symptoms and conditions associated with gaining weight (e.g., anxiety, abdominal pain, constipation) are required. Once weight is in an acceptable range, the team can work on establishment of healthy target weights, expected rates of controlled weight gain, advancing intake levels, and appropriate levels of physical activity. ICF codes being treated include b410 Heart Functions, b420 Blood Pressure Functions, b545 Water, Mineral, and Electrolyte Balance Functions, b550 Thermoregulatory Functions, d250 Managing One's Own Behavior, d550 Eating, d560 Drinking, d570 Looking After One's Health, b455 Exercise Tolerance Functions and b730 Muscle Power Functions.

Psychosocial interventions: These interventions aim at reconnecting the patient to others in his or her community. They include family psychotherapy for children and adolescents, family group psychoeducation for adolescents, cognitive behavioral therapy (CBT) for adults, and interpersonal therapy (IPT) and/or psychodynamically orientated individual or group psychotherapy for adults. There may also be psychosocial interventions based on addiction models, support groups led by professionals or advocacy organizations, internet-based support, and non-verbal therapeutic methods, such as creative arts and movement therapy. ICF codes being treated include b125 Dispositions and Intra-Personal Functions, b126 Temperament and Personality

Functions, b160 Thought Functions, b164 Higher-Level Cognitive Functions, b180 Experience of Self and Time Functions, d710 Basic Interpersonal Interactions, d720 Complex Interpersonal Interactions, d750 Informal Social Relationships, and d760 Family Relationships.

Major outcomes: Treatment success is measured by the amount of weight gained within specified time intervals, proportion of patients achieving a specified percentage of expected body weight, return of menses, and measures of severity or frequency of eating disorder behaviors.

BN Treatment and Major Outcomes

Nutritional rehabilitation counseling: Treatment includes development of structured meal plans, assessment of nutritional intake, and nutritional counseling. ICF codes d250 Managing One's Own Behavior, d550 Eating, d560 Drinking, and d570 Looking After One's Health are the basis for this treatment.

Psychosocial interventions: Treatment modalities include CBT, IPT, psychodynamically oriented therapy, group psychotherapy, family and marital therapy, support groups, and 12-step programs. ICF codes being treated include b125 Dispositions and Intra-Personal Functions, b126 Temperament and Personality Functions, b160 Thought Functions, d710 Basic Interpersonal Interactions, d720 Complex Interpersonal Interactions, d750 Informal Social Relationships, d760 Family Relationships, and d770 Intimate Relationships.

Major outcomes: Treatment success is measured by reduction in the frequency or severity of eating disorder behaviors, such as binge eating, vomiting, or laxative use, and the proportion of patients achieving remission from or a specific reduction in eating disorder behaviors.

Other Eating Disorders

Treatment: Treatment modalities include nutritional rehabilitation counseling, behavioral weight control programs, combinations of diet and psychosocial treatments, other psychosocial treatment, individual or group CBT, IPT, and dialectical behavior therapy. ICF codes being treated include b125 Dispositions and Intra-Personal Functions, b126 Temperament and Personality Functions, b160 Thought Functions, b164 Higher-Level

Cognitive Functions, b180 Experience of Self and Time Functions, d250 Managing One's Own Behavior, d550 Eating, d560 Drinking, d570 Looking After One's Health, d710 Basic Interpersonal Interactions, and d720 Complex Interpersonal Interactions.

Recreational Therapy Interventions

Recreation and leisure can play a unique role in the treatment and recovery of clients with eating disorders. However, as previously stated, little research has been done in this area. The following recommendations compiled from Porter & burlingame (2006), Miller & Jake (2001), and clinical experience of the authors, although not evidence-based, are recommended for consideration by recreational therapists. It is also strongly recommended that more research is conducted in this area.

Leisure education and counseling: Given the excessive amounts of time, thought process, and activity on attention to food, self-image, and exercise, the client will traditionally lack a balanced repertoire of healthy leisure activities. Clients will most likely need assistance in choosing alternative healthy activities that are non-food centered and developing a healthy activity pattern for participation that aids in recovery. The primary ICF code is d920 Recreation and Leisure, but this also affects b125 Dispositions and Intra-Personal Functions, b126 Temperament and Personality Functions, b130 Energy and Drive Functions, and b180 Experience of Self and Time Functions.

Social skills training and development of interpersonal relationships: Social isolation, anxiety, and underlying depression are critical areas to address by teaching new, concrete social skills. Often the client has spent an inordinate amount of time obsessing on his/her body image and isolated himself/herself from activities that involve food. Because of this, basic skills needed to create and nurture friendships may be lacking (b125 Dispositions and Intra-Personal Functions, b126 Temperament and Personality Functions, b180 Experience of Self and Time Functions, d250 Managing One's Own Behavior, and d7 Interpersonal Interactions and Relationships, especially d710 Basic Interpersonal Interactions and d720 Complex Interpersonal Interactions). Wanting to help others, a common social pattern for clients with eating disorders, is often not the type of social skill that needs to be developed. Instead, working on the basic skills of mutual respect and assistance (accepting help while also offering help), basic give and take during conversation ("us" centered conversations), and being sensitive to the feelings of others are good places to begin developing appropriate social skills. The patient needs to learn to correctly read the other person's body language and spoken word instead of wondering how the other person perceives the patient. It is especially important for the patient to stop worrying about how other people perceive the patient's body. Helping clients to develop positive leisure and social skills is essential for lasting recovery from an eating disorder. Walter and Van Puymbroeck (2013) recommend that recreational therapists consider the theory of Symbolic Interactionism (SI) to better understand how individuals with eating disorders process social interactions. According to Blumer (1986, as cited by Walter & Van Puymbroeck, 2013), SI rests on the following three premises: (1) individuals ascribe meaning to objects in their environment and act toward these objects based on the meaning they perceive, (2) individuals ascribe these meanings based on interactions with others, and (3) individuals merge the meanings from the objects, based on the interactions with others, and interpret them based on the situation. When individuals with eating disorders interact with others, they tend to have dysfunctional associations or perceptions, for example, feelings of being judged. The authors believe that changing such perceptions in social interactions may help to reduce eating disorder thoughts and behaviors; and doing this through participation in non-threatening, enjoyable, intrinsically motivating, self-chosen recreational activities that focus on a specific need, such as interpreting social situations, can increase feelings of enjoyment and control in a social context. This helps to change the engrained dysfunctional associations and perceptions. This type of setting also lends itself to feeling safe because it is not focused on food behavior. Therefore, it might help the person become more open to new ideas and thoughts. Since relationships are often damaged due to one person's self-obsessed thoughts, rather than paying attention to conversations, the authors additionally recommend a strong focus on specific social skills training in mutual respect, basic listening and responding skills, and sensitivity to others to help rebuild friendships

and social support. A final recommendation from the authors is to address "leisure control" (having control over what is happening in their leisure time). This involves helping the person identify and express his/her comfort level in social situations, and then helping the person move towards more leisure time choice and control. Having control in one area of life may be influential in helping the person feel in control of other aspects of life.

Re-socialization: As previously reviewed, increased and prolonged social isolation can weaken social skills. Thus the process of re-socializing with others in making friends, initiating and maintaining conversation, feeling comfortable in social situations, and other social issues commonly needs to be addressed (b125 Dispositions and Intra-Personal Functions, d7 Interpersonal Interactions and Relationships, d9 Community, Social, and Civic Life). Re-socialization can also enhance feelings of being part of a community, helping to strengthen feelings of acceptance. Opportunities to participate in social activities and re-establish social connections in the community should be addressed. One activity that is often effective is helping the client to find volunteer opportunities in the community. In addition to the social benefit, the client is able to experience a sense of purpose, adding to their fragile self-concept.

Anxiety and stress reduction interventions: This involves the identification of unique physiological, emotional, and behavioral responses to increased stress levels and then learning specific, positive stress management techniques to reduce the level of stress and impulsive behavior (d240 Handling Stress and Other Psychological Demands). High levels of anxiety are common among eating disorder clients. Traditional relaxation techniques, however, are not always effective with eating disorder clients, particularly with anorexic clients. This may be due to their compulsive need to constantly move and burn calories. The act of simply lying still can have the opposite effect and actually be stress inducing rather than relaxing for the client. Clients who have a history of trauma or abuse may also have challenges with traditional relaxation activities particularly if the lights are dimmed during the activity. Using a wide range of options including music, art, journaling, expressive writing, and aromatherapy may help the client to find a technique that s/he prefers.

Coping skills and impulse control: It is very common for clients with bulimia nervosa to also have problems with alcoholism and chemical dependency (d570 Looking After One's Health). This may be due to limited coping skills (d240 Handling Stress and Other Psychological Demands) or poor impulse control (b130 Energy and Drive Functions). These are important areas to address during treatment.

Self-worth, self-esteem, and personal boundaries: This includes helping the client develop a sense of "who they are" by working on self-worth and self-esteem through the identification of positive attributes not related to weight or body image (b126 Temperament and Personality Functions) and strengthening personal boundaries (d720 Complex Interpersonal Interactions).

Enhancing body image: Body image disturbance is a central factor in the development and maintenance of an eating disorder. Recreational therapists help clients change entrenched and distorted views of appearance through activities that (1) increase the client's skills of observation (e.g., drawing a simple still life that requires the client to realistically see an object and then attempt to recreate the image through fine motor activity), (2) develop an awareness and appreciation of the body and its functions, (3) aid in identifying and overcoming negative body images, and (4) provide pleasant body experiences (b180 Experience of Self and Time Functions, especially b1801 Body Image). It is additionally recommended that recreational therapists structure positive activities with the long-term goal that clients will continue to seek out positive leisure activities after discharge and will develop a renewed sense of appreciation for their body.

Community integration training: Community integration activities may be planned to allow the client to practice normal healthy eating behaviors in a community setting by making food choices, participating in appropriate mealtime conversation, and observing restaurant etiquette (d710 Basic Interpersonal Interactions, d720 Complex Interpersonal Interactions, d9 Community, Social, and Civic Life). Collaborating with the client's dietician is recommended to optimize planning. Community integration training can also be helpful to address additional psychosocial issues, such as socialization and public appearance.

Food fears: Food fears can be addressed through recreation activities including food-related art projects and making environmental tools like a healthy affirmation placemat for mealtimes. In addition, the recreational therapist may work with the dietician in offering the client opportunities to practice recreation-based meal planning and preparation (d550 Eating).

Leisure skills building: Since the eating disorder can become all-powerful in a person's life, social relationships become impaired, isolative behavior grows, and leisure time becomes consumed with eating disorder behavior. As a result, leisure experiences are limited, stunting the development of leisure skills, interests, and abilities. Consequently, leisure skill building may be necessary to address delayed leisure skills or remediate dysfunctional leisure skills related to the eating disorder (d920 Recreation and Leisure).

Positive social and leisure opportunities: According to the Broaden-and-Build Theory of Positive Emotions (Fredrickson, 2004), when people experience positive emotions, they are more open to trying new things and thinking in new ways. With the experience of trying new things and thinking in new ways, people gain new and different resources, such as new skills and new social supports. This broadening, in turn, creates more positive feelings and the positive feedback continues. Engaging in positive social and leisure activities can play a vital role in this process. Document this modality as improving b125 Dispositions and Intra-Personal Functions, b126 Temperament and Personality Functions, and b130 Energy and Drive Functions.

Opportunities for creative expression: Individuals with eating disorders often have psychological or emotional issues that might be expressed through the eating disorder. Interventions aimed at creative expression can be helpful in coping with, releasing, sharing, or just contemplating underlying thoughts and feelings, which can contribute to the healing process (b152 Emotional Functions, d240 Handling Stress and Other Psychological Demands).

Healthy physical activity: Healthy forms of physical activity in appropriate frequency, intensity, and duration should be encouraged and modeled by the therapist and peers (d570 Looking After One's Health).

Resources

Gürze Books
www.bulimia.com
A publishing company specializing in resources for eating disorders recovery.

International Association for Eating Disorder Professionals (IAEDP)
www.iaedp.com
Offers certifications to promote standards within the field of eating disorders (Certified Eating Disorders Specialist — CEDS in mental health, Certified Eating Disorders Registered Dietician — CEDRD, and Certified Eating Disorders Registered Nurse — CEDRN).

References

Academy of Eating Disorders. (2014). About eating disorders. Retrieved from http://www.aedweb.org/Eating_Disorders_Information.htm#.Uuf1cfYo5pg.

American Psychiatric Association. (2013). *Diagnostic and statistical manual of mental disorders, 5th edition*. American Psychiatric Association: Washington, DC.

American Psychiatric Association. (2006). *Practice guideline for the treatment of patients with eating disorders, 3rd edition*. Washington, DC: American Psychiatric Association. Accessed via website http://www.guideline.gov/content.aspx?id=9318.

Bailer, U. F. & Keye, W. H. (2010). Serotonin: Imaging findings in eating disorders. Retrieved from http://eatingdisorders.ucsd.edu/research/pdf_papers/2011/BailerKaye2011_PMID21243470.pdf.

Blumer, H. (1986). *Symbolic interactionism: Perspective and method*. Berkeley, CA: University of California Press.

Eating Disorders Coalition. (2008). Facts about eating disorders. Retrieved from http://www.eatingdisorderscoalition.org/facts-about-eating-disorders.htm.

Eating Disorder HOPE. (2012). Eating disorders in men. Retrieved from http://www.eatingdisorderhope.com/treatment-for-eating-disorders/special-issues/men.

Eating Disorder HOPE. (2012a). Athletes and eating disorders. Retrieved from http://www.eatingdisorderhope.com/treatment-for-eating-disorders/special-issues/athletes.

Eating Disorder HOPE. (2013). Middle-aged women and eating disorders. Retrieved from http://www.eatingdisorderhope.com/treatment-for-eating-disorders/special-issues/older-women.

Eating Disorder HOPE. (2013a). Eating disorders and pregnancy. Retrieved from http://www.eatingdisorderhope.com/treatment-for-eating-disorders/special-issues/pregnancy.

Eating Disorder HOPE. (2013b). Diabetes and eating disorders. Retrieved from http://www.eatingdisorderhope.com/treatment-for-eating-disorders/special-issues/diabetes.

Fredrickson, B. L. (2004). The broaden-and-build theory of positive emotions. *Philosophical Transactions of the Royal Society Biological Sciences, 359*(1449), 1367-1378.

Hood, C. D. (1997). Alcohol and women: The unique role of leisure in recovery. ATRA Annual Conference.

Hornyak, L. M. & Baker, E. (1989). *Experiential therapies for eating disorders*. New York: Guilford Press.

Miller, D. & Jake, L. (2001). *Eating disorders: Providing effective recreational therapy interventions*. Ravensdale, WA: Idyll Arbor, Inc.

National Association of Anorexia Nervosa and Associated Disorders. (2014). About eating disorders. Retrieved from http://www.anad.org/get-information/about-eating-disorders/.

National Eating Disorders Association. (2012). Diabulimia. Retrieved from http://www.nationaleatingdisorders.org/diabulimia-5.

National Eating Disorders Association. (2014). Factors that may contribute to eating disorders. Retrieved from http://www.nationaleatingdisorders.org/factors-may-contribute-eating-disorders.

Porter, H. R. & burlingame, j. (2006). *Handbook of recreational therapy practice: ICF-based diagnosis and treatment*. Idyll Arbor, Inc.: Enumclaw, WA.

Shaw, A. & Favazza, A. (2010). Deliberate insulin underdosing and omission should be included in the *DSM-5* criteria for bulimia nervosa. *The Journal of Neuropsychiatry and Clinical Neurosciences, 22*(352), e13.

Walter, A. A. & Van Puymbroeck, M. (2013). Using symbolic interactionism to improve recreational therapy practice for individuals with eating disorders. *American Journal of Recreation Therapy, 12*(2), 27-32.

Woodside, D. B. (2008). Substance abuse in women with bulimia nervosa. *Psychiatric Times*. Retrieved from http://www.psychiatrictimes.com/articles/substance-abuse-women-bulimia-nervosa.

Zerbe, K. (1993). *The body betrayed: A deeper understanding of women, eating disorders and treatment*. Gurze books.

14. Fibromyalgia and Juvenile Fibromyalgia

Heather R. Porter

Fibromyalgia (FM)

Fibromyalgia (FM) is a form of soft-tissue rheumatism in adults. The word "fibro" is the Latin term for fibrous tissue, the word "myo" is the Greek term for muscle, and the word "algia" is the Greek term for pain. It is characterized by widespread pain for at least three months and pain and tenderness in at least seven of 19 body areas (National Institute of Arthritis and Musculoskeletal and Skin Diseases [NIAMS], 2012; Centers for Disease Control and Prevention [CDC], 2012). Within these tender body areas, individuals typically have tender points about the size of a quarter that produce pain when pressure is applied. Because the tender spots are small, many people are only aware of a few tender points, although more are identifiable through digital palpation (applying pressure with the fingers). In addition to pain, there may be disturbances in sleep patterns, anxiety and depression, cognitive problems, irritable bowel syndrome, and other muscle and nerve dysfunctions.

Although the FM diagnosis falls within the arthritis diagnostic family, it is not truly a form of arthritis because inflammation is not present and damage does not occur to joints, muscles, or other tissues (NIAMSD, 2012). Like arthritis, however, it does cause significant pain and fatigue and can impair ability to complete daily activities (NIAMSD, 2012).

Juvenile Fibromyalgia (JFM)

In children, FM is commonly referred to as juvenile fibromyalgia (JFM), diffuse idiopathic pain syndrome (DIPS), or amplified musculoskeletal pain syndrome (AMPS) (Clinch & Eccleston, 2009; Children's Hospital of Philadelphia [CHOP], 2014). JFM is different from FM in that symptoms may present differently and can't be measured using adult FM assessment tools. The clinical features of childhood musculoskeletal pain are described by Clinch and Eccleston (2009).

> It is not unusual for pain to start in a localized area of the body. The pain may intensify and radiate to other areas. It is associated often with a reluctance to mobilize, an avoidance of movement. Discomfort and pain intensity increase and become constant. As discrete pains multiply and continue, the young person may avoid contact with, or use of, an area of the body affected, which can lead to muscular spasms, abnormal posture and gait, and with chronic avoidance a greatly reduced fitness. Such a pattern of avoidance can lead to fear of pain and movement, and a resultant amplification of pain. (p. 466)

Incidence/Prevalence in U.S.

FM affects approximately five million Americans (CDC, 2012), or about eight percent of the adult population (National Fibromyalgia Association [NFA], 2009). Women are seven times more likely to develop FM than men (CDC, 2012). FM has also been found to co-occur (up to 25-65%) with other rheumatic diseases, such as systemic lupus erythematosus, rheumatoid arthritis, and ankylosing spondylitis (CDC, 2012).

In regards to children, a true indication of incidence/prevalence of JFM has not been determined, however several studies have found that approximately 30% of children and adolescents experience pain lasting more than six months, of which approximately two-thirds is musculoskeletal pain; and that approximately one to two percent of the pediatric population are experiencing severe and disabling chronic pain (Clinch & Eccleston, 2009).

Predominant Age

FM is usually diagnosed from 20 to 50 years of age; however symptoms may be present earlier in life, including childhood (NIAMSD, 2012; NFA, 2009). JFM is more prominent in girls then boys (however the incidence in boys is increasing) and peaks at the age of 14 (Clinch & Eccleston, 2009).

Causes

A primary cause of FM has not been identified. It may be caused by different factors, alone or in combination, such as an infectious illness, physical trauma, emotional trauma, repetitive injuries, abnormal sensory processing within the central nervous system, and genetics. There may be a gene that causes a strong reaction to stimuli that others would not perceive as being painful (NIAMSD, 2012; NFA, 2012; CDC, 2012). Obesity and certain diseases, including lupus, rheumatoid arthritis, and chronic fatigue syndrome, have also been found to associate with FM (CDC, 2012). Other conditions that may be seen with FM or mimic its symptoms include chronic neck and back pain, chronic fatigue syndrome, depression, hypothyroidism, Lyme disease, and sleep disorders (NLM, 2012). There is no known prevention for FM (NLM, 2012).

Clients with FM show elevated levels of substance P, which initiates pain signals after injury, and low levels of serotonin, which tones down the intensity of pain signals (NFA, 2012). The stress response, a communication mechanism between the brain and body that helps a client respond to physical and emotional challenges, is also impaired (NFA, 2012). Whether these abnormalities are a cause or a result of FM is unknown.

Stress often precipitates FM and exacerbates FM symptoms. Stress "causes localized arterial spasm that interferes with perfusion of oxygen in the affected areas" (Sadock & Sadock, 2003, p. 837) resulting in pain. In other words, when stress occurs, an area or areas of the body respond with arterial spasm. The artery, which carries oxygenated blood to the muscles, carries less oxygen. The muscle, when deprived of oxygen, is damaged, often showing up as a muscle spasm, and pain ensues.

The cause of JFM is also unknown; however pediatric chronic pain in general is believed to be singularly, or in combination, related to illness, injury, psychological distress, genetics, developmental influences, and environmental factors (Clinch & Eccleston, 2009). Additionally, children who live in low-educated, low-income families have an approximate 1.4-fold increase in the odds of having pain (Clinch & Eccleston, 2009).

Systems Affected

Fibromyalgia (FM)

FM affects the muscular system and central nervous system, although other systems could possibly be involved including psychological-emotional, circadian rhythm, and the hormonal system (CDC, 2012). Pain is the primary symptom (b280 Sensation of Pain).

Juvenile Fibromyalgia (JFM)

As with FM, JFM affects the muscular system and central nervous system, although other systems could possibly be involved including psychological-emotional, circadian rhythm, and the hormonal system (CDC, 2012). Pain is the primary symptom of juvenile fibromyalgia, although the pain pattern is significantly different from FM and should be documented accurately in the patient's records (b280 Sensation of Pain).

Secondary Problems

Fibromyalgia (FM)

In addition to pain and tender points, people with FM typically experience many other symptoms in different severities, although some people with FM do not experience these symptoms. The secondary problems associated with FM vary greatly depending on the severity of FM symptoms, the perception of control that the person has in managing the symptoms, and the client's initiation and maintenance of proactive steps in managing the symptoms (b126 Temperament and Personality Functions, d570 Looking After One's Health).

Symptoms include profound fatigue (b455 Exercise Tolerance Functions), sleep disturbances related to and sometimes unrelated to pain (b134 Sleep Functions), and feelings of anxiety and depression (b152 Emotional Functions) (CDC, 2012; NIAMS, 2012). It is unknown if these symptoms are related to the FM process or if they are a result of coping with FM. For example, feelings of anxiety and depression could arise from struggling to cope with FM. Poor sleep could be caused by anxiety or pain and profound fatigue could be attributed to constant lack of quality sleep. Whether or not these symptoms are part of the disease or are secondary problems is difficult to determine. However, the high percentage of people who experience these problems shows that they are probably connected to the syndrome of FM.

Individuals with FM have been found to have lower levels of health-related quality of life in seven of the eight subscales on the *SF-36* compared to individuals with other chronic diseases. Role-emotional is the exception. On average they reported a 4.8 on a 1-10 scale (1 lowest, 10 highest) on perceived quality of life (CDC, 2012). Adults with FM are also 3.4 times more likely to have major depression than those without FM (CDC, 2012).

Another common problem associated with FM is referred to as "fibro-fog." Fibro-fog describes a group of cognitive problems that are typically experienced by people with FM. These include feelings of confusion, lapses in memory, especially short-term memory, word-finding problems, word or name mix-ups, and difficulty concentrating (b140-b189 Specific Mental Functions) (CDC, 2012). These problems, like the ones previously discussed, could be caused by anxiety, depression, and lack of sleep. They could also be directly connected to the FM process or they could be a separate medical condition.

Irritable bowel syndrome (also referred to as spastic colon) is also seen with FM, characterized by abdominal pain, bloating, and alternating constipation and diarrhea (b525 Defecation Functions) (CDC, 2012). Other common symptoms of FM include morning stiffness (b780 Sensations Related to Muscles and Movement Functions), migraine and tension headaches (b280 Sensation of Pain), tingling or numbness in the hands and feet (b265 Touch Function), restless leg syndrome, temperature sensitivity (b2700 Sensitivity to Temperature), sensitivity to loud noises or bright lights (b270 Sensory Functions Related to Temperature and Other Stimuli), painful menstrual periods (b650 Menstruation Functions), and other pain syndromes

(b280 Sensation of Pain) (CDC, 2012; NIAMSD, 2012; U.S. National Library of Medicine [NLM], 2012).

The number and severity of symptoms can additionally impact the client's ability to participate in life tasks, perform self-care, engage in recreational opportunities, care for others, exercise, and socialize. When compounded, these can give rise to other secondary problems, such as deconditioning, isolation, and reduced quality of life. ICF Activities and Participation codes that are most likely to be affected will be found in d2 General Tasks and Demands, d4 Mobility, d5 Self-Care, d6 Domestic Life, d7 Interpersonal Interactions and Relationships, d8 Major Life Areas, and d9 Community, Social, and Civic Life. Areas should be noted where the pain of FM causes deficits perceived by the patient or therapist.

Juvenile Fibromyalgia (JFM)

Clinch & Eccleston (2009) describe other problems that are associated with JFM.

Hypervigilance and hypersensitivity: Heightened awareness of pain and pain-associated cues, including unbearable pain with minimal skin contact and heightened fear of touch (b280 Sensation of Pain).

Perceived thermodysregulation: Limbs may be cool and mottled, or very red and hot to touch. The child might also have an abnormal perception of temperature with an increase in thermal pain sensitivity (b550 Thermoregulatory Functions, b2700 Sensitivity to Temperature).

Autonomic dysfunction: Continuous pain signals, compromised mobility, and fatigue affect the autonomic system (s1 Structures of the Nervous System). In an environment of physical and emotional anxiety, the sympathetic system is even more active leading to tachycardia, hyperventilation (compounded by panic attacks), cold sweats, blurred vision, abdominal pain, extreme pallor, nausea, dizziness or vertigo, and feeling faint. Score problems with ICF codes under b4 Functions of the Cardiovascular, Hematological, Immunological, and Respiratory Systems and b5 Functions of the Digestive, Metabolic, and Endocrine Systems.

Musculoskeletal disequilibrium: Due to pain, children may hold certain positions that are more comfortable, such as holding knees and hips in a flexed position or making a tight fist and flexing the wrist. Muscles and tendons quickly tighten from being held in maladaptive positions (b7 Neuromusculoskeletal and Movement-Related Functions, d4 Mobility). The maladaptive positions might also be held to overprotect the painful body part for fear of pain. During the peripubertal growth spurt, bones and muscles are growing at a fast rate and holding such maladaptive positions can cause significant problems. For example, holding the knee in a flexed position not only shortens the muscle, but increased force is being placed on the muscle as bones lengthen during the growth spurt, further increasing pain. Maladaptive positions held by the child during the growth spurt can also severely affect gait, resting positions, and loads on the spine and pelvis.

Children who have JFM also typically present with fatigue (b455 Exercise Tolerance Functions), poor sleep patterns (b134 Sleep Functions), and extremely low mood, which is a reaction to the experienced pain, rather than the primary depression seen in adults (b126 Temperament and Personality Functions) (Clinch & Eccleston, 2009). Unlike adult FM, there has been no definitive work to identify specific tender points (Clinch & Eccleston, 2009).

Chronic pain in children, including JFM, affects the muscular and central nervous system as well, and has the potential to affect a wide variety of other systems including social life (d7 Interpersonal Interactions and Relationships), education (d810-d839 Education), sleep (b134 Sleep Functions), fitness (b455 Exercise Tolerance Functions), independence (choose specific Activities and Participation code), moods (b126 Temperament and Personality Functions), appetite (b130 Energy and Drive Functions), eating (b510 Ingestion Functions), and family (d760 Family Relationships) (Clinch & Eccleston, 2009).

School absences or need for home schooling are possible because of difficulties associated with prolonged sitting, concentration and memory difficulties, interpersonal problems in explaining confusing problems to peers, frequent anxiety-provoking "emergency events" associated with pain, and time away for hospital visits. Score with d750 Informal Social Relationships and d810-d839 Education. Parental distress can come from the desire of the parents to relieve pain for their child, comfort their child, and protect their child (d760 Family Relationships) (Clinch & Eccleston, 2009).

Prognosis

Mortality among adults with FM is similar to the general population, however death rates from suicide and injuries are higher among individuals with FM (CDC, 2012). FM is a chronic condition and can therefore last a long time, possibly a lifetime (NIAMSD, 2012). Although chronic, it is not a progressive disease, it is never fatal, and it does not cause damage to joints, muscles, or internal organs (NIAMSD, 2012).

FM may remit spontaneously with decreased stress in milder cases but it can also become chronic or recur at frequent intervals. FM symptoms can last for weeks or months and can be brought on by emotional or physical stress or they can appear without reference to a direct stressor. The functional prognosis related to the ability to participate in life activities and lead a quality life is usually favorable with a comprehensive, supportive program, even when some degree of symptoms tends to persist (Berkow, 1992).

Studies have reported disability rates as high as 44% in people with FM (Arthritis Foundation, 2006). Pain can become disabling leading to problems with walking. Cognitive problems can affect work performance. On a positive note, a Norwegian study followed 33 women who were diagnosed with FM over a period of six to eight years and found that, in the long run, FM is more likely to get better than worse and that women who have had FM "for quite some time" tend to manage quite well (Arthritis Foundation, 2002).

Children with JFM tend to have better outcomes than adults with FM, especially when there is multidisciplinary involvement, including the involvement of parents (Clinch & Eccleston, 2009). Prolonged time to treatment and marked autonomic changes are indicators of a poorer prognosis (Clinch & Eccleston, 2009). Relapses of pain are common. However, if physical and emotional strategies that have been taught during rehabilitation are employed, the impact of pain can be reduced (Clinch & Eccleston, 2009). In some cases, despite a variety of interventions, the pain does not subside and becomes disabling to the child and family (Clinch & Eccleston, 2009).

Assessment

Typical Scope of Team Assessment

For both forms of fibromyalgia, the team needs to assess the issues listed in the secondary problems. Significant issues may need to be addressed along with treatment to reduce the pain (b280 Sensation of Pain). Assessing the level of pain is done differently for FM and JFM as described below. The team must also analyze how well the client is coping with the pain (d240 Handling Stress and Other Psychological Demands).

Fibromyalgia (FM)

There are currently no laboratory tests for FM. Therefore, unfortunately, some physicians may conclude that a person's pain is not real. They may also tell the person that there is nothing that can be done to alleviate the pain since there is no clearly identified underlying cause (NIAMSD, 2012). This is not considered best medical practice because there are ways to assess and alleviate the pain.

The American College of Rheumatology (ACR) 2010 criteria for the clinical diagnosis of FM include (CDC, 2012):

A score of a seven or greater on the *Widespread Pain Index (WPI)* and a score of five or more on the *Symptoms Severity Scale* (SS); or a score of three to six on the WPI and a score of nine or greater on the SS. The WPI scores the number of areas where the person felt pain over the past week from a set of 19 specified body areas. The SS scale consists of two parts (2A and 2B). On the 2A SS scale, the person rates the severity of his/her experienced fatigue, waking unrefreshed, and cognitive symptoms over the past week with a score of 0 = no problem, 1 = slight/mild problem, 2 = moderate problem, 3 = severe problem. The scores for each of the three areas are then tallied for a score of zero to nine. On the 2B SS scale, a list of 40 somatic symptoms is provided. The person checks the symptoms that s/he has experienced over the past week. Depending on the number of symptoms identified by the person, the person receives a score (0 = no symptoms, 1 = few symptoms, 2 = moderate symptoms, 3 = a great deal of symptoms). The 2A and 2B scores are added together to obtain the overall SS score ranging from zero to 12. A free copy of the WPI and SS are available at http://fmmgmt.com/pdf/Quiz/ACR.pdf.

To be diagnosed as FM, the symptoms must have been present at a similar level for at least three months and there must be no other disorder that can account for the symptoms. The pain may feel like a deep ache or a shooting, burning pain (NLM, 2012). It often seems to improve during the day and worsen at night, and may additionally worsen with activity, cold or damp weather, anxiety, and stress (NLM, 2012).

Juvenile Fibromyalgia (JFM)

The WPI and SS are not appropriate for diagnosing JFM; consequently a different approach for diagnosis is needed. A detailed history is taken, along with a physical exam, to rule out other diagnoses, identify key issues, and build a therapeutic relationship with the client and family. The history includes onset of pain; characteristics of pain; other symptoms, such as fever, bowel problems, or fatigue; effect of pain on daily living; past and family history of illness; and family, emotional, and social circumstances, such as living situation and stressors (Clinch & Eccleston, 2009 — see the article for a detailed outline of history questions). The child may have also had a history of extensive medical care, feelings of being doubted, and a history of failed and pain-provoking interventions (Clinch & Eccleston, 2009). Assessment tools that may be helpful include the *Visual Analog Scale (VAS),* the *Varni/Thompson Paediatric Pain Questionnaire*, the *Functional Disability Index*, the *Bath Adolescent Pain Questionnaire* and the *Bath Adolescent Pain Questionnaire for Parents* (Clinch & Eccleston, 2009).

Areas of Concern for RT Assessment

The RT assessment should first describe the current issues related to pain and the pain variations throughout the day and week. This will point out treatment options related to best times for treatment and limitations related to pain (b280 Sensation of Pain). Many of the related ICF codes that the recreational therapist should consider were listed in the Systems and Secondary Problems sections. Other codes that often affect RT treatments include b126 Temperament and Personality Functions, b152 Emotional Functions, b455 Exercise Tolerance Functions, b140-b189 Specific Mental Functions (related to fibro-fog), b510 Ingestion Functions, b525 Defecation Functions, b270 Sensory

Functions Related to Temperature and Other Stimuli, and b550 Thermoregulatory Functions. The assessment should also look at codes in b4 Functions of the Cardiovascular, Hematological, Immunological, and Respiratory Systems and b7 Neuromusculoskeletal and Movement-Related Functions.

Often people with FM or JFM will withdraw from or drive away family and friends because of their pain or other related symptoms. The RT assessment should check for this by looking at ICF codes under d7 Interpersonal Interactions and Relationships and e3 Support and Relationships.

ICF Core Set

ICF Core Sets that might be helpful in identifying relevant ICF codes, depending upon the client's fibromyalgia-related complications, include Arthritis, Chronic Pain, and Musculoskeletal Conditions.

Treatment Direction

Whole Team Approach

In treating FM, a multidisciplinary treatment approach is recommended to help relieve pain (b280 Sensation of Pain) and other symptoms, as well as cope with the symptoms (d240 Handling Stress and Other Psychological Demands) (NLM, 2012; CDC, 2012). Such interventions may including screening and treatment for depression; pharmacotherapy using antidepressants, muscle relaxants, pain relievers, and/or sleeping aids; aerobic exercise that has been found to improve global well-being and reduce tender point counts; muscle strengthening exercises; education and relaxation therapy that has been shown to improve physical impairments and reduce days not feeling well, general and morning fatigue, stiffness, anxiety, and depression; support groups and cognitive behavioral therapy to change negative thoughts, track pain and related symptoms, and identify triggers; and seeking out and participating in enjoyable activities (CDC, 2012; NLM, 2012). Complementary and alternative therapies may also be helpful, including massage, movement therapies, chiropractic treatment, water therapy, relaxation exercises and deep breathing, aromatherapy, biofeedback, and acupressure or acupuncture (NIAMSD, 2012; NLM, 2012; NFA, 2009). Other things that may be helpful include getting enough sleep and eating a healthy diet to maximize energy, prevent other health problems, and

promote a general sense of feeling better (NIAMSD, 2012). Each of these therapies can be tied directly to problems described in the team assessment, including b126 Temperament and Personality Functions, b130 Energy and Drive Functions, b134 Sleep Functions, b140-b189 Specific Mental Functions, b455 Exercise Tolerance Functions, b7 Neuromusculoskeletal and Movement-Related Functions, d4 Mobility, d570 Looking After One's Health, and d7 Interpersonal Interactions and Relationships.

Treatment interventions for JFM, like FM, focus on symptom management and psychosocial rehabilitation through (Clinch & Eccleston, 2009): education about anatomy and physiology of JFM to reduce fear; pharmacotherapy; and psychological therapies, such as cognitive behavioral therapy that focuses on relaxation, habit reversal, and attention-based interventions. Therapies should also focus on engagement in life activities, with measured outcomes relating to return to school, participation in enjoyable activities, and reduced depression and anxiety. High doses of exercise increase activity of the musculoskeletal system, which reduces muscle spasms and tightening, improves proprioception, and lessens autonomic changes. Whenever possible, children should be encouraged to devise their own constant and paced fitness plan outside of the hospital environment to promote community engagement and maximize motivation. Interventions that provide psychological and emotional support and aid in goal setting, pain communication, maintaining motivation, managing low mood, coping with anger and frustration, and overcoming fears should also be provided if there were related problems noted in the client's assessment. The extent of the above interventions will vary depending on the severity of pain and the kinds of dysfunction that were assessed. The ICF codes for JFM are similar to the codes for FM described above with the addition of d810-d839 Education, d880 Engagement in Play, and d9 Community, Social, and Civic Life.

Recreational Therapy Approach

RT predominantly focuses on four areas: (1) helping people with FM make lifestyle changes that affect the severity of all of the symptoms, although the amount or relief from lifestyle changes will vary; (2) working on finding activities that the clients enjoy to promote healthy exercise and active participation in social and community life; (3) providing techniques to help the client cope with and manage pain; and (4) alleviating relationship and support issues, if possible. Relevant ICF codes are listed in the team approach.

Recreational Therapy Interventions

According to Busse and colleagues (2013), "no review has evaluated all interventional studies for fibromyalgia, which limits attempts to make inferences regarding the relative effectiveness of treatments" (p. 18). As a result, Busse and colleagues (2013) have designed a research protocol to conduct a network meta-analysis of all randomized controlled trials evaluating therapies for FM and patient-reported outcomes to facilitate evidence-based practice and identify future research needs. The outcomes will be classified into nine domains, including pain, physical and emotional functioning (including quality of life), participant rating of improvement and satisfaction with treatment, adverse events, participant disposition, role functioning (including work, education, social and recreational activities, home and family care), interpersonal functioning (interpersonal relationships, sexual activities), sleep, and fatigue. A timeline for publication wasn't noted; however recreational therapists who work with this population should follow this study closely.

In the meantime, recreational therapists should employ traditional interventions aimed at lifestyle changes to aid in pain relief (b280 Sensation of Pain). RTs should also teach skills that were found to be deficient during the RT assessment. These might include coping with stress (b126 Temperament and Personality Functions, b152 Emotional Functions, d240 Handling Stress and Other Psychological Demands), and increasing energy levels (b455 Exercise Tolerance Functions). Adaptations to activities can be provided to promote a more active lifestyle, which will improve areas diagnosed as problems in b4 Functions of the Cardiovascular, Hematological, Immunological, and Respiratory Systems and b7 Neuromusculoskeletal and Movement-Related Functions. Education should be provided to the client, family members, and other support people to improve their interactions and reduce the stress caused by FM or JFM (d7 Interpersonal Interactions and Relationships, e3 Support and Relationships).

Treating JFM can include multi-disciplinary comprehensive day treatment programs specifically for JFM. In these programs, therapists treat the deficits noted in the assessment process with a variety of recreational activities. They can increase engagement in physical activity with activities like active games and swimming and improve coping with activities like art and music. This is a key setting for providing recreational therapy.

Resources

Advocates for Fibromyalgia Funding, Treatment, Education, and Research
www.affter.org
A non-profit organization that helps educate patients, their families, and the medical community by providing support groups, seminars, and various printed and electronic materials. They also conduct, publish, and fund fibromyalgia research.

Arthritis Foundation
www.arthritis.org
A non-profit organization that supports people with the more than 100 types of arthritis and related conditions.

Fibromyalgia Network
www.fmnetnews.com
Provides advocacy, awareness, and education for people with fibromyalgia.

National Fibromyalgia Association
www.fmaware.org
A non-profit organization whose mission is to develop and execute programs dedicated to improving the quality of life for people with fibromyalgia.

National Fibromyalgia Partnership, Inc.
www.fmpartnership.org
Provides high quality, medically accurate information on fibromyalgia symptoms, diagnosis, treatment, and research.

References

Arthritis Foundation. (2006). Delivering on the promise in fibromyalgia. http://www.arthritis.org/research/ Research_Program/Fibromyalgia/default.asp.

Arthritis Foundation. (2002). Fibromyalgia: Long-term outcome looks up. *Journal of Rheumatology, 28*(9), http://www.arthritis.org/resources/arthritistoday/ 2002_archives/2002_03_04_Research_Fibro.asp.

Berkow, R. (1992). *The Merck manual of diagnosis and therapy.* Rahway, NJ: Merck & Co, Inc.

Busse, J. W., Ebrahim, S., Connell, G., Coomes, E. A., Bruno, P., Malik, K., Torrance, D., Ngo, T., Kirmayr, K., Avrahami, D., Riva, J. J., Struijs, P., Brunarski, D., Burnie, S. J., LeBlanc, F., Steenstra, I. A., Mahood, Q., Thorlund, K., Montori, V. M., Sivarajah, V., Alexander, P., Jankowski, M., Lesniak, W., Faulhaber, M., Bala, M. M., Schandelmaier, S., & Guyatt, G. H. (2013). Systematic review and network meta-analysis of interventions for fibromyalgia: A protocol. *Systematic Reviews, 2,* 18.

Centers for Disease Control and Prevention. (2012). Fibromyalgia. Retrieved from http://www.cdc.gov/arthritis/basics/fibromyalgia.htm.

Clinch, J. & Eccleston, C. (2009). Chronic musculoskeletal pain in children: Assessment and management. *Rheumatology, 48,* 466-474.

Children's Hospital of Philadelphia. (2014). About amplified musculoskeletal pain syndrome. Retrieved from http://www.chop.edu/service/amplified-musculoskeletal-pain-syndrome/about-amps/.

National Fibromyalgia Association. (2009). About fibromyalgia. Retrieved from http://fmaware.org/PageServerded3.html?pagename=fibromyalgia.

National Institute of Arthritis and Musculoskeletal and Skin Diseases. (2012). Fibromyalgia. Retrieved from http://www.niams.nih.gov/Health_Info/Fibromyalgia/.

Sadock, B. & Sadock, V. (2003). *Kaplan & Sadock's synopsis of psychiatry.* Philadelphia, PA: Lippincott Williams & Wilkins.

U.S. National Library of Medicine. (2012). *Fibromyalgia.* Retrieved from http://www.ncbi.nlm.nih.gov/pubmedhealth/PMH0001463/.

15. Gambling Disorder

Anne-Marie Sullivan

During the last three decades, gambling has grown in popularity and is now commonly accepted as a pastime for a number of youth and adults. It has been suggested that much of this gambling can be described as social and non-problematic. For some, however, gambling can become a compulsion, an activity that is carried out despite negative consequences or a desire to stop. Pathological gambling (PG) was first included as a mental disorder by the American Psychiatric Association (APA) in the *Diagnostic and Statistical Manual of Mental Disorders* in 1980; it has been renamed from pathological gambling to gambling disorder (GD) in the *DSM-5* (APA, 2013).

Gambling disorder has been shown to be associated with problems in health, social isolation or altered social roles, depression, suicide ideation and suicide, and limited preparation for adulthood and work (Derevensky & Gupta, 2000). As gambling availability and diversity of options increases, there is concern that there may be an increase in problem gambling as well (Volberg, 1996).

It is important to point out that, in addition to GD, a number of other terms are used when referring to problematic gambling including compulsive gambling, gambling addiction, and problem gambling. Compulsive gambling is a term that is used but it is not preferred by clinicians because many clients do not describe the behaviors as compulsive, even though the behavior presents as compulsive. Gambling is often referred to as a process addiction in the recovery movement (Eades, 2003) and Gamblers Anonymous follows a 12-step program similar to those seen in other recovery programs, such as Alcoholics Anonymous or Narcotics Anonymous.

In the *DSM-IV-TR*, gambling was included as an impulse control disorder, not an addiction. One of the changes for the *DSM-5* is that gambling disorder is now included as part of substance-related and addictive disorders since evidence suggests that gambling affects the brain reward system in a way that is similar to substance abuse. Further, in the *DSM-5*, internet gaming is included as a condition to be further researched. This research will determine whether internet gaming should be added as a formal disorder (APA, 2013). While only a small portion of the population (one to five percent) has been identified as pathological gamblers, studies show that as many as 23% of the population may have some level of problems with gambling (Shaffer, Hall, & Vander Bilt, 1997). It is vital that those with gambling problems be acknowledged as potential candidates for treatment.

Both PG and GD will be used in this chapter. GD will be used with the most recent information. PG will be used when discussing older literature reviewed for this chapter where the term PG was used. It is anticipated that future scales and writing will be modified to reflect the changes in the *DSM-5*.

Incidence/Prevalence in U.S.

Since 1990, there has been a great deal of focus on prevalence-based research employing telephone surveys using random population sampling techniques and the *South Oaks Gambling Screen* (SOGS). The SOGS (Lesieur & Blume, 1987) was developed for use in a clinical setting but has been employed at the community level. There has been some criticism for doing this mainly because the SOGS performance in a community population is not well understood (Wiebe, Single, & Falkowski-Ham, 2001). This research has shown a lifetime prevalence of gambling disorders from 2.8% to 6.3%. Similarly, a meta-analysis showed a lifetime prevalence of problem gambling of 5.2% in adults and a past year prevalence of 3.9% (Shaffer et al., 1997). Shaffer et al. (1997) identified 120 prevalence studies of disordered gambling, but there were virtually no incidence studies conducted in the field. They went on to suggest that prevalence and incidence were commonly used interchangeably in the studies included in the meta-analysis, so incidence figures are unavailable. Because of the challenges with the instruments used (many were developed for clinical populations but are used in general populations), true prevalence estimates are difficult to establish (Shaffer et al., 1997).

What is known about problem gambling is that men are more likely to be identified as problem gamblers by approximately a ratio of 2:1 (Potenza et al., 2001; Shaffer et al., 1997). This figure may be inaccurate, however, as there is more social stigma attached to gambling for women and consequently there are fewer women in treatment for problem gambling (Fong, 2005). In general, men who are problem gamblers begin gambling as teenagers, while women tend to start compulsive gambling at a later age (Black & Shaw, 2008). It is also more common to see higher rates of problem gambling in minority groups and in people with lower socioeconomic status (Fong, 2005). Further, there appears to be comorbidity with other mental health problems including substance-related disorders, mood and anxiety disorders, or personality disorders (Black & Shaw, 2008).

Predominant Age

Problem gamblers tend to report gambling behaviors at an earlier age than their counterparts who gamble socially. According to Moore and Jadlos (2002), males who are considered problem gamblers reported their first experience gambling at a much earlier age (10.0 years) than females who are considered problem gamblers (17.2 years). Male social gamblers reported their first gambling experience at 22.6 years.

Using the SOGS to determine presence of problem gambling, level 2 refers to probable pathological gambling and level 3 refers to pathological gambling. According to Shaffer et al., (1997), "Adolescents consistently have higher rates of level 3 and level 2 time frames gambling for both lifetime and past year than their adult general population counterparts" (p.54).

In addition to this group, "College students and adults in treatment or prison consistently had significantly higher rates of lifetime level 3 gambling than adults surveyed from the general population" (Shaffer et al., 1997, p.54). Age then, as well as membership in one of the groups noted, is an important factor that may contribute to the development of GD.

Causes

There has been much debate regarding the causes of gambling. As with many illnesses, researchers have looked to psychological, biological, and social explanations to describe the development and progression of the disease. Although there is little agreement on what specifically causes problem gambling, it seems to be consistently thought that problem gambling is not a disease in and of itself, but a symptom of a larger or more complex mental process (Ferris, Wynne, & Single, 1999). The training of the researcher clearly plays a role in his/her approach to understanding the gambling process with social scientists focusing on family, social, and environmental factors while clinicians and psychologists tend to focus more on internal factors including biological, emotional, cognitive, and behavioral. For a more detailed review of the development of problem gambling see Abbott & Clarke (2007).

Blaszczynski and Nower (2002) proposed three major subgroups of gamblers:

Behaviorally conditioned problem gamblers: Almost all problem gamblers have access to gambling options, particularly those more strongly associated with gambling problems such as slot machines. For many, they're able to recall their first big win and they become conditioned to "chase losses" meaning they lose but believe they will be able to win their money back and so begins the cycle. This cycle continues as the gambler experiences cognitive distortions such as believing s/he somehow has control over the outcome or viewing losses as near wins or almost winning so there is an uncontrollable desire to continue trying. It is also important to note that many people in this subgroup often experience anxiety, depression, and substance use and abuse. It is unknown whether these are factors contributing to or resulting from problem gambling. Further, people in this subgroup tend to have lower levels of gambling problems and are more likely to comply with treatment than those in either of the other two subgroups (Blaszczynski & Nower, 2002).

Emotionally vulnerable problem gamblers: This group often develops similarly to the behaviorally conditioned group; that is, similar conditioning, environmental, and psychological factors are seen in both groups. The emotionally vulnerable subgroup differs in that these gamblers are characterized by pre-existing vulnerabilities, such as anxiety and/or depression, poor coping, and problem-solving skills, as well as negative family experiences and life events (Blaszczynski & Nower, 2002). Such individuals are attracted to gambling to meet psychological needs and reduce emotional states. They are also more likely to have other mental health disorders including addictive behaviors and affective disorders. They are less likely to respond to treatment and are unlikely to be able to gamble in non-problematic ways (Abbott & Clarke, 2008).

Antisocial, impulsive problem gamblers: This group, like the emotionally vulnerable group, is more likely to have predisposing psychological and biological factors contributing to problem gambling. In addition to these factors, they are also believed to have "neurological and neurochemical dysfunctions, as well as features of impulsivity, attention deficit disorder and antisocial personality" (Blaszczynski & Nower, 2002, as cited in Abbott & Clarke, 2008, p. 128). Members of this group tend to have more psychopathology, are much more likely to report parents with substance abuse and antisocial problems, and are more likely to report early exposure to substance and gambling behaviors. This group appears to be unlikely to seek treatment options and does not comply with treatment.

While this categorization is useful, it is still not clearly understood how these subgroups will be employed at the clinical level. Substance use and abuse is better understood in the clinical literature and it is important to look to this material to better understand how to help those with gambling problems given there appears to be a strong relationship between substance misuse and problem gambling.

Systems Affected

GD includes preoccupation with gambling activity, often to the extent of interfering with occupational and/or social functioning (APA, 1994; 2013). Code these problems using d2 General Tasks and Demands, especially d240 Handling Stress and Other Psychological Demands and d250 Managing One's Own Behavior, d7 Interpersonal Interactions and Relationships, and d8 Major Life Areas.

It is not uncommon for gamblers to participate in "chasing" behavior which refers to betting larger sums of money or taking greater risks in order to undo or make up for previous losses (Brown, 1987; Walker, 1992). The person's cognitive processes become irrational as they come to believe they have control over the gambling behavior and outcomes (Walker, 1992). It is also common for the gambler's thoughts to become preoccupied with various elements of gambling including memories of past experiences, as well as anticipation of future gambling (Rosenthal, 1992). For some, this preoccupation impacts all other domains of life including, self, family, and work (National Research Council, 1999). Code the cognitive issues with b126 Temperament and Personality Functions and b164 Higher-Level Cognitive Functions and the relationship issues with d7 Interpersonal Interactions and Relationships, and d8 Major Life Areas.

As a result of these cognitive disturbances, GD frequently has a significant impact on relationships. The person may lie about the gambling and, in many cases, may resort to a variety of antisocial behaviors such as stealing, fraud, forgery, and/or embezzling, in order to obtain more money to support the gambling behavior (Lesieur & Rosenthal, 1991). Such behaviors negatively impact family and social relationships. Loved ones begin to recognize that they can no longer trust the gambler and will often become fearful of the extent of the problem and what may happen to their financial situation if they remain involved with the gambler. Code with b130 Energy and Drive Functions, d250 Managing One's Own Behavior, and d7 Interpersonal Interactions and Relationships.

For many gamblers, there are emotional difficulties that contribute to the gambling problem. As previously noted, for some it is unclear whether these difficulties are contributing factors or result from the gambling behavior. It is likely that some have emotional difficulties, such as depression and inability to cope, that predispose them to GD; while others have these emotional problems because of the gambling behavior and the feeling that they are spiraling out of control (Shaffer & LaPlante, 2005). Code with b125 Dispositions and Intra-Personal

Functions, b126 Temperament and Personality Functions, and b130 Energy and Drive Functions.

Finally, as noted above, there appears to be a strong connection between substance misuse and GD. Again, as with emotional difficulties, it is unclear which causes which. It is important, however, to recognize that the relationship between substance misuse and GD exists and needs to be addressed in clinical settings. Code with d570 Looking After One's Health, especially d57022 Avoiding Risks of Abuse and Drugs or Alcohol.

Secondary Problems

Other problems that are often associated with GD may include, but are not limited to, social/relationship difficulties, including separation and divorce, occupational difficulties, criminal behavior, antisocial behavior, financial troubles, affective and/or substance-related disorders, and suicide (Ladouceur et al., 1994). Applicable ICF codes can be found in the System Affected section. Also see the chapter on Substance-Related Disorders for more information about addictive behavior.

Prognosis

Like alcohol and other substance use problems, GD is chronic and is likely to worsen without intervention (Blaszczynski & Silove, 1995). Even with intervention, it is common for the person to relapse and return to gambling. As previously noted, the subgroup the gambler belongs to will influence the prognosis. For those in the behaviorally conditioned group, treatment options are often successful (Blaszczynski & Nower, 2002). For many of these individuals, gambling is used as escape and to help cope with life stressors. For some, gambling problems result as the person attempts to "chase" losses and becomes preoccupied with the activity. By addressing social and/or emotional difficulties, gambling behaviors will often return to a social activity without the need for further intervention (Blaszczynski & Nower, 2002).

For those in the other two subgroups, treatment is often not as successful. Those who are emotionally vulnerable are more likely to have predisposing factors that will need to be addressed and somehow resolved in treatment if the person is to overcome GD (Blaszczynski & Nower, 2002). For these individuals, it is unlikely that they can return to gambling without

the risk that the gambling may escalate to a pathological level again. For antisocial gamblers, treatment is rarely effective and it is unlikely that they will ever be able to manage non-problematic gambling (Blaszczynski & Nower, 2002). These individuals are less likely to seek treatment and tend to be unwilling to comply with treatment expectations.

Because of the high rates of comorbidity with other mental health issues, it is important that treatment options are provided to address emotional disorders as well as substance abuse disorders. Without some acknowledgement of other issues that may be contributing to GD, treatment compliance will be difficult (Blaszczynski & Nower, 2002).

Assessment

Typical Scope of Team Assessment

The first assessment is to see if the person meets the *DSM-5* criteria for gambling disorder (APA, 2013). This includes seeing if there is a persistent and recurrent problem of at least 12 month's duration. The person must exhibit at least four out of eight traits: a need to gamble with increasing amounts of money, restlessness when not gambling, repeated attempts to stop gambling, preoccupation with gambling, gambling as a way to handle distress, lying about the extent of gambling, risks to relationships or career caused by gambling, and reliance on others to finance the gambling. The team must rule out the possibility that the gambling is better explained as a manic episode. The *ICD-10* code is F63.0 Pathological Gambling.

The team then will have to assess the extent of the problem, as well as any secondary problems that are contributing to or resulting from the gambling behaviors. ICF codes for documenting the deficits were described earlier in the chapter.

Areas of Concern for RT Assessment

The findings will vary depending on the extent of gambling involvement and the existence of any comorbid psychopathology. Generally, recreational therapists can expect to see unhealthy leisure choices with deficits in positive leisure activities (d920 Recreation and Leisure), preoccupation with gambling at the expense of other forms of leisure participation, maladaptive coping (d240 Handling Stress and Other Psychological Demands), and impaired work/school, social, and family relations (d7 Interpersonal Interactions and Relationships, d8 Major Life Areas, d9 Community, Social, and Civic Life) (Carruthers, 1999).

ICF Core Set

No ICF Core Set for Gambling Disorders has been published.

Treatment Direction

The first step toward recovery is recognizing the problem, as GD is strongly associated with denial. Most individuals with GD do not willingly participate in treatment even though they are frequently pressured to seek treatment by others in their lives. Admitting to any of the deficits or problems noted in the assessment process can provide the patient with a motivation for complying with treatment.

Whole Team Approach

There are a number of individual and group-based approaches to treatment that have some success for gambling problems.

Gamblers Anonymous (GA): GA was started in 1957 and is one of the best known interventions for GD. GA is a fellowship of men and women who want to stop gambling. It is a 12-step program following closely the steps of AA. One aspect of the approach is to work on issues in the ICF codes under d7 Interpersonal Interactions and Relationships. Although it is a popular approach, there is not a lot of research examining the effectiveness of GA in reducing GD.

Cognitive behavioral therapy (CBT): As noted, pathological gamblers are preoccupied with thoughts about gambling and often have irrational thoughts regarding their ability to control outcomes. CBT is currently "the primary psycho-therapeutic modality for the treatment of disordered gambling" with strong clinical trials evidence supporting its use in the treatment of PG [now GD] (Korn & Shaffer, 2004, p. 19). This approach is based on social learning theory (Bandura, 1986) and attempts to change the irrational thoughts and behaviors. It reduces problems noted with ICF codes b164 Higher-Level Cognitive Functions, d240 Handling Stress and Other Psychological Demands, and d250 Managing One's Own Behavior.

Psychodynamic psychotherapy: According to Korn and Shafer (2004) this approach, which was widely used before CBT, is used to determine whether there are any underlying psychological factors that may trigger gambling behavior. For those who use gambling as an escape, this approach may be useful in identifying what the person is trying to avoid and discovering more appropriate coping strategies. It is also useful for individuals dealing with dual diagnoses as it may help shed light on other issues that also require intervention. For a detailed account of psychodynamic approaches to gambling treatment, see Rosenthal and Rugle (1994). It aims to understand and treat issues associated with b126 Temperament and Personality Functions, b130 Energy and Drive Functions, and d240 Handling Stress and Other Psychological Demands

Marital and family therapy: Couples treatment is often used as gambling has the potential to wreak havoc on the family unit (Korn & Shaffer, 1999). As well, many pathological gamblers come from turbulent family environments. A key to reducing gambling behavior lies in understanding the family relationships and ensuring the gambler has social support. This also parallels GA which offers Gambling Anon for family members of pathological gamblers (Korn & Shaffer, 2004). All aspects of d7 Interpersonal Interactions and Relationships may be treated, especially d760 Family Relationships and d770 Intimate Relationships.

Pharmacological approaches: Pharmacology is a relatively new approach to treatment of gambling disorder. For a detailed review of pharmacological approaches, see Grant, Kim, and Potenza (2003). Research suggests that the effectiveness of certain medications, including mood stabilizers, serotonin and serotonin reuptake inhibitors (SRIs), selective serotonin reuptake inhibitors (SSRIs), opioid receptor antagonists, and atypical antipsychotics is promising, but additional research is needed to better understand many aspects of GD treatment. Many of the pharma-cological approaches have been tested because of the similarities of gambling disorder to other addictions. For example, naltrexone, an opioid receptor antago-nist, has been tested with substance misuse and results suggest that naltrexone combined with structured behavioral therapy is effective in reducing substance abuse (Swift, 2000, as cited in Grant et al., 2003). Medications may reduce problems noted with

ICF codes b164 Higher-Level Cognitive Functions, d240 Handling Stress and Other Psychological Demands, and d250 Managing One's Own Behavior.

Clearly, further research is needed to determine the efficacy of the treatment approaches available for GD. It is also likely that understanding treatment options will allow for improved insight into the development of GD.

Recreational Therapy Approach

Recreational therapists who work with GD will be working in either an addiction or psychiatric facility. It is likely that they will be working with both populations since GD has a high rate of comorbidity with other psychiatric diagnoses. These programs will most likely include a combination of inpatient and outpatient options for individuals and groups.

Carruthers (1999) recommends that cognitive behavioral models of treatment include cognitive therapy (Blaszczynski & Silove, 1995), stress management (McCormick, 1994, as cited in Carruthers, 1999), relationship and communication skills, and the establishment of a non-gambling lifestyle. A recreational therapist has a great deal to contribute to the overall treatment for gamblers. Below are some common recreational therapy interventions that are used in the treatment in GD.

Recreational Therapy Interventions

Common RT interventions for clients with GD include:

Stress management (b130 Energy and Drive Functions, d240 Handling Stress and Other Psychological Demands): Since escape is a common motivation for gambling behavior, it is important that the individual learn how to better manage stress. The individual needs to learn better coping strategies to manage daily struggles. RT can help clients better understand their stressors and learn how to identify these and cope without gambling behavior (Carruthers, 1995, as cited in Carruthers, 1999). While there is no empirical evidence readily available, adventure-based activities may also be offered as a more acceptable form of risk-taking and/or escape.

Self-esteem interventions (b126 Temperament and Personality Functions): Poor self-esteem is often thought of as an important issue for treatment of GD.

It is necessary to explore feelings of inadequacy and self-worth to better understand why the individual resorts to gambling. According to Austin (1999), recreational therapists can provide opportunities for clients to experience mastery and consequently develop a sense of competence. Gambling provides excitement, a sense of accomplishment, and feelings of self-worth. It is important that these feelings be achieved through less harmful and more meaningful leisure opportunities (Mannell & Kleiber, 1997).

Relationship building (b126 Temperament and Personality Functions, d710 Basic Interpersonal Interactions, d720 Complex Interpersonal Interactions): Relationship and social skills are vital parts of recovery for GD. Skills that need to be emphasized include refusal skills, conversation skills, conflict resolution, and assertiveness. It is important that the individual has the skills to develop non-gambling relationships and the ability to rely on others for support in recovery. RT interventions often focus on social skills training and assertiveness training (Austin, 1999). Social skills training focuses on various elements of verbal and non-verbal communication, as well as proper social etiquette. Assertiveness training emphasizes the importance of conflict resolution, identification and appropriate verbalization of feelings, and refusal skills. According to McCormick (1994), social skills and assertiveness are essential skills to be addressed in treatment programs for GD.

Leisure education and counseling (b126 Temperament and Personality Functions, b130 Energy and Drive Functions, d240 Handling Stress and Other Psychological Demands, d910 Community Life, d920 Recreation and Leisure): Leisure education is a primary focus of RT interventions when working in GD. Leisure activities are a vital part of emotional and physical wellness. They can help manage stress, prevent boredom, and maintain physical and mental health. Leisure activities offer coping strategies and increase self-confidence (Hood & Carruthers, 2002). Often times, those with GD need to learn about alternative leisure opportunities in order to replace gambling. Leisure education will help by offering information about leisure values and attitudes, as well as the importance of leisure as part of well-being. Practical information regarding the availability of leisure resources that do not involve gambling is also shared during leisure education sessions. Leisure education is a vital part of recovery in that it addresses issues related to relapse prevention, coping skills, and community reintegration (Hester & Miller, 1995, as cited in Carruthers, 1999). It is also important to note that while identifying alternate leisure opportunities, the recreational therapist considers whether the gambler's addictive tendencies will cause the new activities to become addictive (Coyle & Kinney, 1990). For example, proposing video games as a substitute for gambling would probably not be a good idea.

Resources

Gamblers Anonymous

www.gamblersanonymous.org/ga/

References

Abbott, M. W. & Clarke, D. (2007). Prospective problem gambling research: Contribution and potential. *International Gambling Studies, 7,* 123-144.

American Psychiatric Association. (1980). *Diagnostic and Statistical Manual of Mental Disorders* (3rd ed.). Washington, DC: Author.

American Psychiatric Association. (1994). *Diagnostic and Statistical Manual of Mental Disorders* (4th ed.). Washington, DC: Author.

American Psychiatric Association. (2000). *Diagnostic and Statistical Manual of Mental Disorders* (4th ed. Text revision). Washington, DC: Author.

American Psychiatric Association. (2013). *Diagnostic and Statistical Manual of Mental Disorders* (5th ed.). Washington, DC: Author.

Austin, D. (1999). *Therapeutic recreation: Processes and techniques.* Champaign, IL Sagamore Publishing.

Bandura, A. (1986). *Social foundations of thought and action: A social cognitive theory.* Englewood Cliffs, NJ: Prentice-Hall, Inc.

Black, D. W. & Shaw, M. (2008). Psychiatric comorbidity associated with pathological gambling. *Psychiatric Times, 25*(12), electronic version: http://www.psychiatrictimes.com/display/article/10168/1342537.

Blaszczynski, A. & Nower, L. (2002). A pathways model of problem and pathological gambling. *Addiction, 97,* 489-499.

Blaszczynski A. & Silove D. (1995). Cognitive and behavioral therapies for pathological gambling. *Journal of Gambling Studies, 11,* 195220.

Brown, R. I. (1987). Classical and operant paradigms in the management of gambling addictions. *Behavioral Psychotherapy, 15*(2), 111-122.

Carruthers, C. (1995). Model leisure education program for people with addictions. *The Counselor, 13*(4), 35-39.

Carruthers, C. (1999). Pathological gambling: Implications for therapeutic recreation practice. *Therapeutic Recreation Journal, 33,* 287-303.

Coyle, C. & Kinney, T. (1990). A comparison of leisure and gambling motives of compulsive gamblers. *Therapeutic Recreation Journal, 24,* 33-39.

Derevensky, J. L. & Gupta, R. (2000). Prevalence estimates of adolescent gambling: A comparison of the SOGS-RA, DSM-IV-J, and the GA 20 Questions. *Journal of Gambling Studies, 16,* 227-251.

Eades, J. M. (2003). *Gambling addiction: The problem, the pain and the path to recovery.* Ventura, CA: Gospel Light Publications.

Ferris, J., Wynne, H., & Single, E. (1999). *Measuring problem gambling in Canada: Phase 1.* Ottawa, ON: Canadian Centre on Substance Abuse.

Fong, T. (2005). The vulnerable faces of pathological gambling. *Psychiatry, 2*(4), 34-42.

Grant, J. E., Kim, S. W., & Potenza, M. N. (2003). Advances in the pharmacological treatment of pathological gambling. *Journal of Gambling Studies, 19,* 85-109.

Hester, R. & Miller, W. (1995). *Handbook of alcoholism treatment approaches: Effective alternatives* (2nd edition). Boston, MA: Allyn & Bacon.

Hood, C. D. & Carruthers, C. P. (2002). Coping skills theory as an underlying framework for therapeutic recreation services. *Therapeutic Recreation Journal, 36,* 137-153.

Korn, D. A. & Shaffer, H. J. (1999). Gambling and the health of the public: Adopting a public health perspective. *Journal of Gambling Studies, 15,* 289-365.

Korn, D. A. & Shaffer, H. J. (2004). *Massachusetts Department of Public Health's practice guidelines for treating gambling-related problems: An evidence-based treatment guide for clinicians.* Boston, MA: Massachusetts Council on Compulsive Gambling.

Ladouceur, R., Boisvert, J. M., Pepin, M., Loranger, M., & Sylvain, C. (1994). Social cost of pathological gambling. *Journal of Gambling Studies, 10,* 399-409.

Lesieur, H. R. & Blume, S. B. (1987). The South Oaks Gambling Screen (SOGS): A new instrument for the identification of problem gamblers. *American Journal of Psychiatry, 144*(9), 1184-8.

Lesieur, H. R. & Rosenthal, R. J. (1991). Pathological gambling: A review of the literature. *Journal of Gambling Studies, 7,* 5-39.

Mannell, R. C. & Kleiber, D. A. (1997). *A social psychology of leisure.* State College, PA: Venture Publishing.

McCormick, R. (1994). The importance of coping skill enhancement in the treatment of the pathological gambler. *Journal of Gambling Studies, 10,* 77- 86.

Moore, T. & Jadlos, T. (2002). *The etiology of pathological gambling: A study to enhance understanding of causal pathways as a step towards improving prevention and treatment.* Wilsonville, OR: Oregon Gambling Addiction Treatment Foundation.

National Research Council. (1999). *Pathological gambling: A critical review.* Washington, DC: National Academy Press.

Potenza, M. N., Steinberg, M. A., McLaughlin, S. D., Wu, R., Rounsaville, B. J., & O'Malley, S. S. (2001). Gender-related differences in the characteristics of problem gamblers using a gambling helpline. *American Journal of Psychiatry, 158,* 1500-1505.

Rosenthal, R. J. (1992). Pathological gambling. *Psychiatric Annals, 22*(2), 72-78.

Rosenthal, R. J. & Rugle, L. J. (1994). A psychodynamic approach to the treatment of pathological gambling: I. Achieving abstinence. *Journal of Gambling Studies, 10*(1), 21-42.

Shaffer, H. J., Hall, M. N., & Vander Bilt, J. (1997). *Estimating the prevalence of disordered gambling behavior in the United States & Canada: A meta-analysis.* Boston, MA: Harvard Medical School Division on Addictions.

Shaffer, H. J. & LaPlante, D. A. (2005). Treatment of gambling disorders (pp. 276-332). In G. A. Marlatt & D. M. Donovan (Eds.). *Relapse prevention: Maintenance strategies in the treatment of addictive behaviors.* New York: Guilford Press.

Swift, R. M. (2000). Opioid antagonists and alcoholism treatment. *CNS Spectrums, 5,* 49-57.

Volberg, R. A. (1996). Prevalence studies of problem gambling in the United States. *Journal of Gambling Studies, 12*(2), 111-128.

Walker, M. B. (1992). Irrational thinking among slot machine players. *Journal of Gambling Studies, 8*(3), 245-261.

Wiebe, J., Single, E., & Falkowski-Ham, A. (2001). *Measuring gambling and problem gambling in Ontario.* Toronto, ON: Canadian Centre on Substance Abuse and Responsible Gambling Council.

16. Generalized Anxiety Disorder

Heather R. Porter

Generalized anxiety disorder (GAD) is one of ten anxiety disorders classified by the American Psychiatric Association in the *Diagnostic and Statistical Manual of Mental Disorders, 5th Edition* (American Psychiatric Association [APA], 2013). It is characterized by excessive and uncontrollable worry about everyday things more days than not for at least six months. "The intensity, duration and frequency of the worry are disproportionate to the issue and interfere with the performance of tasks and ability to concentrate" (Anxiety and Depression Association of America, 2014b). The anxiety also manifests in physical symptoms, often including muscle tension, sweating, nausea, gastrointestinal problems, jumpiness, fidgeting, trembling, inability to relax, being easily startled, trouble sleeping, and feeling on edge. The sources of worry can vary but often include issues with finances, jobs, responsibilities, and relationships.

Some anxiety is normal. In fact, it is a healthy emotion that alerts us to internal or external threats. "It prompts a person to take the necessary steps to prevent the threat or to lessen its consequences" (Sadock & Sadock, 2003, p. 592). Some examples of everyday events that increase anxiety are running to catch the last bus, trying to find the car keys when you're late for an appointment, or preparing for a tough exam. Whether or not an event is perceived as stressful, thus heightening feelings of anxiety, "depends on the nature of the event and on the person's resources, psychological defenses, and coping mechanisms" (Sadock & Sadock, 2003, p. 592).

Anxiety, not GAD, can be described as being mild, moderate, or severe (Pary et al, 2003). Mild anxiety, as previously discussed, is normal and healthy. However, moderate or severe anxiety interferes with daily functioning and, if it persists more days than not over a period of six months, may warrant a diagnosis of GAD. Pary et al (2003) delineates the severity of anxiety through these definitions:

Mild anxiety sharpens the senses and expands the perceptual field, preparing us for action. Learning and problem-solving skills are enhanced.

Moderate anxiety decreases the perceptual field. Sight, hearing, touch, taste, and smell are limited and the ability to think is impaired. Problem solving and the ability to mobilize resources can be hindered.

Severe anxiety constricts the perceptual field so that an individual's focus is limited to one specific detail. Completing a task or processing new information is compromised, and behavior and attention are directed toward the anxiety.

People who have GAD feel like they are losing control of themselves and/or the situation during periods of extreme anxiety. For example, Sarah states that when she is trying to get out of the dorm building to get to class on time, her friends often delay her with conversation. When this occurs, her anxiety begins to heighten and she experiences somatic symptoms (heart pounding, shaking). She then becomes hyper-fixated on "getting out the door" and becomes short-fused and easily agitated. Because this situation occurs frequently, Sarah starts worrying about this problem hours before her class ("I know what's going to happen as soon as I step out of my room. Jim is going to be out there and will start asking me a ton of questions about the weekend."). This "negative running tape" is destructive because it heightens anxiety about a situation before it even occurs.

Negative and anxious thinking also heighten somatic symptoms, which, in turn, increase anxiety until the feedback between the way the body feels and the anxiety it causes spirals out of control. Anxious thoughts and feelings do not have to be in the context of an interaction with another person, they can result from completely internal cues.

Incidence/Prevalence in U.S.

GAD is one of the most prevalent anxiety disorders. It affects about 6.8 million adults, or 3.1% of the U.S. population (Anxiety and Depression Association of America [ADAA], 2014a). Women are twice as likely as men to have GAD (ADAA, 2014a).

Predominant Age

In most people, GAD develops gradually during adolescence and reaches clinical significance during young adulthood (Leger et al., 2003). A diagnosis of GAD, however, is generally uncommon before the age of 25 (Carter et al., 2001). Approximately 10% of women older than 39 years of age will have GAD over the course of their lifetime (Wittchen & Hoyer, 2001).

Causes

Anxiety disorders may develop from a complex set of risk factors, including genetics, brain chemistry, personality, and life events (ADAA, 2014b). About 25% of first-degree relatives of people with GAD are also affected (Sadock & Sadock, 2003). Cognitive behavioral therapy believes that people with GAD incorrectly or inaccurately perceive dangers. "The inaccuracy is generated by selective attention to negative details in the environment. This is caused by distortions in information processing and by an overly negative view of the person's own ability to cope. Psychoanalytic therapy believes that anxiety is a symptom of unresolved unconscious conflicts" (Sadock & Sadock, 2003, p. 632). Psychological trauma occurring in childhood and other stressful life events may also trigger or contribute to the development of GAD.

Systems Affected

GAD affects the mental functions of the patient including mood, cognition (trouble concentrating, difficulty learning new information and behaviors, misperception of events and situations, poor short-term memory, difficulty with abstract thinking), and social functioning. The primary ICF code for GAD is b152 Emotional Functions, especially b1520

Appropriateness of Emotion. The other emotional effects of GAD can be scored using ICF codes b125 Dispositions and Intra-Personal Functions, b126 Temperament and Personality Functions, b160 Thought Functions, b164 Higher-Level Cognitive Functions, b180 Experience of Self and Time Functions, d160 Focusing Attention, and d163 Thinking. The whole set of codes under d2 General Tasks and Demands, especially d240 Handling Stress and Other Psychological Demands, d7 Interpersonal Interactions and Relationships, and d9 Community, Social, and Civic Life need to be considered. Other areas that may be affected include b134 Sleep Functions.

GAD also affects various systems in the body through the influence of the client's emotional state. When anxiety is resolved or minimized, systems typically recover. Anxiety affects the client's motor functioning by causing shakiness, restlessness, and headaches; the gastrointestinal system with diarrhea, constipation, pain, nausea, feeling of "butterflies in the stomach"; cardiovascular system; heart palpitations; respiratory system, shortness of breath; autonomic nervous system, excessive sweating. ICF codes that look at the possible physical deficits include b410 Heart Functions, b440 Respiration Functions, b535 Sensations Associated with the Digestive System, and b765 Involuntary Movement Functions. When using these codes, it's important to compare functional levels between an anxious state and a non-anxious state.

Secondary Problems

A fundamental characteristic of GAD is comorbidity with other psychiatric conditions (Pary et al., 2003): 62.4% major depression, 39.5% dysthymia, 37.6% alcoholism, 35.1% simple phobia, 34.4% social phobia, 27.6% drug abuse, and 23.5% panic disorder.

Comorbid GAD in elderly patients is associated with a more severe presentation of depressive illness and possible suicidal preoccupation (Lenze et al., 2000).

Prognosis

Because of the high incidence of comorbid mental disorders in clients with GAD, the clinical course and prognosis of the disorder are difficult to predict. However, GAD is a chronic condition that may well be lifelong (Sadock & Sadock, 2003). Pharmacological treatment of GAD is typically a six- to twelve-month treatment. About 25% of clients relapse in the first month after discontinuing medication, and 60-80% relapse over the course of the next year. Therefore, if pharmacological interventions are successful in managing GAD, long-term use of medication may be necessary (Sadock & Sadock, 2003). Many individuals who undergo psychotherapy for GAD report that they continue to have anxiety after discharge. However, they are better able to "use the anxiety symptoms as a signal to reflect on internal struggles and to expand their insight and understanding" (Sadock & Sadock, 2003, p. 634-35).

Assessment

Scope of Team Assessment

The criteria for GAD are defined in the *DSM-5*. They include excessive anxiety and worry about a number of events with the worry occurring more days than not for at least six-months. It is difficult for the client to control the worry and it is associated with physical and mental symptoms including being keyed up, fatigued, irritable, and tense. The client may have difficulty sleeping and concentrating. The anxiety may be about anything and must cause the client significant distress in some function. Anxiety caused by substances, a medical condition, or some other defined disorder is not considered GAD. The *GAD-7*, a seven-item screening tool for GAD, will help determine whether or not a full assessment for anxiety is needed. The *GAD-7* can be accessed for free at http://www.integration.samhsa.gov/clinical-practice/screening-tools#anxiety.

Even if anxiety is not classified as GAD, it can still be treated with some of the techniques shown below. Some of the medical conditions that may cause symptoms of anxiety include adrenal tumor, AIDS, alcoholism, carcinoid syndrome (symptoms including flushing, labored breathing, and heart palpitations as a result of a carcinoid tumor), central nervous system degenerative diseases, chronic obstructive pulmonary disease, coronary insufficiency, Cushing's disease, delirium, diabetes, fibromyalgia, hyperthyroidism, hypoglycemia, early stages of Meniére's disease, mitral valve prolapse, and postconcussion syndrome (a group of problems

that occur after a head injury including dizziness, poor concentration, and anxiety) (Longe, 2001).

Medication and other substances can also induce anxiety including excessive caffeine use, drug or alcohol withdrawal, substance abuse, and some prescription medications including antihistamines, antidepressants, and benzodiazepines (Longe, 2001).

Anxiety may be a symptom of another psychiatric disorder. The treatment team will want to determine if the symptoms of anxiety are because of a mood disorder, such as depressive disorder with anxiety, phobias, panic disorder, obsessive-compulsive disorder, adjustment disorder with anxiety, hypochondriasis, adult attention-deficit/hyperactivity disorder, somatization disorder, or any other personality disorder.

If an anxiety disorder is thought to be present, an evaluation from a mental health professional is sought. The general clinician may explore the nature and extent of the anxiety to better understand its impact on life tasks by asking questions about what situations or memories cause anxiety, how the anxiety feels, and what helps to relieve the anxiety.

People experiencing severe anxiety can be at increased risk for suicide. Therefore, it is important to ask highly anxious individuals about suicidal and/or homicidal ideation (Pary et al, 2003).

Along with checking for anxiety and seeing if there is a formal diagnosis of GAD from the *DSM-5*, which could also be noted using the ICF code b152 Emotional Functions, the team will look at problems the GAD is causing in the client's life as described by the ICF codes listed in the Systems Affected section.

Areas of Concern for RT Assessment

In addition to the symptoms mentioned earlier, the recreational therapist might additionally find the following:

Heightened and prolonged anxiety can affect learning and development of healthy coping mechanisms, so maladaptive coping strategies may be apparent (d240 Handling Stress and Other Psychological Demands). The assessment may also find deficits in d920 Recreation and Leisure.

A client with GAD is typically easily discouraged, indecisive, mildly depressed, apprehensive, impatient, irritable, easily distracted, and spends a considerable amount of time worrying about impending disasters (b160 Thought Functions)

(Mobily & MacNeil, 2002). Consequently, some clients may manage the anxiety by reducing their involvement in life tasks leading to social isolation and loss of a social support system (d7 Interpersonal Interactions and Relationships). Other clients may try to take on too many tasks, trying to handle everything they worry about, leading to exhaustion and perceived loss of control (d230 Carrying Out Daily Routine, d240 Handling Stress and Other Psychological Demands, d250 Managing One's Own Behavior).

ICF Core Set

No ICF Core Set for Anxiety in general or for particular anxiety disorders, such as GAD, has been published.

Treatment Direction

Whole Team Approach

A combination of therapy techniques is more effective than using a single technique when treating GAD. Techniques that are commonly used in addition to pharmacology include identification and alteration of anxiety producing thoughts, changing distorted thinking through cognitive behavioral therapy techniques, acceptance and commitment therapy (uses strategies of acceptance and mindfulness, along with commitment and behavior change, as a way to cope with unwanted thoughts, feelings, and sensations), dialectical behavioral therapy (combines cognitive behavioral techniques with mindfulness meditation, along with the development of interpersonal skills, ability to tolerate distress, and ability to regulate emotions) and modeling. Other techniques include development of healthy coping strategies, teaching relaxation training, gradual exposure to anxiety provoking situations, and opportunities to talk about the anxiety (ADAA, 2014b). ICF codes that may be improved with these therapies include b125 Dispositions and Intra-Personal Functions, b126 Temperament and Personality Functions, b152 Emotional Functions, b160 Thought Functions, b164 Higher-Level Cognitive Functions, b180 Experience of Self and Time Functions, and d240 Handling Stress and Other Psychological Demands.

Recreational Therapy Approach

Recreational therapy utilizes the same approach as the whole team approach. However, RT focuses on control of GAD within functional activities, such as eating in a crowded restaurant or getting on an elevator.

Recreational Therapy Interventions

Recreational therapy utilizes all of the non-pharmacological interventions as discussed in the Whole Team Approach. Recreational therapists also have the opportunity to take clients into real-world situations, so they can work on the identified areas in d7 Interpersonal Interactions and Relationships and d9 Community, Social, and Civic Life. Some additional possibilities for therapy include:

Modeling: When a client exhibits signs of anxiety, the therapist listens empathetically and models calm, confident behavior. The simple act of listening is very effective in deescalating a highly anxious client. Reflecting behaviors that the therapist desires to instill in the client can be an effective tool in modifying behavior (b152 Emotional Functions, d240 Handling Stress and Other Psychological Demands).

Reducing anxiety-evoking events and thoughts: Some clients are able to verbalize specific situations that increase their anxiety, but individuals with GAD generally are anxious in many situations and are unable to identify specific triggers that increase their anxiety to an unhealthy level ("I just feel anxious all the time."). For those that are able to identify specific anxiety provoking events, therapists assist clients in problem solving to lessen the anxiety of the specific situation. Examples include allowing extra time to get to destinations and listening to soft music through headphones while in a noisy environment. ICF codes that may be improved include d175 Solving Problems and d240 Handling Stress and Other Psychological Demands. When a specific situation or event cannot be identified, general coping strategies beyond those reviewed in the Whole Team Approach can be taught, such as mindfulness, deep breathing, catching and subsequently rephrasing distorted thinking, expressing feelings through leisure activities such as art, using recreation and leisure including physical activity to cope and lessen feelings of anxiety, decreasing the focus on anxiety and increasing the focus on mastery and success to foster and strengthen the client's internal locus of control, and training family members or caregivers on how to assist their family member in managing GAD (b160 Thought Functions, d240 Handling Stress and Other Psychological Demands, d920 Recreation and Leisure).

Specific activities: Activities that promote abdominal breathing; noncompetitive, process-oriented activities; and self-paced, repetitive, and rhythmical activities can be helpful in reducing stress (b410 Heart Functions, b440 Respiration Functions, b535 Sensations Associated with the Digestive System, d240 Handling Stress and Other Psychological Demands) (Mobily & MacNeil, 2002).

Exposure to anxiety-evoking situations: Therapists seek to gradually expose the client to anxiety-provoking situations so s/he can apply and continue to build techniques to handle a variety of situations (b152 Emotional Functions, d240 Handling Stress and Other Psychological Demands). The success experienced at each step helps to strengthen internal locus of control and self-confidence, bolstering internal resources to overcome the next challenging step. Depending upon the context of treatment, the likelihood of experiencing anxiety-provoking events in the presence of the therapist will vary. Consequently, experiences may need to be therapeutically designed to foster gradual exposure. The strength of the anxiety-provoking situation will vary by client. In general, being further away from actual involvement by talking about it, watching a video about it, or reading about it is less stressful. Full participation in the actual event through role-playing or community integration is more stressful (d7 Interpersonal Interactions and Relationships, d9 Community, Social, and Civic Life).

In all of these interventions, the goal is to work with the client when the anxiety level is under control. Communication with a severely anxious person must be brief, simple, and direct. At panic level, the perceptual field is so diminished that people no longer effectively interpret outside stimuli. Communication and activities are dysfunctional and self-absorbed. Feelings of anger, fear, and helplessness may emerge explosively and be directed toward self or others in a fight-or-flight reaction. When severe anxiety is present, the therapist must get the client to a safe place physically and emotionally before continuing with therapeutic interventions.

Resources

Anxiety and Depression Association of America
www.adaa.org
A leader in education, training, and research for anxiety, obsessive-compulsive disorder, posttraumatic stress disorder, depression, and related disorders.

References

American Psychiatric Association. (2013). *Diagnostic and statistical manual of mental disorders* (5th ed.). Washington, DC: American Psychiatric Association.

Anxiety and Depression Association of America. (2014a). Facts and statistics. Retrieved from http://www.adaa.org/about-adaa/press-room/facts-statistics.

Anxiety and Depression Association of America. (2014b). Generalized anxiety disorder. Retrieved from http://www.adaa.org/understanding-anxiety/generalized-anxiety-disorder-gad.

Carter, R. M., Wittchen, H. U., Phister, H., & Kessler, R. C. (2001). One-year prevalence of subthreshold and threshold DSM-IV generalized anxiety disorder in a nationally representative sample. *Depression and Anxiety 13*, 78-88.

Leger, E., Ladouceur, R., Dugas, J., & Freeston, M. (2003). Cognitive-behavioral treatment of generalized anxiety disorder among adolescents: A case series. *Journal of the American Academy of Child and Adolescent Psychiatry, 42*(3), 327-330.

Lenze, E. J., Mulsant, B. H., Shear, M. K., Schulberg, H. C., Dew, M. A., & Begley, A. E. (2000). Comorbid anxiety disorders in depressed elderly patients. *American Journal of Psychiatry, 157*, 722-728.

Longe, J. (2001). *The Gale encyclopedia of medicine* (2nd ed.). Farmington Hills, MI: Gale Group.

Mobily, K. & MacNeil, R. (2002). *Therapeutic recreation and the nature of disabilities*. State College, PA: Venture Publishing, Inc.

Pary, R., Matsuchka, P., Lewis, S., Caso, W., & Lippmann, S. (2003). Generalized anxiety disorder. *Southern Medical Journal, 96*(6).

Sadock, J. & Sadock, V. (2003). *Kaplan & Sadock's synopsis of psychiatry* (9th ed.). Philadelphia, PA: Lippincott Williams & Wilkins.

Wittchen, H. U. & Hoyer J. (2001). Generalized anxiety disorder: Nature and course. *Journal of Clinical Psychiatry, 62*(Suppl 11), 15-19.

17. Guillain-Barré Syndrome

Heather R. Porter

Guillain-Barré (ghee YAN bah RAY) syndrome (GBS) is an illness in which the body attacks its own nerve cells. GBS affects the peripheral nervous system — the nerve roots that exit the vertebral column to muscles and organs — and not the nerves in the brain or spinal cord (National Institute of Neurological Disorders and Stroke [NINDS], 2011). It is characterized by symmetrical muscle weakness and/or paralysis that begins in the legs and rises upward (ascending paralysis) (NINDS, 2011).

Reflexes are absent and autonomic dysfunction is frequently affected with fluctuations in heart rate and blood pressure (NINDS, 2011). In severe cases, weakness can progress into the respiratory, facial, and esophageal muscles leading to problems with respiration, speech, and swallowing (NINDS, 2011). Weakness and paralysis are usually at their maximum three to four weeks after initial symptoms (NINDS, 2011).

Weakness typically begins to surface from five days to three weeks after an infectious illness, surgery, or immunization (Beers & Berkow, 2004). The most common bacterium associated with GBS is *Campylobacter jejuni*, which normally only causes diarrhea. Although the connection to these events is unclear, there appears to be a significant correlation.

GBS has many other names including acute inflammatory demyelinating polyneuropathy, acute febrile polyneuritis, acute idiopathic polyneuritis, infections polyneuritis, and Landry's ascending paralysis. There have been numerous underlying illnesses or infections identified as leading to GBS, which may be one of the reasons this disease is known by so many different names.

Incidence/Prevalence in U.S.

In the United States, approximately one out of every 100,000 people is diagnosed with GBS (NINDS, 2011). The percentage of people who experience respiratory failure and require intubation is unclear. Findings indicate anywhere from 5-30% (Beers & Berkow, 2004; Mack, 2004; Cha-Kim, 2004).

Predominant Age

GBS affects both males and females at any age and without regard to race or ethnicity. However, it does appear that there are a greater percentage of older people than younger people diagnosed with GBS (Mack, 2004).

Causes

The cause of GBS is unknown; however it is believed that the mechanism of the disease involves an abnormal T-cell response precipitated by a preceding infection (Mack, 2004).

Systems Affected

GBS affects motor and sensory functioning. The number of systems affected depends upon the progression of the disease and the time lapse before medical intervention stops the disease from progressing higher in the body. At the very least the peripheral nervous system (b730 Muscle Power Functions, b760 Control of Voluntary Movement Functions, b1564 Tactile Perception, b840 Sensation Related to the Skin), the muscular system (b730-b749 Muscle Functions, especially b730 Muscle Power Functions), autonomic functioning (b410 Heart Functions, b420 Blood Pressure Functions), and reflexes (b750 Motor Reflex Functions) are affected. People often report feelings of weakness (b730 Muscle Power Functions), loss of balance or feeling unsteady (b235 Vestibular Functions, d415 Maintaining a Body Position), pain (b280 Sensation of Pain), and/or paresthesia (b265 Touch Function, b1564 Tactile Perception, b840

Sensation Related to the Skin) (NINDS, 2011). In children, pain is often the most prominent symptom. If the disease is severe, it can additionally affect bowel (b515 Digestive Functions, b525 Defecation Functions) and bladder functioning (b620 Urination Functions), speech (b310 Voice Functions, b320 Articulation Functions), respiration (b445 Respiratory Muscle Functions), swallowing (b510 Ingestion Functions), and vision (b210 Seeing Functions) (NINDS, 2011).

Secondary Problems

Complications from inactivity and bed rest, such as deep vein thrombosis, skin breakdown, muscle contractures (b4 Functions of the Cardiovascular, Hematological, Immunological, and Respiratory Systems, b7 Neuromusculoskeletal and Movement-Related Functions, b8 Functions of the Skin and Related Structures), and issues related to pain management, such as medication, heat, transcutaneous electrical nerve stimulation, relaxation training (b280 Sensation of Pain) are common areas that require attention in addition to the ones already reviewed.

GBS, although typically improving over time, often continues to have a residual impact on various life areas. For example, a study of 76 individuals who had GBS with a median time since GBS of six years and a range of one to 14 years showed that although good functional recovery was seen, 16% reported moderate to extreme impact on their ability to participate in work, family, and social activities, and 22% reported substantial impact on mood, confidence, and ability to live independently (b125 Dispositions and Intra-Personal Functions, b126 Temperament and Personality Functions, d2 General Tasks and Demands, d4 Mobility, d9 Community, Social, and Civic Life) (Khan, Pallant, & Bhasker, 2010). The study also found that they had higher rates of extreme depression, anxiety, and stress compared to the norm population (b152 Emotional Functions, d240 Handling Stress and Other Psychological Demands, d7 Interpersonal Interactions and Relationships). The authors concluded that GBS is a complex diagnosis that requires "long-term management of psychological sequelae impacting activity and participation" (p. 2024).

Prognosis

After a client reaches maximum weakness at approximately three weeks post initial onset, symptoms stabilize at this level for days to months (NINDS, 2011). The recovery period can take several weeks to several years (NINDS, 2011). Approximately 40% of all GBS cases require inpatient rehabilitation of three to six weeks, followed by three to four months of home or outpatient therapy (Kahn, 2004). On average, 75-85% of individuals who have GBS have complete or good recovery, 15-20% have moderate residual impairments, and 1-10% have significant permanent disability (Cha-Kim, 2004). Additionally, about three percent may experience a relapse in muscle weakness and tingling sensations years after the initial attack (NINDS, 2011). Some people may continue to have chronic reoccurrences of GBS, referred to as chronic inflammatory demyelinating polyradiculoneuropathy (CIDP).

Mortality rates range from 2-12%. Deaths are typically a result of autonomic instability, pneumonia, respiratory distress, and pulmonary emboli. People who are over the age of 40 and who have rapid progression to quadriparesis or underlying malignancy have a poorer prognosis (Mack, 2004).

Assessment

Typical Scope of Team Assessment

A diagnosis of GBS is made mostly by observing symptoms, such as ascending tract weakness and areflexia, and taking a history of recent infectious illnesses, surgeries, or immunizations (NINDS, 2011). Various lab work, imaging studies, and tests including a nerve conduction velocity test and cerebrospinal fluid collection are used to confirm the diagnosis. Structural findings can be documented with s1201 Spinal Nerves. Once the client is stabilized in the acute care setting, s/he may be transferred to an inpatient acute care rehabilitation center. The rehabilitation team assesses the client's baseline level of functioning using discipline-specific diagnostic tools to assess muscle strength, range of motion, sensation, mobility, speech, swallowing, respiration, autonomic functioning, and ability to perform specific daily activities like transfers, dressing, and eating. Findings can be documented using the ICF codes discussed in the Systems Affected section.

Areas of Concern for RT Assessment

The anticipated findings will vary depending upon the extent of the dysfunction, the age of the person, and the person's prior medical history. The most relevant findings for recreational therapy include:

Anxiety: The person is commonly in an anxious state (b126 Temperament and Personality Functions). People with GBS often report that the weakness seemed to "come out of nowhere" and progress rapidly. There is often little time to prepare for hospitalization, so affairs are often in disarray, causing anxiety and loss of internal locus of control. Anxiety, worry, and fear of the prognosis are common for an adult with GBS and for the parents of a child with GBS. If the client is a child, anxiety is often expressed in relation to the child's developmental level.

Pain: Complaints of pain and need for pain management interventions are common (b280 Sensation of Pain).

Autonomic dysfunction: The client may have orthostatic hypotension, high blood pressure, tachycardia, trouble breathing, perhaps requiring a ventilator, and absent reflexes. Code as described in the Systems Affected section.

Lack of leisure: Leisure is often not a voiced priority for adults, compared to children who often desire to play. However, participation in leisure activities may help reduce the perceived level of pain (b280 Sensation of Pain) and re-direct the client from anxiety-producing thoughts (b160 Thought Functions). Deficits in the ability to participate in leisure activities can be coded with d9 Community, Social, and Civic Life.

Lower extremity weakness: In order to be admitted to an inpatient rehabilitation hospital, the extent of weakness or paralysis must significantly impair the person's functioning. The client will have at least moderate to severe weakness or paralysis of the lower extremities (b730 Muscle Power Functions, b735 Muscle Tone Functions, b750 Motor Reflex Functions, b760 Control of Voluntary Movement Functions).

Environment: The recreational therapist evaluates the client's environment to note changes that may be needed if the recovery is not complete. All aspects of the physical and social environment should be documented using the appropriate Environmental Factors codes.

ICF Core Set

No ICF Core Set for GBS has been published. ICF Core Sets that might be helpful in identifying relevant ICF codes include Chronic Pain, Depression, and Neurological Conditions.

Treatment Direction

Whole Team Approach

Plasmapheresis or intravenous immunoglobulin (IVIG) is typically administered in the early stages of the disease because it can shorten the course of the disease and hospitalization, as well as reduce mortality and incidence of permanent paralysis (Beers & Berkow, 2004). Vital signs are taken frequently to monitor the need for assisted breathing. Fluids are pushed to decrease risks of urinary tract infection and kidney stones. Precautions are adopted to decrease risks of developing skin breakdown. Passive range-of-motion exercises are necessary to prevent contractures and activity is encouraged within safe parameters. Heparin is commonly prescribed to prevent blood clots from forming as a secondary complication from increased bed rest. Paralyzed extremities are protected from trauma (e.g., bed rails to protect the arm from falling off the side of the bed) (NINDS, 2011). ICF codes related to these treatments include b410 Heart Functions, b420 Blood Pressure Functions, b445 Respiratory Muscle Functions, b510 Ingestion Functions, b515 Digestive Functions, b525 Defecation Functions, and b620 Urination Functions.

In general, therapy aims to improve the muscular system (b730 Muscle Power Functions, b735 Muscle Tone Functions, b750 Motor Reflex Functions, b760 Control of Voluntary Movement Functions); enhance ability to perform life tasks (d2 General Tasks and Demands); and educate the person and the family about the disease, the anticipated course that it will take, and how to prevent secondary complications that are caused by a decreased level of activity.

For those that require intensive inpatient rehabilitation, an interdisciplinary team approach is best to address the following issues (Kahn, 2004):

Respiratory complications: These include clearing respiratory secretions to reduce the work of breathing (b440-b449 Functions of the Respiratory System).

Deep vein thrombosis prevention: The patient is encouraged to be active and wear compression stockings. The team implements progressive mobilization protocols (b410-b429 Functions of the Cardiovascular System).

Dysautonomia management: The team implements interventions to control malfunction of the autonomic nervous system, such as postural hypotension and bowel/bladder function (b525 Defecation Functions, b620 Urination Functions).

Mobilization: Treatment includes posture training, range of motion, orthoses or splints to prevent contractures, endurance training through repetitive exercises with low resistance, strengthening exercises, flexibility exercises, progressive ambulation and mobility, special attention to correct positioning for compression nerve palsies, education and care regarding pressure ulcers, and aggressive joint range of motion to prevent heterotopic ossification (b7 Neuromusculoskeletal and Movement-Related Functions, b8 Functions of the Skin and Related Structures).

Fatigue and pain: Modalities include desensitization therapy to help the client tolerate activities and sensations, pharmacology, energy conservation techniques, adaptive equipment, and activity modifications (d2 General Tasks and Demands, b280 Sensation of Pain).

Psychological and social issues: Depression, mental fatigue, family education, self-worth, self-image, role within the family, coping, stress management, community participation, respite needs, support groups, and/or resources may need to be covered (b125 Dispositions and Intra-Personal Functions, b126 Temperament and Personality Functions, d2 General Tasks and Demands, d7 Interpersonal Interactions and Relationships).

Recreational Therapy Approach

The approach used by the recreational therapist focuses on four areas: aspects of the client's lifestyle that will reduce long-term secondary impacts, psychosocial adjustment, adaptation of activity to allow a more normal lifestyle, and addressing specific symptoms that result from GBS.

Recreational Therapy Interventions

Interventions that are frequently implemented with clients who have GBS include:

Psychosocial adjustment: Participation in recreation, leisure, play, and community activities can help with psychosocial adjustment (d920 Recreation and Leisure, b125 Dispositions and Intra-Personal Functions, b126 Temperament and Personality Functions, b455 Exercise Tolerance Functions, d2 General Tasks and Demands, d7 Interpersonal Interactions and Relationships). Consider referring and helping clients integrate into formal and informal community groups to aid with social support. Cha-Kim (2004) notes that "psychosocial functional health status can be impaired even years after the GBS event [and that] psychosocial performance does not seem to correlate with the severity of residual physical function. Poor conditioning and easy fatigability may be contributory factors. Therefore, providing long-term attention and support is important" (p. 8).

Movement and mobility: Recreational therapy seeks to improve areas of difficulty and promote engagement in enjoyable forms of physical activity (d920 Recreation and Leisure). These will vary from client to client although most revolve around the muscular system (e.g., b455 Exercise Tolerance Functions, d410 Changing Basic Body Position, d415 Maintaining a Body Position, d420 Transferring Oneself, d440 Fine Hand Use, d445 Hand and Arm Use, d450 Walking, and d460 Moving Around in Different Locations).

Pain: Therapists use the anxiety and stress management interventions reviewed previously to help with pain management (b280 Sensation of Pain).

Lifestyle and secondary impacts: Therapists educate clients about the role of their leisure lifestyle on health and recovery (d570 Looking After One's Health).

Adaptation: Recovery from GBS can range from several weeks to several years, so in many cases the recreational therapist teaches the client how to adapt for areas of impairment and difficulty to promote independence and functioning within activities and life situations (d2 General Tasks and Demands, d4 Mobility, d7 Interpersonal Interactions and Relationships, and appropriate Environmental Factor codes).

Resources

Guillain-Barré Syndrome/Chronic Inflammatory Demyelinating Polyneuropathy Foundation International (GBS/CIDP Foundation International)

www.gbs-cidp.org

A foundation committed to support those with GBS/CIDP so that every patient experiences an early diagnosis, proper treatment, and the opportunity for a full recovery.

References

Beers, M. & Berkow, R. (2004). Guillain-Barré syndrome. Retrieved from www.merck.com.

Cha-Kim, A. (2004). Guillain-Barré syndrome. Retrieved from www.emedicine.com.

Kahn, F. (2004). Rehabilitation in Guillain-Barré syndrome. *Australian Family Physician, 33*(12), 1013-1017.

Kahn, F., Pallant, J. F., Ng, L., & Bhasker, A. (2010). Factors associated with long-term functional outcomes and psychological sequelae in Guillain-Barré Syndrome. *Journal of Neurology, 257,* 2024-2031.

Mack, K. (2004). Guillain-Barré syndrome in childhood. Retrieved from www.emedicine.com.

National Institute of Neurological Disorders and Stroke. (2011). Guillain-Barré syndrome fact sheet. Retrieved from http://www.ninds.nih.gov/disorders/gbs/detail_gbs.htm.

18. Hearing Loss

Jo Ann Coco-Ripp

Hearing loss occurs across the population in varying degrees. A small percentage of children are born deaf or hard of hearing. Later in life children, adolescents, and adults lose hearing to some degree through accidents, disease, or lifestyle activities. As a person ages, hearing loss is more common and is more likely among men than women. There are several views to hearing loss. Some individuals view the loss as a problem to be fixed. Others, especially those who have a significant hearing loss, feel that being deaf makes them part of a separate culture. A discussion on the varying views is not appropriate for this text. However, understanding that there is a continuum of views is important when working with a person with a hearing loss.

Another important fact to keep in mind when working with a person with a hearing loss is the length of time the person has had the loss. In a person who loses hearing suddenly, the change is dramatic. The difference between a person with a sudden hearing loss and a person who was born deaf is drastic. However, often in older persons, the loss is gradual and the difference is incremental. Age is another factor that impacts hearing loss to a great extent. If a person experiences the loss after acquiring communication skills, that has quite a different impact than a child who is born deaf or experiences hearing loss before developing functional communication.

Incidence/Prevalence in U.S.

Statistics compiled by the National Institute on Deafness and Other Communication Disorders (NIDCD, n.d.) provides a profile of those who have hearing loss:

- Men are more likely to experience hearing loss than women.

- Roughly 25 million Americans have experienced tinnitus. Of adults ages 65 and older in the United States, 12.3% of men and nearly 14% of women are affected by tinnitus. Tinnitus is identified more frequently in white individuals and the prevalence of tinnitus is almost twice as frequent in the South as in the Northeast.

- Approximately 17% (36 million) of American adults report some degree of hearing loss.

- There is a strong relationship between age and reported hearing loss: 18% of American adults 45-64 years old, 30% of adults 65-74 years old, and 47% of adults 75 years old or older have a hearing loss.

- Two to three out of every 1,000 children in the United States are born deaf or hard-of-hearing. Nine out of every 10 children who are born deaf are born to parents who can hear.

- The NIDCD estimates that approximately 15% (26 million) of Americans between the ages of 20 and 69 have high frequency hearing loss due to exposure to loud sounds or noise at work or in leisure activities.

- Only one out of five people who could benefit from a hearing aid actually wears one.

- Three out of four children experience ear infection (otitis media) by the time they are three years old.

- Approximately 4,000 new cases of sudden deafness occur each year in the United States. Hearing loss affects only one ear in nine out of ten people who experience sudden deafness. Only 10-15% of individuals with sudden deafness know what caused their loss.

- Approximately 615,000 individuals have been diagnosed with Ménière's disease in the United States. Another 45,500 are newly diagnosed each year.

- Approximately three to six percent of all deaf children and perhaps another three to six percent of hard-of-hearing children have Usher syndrome. In developed countries such as the United States, about four babies in every 100,000 births have Usher syndrome.
- One out of every 100,000 individuals per year develops an acoustic neurinoma (vestibular schwannoma).

According to the U.S. Food and Drug Administration, which tracks cochlear implant device use, in December 2010 approximately 219,000 people worldwide have received cochlear implants, including approximately 42,600 adults and 28,400 children in the United States. Roughly 40% of children who are born profoundly deaf now receive a cochlear implant (NIDCD, 2012).

The 2010 Annual Data for Early Hearing Detection and Intervention (EHDI) Program lists the prevalence rate for hearing loss in screenings of about 97% of infants in the United States by three months at 1.4 per 1,000 screened (Centers for Disease Control and Prevention, 2012). It also reports from each state and territory the number of monitoring or early intervention services for screened infants. The overall rate of follow up is listed at 66.5%. In a national health survey, parents reported that 4.5 per 1,000 children ages three through seventeen in the United States were deaf or had a lot of trouble hearing without a hearing aid (Boulet, Boyle, & Schieve, 2009). The survey also showed these areas to be high co-occurrences for children who reported being deaf or hard of hearing: varied developmental delays, ADHD/ADD, and learning disabilities.

Predominant Age

The percentage distribution by sex and age, based on subjects' reports of any permanent hearing loss (NIDCD, n.d.), are

Age	Female	Male
Birth	3	2
0-2 years	2	1
3-5 years	3	2
6-18 years	9	10
19-44 years	27	39
45-64 years	27	29
65+ years	29	17

Causes

Hearing loss is caused by noise, aging, disease, and heredity. Additionally, illnesses and certain medications can cause individuals to lose hearing (Centers for Disease Control, 2012). The cause is unknown for about 25% of babies born with a detectible hearing loss. For another 25%, the cause is believed to be due to maternal infections during pregnancy, complications after birth, and head trauma. For 50%, the cause is due to genetics. Of this group, about one third is attributed to a specific syndrome such as Down or Usher (Hearing loss, 2012). Usher syndrome is a progressive vision loss present in approximately 3-10% of adults who have been deaf since birth or early childhood. Usher syndrome is a combination of retinitis pigmentosa and hearing loss; retinitis pigmentosa affects one in 4,000 in the general population and 3-10% or 120-400 times higher in persons who are deaf since birth or early childhood (Barnett et al., 2011).

Hearing is a complex sense involving both the ear's ability to detect sounds in the environment and the brain's ability to interpret the sounds of speech. Major determinants of the impact of hearing loss on members of a population include (Gates & Hoffman, n.d.) degree of hearing loss; configuration or pattern of hearing loss across frequencies; laterality/bilaterality of hearing loss (one or both ears affected); the area(s) of abnormality in the auditory system, such as the middle ear, inner ear, auditory neural pathways, or brain; speech recognition ability; age; and history of exposures to loud noise and environmental or pharmacologic toxicants that damage hearing.

Systems Affected

The main biological systems impacted by a hearing loss are the auditory systems including the inner, middle, and outer ears as well as the acoustic nerve and auditory processing areas of the brain. In addition to the ear, in some cases, other systems are affected. For example, hearing loss is part of Usher syndrome, a genetic disorder that impacts both sight and hearing. ICF codes specific to the hearing loss include b1560 Auditory Perception, b230 Hearing Functions, b235 Vestibular Functions, b240 Sensations Associated with Hearing and Vestibular Functions, s110 Structure of Brain, s240 Structure of External Ear, s250 Structure of Middle Ear, s260

Structure of Inner Ear, and s710 Structure of Head and Neck Region.

Medical specialists (Centers for Disease Control and Prevention, 2011) categorize hearing loss into four types, by progressive degrees, and using other descriptors. The four types are

Conductive hearing loss: Hearing loss caused by something that stops sounds from getting through the outer or middle ear. This type of hearing loss can often be treated with medicine or surgery.

Sensorineural hearing loss: Hearing loss that occurs when there is a problem in the way the inner ear or hearing nerve works.

Mixed hearing loss: Hearing loss that includes both a conductive and a sensorineural hearing loss.

Auditory neuropathy spectrum disorder: Hearing loss that occurs when sound enters the ear normally, but because of damage to the inner ear or the hearing nerve, sound isn't organized in a way that the brain can understand.

The degrees of hearing loss are

Mild hearing loss: A person with a mild hearing loss may hear some speech sounds but soft sounds are hard to hear.

Moderate hearing loss: A person with a moderate hearing loss may hear almost no speech when another person is talking at a normal level.

Severe hearing loss: A person with severe hearing loss will hear no speech when a person is talking at a normal level and only some loud sounds.

Profound hearing loss: A person with a profound hearing loss will not hear any speech and only very loud sounds.

Additional descriptors for hearing loss include:

Unilateral or bilateral: Hearing loss is in one ear (unilateral) or both ears (bilateral).

Pre-lingual or post-lingual: Hearing loss happened before a person learned to talk (pre-lingual) or after a person learned to talk (post-lingual).

Symmetrical or asymmetrical: Hearing loss is the same in both ears (symmetrical) or is different in each ear (asymmetrical).

Progressive or sudden: Hearing loss worsened over time (progressive) or happened quickly (sudden).

Fluctuating or stable: Hearing loss gets either better or worse over time (fluctuating) or stays the same over time (stable).

Congenital or acquired/delayed onset: Hearing loss is present at birth (congenital) or appears later in life (acquired or delayed onset).

Even though hearing loss primarily impacts auditory systems, secondary influences from the effect on communication should be kept in mind. Use of assistive devices such as a cochlear implant or hearing aid, as well as support from various services such as a note taker or interpreter, also impact social and emotional growth and functioning. Young children are impacted during crucial language development times and older people may experience isolation due to consequences of a hearing loss. Each person may be impacted in a very individual way despite the diagnosis similarity.

Secondary Problems

A typical symptom associated with hearing difficulties is tinnitus. It is a symptom that something is wrong in the auditory system, which includes the ear, the auditory nerve that connects the inner ear to the brain, and the parts of the brain that process sound. Something as simple as a piece of earwax blocking the ear canal can cause tinnitus. But it can also be the result of a number of health conditions, such as noise-induced hearing loss, ear and sinus infections, diseases of the heart or blood vessels, Ménière's disease, brain tumors, hormonal changes in women, or thyroid abnormalities.

Tinnitus is sometimes the first sign of hearing loss in older people. It also can be a side effect of medications (NIDCD, n.d.).

Other complications with hearing loss vary with the cause of the loss. For instance, Ménière's disease is a disorder of the inner ear and severe dizziness is common along with the hearing loss. As mentioned earlier, Usher syndrome affects vision as well as hearing. The visual aspects of Usher's include limited peripheral vision, balance problems, and gradual degeneration of the retina. The health condition of retinitis pigmentosa that has a high prevalence among people who have been deaf since birth is up to 10% more likely to occur than within the general population (Barnett et al., 2011).

There are many functional and social problems that may be caused by hearing loss. These problems and the associated ICF codes will be discussed in the assessment section.

Prognosis

The outcome of a hearing loss is very individual and depends on age, cause of loss, and a range of other factors. Some approaches are designed to restore hearing, such as a hearing aid or cochlear implant. Other approaches seek to support alternative communication systems such as learning sign language or using visual methods. Some hearing loss may be temporary, such as a blockage from a tumor or an infection. Most hearing loss is permanent, often only in one ear, and may grow worse after initial diagnosis, so ongoing testing is suggested.

Early screening of infants is highly recommended to increase opportunities for early interventions (Centers for Disease Control, 2012; NIDCD, 2012). Similarly, it is suggested that youth and adults who experience hearing loss, whether gradual or sudden, be tested so adaptations and interventions can be implemented before other problems develop.

Assessment

A child or adult with a hearing loss will have screening results from auditory tests. These describe the level of loss and the tests used. The functional results from loss of communication may not be part of what is routinely done for all persons with a hearing loss. However, the American Academy of Pediatrics (2006) and others (Jackson, Wegner, & Turnbull, 2010; Schein & Miller, 2008) suggest that screening and diagnostic information be extensive so that proper services can begin early in the child's life. Concerns about missing other genetically linked physical areas, such as vision or kidney, compel more careful scrutiny and heightened awareness for children and youth with hearing loss. Addition areas of concern for assessment are focused on structure of the instruments and use of culturally sensitive instruments or methods, especially for persons who consider themselves members of the Deaf community or non-English users (Borum, 2012; Graybill et al., 2010). Golos, Moses, and Wolbers (2012) examine this issue in relation to young children and identity development and Graybill et al. (2010) suggest development of assessment tools that reflect the needs of American Sign Language users is critical for gathering reliable, valid information.

Typical Scope of Team Assessment

Hearing screenings are now being recommended for infants at one month in a majority of the states and by many professionals (NIDCD, 2012). In addition to measuring actual hearing loss, some assess whether assistive devices, such as hearing aids, are needed. Other assessment approaches look at broader technology needs such as alternate communication devices if speech is limited or there are multiple diagnostic codes. As the population changes and increased numbers of older adults are deaf or lose their hearing as they age, unique needs for those groups are being uncovered. Gerich and Fellinger (2012) suggest increased self-efficacy and communication skills would offset other difficulties related to hearing loss; thus, the scope of assessment may need to extend to coping, self-efficacy, and other areas beyond functional hearing loss measures.

Zheng, Caissie, and Comeau (2003) recommend exploring the perceptions of the impact of the hearing loss on communication by surveying all those involved with adolescents who have a hearing loss. This includes parents, caregivers, teachers, the adolescents, and others. Marschark et al. (2012) suggests there is a connection to reading and other skill areas that is particular to young adults who are deaf. Other researchers strongly suggest viewing the child or adolescent from a systems perspective. Belzner and Seal (2009) report on cochlear implants since they were first used in 2000 in the United States. Family dynamics is a relatively new element due to the issues involved in the decisions involving implants as well as language choices (Borum, 2012; Jackson, Wegner, & Turnbull, 2010). In addition to communication choice and use, Borum (2012) stresses that cultural implications are another area for consideration within families and communities for assessing needs of children and adolescents with hearing loss.

When assessing the impact of hearing loss on other aspects of life, the team should look for deficits in ICF Body Functions codes b117 Intellectual Functions, b126 Temperament and Personality Functions, b130 Energy and Drive Functions, b140 Attention Functions, b152 Emotional Functions, b164 Higher-Level Cognitive Functions, b167 Mental Functions of Language, b310 Voice Functions, b320 Articulation Functions, and b330 Fluency and Rhythm of Speech Functions. They should also assess whether assistive technology is required (e1 Products and Technology).

Areas of Concern for RT Assessment

Recreational therapy assessment focuses on functional communication in groups, social situations, and other social interaction needs. Results from chart or record reviews should focus on the preferred communication mode, such as sign language or written or verbal, and what the client needs to do to increase effective communication across a variety of environments. In addition, the therapist should review or assess any assistive technology needs, such as use of video relay or captioning for television. Oliva and Simonsen (2000) and Riddick (2011) recommend that the appropriate framework for viewing persons with hearing loss can increase successful outcomes across most settings.

Outcomes from assessments in academic areas, such as an Individualized Education Plan (IEP), may provide information for the recreational therapist. Lollis and LaSasso (2009) reveal the discrepancies in state mandated reading competency tests for some high school students who are deaf. Recreational therapists may need to interpret standardized tests to provide advocacy and support for families and students. Communication needs for independent living can also be an area of focus for young adults who have transitioned from high school (Appelman et al., 2012). Rieffe (2012) suggests an area of particular concern for children who are deaf or have significant hearing loss is awareness and regulation of emotion. Results from assessments related to affective domain or coping skills will be helpful for this concern.

Results from assessments in settings where older adults are being served may show behavioral tendencies related to hearing loss (Smith & Kampfe, 1997). Gradual hearing loss or loss of friends who communicate in sign language may impact the person negatively. Decreased social interaction or mental health issues may arise due to isolation, frustration, or other tendencies. The recreational therapist should be alert to these secondary outcomes related to hearing loss. Systematic observation (Coco-Ripp, 2005) is often a method to uncover needs related to communication difficulties. Many older adults are reluctant to seek mental health services (Feldman &

Gum, 2007) and referrals from an assessment for hearing loss issues may be a path that is beneficial.

Social skills, which are dependent on the developmental level of the person, should also be assessed to determine the impact the hearing loss or obstacles to effective communication have on optimal social interactions and maintenance of healthy relationships. This assessment may yield deficits or need areas in social skills (b126 Temperament and Personality Functions, d710 Basic Interpersonal Interactions, d720 Complex Interpersonal Interactions). A few typical areas are listed below.

- Awareness of how their hearing loss impacts them in a variety of social situations.
- Ability to identify how other people feel and express empathy.
- Willingness to admit when they do not know or hear the information, as opposed to bluffing.
- Respect for others' opinions and points of view even if different from their own.
- Understanding of various levels of friendships from acquaintances to close friends.

Different age groups will have different sets of deficits in ICF Activities and Participation codes. Some specific codes that recreational therapists should consider include d230 Carrying Out Daily Routine, d240 Handling Stress and Other Psychological Demands, d310 Communicating with — Receiving — Spoken Messages, d330 Speaking, d350 Conversation, d360 Using Communication Devices and Techniques, d460 Moving Around in Different Locations, d470 Using Transportation, d475 Driving, d7 Interpersonal Interactions and Relationships, d8 Major Life Areas, and d9 Community, Social, and Civic Life. Cultural sensitivity is required when the therapist is considering whether an observation represents a deficit for the particular client in these codes and also in any applicable environmental factors related to support, interpersonal relationships, and services available.

ICF Core Set

A brief and comprehensive ICF Core Set for Hearing Loss is available.

Treatment Direction

When hearing loss is the primary diagnosis, the team focuses on correcting the Body Structure problems that were diagnosed. Then they work on associated functional and participation issues.

Hearing loss is also a concern when a person is being treated for another issue or problem. For example, the person is diagnosed with diabetes or obsessive-compulsive disorder and has a hearing loss. Groff, Lawrence, and Grivna (2006) report on a case of a young person with cerebral palsy who is also deaf. Communication was a challenge for successful treatment. Even though the individual used American Sign Language, some practitioners providing his treatment were not able to communicate with him. The authors (Groff, Lawrence, & Grivna, 2006) recommend either budgeting for an interpreter or practitioners learning basic sign language skills.

Working with a person with a hearing loss influences the outcome of the primary problem in several ways (Steinberg et al., 2005). First, the primary means of communication should be determined and respected in all aspects of the treatment process. Second, assessment of the impact of the hearing loss on the outcomes of the primary problem, as well as other quality of life indicators, should be determined. The communication obstacles may influence the standard treatment protocols. Third, support systems for the person with a hearing loss should be determined to improve the success of the treatment. For example, providing a companion during surgery for a person who is older and has a hearing loss gives a sense of security and continuity throughout. Finally, providing appropriate sign language interpreters or other requested accommodations for all levels of the treatment process are important not just for critical meetings or treatment sessions but throughout the milieu (e340 Personal Care Providers and Personal Assistants, e355 Health Professionals).

Whole Team Approach

The whole team approaches the needs of the person with a hearing loss with the primary problem in mind. Yet parallel to this is the confounding issue surrounding communication or other issues that result from the hearing loss. Communication is so integral to the success of the treatment that the needs of the person should be considered at each step in the process. Not taking into account the impact of a hearing loss on communication can lead to less effective outcomes from the treatment. Use of visual communication strategies, such as written notes or amplification for telephones, can assist communication. Each person is unique in preferred mode of communication, so finding out preferences at the beginning is important because it allows the team to be prepared. Use of video relay or voice to text may need some prior arrangements, yet will be helpful for the individual receiving treatment. Barak and Sadovsky (2008) found adolescents expressed empowerment when participating in computer-based activities because the communication barriers did not limit interactions as much.

Allied health professionals who focus on an aural rehabilitation approach, such as audiologists, speech-language pathologists, and speech, language, and hearing scientists (American Speech-Language-Hearing Association, 2011), target services such as improved speech or procurement of hearing aids and speech-generating devices as part of meeting the needs of persons with a hearing loss. Thibodeau and Alford (2010) report successful benefits for intensive auditory training with certain individuals. This approach provides some helpful services, and is within the scope of practice for recreational therapy. The whole team should be aware of assessed deficits in functions and work toward providing coping strategies for dealing with the hearing loss, especially when it is a new problem. The cultural approach should be emphasized to provide interventions and services that assist persons with a hearing loss or the person who is deaf or hard of hearing to lead a productive and healthy life or improve the quality of life. Some of the ICF codes that are treated with these approaches include b117 Intellectual Functions, b126 Temperament and Personality Functions, b130 Energy and Drive Functions, b140 Attention Functions, b152 Emotional Functions, b164 Higher-Level Cognitive Functions, b167 Mental Functions of Language, b310 Voice Functions, b320 Articulation Functions, and b330 Fluency and Rhythm of Speech Functions.

Persons who experience both hearing loss and visual problems receive specific services and present unique needs. Berry, Kelley-Bock, and Reid (2008) describe a two-week program, Confident Living, designed to foster increased independence for older persons with dual sensory impairments. One specific aspect of the program targets social and emotional issues unique to the individuals, then helps them to connect back to their community upon completion of the training. Many professionals recommend recreation as the ideal venue for adolescents to develop self-determination skills and other strategies for becoming more independent (Lieberman & MacVicar, 2003; Lieberman & Stuart, 2002; Tutt, 2007).

Recreational Therapy Approach

The recreational therapist follows the whole team approach and extends the communication accessibility to the recreational therapy sessions as well as all other areas the person may access, such as the swimming pool, art room, or dining area. Making sure the noise level is taken into account for a person who is deaf or hard of hearing will facilitate successful communication. Another environmental issue is lighting. Someone who relies on visual cues for communication will generally need well-lit areas to do activities or sessions. An individual or small group format can focus on approaches that include use of adaptations, compensatory strategies, coping techniques, social skills training, community integration programs, or lifelong leisure and recreation skill development (e1 Products and Technology, e580 Health Services, Systems, and Policies).

Recreational Therapy Interventions

The type of intervention depends on the setting and primary problem. Often the therapist will choose small group or individual interventions to minimize the difficulties that larger groups pose for a person who is deaf or hard of hearing. Another general guideline in choosing interventions is to learn about the community resources that the person will have upon discharge or transition from a more structured setting (d9 Community, Social, and Civic Life, e1 Products and Technology, e3 Support and Relationships). Resources in the community related to recreation or communication support may impact involvement by the person once they leave the hospital, rehabilitation center, or other facility. For example, are there clubs or advocacy organizations in a community where a person lives that might be beneficial and increase quality of life for that person? DeForge, Regan, and Gutmanis (2008) report on a program to involve frail elders in a community center. Two national organizations with different perspectives are the National Association of the Deaf and the Hearing Loss Association of America. Both

have local chapters and would be good resources for a person needing local support. Coco-Ripp (2003) found that contact for persons who are deaf and use sign language with others who do not will provide positive effects for both groups. Therefore, community programs that provide support for persons with hearing loss can be beneficial beyond the individual being served (d9 Community, Social, and Civic Life).

Interventions that focus on enhancing adaptations for communication in various settings might use role-play, outings, or family sessions to accomplish short- and long-term goals. Mathews et al. (2011) describe a successful role-play program called Deaf Strong Hospital using role reversal that includes a focus on communication and cultural aspects of being a member of the Deaf community. Compensatory strategies, coping techniques, social skills training, community integration programs, or lifelong leisure and recreation skill development are other areas of intervention programs that have been used (Lane & Clark, 2012; Luckner, 1989; Wachter, 1994).

The forensic or prison setting is reported to be quite problematic for individuals with hearing loss. Vernon (2010) details the many roadblocks that ineffective communication can have for a person who uses sign language or has a significant hearing loss. Often the person does not have necessary skills, knowledge, or understanding to ask for support, assistance, or request an interpreter. Recreational therapists who work in this setting can include assertiveness training, coping skills, and other relevant programs based on the needs of the population group (d230 Carrying Out Daily Routine, d240 Handling Stress and Other Psychological Demands, d7 Interpersonal Interactions and Relationships, d8 Major Life Areas, and d9 Community, Social, and Civic Life).

Functional Skills

Functional skill interventions for persons who are deaf or hard of hearing usually focus on these three areas: communication (d3 Communication), social skills and relationships (d7 Interpersonal Interactions and Relationships), and use of assistive technology (e1 Products and Technology). Communication access impacts major areas of an individual's life including work or career (d8 Major Life Areas) and leisure or recreation (d920 Recreation and Leisure). Enhancing functional skills in these three areas using a comprehensive approach is most effective.

Communication skill development (d3 Communication) and improvement may include expressive and receptive skills as well as increased awareness of environmental needs. Expressive skills could focus on expanding a person's vocabulary for communicating emotions; increasing ways to communicate, such as writing or electronic devices; or enhancing comfort level in dialogue with persons who use other linguistic communication systems. For example, an ASL user may gain more confidence communicating with a professional who uses spoken English. Receptive skill development may focus on learning to correctly interpret facial or other non-verbal gestural modes of communication; increasing time on focus in a dialogue; matching appropriate levels of disclosure in a conversation; or accuracy in vocabulary comprehension. Environmental awareness could mean combining expressive and receptive skills to state needs, such as letting the teacher know that a front row seat is needed; increasing personal understanding of needs in a variety of facilities or spaces; or learning to self-advocate for more effective communication spaces at work, school, and home or in other places (d240 Handling Stress and Other Psychological Demands, d710 Basic Interpersonal Interactions, d720 Complex Interpersonal Interactions).

Functional skills in the area of assistive technology may include training the individual in selection or use of devices such as a video relay for telephone use. Skill development may also focus on improved use of personal technology, such as hearing aids. Other functional skill enhancement might be use of technology in varied environments, such as a voice to text application on a device in a movie or lecture. Some assistive technology changes rapidly, yet the needs of the individual must be the primary goal in this area. Therefore, sensitivity to the individual's communication and social skill needs is a consideration for assistive technology use.

Education, Training, and Counseling

Typical training programs for persons who are deaf or hard of hearing include services such as these offered at the transitional unit at the National Deaf Academy (n. d.).

Domestic and life skills (d5 Self-Care): Training in a variety of skill areas ensures the individual makes progress to become as independent in living in the community as possible upon discharge. Increased confidence in self-care can have a positive impact on other areas of treatment. For many children or adolescents, increased time on communication issues has taken time from other life areas.

Money management (d860 Basic Economic Transactions, d865 Complex Economic Transactions, d870 Economic Self-Sufficiency): Gaining the needed ability to manage money and resources may be a priority for success upon discharge. Objectives can vary from learning the cost of services to budgeting for a high cost item to understanding the information on a bank statement.

Job skills (d840-d859 Work and Employment): Prevocational training can begin at an early age and increase confidence for the child with a hearing loss. Incorporating communication development with vocational skill development can enhance the career success as well as provide motivation to continue learning upon discharge.

Communication, social and interpersonal skills (d3 Communication, d7 Interpersonal Interactions and Relationships): These are key areas for an individual with hearing loss, as previously discussed. Combining these areas with other training can improve the learning outcomes.

Advanced self-care skills (d5 Self-Care, d230 Carrying Out Daily Routine): Often a child who experiences frustration with communication, socialization, or being understood in certain environments, such as school or recreation, will need to have additional focus on areas of personal care and hygiene. This may be due to lack of awareness, neglect, or more time spent on other life skills. Becoming independent in self-care can include skills such as laundry, arranging for a haircut, or selecting shoes. Again, combining communication and social skills training within self-care training is suggested.

Leadership (b126 Temperament and Personality Functions): Improved assertiveness skills apply across diverse settings and help the person use facts to advocate for self and others.

Leisure skills (d155 Acquiring Skills, d920 Recreation and Leisure, d880 Engagement in Play): Development of a variety of recreation or play interests, abilities, and skills related to a healthy leisure lifestyle using a developmental approach may be needed. Depending on the age or needs of the person with a hearing loss, communication and social skills will be a major focus to acquire new interests, plan social events, or maintain participation in preferred leisure.

Meal preparation and cooking (d630 Preparing Meals): It is important to acquire skills and knowledge related to nutrition, as well as safe food handling procedures.

Communication awareness and reintegration (d9 Community, Social, and Civic Life): Learning how to be involved in multiple community settings with varied environmental needs for communication is required for successful inclusion. Awareness of rights such as alternate communication modes, interpreter scheduling, sitting in the front row at a meeting or class, and many other skills that support effective communication may be part of a training program for adults and adolescents to be independent upon discharge.

Community Integration

A model program for people who are deaf or hard of hearing with behavioral health needs is located in Fairview, MN. The Minnesota Chemical Dependency Program (n.d.) offers a specialized program designed to meet the communication and cultural needs of persons in chemical dependency treatment who are deaf and hard-of-hearing. Another program focuses on children and young adults who are deaf or hard of hearing with behavioral health needs is the National Deaf Academy in Florida. This facility provides residential treatment and transitional services. The North Carolina School for the Deaf (n.d.) is a state school that provides recreational therapy as part of the residential services for students attending the facility. All three of these programs provide specialized services designed to meet the communication and other specific needs of persons who are deaf or hard of hearing. All of the programs highlight the use of American Sign Language and various communication technologies, such as video or listening devices.

In communities, other services are offered through municipal parks and recreation departments in the inclusion sections. Various methods of support are provided to meet the needs of a resident who wants to participate in recreation. In addition, schools and community recreation providers collaborate to meet the needs of children in the area with spe-

cialized programs that range from leisure education to recreation participation. Services may include individual treatment, usually as part of the Individualized Education Plan for the child. The therapist may work for the school or for the community service provider.

Barriers and obstacles to community participation, as well as active engagement in regularly occurring events, is another focus area. Tsai and Fung (2005) found perceived constraints for students to be involved in leisure time physical activity and suggested intentional efforts to change perceptions as well as provide support to overcome the challenges of the barriers. Kurkova, Scheetz, and Stelzer (2010) reported that decreasing constraints in physical education programs can enhance activity involvement. Generally these issues fall under one of the codes in e5 Services, Systems, and Policies

Health Promotion

Prevention of hearing loss is a focus of many organizations and agencies (Felzien, 2010; Centers for Disease Control and Prevention, 2012). Recreational noise exposure, decreasing problems from job-related hearing loss, and targeting adolescents who use portable entertainment devices are areas of recent research studies targeting prevention of hearing loss (Biassoni et al., 2005; Fligor, 2010; Serra et al., 2005; Shah et al., 2009). The consensus is to retain the level of hearing and prevent further loss by minimizing exposure that has been shown to cause damage. These changes are covered in ICF code e5 Services, Systems, and Policies.

Among people with hearing loss or people who are deaf or hard of hearing, the main need is often behavioral health (Feldman & Gum, 2007). Recognition of mental illness in a person who has difficulty communicating provides an additional obstacle. Mental health issues are often overlooked in persons who age and lose their hearing. Increasing awareness of healthcare providers to be alert to signs and symptoms, as well as training for the unique needs of the person's communication issues, remains a priority.

Overall health of persons who are deaf is a concern of researchers. Margellos-Anast et al. (2005) suggest they are a unique group and more focus on including persons with hearing loss or who are culturally deaf needs to be done across the healthcare continuum. Barnett et al. (2011) strongly recommend policy and procedure changes to minimize the disparities among persons who use sign language in the field of healthcare.

Resources

Beginnings of North Carolina

ncbegin.org/

This is a non-profit agency that provides information for parents, caregivers, and service providers. A list of helpful links is available as well as a handy communication choices chart. The site gives a broad spectrum of sources so parents can have information to make decisions and have access to help.

Camp Mark Seven

campmark7.org/

This outdoor camp serves children and adults who are deaf, hard of hearing, and hearing impaired. Programs include retreats, educational or leadership seminars, sign language training, sessions for KODA (kids of deaf adults), and senior citizens.

CapVidio

www.capvidio.com/

A service provider for real time transcription needs such as classrooms, lectures, or meetings.

Clear Captions

www.clearcaptions.com/

A service for individuals with a hearing loss who need support in using the phone. It is a free service for qualified persons.

Communication Services for the Deaf, Inc.

www.c-s-d.org/

This private, nonprofit, multi-national organization believes their mission is to enhance the opportunities for individuals who are deaf and hard of hearing through innovative technology and services. Some of their services are relay services, national interpreter referral services, CapTel (phone transcription service), and a variety of other support for communication. Among the expansion of the services are advocacy and educational approaches such as the Deaf Domestic Violence Programs. Another training program, Project Endeavor, has a variety of resources such as health-focused videos on diabetes and mental health with sign language as the primary communication mode. Camp Lakodia is a special project

completed by an all-Deaf crew. It is an outdoor retreat center in South Dakota.

Deaflympics

www.deaflympics.com

International sports competition with summer and winter events for deaf and hard of hearing athletes.

Deaf and Hard of Hearing Consumer Advocacy Network (DHHCAN)

Nineteen organizations are members of this national coalition of, for, and by the deaf and hard of hearing: American Association of the Deaf-Blind (AADB), American Deafness and Rehabilitation Association (ADARA), American Society for Deaf Children (ASDC), Association of Late-Deafened Adults (ALDA), Communication Services for the Deaf (CSD), Conference of Educational Administrators of Schools and Programs for the Deaf (CEASD), CSDVRS, Deaf Seniors of America (DSA), Gallaudet University, Gallaudet University Alumni Association (GUAA), National Association of the Deaf (NAD), National Black Deaf Advocates (NBDA), National Center for Accessible Media/WGBH-Boston (NCAM/WGBH), National Deaf Business Institute (NDBI), Purple Communications, Registry of Interpreters for the Deaf, Inc. (RID), Sorenson Communications, Telecommunications for the Deaf and Hard of Hearing, Inc. (TDI) and United States Deaf Sports Federation (USADSF).

Deaf Seniors of America

www.deafseniorsofamerica.org/

An advocacy and awareness group that serves elder deaf and hard of hearing through conferences, seminars, and other activities.

Deaf Studies Digital Journal

dsdj.gallaudet.edu/

Articles and information are presented using a visual approach; excellent introduction into visual communication and sign language use.

Gallaudet University

www.gallaudet.edu/

The school is the world leader in liberal education and career development for deaf and hard of hearing undergraduate students. The university enjoys an international reputation for the outstanding graduate programs it provides deaf, hard of hearing, and hearing students, as well as for the quality of the research it conducts on the history, language, culture, and other topics related to Deaf people. In addition, the University's Laurent Clerc National Deaf Education Center serves Deaf and hard of hearing children at its two demonstration schools and throughout the nation by developing, implementing, and disseminating innovative educational strategies.

Gallaudet University Camp List

www.gallaudet.edu/clerc_center/information_and_re-sources/info_to_go/resources/summer_camps.html. A list of camp opportunities.

Mental Health Resources

research.gallaudet.edu/resources/mhd/

An online listing of mental health resources for persons who are deaf.

National Center for Deaf Health Research

www.urmc.rochester.edu/ncdhr/

www.urmc.rochester.edu/ncdhr/links/

A center funded by the Centers for Disease Control and Prevention through Prevention Research Centers and hosted by the University of Rochester Medical Center. This site has current information on events, research, and other sources for persons interested in health for deaf or hard of hearing population groups. NCDHR goals are guided by a cultural model that says Deaf people are a minority group who share a common language — the American Sign Language (ASL) — and culture. The goals are not guided by a clinical model that says deafness is a condition that should be prevented or treated. At the site there are many links for health-related topics, sign language, and culture with many sites offered in ASL.

National Institute on Deafness and Other Communication Disorders

www.nidcd.nih.gov/staticresources/health/hearing/FactSheetCochlearImplant.pdf

Information on cochlear implants can be found here.

National Technical Institute for the Deaf at Rochester Institute for Technology

www.ntid.rit.edu/

Outstanding support for undergraduate and graduates in getting degrees in a wide range of areas of technology. Also, integrated research program of national and international prominence, focusing on teaching and learning; access, support services, and related technology; and communication in personal, learning, and working environments.

Purple Communications

www.purple.us/

A company focused on communication for Deaf and hard-of-hearing individuals and businesses. They provide on-site interpreting services, video relay services, text relay services, and video remote interpreting. Purple develops products and services that open communications between all people, regardless of differences in abilities, languages, and locations.

Rochester Recreation Club of the Deaf

www.rochesterdeafclub.com/

This is an example of one club, but there are many different cities that have similar clubs for Deaf to gather and serve as a center for recreation and social activities.

Sertoma Organization

www.sertoma.org/

A national service organization with primary focus on assisting the more than 50 million people with hearing health issues and educating the public on the issues surrounding hearing health.

Sorenson Communications

www.sorensonvrs.com/

Video relay and other communication products and services.

Video Caption Corporation

www.vicaps.com/

The company provides high quality captioning and subtitling services for multiple needs.

References

American Academy of Pediatrics. (2006). Developmental screening tools. Retrieved from http://www.medicalhomeinfo.org/downloads/pdfs/DPIPscreeningtoolgrid.pdf.

American Speech-Language-Hearing Association. (2011). Mission statement. Retrieved from http://www.asha.org/.

Appelman, K. I., Callahan, J. O., Mayer, M. H., Luetke, B. S., & Stryker, D. S. (2012). Education, employment and independent living of young adults who are deaf and hard of hearing. *American Annals of the Deaf, 157*(3), 264-275.

Barak, A. & Sadovsky Y. (2008). Internet use and personal empowerment of hearing-impaired adolescents. *Computers in Human Behavior, 24*, 2311-2324.

Barnett, S., McKee, M., Smith, S., & Pearson, T. A. (2011). Deaf sign language users, health inequities, and public health: Opportunity for social justice. *Preventing Chronic Disease: Public Health Research, Practice, and Policy, 8*(2) 1-6.

Belzner, K. A. & Seal, B. C. (2009). Children with cochlear implants: A review of demographics and communication disorders. *American Annals for the Deaf, 154*(3), 311-333.

Berry, P., Kelley-Bock, M., & Reid, C. (2008). Confident Living Program for senior adults experiencing vision and hearing loss. *Care Management Journals, 9*(1), 31-35.

Biassoni, E. C., Serra, M. R., Richter, U., Joekes, S., Yacci, M. R., ... Franco, G. (2005). Recreational noise exposure and its effects on the hearing of adolescents. Part II: Development of hearing disorders. *International Journal of Audiology, 44*(2), 74-85.

Borum, V. (2012). Perceptions of communication choice and usage among African American hearing parents: Afrocentric cultural implications for African American Deaf and hard of hearing children. *American Annals of the Deaf, 157*(1), 7-15.

Boulet, S. L., Boyle, C. A., & Schieve, L. A. (2009). Health care use and health and functional impact of developmental disabilities among U.S. children, 1997-2005. *Archives of Pediatric & Adolescent Medicine, 163*(1), 19-26.

Centers for Disease Control and Prevention. (2011). Types of hearing loss. Retrieved from http://www.cdc.gov/ncbddd/hearingloss/types.html.

Centers for Disease Control and Prevention. (2012). 2010 annual data Early Hearing Detection and Intervention (EHDI) Program. Retrieved from http://www.cdc.gov/ncbddd/hearingloss/ehdi-data2010.html.

Centers for Disease Control and Prevention. (2012). Hearing loss in children: Facts. Retrieved from http://www.cdc.gov/ncbddd/hearingloss/facts.html.

Coco-Ripp, J. A. (2003). The effect of awareness training and planned contact on the provision of an inclusive environment for persons who are deaf. (Doctoral dissertation). Retrieved from ProQuest Nursing & Allied Health Source, AAT 3094280.

Coco-Ripp, J. A. (2005). Research update: Including people who are deaf in recreation. *Parks & Recreation, 40*(2). 26-32.

DeForge, R., Regan, B., & Gutmanis, I. (2008). Lean on Me: Building volunteer capacity to support frail seniors' participation in community seniors' centre programs: A pilot project evaluation report. *Therapeutic Recreation Journal, 42*(3), 172-180.

Feldman, D. M. & Gum, A. (2007). Multigenerational perceptions of mental health services among deaf adults in Florida. *American Annals for the Deaf, 152*(4), 391-399.

Felzien, M. (2010). AG Bell Chapters: Community building. *Volta Voices, 17*(3), 26-29.

Fligor, B. (2010). Recreational noise and its potential risk to hearing. *The Hearing Review, 17*, 48-54.

Gates, G. A. & Hoffman, H. (n. d.). What the numbers mean: An epidemiological perspective on hearing. National Institute on Deafness and Other Communication Disorders. Retrieved from http://www.nidcd.nih.gov/health/statistics/measuring.htm.

Gerich, J. & Fellinger, J. (2012). Effects of social networks on the quality of life in an elder and middle-aged deaf community sample. *Journal of Deaf Studies and Deaf Education, 17*(1), 102-115.

Golos, D. B., Moses, A. M., & Wolbers, K. A. (2012). Culture or disability? Examining deaf characters in children's book illustrations. *Early Childhood Education Journal, 40*, 239-249.

Graybill, P., Aggas, J., Dean, R. K., Demers, S., Finnagan, E. G., & Pollard, R. Q. Jr. (2010). A community-participatory approach to adapting survey items for deaf individuals and American Sign Language. *Field Methods, 22*(4), 429-448.

Groff, D., Lawrence, E., & Grivna, S. (2006). Effects of a therapeutic recreation intervention using exercise: A case study with a child with cerebral palsy. *Therapeutic Recreation Journal, 40*(4), 269-283.

Hearing Loss Association of America. (n. d.). States and chapters. Retrieved from http://www.hearingloss.org/chapters/index.asp.

Jackson, C. W., Wegner, J. R., & Turnbull, A. P. (2010). Family quality of life following early identification of deafness. *Language, Speech, and Hearing Services in Schools, 41*, 194-205.

Kurkova, P., Scheetz, N., & Stelzer, J. (2010). Health and physical education as an important part of school curricula: A comparison of schools for the deaf in the Czech Republic and the United States. *American Annals of the Deaf, 155*(1), 78-95.

Lane, K. R. & Clark, M. K. (2012). Working with hearing-impaired clients: Techniques to optimize communication. *American Journal of Recreation Therapy, 11*(3), 26-30.

Lieberman, L. & MacVicar, J. M. (2003). Play and recreational habits of youths who are deaf-blind. *Journal of Visual Impairment & Blindness, 97*, 755-768.

Lieberman, L. & Stuart, M. (2002). Self-determined recreational and leisure choices of individuals with deaf-blindness. *Journal of Visual Impairment & Blindness, 96*, 724-735.

Lollis, J. & LaSasso, C. (2009). The appropriateness of the NC state-mandated reading competency test for deaf students as a criterion for high school graduation. *Journal of Deaf Studies and Deaf Education, 14*(1), 76-98.

Luckner, J. L. (1989). Altering locus of control of individuals with hearing impairments by outdoor-adventure courses. *Journal of Rehabilitation, 11*, 62-67.

Margellos-Anast, H., Hedding, T., Perlman, T., Miller, L., Rodgers, R., ... Whitman, S. (2005). Developing a standardized comprehensive health survey for use with deaf adults. *American Annals for the Deaf, 150*(4), 388-396.

Marschark, M., Sarchet, T., Convertino, C. M., Borgna, G., Morrison, C., & Remelt, S. (2012). Print exposure, reading habits, and reading achievement among deaf and hearing college students. *Journal of Deaf Studies and Deaf Education, 17*(1), 61-74.

Mathews, J. L., Parkhill, A. L., Schlehofer, D. A., Starr, M. J., & Barnett, S. (2011). Innovations in teaching: Role-reversal exercise with Deaf Strong Hospital to teach communication competency and cultural awareness. *American Journal of Pharmaceutical Education, 75*(3), 1-10.

Minnesota Chemical Dependency Program for Deaf and Hard-of-Hearing Individuals. (n.d.). Behavioral health. Retrieved from http://www.fairview.org/Services/BehavioralHealth/Chemi-calDependency/DeafandHard-of-HearingChemicalDependency/BVR-DEAF.

National Association for the Deaf. (n.d.). State association affiliations. Retrieved from http://www.nad.org/community/state-association-affiliates.

National Deaf Academy. (n.d.). Our history. Retrieved from http://nda.com/about/history.php.

National Institute on Deafness and Other Communication Disorders (NIDCD). (n.d.). Quick statistics. Retrieved from http://www.nidcd.nih.gov/health/statistics/quick.htm.

National Institute on Deafness and Other Communication Disorders (NIDCD). (2012). NIDCD 2012-2016 Strategic Plan. Retrieved from http://www.nidcd.nih.gov/staticresources/about/plans/strategic/2012-2016NIDCDStrategicPlan.pdf.

North Carolina School for the Deaf. (n.d.). Education services. Retrieved from http://www.ncoes.net/NCSD.shtml.

Oliva, G. & Simonsen, A. (2000). Re-thinking leisure services for deaf and hard of hearing persons: A new paradigm. *Parks & Recreation, 35*(5), 78-85.

Riddick, C. C. (2011). The reliability and norms of the Leisure Diagnostic Battery for undergraduate recreation majors who are deaf. *International Journal on Disability and Human Development, 10*(2), 150-165.

Rieffe, C. (2012). Awareness and regulation of emotions in deaf children. *British Journal of Developmental Psychology, 30*, 477-492.

Schein, J. D. & Miller, M. H. (2008). Genetics and deafness: Implications for education and life care of deaf students. *American Annals of the Deaf, 153*(4), 408-10.

Serra, M. R., Biassoni, E. C., Richter, U., Minolda, G., Franco, G., ….Yacci, M. R. (2005). Recreational noise exposure and its effects on the hearing of adolescents. Part I: An interdisciplinary long term study. *International Journal of Audiology, 44*(2), 65-73.

Shah, S., Gopal, B., Reis, J., & Novak, M. (2009). Hear today, gone tomorrow: An assessment of portable entertainment player use and hearing acuity in a community sample. *Journal of the American Board of Family Medicine, 22*(1), 17-23.

Smith, S. M. & Kampfe, C. M. (1997). Interpersonal relationship implications of hearing loss in persons who are older. *Journal of Rehabilitation, 63*, 15-21.

Steinberg, A. G., Barnett, S., Meador, H. E., Wiggins, E. A., & Zazove, P. (2005). Health care system accessibility: Experiences and perceptions of deaf people. *American Annals of the Deaf, 138*(1), 260-66.

Thibodeau, L. M. & Alford, J. A. (2010). Benefits of intensive auditory rehabilitation training. *Perspectives on Aural Rehabilitation & Its Instrumentation, 17*(1), 4-18.

Tsai, E. & Fung, L. (2005). Perceived constraints to leisure time physical activity participation of students with hearing impairment. *Therapeutic Recreation Journal, 39*(3), 192-206.

Tutt, L. M. (2007) This mattered to me. [Review of Play and recreation habits of youths who are deaf-blind by L. J. Lieberman and J. M. MacVicar in *Journal of Visual Impairment & Blindness, 97*(12), 755-768]. *Journal of Visual Impairment & Blindness, 101*(7), 435-6.

Vernon, M. (2010). The horror of being deaf and in prison. *American Annals for the Deaf, 155*(3), 311-321.

Wachter, C. J. (1994). The influence of communication mode on the leisure behavior of adults who are deaf. *Therapeutic Recreation Journal, 28*(4), 213-220.

Zheng, Y., Caissie, R., & Comeau, M. (2003). Perceptions of hearing difficulties by adolescents who are deaf or hard of hearing and their parents, teachers, and peers with normal hearing. *The Volta Review, 103*(3), 183-202.

19. Heart Disease

Heather R. Porter

Heart disease is an umbrella term that includes a range of medical conditions that involve the heart in one way or another (Mayo Clinic, 2014; American Heart Association, 2012). Examples of the most frequently seen conditions include:

Blood vessel diseases (cardiovascular disease): Narrowed, blocked, or stiffened blood vessels that impair circulation. Symptoms include angina (chest pain); shortness of breath; and pain, numbness, weakness, or feelings of coldness in extremities.

Heart arrhythmias: An abnormal heartbeat, which can be quick, slow, or irregular. Symptoms include fluttering in the chest, tachycardia (racing heartbeat), bradycardia (slow heart beat), angina, shortness of breath, vertigo, feeling lightheaded, and syncope (fainting).

Congenital heart defects: Structural problems of the heart or major blood vessels — over 18 types of congenital heart defects are recognized. These defects are usually seen in babies. Symptoms vary depending upon the abnormality or defect. Common symptoms include cyanosis (pale gray or blue skin color); swelling in the hands, ankles, feet, abdomen, or the areas around the eyes; shortness of breath during feedings leading to poor weight gain; tiring easily; and excess fluid in the heart or lungs.

Cardiomyopathy: Thickening and stiffening of the heart muscle. Symptoms include shortness of breath; swelling in the legs, ankle, or feet; bloating of the abdomen; fatigue; irregular heartbeats that feel rapid or pounding; vertigo; feeling of lightheadedness; and syncope.

Heart infections: There are three types of heart infections: pericarditis (infection of the tissue surrounding the heart), myocarditis (infection of the muscular middle layer of the heart walls), and endocarditis (infection of the inner membrane that separates the chambers and heart valves). Symptoms include fever, shortness of breath, fatigue, weakness, swelling in the legs or abdomen, heart rhythm changes, a dry or persistent cough, and skin rashes or unusual spots.

Valvular heart disease: Functions of one or more heart valves are damaged leading to stenosis (narrowing), regurgitation (leaking), or prolapse (improper closing). General symptoms include fatigue, shortness of breath, irregular heartbeat or heart murmur, swollen feet or ankles, angina, and syncope.

Incidence/Prevalence in U.S.

Heart disease is the leading cause of death in the U.S. for both men and women. Coronary artery disease is the most common (CDC, 2013). Congenital heart defects are the most common birth defect, affecting one percent (or about 40,000 births) per year, of which ventricular septal defect is most prevalent (CDC, 2011).

Predominant Age

Heart disease can affect anyone at any age; however the risk of cardiovascular disease increases with age. Risk significantly increases at age 45 for men and 55 for women (Seconds Count, 2013). Congenital heart defects are usually found and treated, if possible, in infancy. The epidemic of obesity in youth has put them more at risk. In a population-based sample of obese youth age five to 17, 70% had at least two cardiovascular disease risk factors (Seconds Count, 2013).

Causes

The causes of heart disease vary by the type of heart disease (Mayo Clinic, 2013; CDC, 2011):

Blood vessel disease (cardiovascular disease): Caused by atherosclerosis, a buildup of plaque in the arteries, from unhealthy diet, lack of exercise, being overweight, and smoking.

Heart arrhythmia: Commonly a result of congenital heart defects, coronary artery disease, hypertension, diabetes, smoking, excessive alcohol or caffeine use, drug abuse, stress, some medications, including supplements and herbal remedies, and valvular heart disease.

Congenital heart defects: At least 15% of congenital heart defects are associated with genetic conditions that develop in the womb; however, abnormalities in the structure of the heart can also occur as one ages.

Cardiomyopathy: The cause is currently unknown.

Heart infection: Caused by bacteria, viruses, parasites, medications that cause an allergic or toxic reaction, and certain autoimmune diseases, such as lupus, connective tissue disorders, vasculitis, and other rare inflammatory conditions.

Valvular heart disease: Caused by a congenital heart defect or damage to the valves from certain conditions, such as rheumatic fever, infections, connective tissue disorders, certain medications, or radiation treatments.

Heart disease risk factors include (CDC, 2009):

Specific health conditions: Bad cholesterol levels (too much LDL and not enough HDL) lead to plaque build-up and subsequent narrowing of the arteries. High blood pressure places increased stress on the arteries contributing to the risk of a heart attack. Uncontrolled diabetes results in increased glucose levels in the blood that cause organ damage. About three-fourths of people with diabetes die from heart or blood vessel disease.

Behavior: Cigarette smoking promotes atherosclerosis and increases levels of blood clotting factors. Nicotine raises blood pressure and carbon monoxide reduces the amount of oxygen that blood can carry. Diets high in saturated fat and cholesterol may raise cholesterol levels and cause atherosclerosis. For some people diets high in sodium raise blood pressure. Physical inactivity impairs the health of body structures and functions and is a risk factor for obesity, high blood pressure, bad cholesterol levels, and diabetes, all of which are risk factors for heart disease. Obesity is associated with bad cholesterol levels, high blood pressure, and diabetes, again, all of which are risk factors for heart disease. Excessive

alcohol use increases blood pressure and high triglycerides that contribute to atherosclerosis.

Heredity: Heart disease tends to run in families, indicating that there might be a genetic component. It could also be the result of living in a common environment and adopting similar behavioral patterns that contribute to heart disease, such as poor eating habits.

Systems Affected

Heart disease affects the circulatory system. Structural issues may be documented with ICF code s410 Structure of Cardiovascular System. Functional issues may be coded with b410 Heart Functions, b415 Blood Vessel Functions, b420 Blood Pressure Functions, and b460 Sensations Associated with Cardiovascular and Respiratory Functions. Depending on the cause and extent of the problem, many other systems in the body can be affected directly or indirectly. Other ICF codes that may be involved include b130 Energy and Drive Functions, b152 Emotional Functions, b280 Sensation of Pain, b730 Muscle Power Functions, and b735 Muscle Tone Functions.

Secondary Problems

Secondary problems will vary depending upon the type of heart disease. A few of the more general problems are listed below:

About 20-30% of individuals with congenital heart defects have other physical, developmental, or cognitive disorders (CDC, 2011).

Five to 10% of people with cardiac problems have anxiety disorders, particularly panic attacks and phobias, and 10-15% have mood disorders, predominantly depressive episodes, minor depression, or dysthymia (b126 Temperament and Personality Functions) (Sadock & Sadock, 2003). The risk of depression is up to 25% for individuals who have cardiovascular disease and diabetes, resulting in poorer medical outcomes, poorer glycemic control, increased diabetic symptoms, and greater all-cause mortality due to both biological and psychological processes (Fenton & Stover, 2006).

Sexual activity (b640 Sexual Functions) may be contraindicated due to increased stress on the cardiovascular system. See Levine and colleagues (2012) for specific recommendations set forth by the American Heart Association for sexual activity by type of heart disease. Stress, medication, depression, and fear of causing a cardiac event may also interfere with sexual ability.

Individuals who have cardiovascular disease related to lifestyle behaviors will most likely have other related secondary problems, such as back problems from being overweight or deconditioning from lack of physical activity (d570 Looking After One's Health).

Heart disease can affect many areas of activities and participation, as discussed in the Assessment section.

Prognosis

In the U.S., about 600,000 people die of heart disease every year, accounting for one fourth of all deaths (CDC, 2013). Death rates due to heart disease tend to be the highest in the south and lowest in the west (CDC, 2013). Prognosis for heart disease will vary depending upon the specific condition and other variables, such as age, health history, and level of support.

Assessment

Typical Scope of Team Assessment

During a cardiac event or a suspected cardiac problem, the medical team aims to stabilize the client and determine the underlying cause of the event. Assessment often includes an evaluation of risk factors, vital signs, blood work, listening to heart sounds with a stethoscope, and tests, such as electrocardiography (ECG), chest x-rays, and ultrasound.

In a rehabilitation setting, therapists receive a written order from the physician indicating the cardiac precautions and parameters that the client must stay within. Limits are often set on systolic and diastolic blood pressure, heart rate, oxygen saturation level, and MET ranges. Using these guidelines, therapists assess the client's ability to engage in functional tasks, such as transferring, walking, and leisure activities. Previously mentioned parameters are monitored during activity. In addition, the therapist watches for feelings of vertigo or dizziness, nausea, skin color changes, level of pain reported by the client using a 0-10 pain scale, client's perceived level of exertion, cool extremities, or feeling faint. Observations of the client's ability to perform tasks

can be documented with ICF codes b110 Consciousness Functions, b130 Energy and Drive Functions, b270 Sensory Functions Related to Temperature and Other Stimuli, b280 Sensation of Pain, b410 Heart Functions, b415 Blood Vessel Functions, b420 Blood Pressure Functions, b455 Exercise Tolerance Functions, d230 Carrying Out Daily Routine, d240 Handling Stress and Other Psychological Demands, d450 Walking, and d455 Moving Around.

A baseline of functioning is determined and goals are established that stay within the cardiac precautions and parameters set by the physician. Individuals with cardiac disease might also be assigned a NYHA Functional Capacity Classification to indicate the severity of functional limitations, along with an Objective Assessment Classification (American Heart Association, 2014).

Functional Capacity

Class I: Ordinary physical activity does not cause undue fatigue, palpitation, dyspnea, or angina.

Class II: Individuals have a slight limitation when engaged in physical activity. They are comfortable at rest; however ordinary physical activity results in fatigue, palpitation, dyspnea, or angina.

Class III: Individuals have a marked limitation when engaged in physical activity. They are comfortable at rest, however less than ordinary activity causes fatigue, palpitation, dyspnea, or angina.

Class IV: Individuals are unable to carry out any physical activity without discomfort. Symptoms of heart failure or the angina syndrome may be present even at rest. If any physical activity is undertaken, discomfort is increased.

Objective Assessment

A: No objective evidence of cardiovascular disease.

B: Objective evidence of minimal cardiovascular disease.

C: Objective evidence of moderately severe cardiovascular disease.

D: Objective evidence of severe cardiovascular disease.

Areas of Concern for RT Assessment

It is difficult to identify common findings among this population due to the diversity of cardiac damage and functioning. However, since the majority of heart disease conditions are due to modifiable lifestyle conditions, risk factors such as poor diet, lack of physical activity, smoking, alcohol use, uncontrolled stress, hypertension, and diabetes are often present (d570 Looking After One's Health). When the therapist sees the client in a rehabilitation facility, the therapist will often find poor endurance (b455 Exercise Tolerance Functions) and strength (b730 Muscle Power Functions) as key indicators for therapy. Cardiac precautions and parameters impose limits on physical exertion. Depression and anxiety (b126 Temperament and Personality Functions, d240 Handling Stress and Other Psychological Demands) may additionally be seen, since these are common psychological issues in this population. All of the ICF codes listed in the team assessment should also be considered, especially those associated with b455 Exercise Tolerance Functions, d230 Carrying Out Daily Routine, d450 Walking, and d455 Moving Around. Other ICF codes include b152 Emotional Functions, d620 Acquisition of Goods and Services, d760 Family Relationships, d770 Intimate Relationships, d850 Remunerative Employment, and d9 Community, Social, and Civic Life.

The recreational therapist should also assess the environment the client will be returning to after treatment, as it pertains to impact on recovery and health promotion. Issues to consider include e110 Products or Substances for Personal Consumption, e140 Products and Technology for Culture, Recreation, and Sport, e310 Immediate Family, e320 Friends, e325 Acquaintances, Peers, Colleagues, Neighbors, and Community Members, and e355 Health Professionals.

ICF Core Set

ICF Core Sets that might be helpful in identifying relevant ICF codes include Cardiopulmonary Conditions and Chronic Ischemic Heart Disease.

Treatment Direction

Whole Team Approach

The team approach will vary depending upon the specific heart disease and may include pharmacological and surgical interventions, such as angioplasty, coronary artery bypass, or heart transplant to treat structural heart issues followed by cardiac rehabilitation (s410 Structure of Cardiovascular System). Cardiac rehabilitation is generally divided into three phases (Roy, Wolf, & Scalzitti, 2012; The American Association of Cardiovascular and Pulmonary Rehabilitation [AACPR], 2014):

Phase One: This occurs during inpatient hospitalization and includes (1) monitoring activity tolerance through vital signs (blood pressure, heart rate, respiratory rate, oxygen saturation levels), perceived exertion (BORG scale), signs and symptoms of intolerance, and ECG monitoring, (2) progression of activity from approximately one to five METs, (3) education on topics, such as adverse symptoms related to activity, identification of cardiovascular risk factors, and signs of activity intolerance and (4) preparing for discharge with an assessment of function related to discharge placement, instruction for home exercise program, etc.

Phase Two: This occurs during outpatient rehabilitation (three to six months) and includes (1) exercise tolerance testing, (2) supervised exercise focused on aerobic and strength training, and (3) education, counseling, behavioral intervention, and goal setting related to nutrition, weight management, blood pressure management, lipid management, diabetes management, tobacco cessation, psychosocial management, exercise training, and physical activity.

Phase Three: This is the long-term maintenance phase that starts after six months and may continue for the rest of the patient's life.

Cardiac rehabilitation for myocardial infarction, percutaneous coronary intervention, coronary artery bypass grafting, angina, heart failure, valvular heart disease, and peripheral arterial disease have been found to yield significant outcomes including a 20-30% reduction in all-cause mortality, decreased mortality up to five years post participation, reduced symptoms, reduction in nonfatal recurrent myocardial infarction over median follow-up of 12 months, improved adherence to use of preventive medications, increased exercise performance, improved lipid panel, increased knowledge about cardiac disease and its management, enhanced ability to perform activities of daily living, improved health-related quality of life, improved psychosocial symptoms including reversal of anxiety and depression and increased self-efficacy, reduced hospitalizations and use of medical resources, and return to work or leisure activities (AACPR, 2014). Improvements are noted with ICF codes b110 Consciousness

Functions, b126 Temperament and Personality Functions, b130 Energy and Drive Functions, b270 Sensory Functions Related to Temperature and Other Stimuli, b280 Sensation of Pain, b410 Heart Functions, b415 Blood Vessel Functions, b420 Blood Pressure Functions, b455 Exercise Tolerance Functions, d230 Carrying Out Daily Routine, d240 Handling Stress and Other Psychological Demands, d450 Walking, d455 Moving Around, d570 Looking After One's Health, d760 Family Relationships, d770 Intimate Relationships, d850 Remunerative Employment, and d9 Community, Social, and Civic Life.

A growing trend in cardiac rehab is the utilization of the Ornish Spectrum Program, a comprehensive lifestyle change program that has demonstrated ability to reverse heart disease without surgery or pharmacology (see Resources). The program consists of healthy eating, engagement in physical activity, handling stress, and love and support. Individuals, as well as healthcare organizations, can become a certified provider. The 72-hour program is reimbursable by Medicare, as well as by many private insurance companies.

Recreational Therapy Approach

Recreational therapy focuses on cardiac recovery, prevention, and general health promotion. Cardiac precautions and parameters as ordered by the physician are monitored during activity to ensure safety. Additionally, the therapist helps the client to identify and change lifestyle habits that increase the risk of further cardiac dysfunction and teaches the client how to adapt activities so an unsafe cardiac load is avoided. Psychosocial issues and other barriers that hinder participation in life activities are also addressed.

Recreational Therapy Interventions

Engagement in play, leisure, recreation, and community activities (d9 Community, Social, and Civic Life) is a vital component of health in this population. Such engagement, if designed appropriately, has the potential to decrease cardiac risk factors by aiding in relaxation, promoting physical activity that can help control diabetes and hypertension, as well as reduce body weight, alleviating depression and anxiety, providing a healthy alternative for non-healthy behaviors such as cigarette smoking and

alcohol use, and improving overall well-being and quality of life. The specific interventions chosen and behavioral strategies utilized will vary based on individual need. Some general interventions for consideration include:

Remediation of reduced functional capacities such as strength and aerobic capacity (b130 Energy and Drive Functions, b410 Heart Functions, b415 Blood Vessel Functions, b420 Blood Pressure Functions, b455 Exercise Tolerance Functions, d450 Walking, d455 Moving Around).

Psychological or emotional interventions aimed at reducing depression and anxiety (b126 Temperament and Personality Functions, d240 Handling Stress and Other Psychological Demands), as well as general strengthening of psychological and emotional health (b126 Temperament and Personality Functions) related to bolstering ability to implement and follow through with lifestyle behavioral interventions (d570 Looking After One's Health).

Education, counseling, and behavioral interventions aimed at reducing risk factors. These interventions include smoking cessation, healthy diet, stress management, increasing physical activity, and reducing or eliminating alcohol intake (d570 Looking After One's Health, d9 Community, Social, and Civic Life). Heart-related education includes (1) self-monitoring heart rate and blood pressure within activity, (2) learning to recognize symptoms of cardiac exertion above limitations during activity, including signs of fatigue, (3) making activity accommodations, (4) knowing the warning signs of a coronary event, and (5) monitoring environmental conditions that could put extra stress on the heart, such as humidity, pollution levels, and temperature extremes (d570 Looking After One's Health).

Problem solving for reducing or eliminating barriers, such as transportation, finances, or lack of social support, that hinder the client's ability to implement positive behavior change and strengthening existing facilitators, such as good family relationships, that support positive behavior change (d760 Family Relationships, d770 Intimate Relationships, e110 Products or Substances for Personal Consumption, e310 Immediate Family, e320 Friends, e325 Acquaintances, Peers, Colleagues, Neighbors, and Community Members)

Activity adaptation or modification and related education as needed to maintain precautions and parameters. There are many possible adaptations to activities including a modified golf swing, lighter weight bowling balls, and education about energy conservation techniques to reduce fatigue (e.g., d570 Looking After One's Health, e140 Products and Technology for Culture, Recreation, and Sport).

Skill development, education, counseling, and community integration training related to engagement in specific forms of play, leisure, recreation, and community activities that aid in health promotion and recovery (d570 Looking After One's Health, d9 Community, Social, and Civic Life).

Resources

American Heart Association

www.heart.org

The nation's oldest and largest volunteer organization devoted to fighting cardiovascular diseases and stroke. Provides resources, education, training, and treatment guidelines.

Ornish Spectrum Program

www.ornishspectrum.com

A comprehensive lifestyle change program for chronic health conditions.

References

American Association of Cardiovascular and Pulmonary Rehabilitation. (2014). About cardiovascular and pulmonary rehabilitation. Retrieved from https://www.aacvpr.org/about/aboutcardiacpulmonaryrehab/tabid/560/default.aspx.

American Heart Association. (2014). Classification of functional capacity and objective measurement. Retrieved from http://my.americanheart.org/professional/StatementsGuidelines/ByPublicationDate/PreviousYears/Classification-of-Functional-Capacity-and-Objective-Assessment_UCM_423811_Article.jsp.

American Heart Association. (2012). Common types of heart defects. Retrieved from http://www.heart.org/HEARTORG/Conditions/CongenitalHeartDefects/AboutCongenitalHeartDefects/Common-Types-of-Heart-Defects_UCM_307017_Article.jsp.

Centers for Disease Control. (2013). Heart disease facts. Retrieved from http://www.cdc.gov/heartdisease/facts.htm.

Centers for Disease Control. (2011). Congenital heart defects: Data and statistics. Retrieved from http://www.cdc.gov/ncbddd/heartdefects/data.html.

Centers for Disease Control. (2009). Heart disease risk factors. Retrieved from http://www.cdc.gov/heartdisease/risk_factors.htm.

Fenton, W. S. & Stover, E. S. (2006). Mood disorders: Cardiovascular and diabetes comorbidity. *Current Opinion in Psychiatry, 19*(4), 421-7.

Levine, G. N., Steinke, E. E., Bakaeen, F. G., Bozkurt, B., Cheitlin, M. D., Conti, J. B., Foster, E., Jaarsma, T., Kloner, R. A., Lange, R. A., Lindau, S. T., Maron, B. J., Moser, D. K., Ohman, M., Seftel, A. D., & Stewart, W. J. (2012). Sexual activity and cardiovascular disease: A scientific statement from the American Heart Association. *Circulation, 125*, 1058-1072. Retrieved from http://circ.ahajournals.org/content/125/8/1058.full.pdf).

Mayo Clinic. (2013). Heart disease: Causes. Retrieved from http://www.mayoclinic.org/diseases-conditions/heart-disease/basics/causes/CON-20034056.

Mayo Clinic. (2014). Heart disease. Retrieved from http://www.mayoclinic.org/diseases-conditions/heart-disease/basics/definition/CON-20034056?p=1.

Roy, S. H., Wolf, S. L., & Scalzitti, D. A. (2012). *The rehabilitation specialist's handbook*. F. A. Davis.

Sadock, B. & Sadock, V. (2003). *Synopsis of psychiatry, 9ᵗʰ edition*. Philadelphia: Lippincott, Williams & Wilkins.

Seconds Count. (2013). The faces of cardiovascular disease. Retrieved from http://www.scai.org/SecondsCount/Heart/WhoIsAffectedByCardiovascularDisease.aspx.

20. Intellectual Disability

Mary Lou Schilling

Intellectual disability is the most common type of developmental disability (CDC, 2005). To be diagnosed with an intellectual disability a person must exhibit significant sub-average intellectual functioning, existing concurrently with deficits in adaptive behavior, manifested during the developmental period (APA, 2013). Until recently, this diagnostic group was referred to as Mental Retardation (AMA, 2009; APA, 2000). Due to a history of negative social stigma caused by the misuse of this term, healthcare professionals, physicians, and most recently diagnostic manuals have replaced the term mental retardation with intellectual disability (AMA, 2013; APA 2013; Sulkes, 2006).

People with intellectual disability (ID) have varying degrees of functioning. While recognizing each person as an individual, physicians and healthcare workers find it helpful to classify this diagnosis based on cognitive functioning. Deficits in intellectual functioning must be two standard deviations below the norm or an intelligence quotient (IQ) of 70-75 or less. There are four recognized levels of cognitive impairment.

Mild intellectual disability: IQ range of 50-69 (AMA, 2009). This category accounts for the majority (85%) of the persons with ID (Reynolds & Dombeck, 2006). Individuals with mild cognitive impairment can be expected to achieve a mental age of 9-12 years (World Health Organization [WHO], 2007).

Moderate intellectual disability: IQ range of 35-49 (AMA, 2009). This category accounts for approximately 10% of the individuals with ID (Reynolds & Dombeck, 2006). Individuals with this diagnosis can be expected to achieve a mental age of 6-9 years (WHO, 2007).

Severe intellectual disability: IQ range of 20-34 (AMA, 2009) Accounts for approximately three to four percent of those with ID (Reynolds & Dombeck,

2006). Individuals with this diagnosis can be expected to achieve a mental age of three to six years and require continuous support throughout their lifetime (WHO, 2007).

Profound intellectual disability: IQ range below 20 (AMA, 2009). Accounts for one to two percent of the population of those with ID (Reynolds & Dombeck, 2006). Individuals with this diagnosis can be expected to achieve a mental age below three years and have severe limitations in communication, self-care, and mobility (WHO, 2007).

Low scores on IQ tests by themselves do not qualify a person to be diagnosed with an intellectual disability. Individuals must show evidence that the lower IQ negatively impacts their ability to perform activities of daily living. These skills, which are known as adaptive behaviors, represent an individual's level of personal independence and social responsibility. Adaptive behaviors are based on cultural expectations of performance at various ages throughout life. For example, in the United States we generally expect two-year-olds to be very busy, three-year-olds to identify all toys as "mine," five-year-olds to tie their shoes, 16-year-olds to drive a car, 18-year-olds to vote, and 21-year-olds to consume alcohol in a responsible manner.

Most individuals with intellectual disability have difficulty acquiring these skills at the same age as their peers. The American Association of Intellectual and Developmental Disabilities (AAIDD) (2008) identify three areas of adaptive behavior skills that challenge individuals with intellectual disability:

Conceptual skills: self-direction, knowledge of money and its value, orientation to time, number concepts, and language.

Social skills: social pragmatics, social responsibilities, interpersonal skills, following rules, social graces, social problem solving, gullibility, and the ability to avoid being victimized.

Practical skills: occupational skills, safety, use of money, use of a telephone, healthcare management, personal care, and activities of daily living.

For diagnostic purposes, an individual's intellectual functioning and assessed deficits in adaptive behaviors must occur during the developmental period or prior to 18 years of age. The purpose of establishing a diagnosis of intellectual disability is to determine eligibility for Social Security benefits, Medicaid benefits, home-based waiver services, special education services, support services, and specialized treatment in the correctional justice system (AAIDD, 2008).

Intellectual disability often occurs in tandem with or as a secondary symptom of other diagnoses. For example, ID is prevalent in 50% of the cases of autism (Accardo & Whitman, 2002), 50% of those with cerebral palsy (Batshaw, Pellegrino, & Roizen, 2007), and nearly all individuals with Down syndrome (Jacobson, Mulick, & Rojahn, 2007). Listed below are some of the diagnoses that are commonly associated with intellectual disability.

Angelman syndrome: Severe intellectual disability; speech and language impairments; noted ataxia causing issues with balance, coordination, and gait; behavioral uniqueness including frequent laughter, happy demeanor, short attention span, and hand "flapping"; microcephaly; seizure disorders; feeding problems; and sleep disturbances (Accardo & Whitman, 2002).

Autism spectrum disorder: Moderate intellectual disability in 75% of those diagnosed with autism, significant deficits noted in social and emotional reciprocity, impaired communication skills, preoccupations with preferred objects, narrow interests, routines, and rituals (Jacobson et al., 2007).

Cerebral palsy: Neuromuscular impairment causing motor planning deficits, 50% of those with cerebral palsy have moderate to profound intellectual disability (Batshaw et al., 2007).

Cornelia de Lange syndrome: Varying degrees of cognitive functioning — from mild to severe intellectual disability, delayed skeletal maturation, craniofacial anomalies, microcephaly, webbing of hands and feet, hearing impairments, cardiac complications, deficits in the upper extremities (Accardo & Whitman, 2002; Cornelia de Lange Syndrome, 2006).

Cri-du-chat syndrome: Severe to profound intellectual disability, microcephaly, facial anomalies (Accardo & Whitman, 2002).

Dandy Walker syndrome: Cognitive impairment, confused thought, challenged memory, hydrocephalus, delayed developmental milestones, gait anomalies, coordination deficits (Elquist & Demchak, 2005).

Down syndrome: Mild to profound intellectual disability; low muscle tone; small stature; facial anomalies; cardiac issues; seizure activity; orthopedic impairments, including hyperflexible joints, hip and knee subluxation, atlantoaxial subluxation, scoliosis, and flat footedness; osteoporosis; hypothyroidism; sleep apnea; eczema (Batshaw et al., 2007).

Fetal alcohol syndrome: Mild intellectual disability or learning disability, poor social skills, behavioral issues, cranio-facial anomalies, microcephaly, epilepsy (Nolen-Hoeksema, 2007).

Fragile X syndrome: Intellectual disability (females are likely to experience mild cognitive impairment whereas males experience moderate to severe cognitive impairment), long narrow face, prominent and protruding ears, hypotonicity, hyperextensible joints, short stature, stereotypic behaviors, seven percent diagnosed with autism (Jacobson et al., 2007).

Hurler syndrome: Severe intellectual disability, short stature, cardiac issues, visual disturbances, deafness, increased body hair, kyphosis, hip dislocation, compromised range of motion in extremities (Accardo & Whitman, 2002).

Hydrocephalus: Intellectual disability, compromised flow of cerebrospinal fluid, tethering of the spinal cord to the vertebral column, occurs in conjunction with spina bifida cystica (Accardo & Whitman, 2007).

Prader-Willi syndrome: Mild intellectual disability, insatiable appetite, issues with pica (consumption of non-edibles), obesity, hypotonicity, osteoporosis, scoliosis, smaller hands and feet, short stature (Jacobson et al., 2007).

Shaken baby syndrome: Varying levels of cognitive and physical disability based upon residual deficits caused by subdural and retinal hemorrhaging (Accardo & Whitman, 2002; National Center for Shaken Baby Syndrome, n.d.).

Turner syndrome: Learning disability; only females affected; short stature (4' 7"); webbed neck;

heart, kidney, and thyroid complications; visual organization problems; diabetes; high blood pressure; infertility (Boyse, 2010).

Williams syndrome: Mild intellectual disability, attention deficit or learning disability, unique and common facial anomalies, cardiac complications, decreased muscle tone, joint laxity, hypersensitivity to sounds, low birth weight, overly social (Batshaw et al., 2007).

Incidence/Prevalence in U.S.

About 2.5% of the population have IQ scores below 70, which is the cutoff to consider a diagnosis of ID. More than half of these people have sufficient skills to perform activities of daily living. When this is taken into account, estimates are that one percent of the population of the U.S. meets the criteria for intellectual disability (Reynolds & Dombeck, 2006; APA, 2013). ID is more prevalent in males than females (1.5:1.0) (APA. 2000).

Predominant Age

Some syndromes associated with ID are recognized at birth. The majority of children with ID, especially those with mild cognitive loss, are not identified until preschool age (Sulkes, 2006).

Causes

There are many different causes of ID that are generally classified by the time and type of insult. The Arc (2009) lists five general categories of causes of intellectual disability:

Genetic conditions: Abnormalities of genetic material that are inherited from the individual's parents: chromosome abnormalities, errors in the combining or grouping of genes, damage to genetic material during pregnancy because of overexposure to X-rays or other factors.

Problems during pregnancy: The use of drugs or alcohol by the expectant mother during pregnancy, malnutrition, and illnesses in the mother during pregnancy, including rubella, syphilis, toxoplasmosis, and AIDS.

Problems at birth: Problems during delivery that cause oxygen deprivation or birth injuries, such as meconium aspiration or intracranial hemorrhage, low birth weight, prematurity.

Problems after birth: Lead or mercury poisoning, near drowning causing oxygen deprivation, head injuries, cerebrovascular accidents in children, shaken baby syndrome causing brain damage, diseases such as meningitis and encephalitis.

Poverty and cultural deprivation: Growing up in extreme poverty places a child at greater risk for malnutrition and disease, as well as exposure to environmental hazards that can lead to intellectual disability. Children in impoverished conditions often lack exposure to healthy, stimulating environments required for proper neurological development.

Systems Affected

Intellectual disability affects the nervous system, although it is common for the individual to have numerous systems affected because of the frequency of secondary problems. The individual with intellectual disability may experience physical anomalies such as delays in motor development, motor planning deficits, balance deficits, hypo- or hypertonicity, as well as issues with obesity. Seizure activity and visual and hearing losses may be present based on the type of syndrome associated with the ID. In addition, some syndromes have characteristic cardiac issues including aortic regurgitation or mitral valve prolapse.

Secondary Problems

Alzheimer's disease: As compared to individuals without disability, individuals with ID have a greater likelihood to acquire Alzheimer's disease (AD) as they age. This is particularly apparent in those with Down syndrome (DS), where it is predicted that nearly all of those with DS will experience the behavioral symptoms and cognitive decline associated with AD (Barr, 1990). The symptoms of AD in persons with ID emerge at a younger age (mid-40s) and progress more rapidly (5-10 years) than those without disability (Prasher, 1995). Behavioral symptoms of this condition differ somewhat from those without disability as evidenced through changes in personality, stereotypic behaviors, verbal and physical aggression, loss of speech, decline in self-care skills, and seizure activity where none were previously present.

Sensory processing deficits: These deficits are noted among many individuals with ID. Sensory processing deficits occur most often in people with severe cognitive loss and involve the inability to make sense of vestibular, proprioceptive, or tactile input. Sensory deficits are evidenced by attention problems, hyperactivity, stereotypic behaviors, self-stimulation, self-injurious behavior (SIB), emotional explosions, avoidance of touch or movement, disregard for others, and an inability to interact with others (Dykens, 2000; WHO, 1996).

Seizure activity: It is estimated that seizure activity occurs in 25% of individuals with ID, 25% of those with autism, 14% of the individuals with Down syndrome, and 13% of those with cerebral palsy (North Pacific Epilepsy Research, 2010). Individuals may experience either grand mal or petite mal seizures.

Physical disability and neuromuscular impairments: Tone anomalies include ataxia, spasticity, athetosis, and rigidity. Motor planning deficits can greatly compromise the individual's functioning in leisure, self-care, and activities of daily living. These disabilities and impairments are common in people with ID (WHO, 1996).

Mental illness: Many individuals with ID have compromised coping skills and have exacerbated family stressors. Reduced self-esteem is common and may lead to bullying and abuse (Perkins, 2007). The rate of mental illness in individuals with ID is many times higher than in normal population (Emerson, 2003). Estimates show that up to two thirds of individuals with ID also qualify for a mental illness diagnosis (Sadock & Sadock, 2003). The types of mental illness include psychosis, depression, and eating disorders (Dykens, 2004; Kerr et al., 2003; WHO, 1996). Symptoms include mood instability, irritability, aggression, and loss of previously learned skills (Dykens, 2000; Perkins, 2007; WHO, 1996).

Criminal behavior: It is estimated that four to ten percent of the prison population have an ID (Davis, 2005). The types of criminal offenses range from minor crimes to thefts, physical assaults, and sexual misconduct.

Prognosis

Mild intellectual disability: Prognosis varies depending on the level of ID and associated handicapping conditions. Individuals with mild intellectual disability should be able to live in the community with supervision for finances, home maintenance, and vocational assistance. Social and language barriers are the primary areas of deficit for the person with mild cognitive impairment (Katz & Lazcano-Ponce, 2007). Their ability to engage in independent leisure skills will be based on past knowledge, availability of leisure partners, and exposure to various recreational activities throughout their lifespan.

Moderate intellectual disability: Individuals with moderate intellectual disability function well in adult foster care or assisted living facilities. They require supervision in home-maintenance, activities of daily living (ADLs), personal safety, vocational pursuits, and economic self-sufficiency (Katz & Lazcano-Ponce, 2007). They require support for community-based leisure participation including set-up, planning, organization, structure, and supervision.

Severe intellectual disability: Individuals with severe intellectual disability function best in adult foster care or other residential settings that provide significant daily support. It is common for persons with severe intellectual disability to experience deficits in physical development, speech and language, ADLs, and play behavior. They may exhibit self-stimulatory or self-injurious behaviors (Katz & Lazcano-Ponce, 2007). They will require significantly greater supervision than those with moderate cognitive impairment; often requiring both verbal and physical assistance to perform simple recreation and leisure activities.

Profound intellectual disability: Individuals with profound intellectual disability function best in adult foster care or residential settings that provide daily and on-going support. Individuals with this level of intellectual disability often have significant medical complications and require nursing or attendant care services 24 hours a day (Katz & Lazcano-Ponce, 2007). They will require significant physical and verbal assistance to follow one-step tasks, attend to tasks, respond to others, manipulate objects with purpose, and respond to environmental stimuli.

The prognosis for all individuals with cognitive impairment is best anticipated by evaluating their functional ability rather than their measured IQ. Due to medical advances and training opportunities, the majority of people with ID live longer than they used to and appear to have greater quality of life (Patja et al., 2001). Individuals with mild ID have similar life expectancy to individuals without disability. Conversely, those with Down syndrome, profound ID, and epilepsy have decreased life expectancy (Patja et al., 2001).

Assessment

Typical Scope of Team Assessment

Team members use a multifaceted approach to determine the needs, interests, and abilities of persons with intellectual disability. Members will assess intellectual functioning, adaptive behavior skills, physical functioning, emotional and behavioral issues, as well as vocational, educational, and leisure pursuits. This information is combined with consumer interests to assure that life planning is consistent with the wishes and aspirations of the individual served. Initial assessments are utilized to determine individual eligibility for support services. Later assessments are to assure that services match the individual's abilities as well as expressed wishes.

The AAIDD (2008) suggest the following process when determining necessary support for the person with intellectual disability:

- Evaluate limitations in cognitive and adaptive behavior functioning.
- Consider differences in culture and linguistics.
- Consider differences in communication, motor, sensory, and behavioral skills.
- Identify individual strengths that coexist with the limitations.
- Develop an individual plan to improve functioning of the person with intellectual disability.

Because there are so many possible issues associated with ID, it is difficult to rule out the need to use any of the ICF codes. ICF codes specifically related to the intellectual part of the diagnosis include most of b1 Mental Functions. Almost all of the ICF codes in Activities and Participation are affected by ID.

Support services are identified to improve individual functioning (b1 Mental Functions), foster self-determination (d230 Carrying Out Daily Routine, d250 Managing One's Own Behavior, d5 Self-Care, d6 Domestic Life), and enhance quality of life (d7 Interpersonal Interactions and Relationships, d8 Major Life Areas, and d9 Community, Social, and Civic Life) for the person with ID. Supports should promote inclusion and lead to improvements in education and training, community living, employment, health, behavior, social skills, and self-determination (e3 Support and Relationships).

Areas of Concern for RT Assessment

Lack of diversity in leisure interests (d920 Recreation and Leisure): The majority of individuals with intellectual disability engage in passive and solitary leisure activities (Buttimer & Tierney, 2005). In addition, when individuals with ID engage in activities with others, their partners are typically family members or the members of their support staff (d710 Basic Interpersonal Interactions, d720 Complex Interpersonal Interactions, d750 Informal Social Relationships) (Abells, Burbidge, & Minnes, 2008). Hoge and Dattilo (1995) found that individuals with intellectual disability participated in passive activities of which 50% were home-based and 50% were community-based. Based on past recreational participation patterns, individuals with ID most frequently engage in television viewing, listening to music, dining out, talking on the phone, working on crafts, going for walks, going for a ride in a car, and shopping (Abells, Burbidge, & Minnes, 2008; Buttimer & Tierney, 2005; Hoge & Dattilo, 1995; Malik, 1990; Sparrow & Mayne, 1990). Barriers to leisure participation include lack of transportation, finances, recreational skill, personal attitudes, the disability itself, lack of partners, and a lack of empowerment or control over leisure time (d230 Carrying Out Daily Routine, d250 Managing One's Own Behavior, e3 Support and Relationships) (Abells, Burbidge, & Minnes, 2008; Germ & Schleien, 1997; Schleien, Germ, & McAvoy, 1996). The recreational therapist may wish to assist in broadening the individual's leisure interests through community-based exposure, barrier negotiation (especially related to leisure partners and fostering friendships), activity skill development, and empowerment to assure individual choice and decision-making through leisure.

Specific leisure skill deficits (choose appropriate Body Function or Activities & Participation ICF codes): Individuals with ID lack specific recreational skills to engage in a wide variety of leisure pursuits. The impact of these skill deficits can lead to sedentary lifestyle, increased secondary illness, boredom, obesity, and social or emotional issues that will negatively impact quality of life as well as health and wellness throughout the lifespan. Schleien (1991) suggests that recreational therapists work on skill development in two areas: increased skills related to interacting with people (e.g., d710 Basic

Interpersonal Interactions, b122 Global Psychosocial Functions) and increased skills related to using and interacting with objects (e.g., b117 Intellectual Functions, b156 Perceptual Functions, d131 Learning Through Actions with Objects). Some clients may take years to learn a few basic leisure skills. The recreational therapist may want to work on one new skill every three to six months, gradually increasing the client's skill level.

Functional skill deficits: Deficits in functional skills will be revealed as the recreational therapist assesses physical, social, emotional, and cognitive behaviors.

- *Physical deficits* often noted when assessing an individual with ID range from deficits in range of motion (b710 Mobility of Joint Functions), strength (b730 Muscle Power Functions), coordination (b760 Control of Voluntary Movement Functions), balance (b755 Involuntary Movement Reaction Functions, d410 Changing Basic Body Position, d415 Maintaining a Body Position), flexibility (e.g., b710 Mobility of Joint Functions), posture (d415 Maintaining a Body Position), endurance (b740 Muscle Endurance Functions, b455 Exercise Tolerance Functions) and weight management (b530 Weight Maintenance Functions, d570 Looking After One's Health) (Hall & Thomas, 2008; Koritsas & Iacono, 2011; Rimmer et al., 2004).

- *Cognitive deficits* are apparent based on the individual's level of intellectual functioning. Those with severe and profound intellectual disability may exhibit deficits in the ability to respond to environmental stimuli (b270 Sensory Functions Related to Temperature and Other Stimuli, b156 Perceptual Functions), manipulate objects (d4402 Manipulating, b1143 Orientation to Objects, d131 Learning Through Actions with Objects), attend to task (b140 Attention Functions, d160 Focusing Attention, d161 Directing Attention), and follow directions (d210 Undertaking a Single Task). Individuals with moderate and mild intellectual disability may exhibit deficits in the ability to organize and plan activities, problem solve, strategize, analyze, and set personal goals or lack executive functioning skills (b164 Higher-Level Cognitive Functions, b1 Mental Functions, d220 Undertaking Multiple Tasks) (Lee et al., 2001).

ADL skill deficits (Choose appropriate Activities & Participation ICF codes, especially d5 Self-Care and d6 Domestic Life): Deficits in skills associated with activities of daily living may be revealed through assessment of the individual's performance as they engage in various community-based recreational activities. These ADL skills are essential to maximize the individual's level of independence in various community-based activities. For example, the individual with moderate intellectual disability may attend a bowling program and demonstrate deficits in the ability to don and doff shoes, identify shoe size, exchange money, use a vending machine, or properly interact with a sales clerk.

Impaired social skills: It is common for individuals with intellectual disabilities to have impaired social skills. Individuals with mild cognitive impairment often have deficits with social pragmatics and advanced social skills, such as proper social graces, expressing feelings, using self-control, and dealing with teasing (d710 Basic Interpersonal Interactions, d720 Complex Interpersonal Interactions, b130 Energy and Drive Functions). Individuals with moderate cognitive impairment often have deficits in social pragmatics and beginning social skills, such as listening, having a conversation, and making introductions (d710 Basic Interpersonal Interactions). People with severe or profound intellectual disability display deficits in prerequisite social behaviors that include the ability to make eye contact, respond to their name (d710 Basic Interpersonal Interactions), and smile socially (d7104 Social Cues in Relationships). The recreational therapist can address social behaviors informally through on-going support of proper social behavior and formally through activity-based interventions or courses that offer training in proper social exchanges.

Age-inappropriate leisure interests: Persons with ID may express an interest in leisure activities (d920 Recreation and Leisure) that are age-inappropriate. (Activities are generally geared toward individuals that are much younger.) This mismatch between age and activity may be attributed to the individual's delayed intellectual level and commercial activity resources that are designed for children. Part of the recreational therapist's challenge is to adapt these activities to match the intellectual and chronological age of the consumer.

Impaired community integration skills: One of the primary barriers to leisure activities for individuals with ID is a lack of skills related to using resources in the community (d9 Community, Social, and Civic Life). These skills may include knowledge of community-based recreational resources, recreational skills necessary to participate, use of community transportation to access recreational resources (d470 Using Transportation), identification of leisure partners who may be interested in the same activity, and self-initiation of the community experience (b126 Temperament and Personality Functions, b130 Energy and Drive Functions). Through a guided leisure education program, the recreational therapist can assist the individual in skill development and problem solving that will allow community integration.

ICF Core Set

No ICF Core Set for Intellectual Disabilities has been published.

Treatment Direction

Whole Team Approach

When working with persons with ID, the team approach differs significantly from the traditional medical approach to service delivery. Since a person with ID has diagnostic features that will remain throughout a lifetime, it is important that the team develop a plan of service that is based on the consumer's expressed wishes, maximizing their level of independence, and empowering them to make educated decisions toward life planning. For this reason the team follows a person-centered planning (PCP) approach to service delivery (Everson & Zhang, 2000). This approach assures that the individual with ID is a primary decision-maker in his/her life planning process. The individual is empowered to direct the plan with the support of a professional coordinator. Professional members of the team are invited by the consumer to become members of the PCP team to assist the consumer in achieving his/her goals and objectives. To that end, the team may include an occupational therapist, physical therapist, vocational specialist, special education or transition teacher, recreational therapist, nutritionist, and a support coordinator from a local community health agency.

Recreational Therapy Approach

The types of services provided depend on the individual's strengths, needs, interests, and age. Possible types of services are identified below.

Mild and moderate intellectual disability: Individuals with mild to moderate cognitive impairment benefit from training opportunities to develop self-determining behaviors and decision-making skills. Critical to independence is the individual's ability to make personal choices and preferences based on educated decision-making. Recreational activity is a perfect venue to encourage individuals to make these personal choices, communicate preferences, and set personal goals (Dattilo, Kleiber, & William, 1998). In fact, it has been demonstrated that the more time spent in recreational activity, the higher the level of individual self-determining behaviors (McGuire & McDonnell, 2008). ICF codes include b126 Temperament and Personality Functions, b130 Energy and Drive Functions, d250 Managing One's Own Behavior, and d710 Basic Interpersonal Interactions.

Individuals with mild to moderate ID also benefit from training to enhance social skills. Such training may include appropriate social interactions and conversational skills (Blacher & Howell, 2008); social knowledge or pragmatic skills (Cory, Dattilo, & Williams, 2006; Dattilo, Williams, & Cory, 2003); establishing friendships (Solish, Perry, & Minnes, 2010); social capital, contributions to others, or valued social roles (Devine & Parr, 2008; Patterson & Pegg, 2009); as well as improved self-concept and self-esteem (Duvdevany, 2002). ICF codes include d710 Basic Interpersonal Interactions and d720 Complex Interpersonal Interactions.

To maximize levels of independence in the community, individuals with mild to moderate ID benefit from leisure education training which focuses on skill development, knowledge and access to community resources, family involvement, and the development of friendships or peer relationships (Hoge, Dattilo, & Williams, 1990). Personal choice and preferences should direct the leisure activities introduced but the activities should also include a repertoire of physical, mental, and social activities. In addition, activities should range from passive to active with the goal of developing home-based and community-based leisure skills. Individuals with ID prefer activity pursuits similar to those preferred by persons without disability. Such activity preferences include dining out, listening to music, watching television, playing video games, exercising, shopping, and playing sports (Glausier, Whorton, & Morgan, 1996). Best practice strategies for inclusion are the use of leisure coaches (Hoge, Dattilo, & Williams, 1999), buddy programs (Sable & Gravink, 1995), and inclusion into generic programs (Wachter & McGowan, 2002). ICF codes include d750 Informal Social Relationships, d760 Family Relationships, d770 Intimate Relationships, d910 Community Life, and d920 Recreation and Leisure.

When compared to individuals without disabilities, those with ID display lower levels of physical fitness, including reduced muscular strength, flexibility, coordination, cardiovascular endurance, and higher levels of body fat (Graham & Reid, 2000). Recreational therapy can reduce the likelihood of such health-related issues by providing training in fitness, sports, and other leisure activities to promote health and wellness. Exercise and weight training programs are found to have a positive effect on weight management, blood pressure levels, resting heart rates (Carter, 2002; Carter et al., 2004), and upper extremity muscular endurance (Shields, Taylor, & Dodd, 2008). Membership and training to use community-based fitness clubs, recreation centers, indoor climbing facilities, YMCAs and YWCAs, horseback riding clubs, as well as Special Olympic programs are encouraged to promote increased participation in recreational activity, which ultimately promotes health and wellness throughout life (Elliott, Funderburk, & Holland, 2008; Hughes & McDonald, 2009). ICF codes include b455 Exercise Tolerance Functions, b730 Muscle Power Functions, b735 Muscle Tone Functions, b740 Muscle Endurance Functions, and d920 Recreation and Leisure.

While teaching leisure skills and promoting social and physical wellness, the recreational therapist has opportunities to provide support training in various activities of daily living. These ADLs may include meal preparation, money management, phone use, mapping and community orientation, personal safety skills (Rider & Scharfenberg, 1999), and work-retirement transition planning (Hodges, Luken, & Hubbard, 2004). ICF codes include d5 Self-Care and d6 Domestic Life.

Severe and profound intellectual disability: Individuals with more severe ID benefit from recreational therapy services that promote physical growth and development, enhance cognitive and social skills, and develop leisure-activity skills through the support of staff or caregivers. ICF codes include aspects of b1 Mental Functions and d1 Learning and Applying Knowledge.

Facilitating inclusion for those with severe ID typically requires either additional staff support (Wachter & McGowan, 2002) or reverse mainstreaming (Zoerink & Rosegard, 1997). Reverse mainstreaming occurs when agencies that typically provide services to individuals with disabilities open their programs to individuals without disabilities. Increased staff support is considered essential to provide training to individuals with severe cognitive impairments. Such staffing, under the direction of the recreational therapist, provides systematic step-by-step instruction, physical assistance and prompting, assistance in the use of adaptive equipment, and assistance facilitating interactions with others (Miller, Schleien, & Bowens, 2010; Wall & Gast, 1997). The improved environment can be coded with support code e355 Health Professionals.

Individuals with severe ID engage primarily in passive leisure activities such as watching television, modified crafts (Specht et al., 2002), listening to music, and going for car rides (Mactavish & Schleien, 2000). The use of virtual reality technology, adaptive switching devices, and other technological aids allows individuals with severe ID to expand leisure options (Yalon-Chamovitz & Weiss, 2008), become an active participant, and even gain greater control over their environment. ICF code d920 Recreation and Leisure.

Individuals with severe to profound cognitive loss often have difficulty processing sensory input (WHO, 1996). Attention problems, difficulty maintaining a relaxed state, avoidance of touch, aggression, self-injury, and stereotypic behaviors may represent a sensory processing problem. For this reason the recreational therapist uses sensory stimulation techniques to facilitate calm or alerting responses (Buettner & Lesovoy, 2009; Potter & Erzen, 2008). Sensory stimulation programs have been found to increase attending and concentration, reduce stereotypic and maladaptive behaviors, and promote relaxation and enjoyment (Patterson, 2004). Document changes with ICF codes in b2 Sensory Functions and Pain.

Recreational Therapy Interventions

Functional Skills

The recreational therapist can address a variety of functional needs while simultaneously teaching recreation and leisure skills. The child with ID, as well as those with severe and profound ID, benefit from activities that address normal physical growth and development patterns. Examples of these functional skills may include head control (b760 Control of Voluntary Movement Functions), upper extremity coordination (b760 Control of Voluntary Movement Functions), sitting balance (d4153 Maintaining a Sitting Position, b755 Involuntary Movement Reaction Functions), and object manipulation (d440 Fine Hand Use, d131 Learning Through Actions with Objects) (Block, Hornbaker, & Klavina, 2006). The person with moderate cognitive impairment would benefit from activities that develop coordination (b760 Control of Voluntary Movement Functions), strength (b730 Muscle Power Functions), and fine motor skills (d440 Fine Hand Use) (Carter, 2002; Carter et al., 2004). The person with mild ID would benefit from social skill training (d710 Basic Interpersonal Interactions) during community integration (d910 Community Life) (Shields, Taylor, & Dodd, 2008).

Since individuals with ID do not acquire knowledge or skills incidentally, social skills should be addressed through recreational activity. Social skills can be formally addressed through role modeling and practice or rehearsal techniques. Social skills addressed may include the ability to engage in appropriate conversation, remain on-topic, include others, take turns, wait in line, share, deal with teasing, and negotiate (Cory, Dattilo, & Williams, 2006; Dattilo, Williams, & Cory, 2003; Siperstein & Rickards, 2004). ICF codes for these skills include d710 Basic Interpersonal Interactions and d720 Complex Interpersonal Interactions.

Cognitive skills may also be addressed to improve the individual's ability to identify objects. In particular, focus should be directed toward knowledge of the equipment used during play (d9200 Play, d880 Engagement in Play), recalling rules (b144 Memory Functions), attending to task (b140 Attention Functions), following directions (d210 Undertaking a Single Task), making decisions (d177 Making Decisions), and problem solving (d175 Solving Problems (Foxx & Bittle, 1989).

Education, Training, and Counseling

Individuals with ID should be empowered to develop leisure skills that are based on their personal interests, wishes, and aspirations. As a member of the PCP team, the recreational therapist may be asked to teach leisure skills that are requested by the consumer. This may include but not be limited to sports, swimming, horseback riding, biking, hobbies and crafts, video games, as well as physical games that promote the development of life-long health and wellness. Document these interventions using d4 Mobility, d880 Engagement in Play, and d920 Recreation and Leisure. Activity and task analysis should be used to separate each skill into tasks for ease of skill development and instruction.

Individuals with ID often lack the skills necessary to initiate leisure activities with others. The recreational therapist should use guided discovery techniques that encourage the individual to explore surroundings and make decisions about what they can do, who they can ask to join in, how they can secure necessary equipment and supplies, and how to identify the best location for the activity (Hoge, Dattilo, & Williams, 1999). Individuals with ID will need prompting and guidance to direct leisure experiences both in their home and in the community (Miller, Schleien, & Bowens, 2010). Document with ICF codes d250 Managing One's Own Behavior, d7 Interpersonal Interactions and Relationships, and d9 Community, Social, and Civic Life

To maximize levels of independence in their homes and communities (including recreational activities) individuals with intellectual disability benefit from training in activities of daily living. Such activities may include meal preparation, baking, and menu planning (d630 Preparing Meals); shopping (d620 Acquisition of Goods and Services); travel (d470 Using Transportation); mobility training (d4 Mobility); money management (d860 Basic Economic Transactions); computer usage (d360 Using Communication Devices and Techniques); and others.

Community Integration

From pedestrian training (d460 Moving Around in Different Locations) to bus and travel training (d470 Using Transportation), the individual with ID should be encouraged to develop the skills necessary to negotiate the community with the greatest possible amount of independence (d910 Community Life) (Cummins & Lau, 2003). Based upon the individual's wishes and aspirations, the recreational therapist should assure that the individual gains knowledge of recreation resources within his/her community (e.g., parks, community centers, movie theaters, bowling alleys), activity rules and equipment, costs associated with activity participation, appropriate clothing and apparel, as well as knowledge of how to access facilities (d5 Self-Care, d620 Acquisition of Goods and Services, d710 Basic Interpersonal Interactions, d920 Recreation and Leisure). For example, if a consumer with mild ID wishes to join a health club, s/he should receive training for bus travel, proper social interactions with club members and employees, use of the locker room, proper apparel, donning and doffing apparel, safety skills when using equipment and moving throughout the facility, use of vending machines, and problem-solving in an emergency.

Health Promotion

Physical exercise and recreation have been found to improve strength (b730 Muscle Power Functions), coordination (b760 Control of Voluntary Movement Functions), and overall health (Carter, 2002; Carter et al., 2004; Shields, Taylor, & Dodd, 2008) in individuals with ID. In addition, such activity is suggested to improve mood (b126 Temperament and Personality Functions), sleep patterns (b134 Sleep Functions), reduce stress (d240 Handling Stress and Other Psychological Demands) (Wilhite, Biren, & Spencer, 2012), and improve nutritional habits (d570 Looking After One's Health) (Kemeny & Arnold, 2012). Furthermore, daily, frequent physical activity is noted to reduce and even eliminate the presence of stereotypic and challenging behaviors in those with severe ID (b125 Dispositions and Intra-Personal Functions) (Cannella-Malone, Tullis, & Kazee, 2011). Finally, opportunities to engage in recreational and community-based activity are considered key components in assuring enhanced quality of life for individuals with ID (d920 Recreation and Leisure) (Duvdevany & Arar, 2004; McIntyre et al., 2011).

However, individuals with ID often lack the motivation (b130 Energy and Drive Functions) or personal body awareness (b180 Experience of Self and Time Functions) for fitness related activities, which aid in promoting wellness throughout the lifespan. For this reason, recreational therapists are encouraged to motivate individuals to take part in Special Olympic programming and other structured opportunities that promote physical activity through both competitive and non-competitive venues (Carter et al., 2004). In addition, persons with ID may enjoy physical activities such as dance, tai chi, yoga, fitness club membership, cross-country skiing, biking, or swimming. The intent of these activities is to foster participation through fun activities that will motivate the individual to develop skills for lifelong cardiovascular wellness and health (d570 Looking After One's Health).

Resources

American Association on Intellectual and Developmental Disabilities (AAIDD)
501 3rd Street, NW Suite 200
Washington, DC 20001
202-387-1968
www.aaidd.org
An advocacy group promoting research, best practices, progressive policies, and universal human rights for people with intellectual and developmental disabilities.

Special Olympics International
Special Olympics Headquarters
202-628-3630 or 800-700-8585
www.specialolympics.org
A non-profit organization supporting recreation and sport participation, training, and competitive opportunities for individuals with intellectual disabilities.

The Arc
1825 K Street W, Suite 1200
Washington, DC 20006
800-433-5255
www.thearc.org
An advocacy and resource group for individuals with intellectual and developmental disabilities and their families.

References

Abells, D., Burbidge, J., & Minnes, P. (2008). Involvement of adolescents with intellectual disabilities in social and recreational activities. *Journal on Developmental Disabilities, 14*(2), 88-94.

Accardo, P. & Whitman, B. (2002). *Dictionary of developmental disabilities terminology* (2nd ed.). Baltimore, MD: Brookes.

American Association of Intellectual and Developmental Disabilities (AAIDD). (2008). FAQ on intellectual disability. Retrieved on October 8, 2010 from http://www.aamr.org/content_104.cfm.

American Medical Association (AMA). (2009). *International classification of diseases* (9th revision). AMA Press.

American Medical Association (AMA). (2013). *International classification of diseases* (9th revision Clinical Modification). AMA Press.

American Psychiatric Association. (2000). *Diagnostic and statistical manual of mental disorders* (IV ed.). Washington, DC: American Psychiatric Press.

American Psychiatric Association. (2013). *Diagnostic and statistical manual of mental disorders* (5th ed.). Arlington, VA: American Psychiatric Publishing.

Autism Society of America. (2008). Characteristics of Autism. Retrieved on October 28, 2010 from http://www.autism-society.org/site/PageServer.

Barr, O. (1990). Down's syndrome and Alzheimer's disease — What is the link, *Professional Nurse, 5*(9), 465-468.

Batshaw, M., Pellegrino, L., & Roizen, N. (2007). *Children with disabilities* (6th ed.). Baltimore: Brookes.

Bigby, C., Fyffe, C., & Ozanne, E. (Eds.). (2007). *Planning and support for people with intellectual disabilities: Issues for case managers and other professionals.* Philadelphia, PA: Jessica Kingsley.

Blacher, J. & Howell, E. (2008). Becoming social: Interventions with youth who have high-functioning autism and Asperger syndrome. *Exceptional Parent, 10,* 56-58.

Block, M., Hornbaker, J., & Klavina, A. (2006). Functional assessment of students with severe disabilities. *Palestra, 22*(4), 25-31.

Boyse, K. (2010). Turner Syndrome. Retrieved on October 28, 2010 from http://www.med.umich.edu/yourchild/topics/turners.htm.

Buettner, L. & Lesovoy, A. (2009). Toddlers with autism: A sensory tree house intervention for recreation therapy. *American Journal of Recreation Therapy, 8*(1), 15-18.

Buttimer, J. & Tierney, E. (2005). Patterns of leisure participation among adolescents with mild intellectual disability. *Journal of Intellectual Disabilities, 9*(1), 25-42.

Cannella-Malone, H. Tullis, C., & Kazee, A, (2011). Using antecedent exercise to decrease challenging behavior in boys with developmental disabilities and an emotional disorder. *Journal of Positive Behavior Interventions, 13*(4), 230-239.

Carter, M. (2002). Inclusive fitness strategies: Building wellness among developmentally disabled adults. *Parks and Recreation, 12,* 55-57.

Carter, M., McCown, K., Forest, S., Martin, J., Wacher, R., Gaede, D., & Fernandez, T. (2004). Exercise and fitness for adults with developmental disability: Case report of a group intervention. *Therapeutic Recreation Journal, 38*(1), 72-84.

Carter, M., Van Andel, G., & Robb, G. (2003). *Therapeutic recreation: A practical approach* (3rd ed.). Prospect Heights, IL: Waveland.

Centers for Disease Control and Prevention (CDC). (2005, October 29). Intellectual disability. Retrieved on October 8, 2010 from http://www.cdc.gov/ncbddd/dd/mr3.htm.

Centers for Disease Control and Prevention (CDC). (2010). Fetal alcohol spectrum disorder diagnosis. Retrieved on October 28, 2010 from http://www.cdc.gov/ncbdd/fasd/diagnosis.html.

Cornelia de Lange Syndrome — USA Foundation. (2006). Diagnostic criteria. Retrieved on October 28, 2010 from http://www.cdlsusa.org/.

Cory, L., Dattilo, J., & Williams, R. (2006). Effects of leisure education program on social knowledge and skills of youth with cognitive disabilities. *Therapeutic Recreation Journal, 40*(3), 144-164.

Cummins, R. & Lau, A. (2003). Community integration or community exposure? A review and discussion in relation to people with an intellectual disability. *Journal of Applied Research in Intellectual Disabilities, 16*(2), 145-157.

Dattilo, J., Kleiber, D., & William, R. (1998). Self-determination and enjoyment: A psychologically-based service delivery model for therapeutic recreation. *Therapeutic Recreation Journal, 32*(4), 258-271.

Dattilo, J., Williams, R., & Cory, L. (2003). Effects of computerized leisure education on knowledge of social skills of youth with intellectual disabilities. *Therapeutic Recreation Journal, 37*(2), 142-155.

Davis, L. (2005). People with intellectual disabilities in the criminal justice system: Victims and suspects. Fact Sheet. Retrieved on October 8, 2010 from http://www.thearc.org/document.doc?id=149.

Devine, M. & Parr, M. (2008). Come on in, but not too far: Social capital in an inclusive leisure setting. *Leisure Sciences, 30*(5), 391-408.

Duvdevany, I. (2002). Self-concept and adaptive behavior of people with intellectual disability in integrated and segregated recreation activities. *Journal of Intellectual Disability Research, 46*(5), 419-429.

Duvdevany, I. & Arar, E. (2004). Leisure activities, friendships, & quality of life of persons with intellectual disability: Foster homes vs. community residential settings. *International Journal of Rehabilitation Research, 27*(4), 289-296.

Dykens, E. (2000). Annotation: Psychopathology in children with intellectual disability. *Journal of Child Psychology and Psychiatry, 41*(4), 407-417.

Dykens, E. (2004). Maladaptive and compulsive behavior in Prader-Willi syndrome: New insights from older adults. *American Journal on Mental Retardation, 109*(2), 142-153.

Elliott, S., Funderburk, J., & Holland, J. (2008). The impact of the "stirrup some fun" therapeutic horseback riding program: A qualitative investigation. *American Journal of Recreation Therapy, 7*(2), 19-28.

Elquist, M. & Demchak, M. (2005). Dandy Walker syndrome fact sheet. Retrieved on October 28, 2010 from http://www.cde.state.co.us/cdesped/download/pdf/blv-DandyWalkerSyndrome.pdf.

Emerson, E. (2003). Prevalence of psychiatric disorders in children and adolescents with and without intellectual disability. *Journal of Intellectual Disability Research, 47*(1), 51-58.

Everson, J. & Zhang, D. (2000). Person-centered planning: Characteristics, inhibitors, and supports. *Education and Training in Mental Retardation and Developmental Disabilities, 35*(1), 36-43.

Foose, A. & Ardovino, P. (2008). Therapeutic recreation and developmental disabilities. In T. Robertson & T. Long. (Eds.). *Foundations in therapeutic recreation: Perceptions, philosophies, and practices for the 21st Century* (pp. 127-144). Champaign, IL: Human Kinetics.

Foxx, R. & Bittle, R. (1989). *Thinking it through: Teaching a problem-solving strategy for community living: Curriculum for individuals with developmental disabilities.* Champaign, IL: Research Press.

Germ, P. & Schleien, S. (1997). Inclusive community leisure services: Responsibilities of key players. *Therapeutic Recreation Journal, 31*(1), 22-37.

Glausier, S., Whorton, J., & Morgan, R. (1996). *A recreation and leisure inventory: Development and application.* U.S. Department of Education, Office of Education Research and

Improvement. (ERIC document reproduction service no. ED 394 763).

Graham, A. & Reid, G. (2000). Physical fitness of adults with and without intellectual disability: A 13-year follow-up study. *Research Quarterly for Exercise and Sport, 71*(2), 152-158.

Hall, J. & Thomas, J. (2008). Promoting physical activity and exercise in older adults with developmental disabilities. *Topics in Geriatric Rehabilitation, 24*(1), 64-73.

Hodges, J., Luken, K., & Hubbard, R. (2004). Supporting the transition of one man with autism from work to retirement. *Therapeutic Recreation Journal, 38*(3), 301-311.

Hoge, G. & Dattilo, J. (1995). Recreation patterns of adults with and without mental retardation. *Education and Training in Mental Retardation and Developmental Disabilities, 30*(4), 283-98.

Hoge, G., Dattilo, J., & Williams, R. (1999). Effects of leisure education on perceived freedom in leisure of adolescents with mental retardation. *Therapeutic Recreation Journal, 33*(4), 320-332.

Hughes, C. & McDonald, M. (2008). The Special Olympics: Sporting or social event? *Research & Practice for Persons with Severe Disabilities, 33*(3), 143-145.

Jacobson, J. W., Mulick, J. A., & Rojahn, J. (2007). *Handbook of intellectual and developmental disabilities.* New York, NY: Springer.

Katz, G. & Lazcano-Ponce, E. (2007). Intellectual disability: Definition, etiological factors, classification, diagnosis, treatment and prognosis. *SaludPublicaMex, 50*(2), 132-141.

Kemeny, E. & Arnhold, R. (2012). "I can do it, you can do it" Collaborative practices for enhancing physical activity. *Therapeutic Recreation Journal, 46*(4), 268-283.

Kerr, A., McCulloch, D., Oliver, K., McLean, B., Coleman, E., Law, T., Beaton, P., Wallace, S., Newell, E., Eccles, T., Prescott, R. (2003). Medical needs of people with intellectual disability require regular reassessment, and the provision of client- and carer-held reports. *Journal of Intellectual Disability Research, 47*(2), 134-145.

King, G., Law, M., King, S., Rosenbaum, P., Kertoy, M., & Young, N. (2003). A conceptual model of the factors affecting the recreation and leisure participation of children with disabilities. *Physical and Occupation Therapy in Pediatrics, 23*(1), 63-89.

Koritsas, S. & Iacono, T. (2011). Secondary conditions in people with developmental disabilities. *American Journal on Intellectual and Developmental Disabilities, 116*(1), 36-47.

Lee, N., Fidler, D., Blakeley-Smith, A., Daunhauer, L., Robinson, C., & Hepburn, S. (2011). Caregiver report of executive functioning in a population-based sample of young children with Down syndrome. *American Journal on Intellectual and Developmental Disabilities, 116*(4), 290-304.

Mactavish, J. & Schleien, S. (2000). Exploring family recreation activities in families that include children with developmental disabilities. *Therapeutic Recreation Journal, 34*(2), 132-153.

Malik, P. (1990). Leisure interests and perceptions of group home residents. *Annual in Therapeutic Recreation, 1*, 67-73.

McGuire, J. & McDonnell, J. (2008). Relationships between recreation and levels of self-determination for adolescents and young adults with disabilities. *Career Development for Exceptional Individuals, 31*(3), 154-163.

McIntyre, L., Kraemer, B., Blacher, J., & Simmerman, S. (2011). Quality of life for young adults with severe intellectual disability: Mothers' thoughts and reflections. *Journal of Intellectual & Developmental Disability, 29*(2), 131-146.

Miller, K., Schleien, S., & Bowens, F. (2010). Support staff as an essential component of inclusive recreation services. *Therapeutic Recreation Journal, 44*(1), 35-49.

Mobily, K. & MacNeil, R. (2002). *Therapeutic recreation and the nature of disabilities.* State College, PA: Venture Publishing, Inc.

National Association for Down Syndrome. (2010). Facts about Down syndrome. Retrieved on October 28, 2010 from http://www.nads.org/pages_new/facts.html.

National Center for Shaken Baby Syndrome. (n.d.). All about SBS/AHT. Retrieved on October 28, 2010 from http://dontshake.org/sbs.php?topNavID=3 & subNavID=317.

Nolen-Hoeksema, S. (2007). *Abnormal psychology* (4th ed.). New York, NY: McGraw-Hill.

North Pacific Epilepsy Research. (2010). Epilepsy facts and figures. Retrieved on November 2, 2010 from https://www.seizures.com/articles-information/epilepsy/epilepsy-facts-figures/.

Patja, K., Livananinen, M., Vesala, H., Oksanen, H., & Puoppila, L. (2001). Life expectancy of people with intellectual disability: A 35-year follow-up study. *Journal of Intellectual Disability Research, 44*(5), 591-599.

Patterson, I. (2004). Snoezelen as a casual leisure activity for people with developmental disability. *Therapeutic Recreation Journal, 38*(3), 289-300.

Patterson, I. & Pegg, S. (2009). Serious leisure and people with intellectual disabilities: Benefits and opportunities. *Leisure Studies, 28*(4), 387-402.

Perkins, C. (2007). Mental illness in people with intellectual disability, *New Zealand Family Physician, 34*(5), 358-362.

Potter, C. & Erzen, C. (2008). A multisensory aquatic environment for individuals with intellectual/developmental disabilities. *Exceptional Parent, 10*, 68-69.

Prasher, V. (1995). Age specific prevalence, thyroid dysfunction and depressive symptomatology in adults with Down syndrome and dementia. *International Journal of Geriatric Psychiatry, 10*, 25-31.

Reid, D., Everson, J., & Green, C. (1999). A systematic evaluation of preferences identified through person-centered planning for people with profound multiple disabilities. *Journal of Applied Behavioral Analysis, 32*(4), 467-477.

Reynolds, T. & Dombeck, M. (2006). Mental retardation (intellectual disabilities). Retrieved on September 24, 2010 from http://www.mentalhelp.net/poc/view_doc.php?type=doc & id=10346 & cn=208.

Rider, B. & Scharfenberg, C. (1999). *The book of activity cards: For DD adults.* Kansas City, KS: Rider.

Rimmer, J., Heller, T., Wang, E., & Valerio, I. (2004). Improvements in physical fitness in adults with Down syndrome. *American Journal on Mental Retardation, 109*(2), 165-174.

Sable, J. & Gravink, J. (1995). Partners: Promoting accessible recreation. *Parks and Recreation, 30*(5), 34-40.

Sadock, B. & Sadock, V. (2003). *Synopsis of psychiatry* (9th ed.). Philadelphia, PA: Lippincott Williams & Wilkins.

Schleien, S. (1991). Severe multiple disabilities. In D. Austin & M. Crawford (Eds.). *Therapeutic recreation: An introduction.* (pp. 189-223). Englewood Cliffs, NJ: Prentice Hall.

Schleien, S., Germ, P., & McAvoy, L. (1996). Inclusive community leisure services: Recommended professional practices and barriers encountered. *Therapeutic Recreation Journal, 30*(4), 260-273.

Shields, N., Taylor, N., & Dodd, K. (2008). Effects of community-based progressive resistance training program on muscle performance and physical function in adults with Down syndrome: A randomized controlled trial. *Arch Phys Med Rehabil, 89*, 1215-1220.

Silka, V. & Hauser, M. (1997). Psychiatric assessment of the person with mental retardation. *Psychiatric Annals, 27*(3), 162-169.

Siperstein, G. & Rickards, E. (2004). *Promoting social skills.* Baltimore, MD: Brookes.

Solish, A., Perry, A., & Minnes, P. (2009). Participation of children with and without disabilities in social, recreational, and leisure activities. *Journal of Applied Research in Intellectual Disabilities, 23*, 226-236.

Sparrow, W. & Mayne, S. (1990). Recreation patterns of adults with intellectual disabilities. *Therapeutic Recreation Journal, 24*(3), 45-49.

Specht, J., King, G., Brown, E., & Foris, C. (2002). The importance of leisure in the lives of persons with congenital physical disabilities. *American Journal of Occupational Therapy, 56*, 436-445.

Sulkes, S. (2006). Mental retardation/intellectual disability. Retrieved on October 8, 2010 from http://www.merck.com/mmhe/sec23/ch285/ch285a.html.

The Arc of the United States. (2009). Causes and prevention of intellectual disabilities. Retrieved on October 24, 2010 from http://www.thearc.org/page.aspx?pid=2453.

Wachter, C. & McGowan, A. (2002). Inclusive practices of special recreation agencies in Illinois. *Therapeutic Recreation Journal, 36*(2), 172-185.

Wall, M. & Gast, D. (1997). Caregivers' use of constant time delay to teach leisure skills to adolescents or young adults with moderate or severe intellectual disabilities. *Education and Training in Mental Retardation and Developmental Disabilities, 32*(4), 340-356.

Wilhite, B., Biren, G., & Spencer, L. (2012). Fitness intervention for adults with developmental disabilities and their caregivers. *Therapeutic Recreation Journal, 46*(4), 245-267.

World Health Organization. (1996). *ICD-10: Guide for mental retardation.* Division of Mental Health & Prevention of Substance Abuse. WHO. Geneva.

World Health Organization. (2007). *International statistical classification of diseases and related health problems* (10th revision). German Institute of Medical Documentation and Information. WHO/DIMDI. German Institute of Medical Documentation.

Yalon-Chamovitz, S. & Weiss, P. (2008). Virtual reality as a leisure activity for young adults with physical and intellectual disabilities. *Research in Developmental Disabilities, 29*, 273-287.

Zoerink, D. & Rosegard, E. (1997). Social justice through inclusive leisure services. In D. Compton (Ed.), *Issues in therapeutic recreation: Toward a new millennium* (2nd ed.), 17-38. Champaign, IL: Sagamore.

21. Major Depressive Disorder

Stephen T. Lewis

According to the American Psychiatric Association (APA), major depressive disorder (MDD) is an Axis I disorder. It may manifest with somewhat diverse symptomatology and occur as a single episode (*DSM-5* codes 296.20-296.26) or as a recurrent condition (*DSM-5* codes 296.30-296.36) and range in intensity from mild to severe (APA, 2013). MDD is a pervasive disorder, and even when the onset is triggered by situational factors, the person with MDD displays symptoms that are more severe than would be expected by such triggers. Because of the excessive response, MDD can be differentiated from mild sadness or a brief response to external stressors (Belmaker & Agam, 2008). MDD lasts at least two weeks while manifesting at least five of the following symptoms that significantly impair functioning:

- Depressed mood most of the day, nearly every day
- Diminished interest or pleasure in most or all activities, nearly every day
- Significant unintentional increase or decrease in weight or appetite
- Lack of sleep or sleeping excessively, nearly every day
- Psychomotor changes noticed by others (agitation or sluggishness), nearly every day
- Fatigue and/or loss of energy, nearly every day
- Feelings of guilt and/or worthlessness, nearly every day
- Diminished cognitive abilities, nearly every day
- Recurrent thoughts of death (APA, 2013)

MDD may also present in different subtypes. The depressive subtypes are listed below with descriptions and related treatment implications (APA, 2013).

Psychotic features: MDD is accompanied by hallucinations or delusions. This subtype is under-diagnosed in treatment. It may indicate a need for more invasive treatment methods.

Catatonic features: At least two of the following are found in conjunction with MDD: immobility, extreme agitation, extreme negativism, peculiarities of voluntary movement, and echolalia or echopraxia. In treatment this subtype must be differentiated from other psychiatric and medical conditions. Catatonic signs may dominate clinical findings and require supportive medical interventions. There may be a need for more invasive treatment methods.

Melancholic features: These are the characteristic somatic symptoms of depression. There will be early morning wakening and intensified morning symptoms. It is often seen with significant anorexia and/or weight loss. In treatment there is a high risk of suicidal behaviors and an increased risk for recurrence despite maintenance pharmacotherapy. Psychotherapy is less effective with this subtype.

Atypical features: There is a pattern of marked mood reactivity and at least two of the following symptoms: leaden paralysis, long-standing pattern of interpersonal rejection sensitivity, increase in appetite and/or weight, and hypersomnia. It is more common in women and has an earlier onset than other types. In treatment it has a higher likelihood for chronic depressive symptoms and a wide range of treatment options. A depressive episode related to bipolar disorder must be ruled out.

Seasonal patterns: There will be a regular relationship with depressive symptoms and remission based on time of year (typically early October to late November onset and mid-February to mid-April remission patterns in North America). Seasonally related psychosocial stressors must be ruled out. Atypical features of hypersomnia and increased weight are common. The entire range of MDD treatments are options including light therapy as adjunctive therapy.

Incidence/Prevalence in U.S.

The twelve-month prevalence rate of MDD is approximately 6.7% in the U.S. adult population, and as high as 17% in lifetime prevalence (Kessler et al., 2003). Persons living in poverty report depression almost twice as often as those possessing higher socioeconomic resources (Lorant et al., 2003; Muntaner et al., 2004). Twins studies indicate a level of heritability in MDD of approximately 37%, which is significantly higher than incidence in the overall general population, but it is at a lower rate than bipolar disorder or schizophrenia (Belmaker & Agam, 2008).

Women are 70% more likely than men to report depression, and non-Hispanic blacks are 40% less likely than non-Hispanic whites to experience MDD (Kessler et al., 2003). Non-white ethnic groups often report MDD at a significantly lower rate than Caucasian-Americans, often due to different cultural conceptualization and presentations of depression combined with lower access to mental health screening (APA, 2010). MDD prevalence in older adults ranges from 7-36% in outpatient settings, but increases to 40-50% or higher in hospitalized patients (APA, 2010; Koenig & Blazer, 1992).

Predominant Age

MDD may occur any time between childhood and late adulthood, but the average age of onset occurs in a person's late 20s to early 30s (APA, 2010; Kessler et al., 2003). However, MDD is increasing in lifetime prevalence within younger generations in the U.S., with a gradually decreasing average age of onset (Craighead et al., 2007).

Causes

Even though MDD is sometimes associated with a level of heritability and/or psychosocial and environmental triggers, anyone can experience MDD, even without a family history or notable external stressors. Causes for depression are not completely understood by researchers. Leading evidence maintains MDD is a disorder of the brain, and it is thought to be caused by differing combinations of genetic, biochemical, psychosocial, and environmental factors (APA, 2013; APA, 2010, Tsuang et al., 2004).

Systems Affected

MDD's pervasive and holistic impact on a person often results in significantly diminished quality of life, lost work productivity (d845 Acquiring, Keeping, and Terminating a Job), cognitive and emotional impairment (b126 Temperament and Personality Functions, b152 Emotional Functions, b160 Thought Functions), and is the leading cause of years lived with disability (Cieza et al., 2004; Kennedy, Eisfeld, & Cooke, 2001; Wang, Simon, & Kessler, 2003).

Symptoms of MDD have the potential to negatively impact short-term and long-term relationships (d350 Conversation, d710 Basic Interpersonal Interactions, d750 Informal Social Relationships, d760 Family Relationships, d770 Intimate Relationships) (Coates & Wortman, 1980) as well as alter one's appraisals of existing social supports (b164 Higher-Level Cognitive Functions) (Elliott & Shewchuk, 1995).

MDD can further disrupt daily activities (d230 Carrying Out Daily Routine, d910 Community Life, d920 Recreation and Leisure, d930 Religion and Spirituality) through symptoms of amotivation and lethargy (b130 Energy and Drive Functions, b140 Attention Functions, b147 Psychomotor Functions), less energy for dealing with issues (d163 Thinking, d175 Solving Problems, d177 Making Decisions, d240 Handling Stress and Other Psychological Demands), and low self-efficacy (b126 Temperament and Personality Functions) (APA, 2010).

Basic self-care can be neglected. Weight gain or loss may also occur as a result of depression. Use ICF codes b180 Experience of Self and Time Functions, d510 Washing Oneself, and d570 Looking After One's Health.

Secondary Problems

MDD frequently co-occurs with many physical and mental health conditions (APA, 2010; 2013). MDD is seen at higher rates among persons with chronic pain, illness, and disability, and cardiovascular disorders are more frequent among persons with chronic MDD (APA, 2010). MDD is frequently co-occurring with anxiety, substance abuse, eating disorders, dementia, and personality disorders, but which causes which is not always clear (APA, 2010). Anxiety is an extremely common comorbidity, as over 60% of persons with MDD may meet criteria for general anxiety disorder, and up to 50% may also qualify for social phobia or PTSD, with slightly lower rates of obsessive-compulsive disorder, panic disorder, and specific phobia (APA, 2010). See relevant chapters for information on how to document any comorbid conditions.

Prognosis

Acute symptoms of MDD are responsive to treatment in most cases, but prognosis differs depending on a variety of variables. These include access to diagnosis and care, availability of healthy social supports, severity and chronicity of symptoms, and response and adherence to treatments (APA, 2010; Holma et al., 2008). Approximately half of those receiving antidepressant and/or psychological interventions are able to experience a full remission of symptoms. Still, approximately one-third of those in treatment fail to fully recover (Malhi et al., 2009). The overall prognosis of MDD can be further complicated by suicidal ideation and impulses and the co-occurrence of other medical and psychiatric symptoms (APA, 2010).

Assessment

The U.S. Preventive Services Task Force (USPSTF) recommends that physicians screen for depression in *all* adult patients, as early detection can lead to better treatment outcomes (Sharp & Lipsky, 2002). Special screening tools are indicated for older adults (Roman & Callen, 2008), and although there is insufficient evidence to warrant regular screening of children and adolescents, care providers are encouraged to watch for warning signs possibly indicating depressive disorder (Sharp & Lipsky, 2002).

Typical Scope of Team Assessment

Persons scoring above the established cutoff in depression screening tools are recommended for formal assessment from a physician or qualified mental health professional with diagnostic abilities, referencing the APA's *Diagnostic and Statistical Manual of Mental Disorders* (APA, 2013; Sharp & Lipsky, 2002). Thorough assessment will help to avoid misdiagnosis, rule out alternative explanations of symptoms, and identify co-occurring conditions. Valid assessment takes context and cultural issues into account, and provides an approximate level of depressive symptoms and their impacts on global

functioning. Attention to safety issues related to possible self-care neglect and suicidal ideation is an important part of the assessment (APA, 2010). Some commonly assessed factors for suicidal risk include:

- History of suicide attempts
- Presence and lethality of suicide plan
- Feelings of acute hopelessness and psychic pain
- Presence of psychotic symptoms
- Active co-occurring substance abuse
- Presence of co-occurring disabling condition
- Higher demographic risk
- Absence of social supports and/or other protective factors
- Family history or recent exposure to suicide (APA, 2010)

There are several common tools used by the broader treatment team and for recreational therapy assessment. It should be noted that persons with acute MDD symptoms may have difficulty completing longer and more complex assessments, especially within one session.

Patient Health Questionnaire (PHQ-9): This is the most common screening tool to identify depression in adults. A modified version is available for adolescents.

Global Assessment of Functioning (GAF): Part of the DSM, and frequently used in mental health and VA settings. GAF is a broad estimate of mental health with a score that ranges from 0-100. Dehn (1995) modified the GAF to apply it directly to leisure functioning with the *Global Assessment of Leisure Functioning*.

Suicide Assessment Five-Step Evaluation and Triage (SAFE-T): Developed in collaboration with the Suicide Prevention Resource Center and Screening for Mental Health to assess risk of suicide.

Suicide Behaviors Questionnaire (SBQ-R): Assesses suicide-related thoughts and behaviors.

Quality of Life-BREF (WHOQoL-BREF): A shorter version of original instrument; developed by the World Health Organization for international and cross-cultural use. It assesses physical, psychological, and social health as embedded in the context of environment, culture, and personal goals, standards, and concerns.

Intake assessment and interview: Varies by setting; recreational therapists will typically complete their own intake for recreational therapy services.

Leisure Motivation Scale: Measures a person's motivation for engaging in leisure activities. It may be especially helpful for clients with MDD who struggle with energy, inertia, and motivation needed to engage in recreation and leisure activities.

Barriers Scale (Scale F in Leisure Diagnostic Battery) (LDB): Measures a variety of constraining factors to leisure participation and enjoyment. A solutions-focused recreational therapist could help the client be more active in the community through negotiation of perceived and real barriers.

Leisure Resources Asset Mapping; Circle of Support/Circle of Friends: These holistic assessments help individuals identify internal and external assets for community participation and types and levels of social support. It may be completed with the individual's social supports and is congruent with a recovery perspective (Anderson & Heyne, 2012, pp. 222-223).

Wellness Recovery Action Plan (WRAP): The development of a Wellness Recovery Action Plan involves a great deal of self-assessment including, but not limited to, personal perspectives on health, mental health, and holistic wellness; personal goals, aspirations, and dreams; coping tools and personal, social, and environmental strengths and supports; personal indicators of health decline and crisis; triggers; and daily maintenance/recovery initiatives.

The team can use these tools to discover deficits in the clients functional levels, which can be recorded using the ICF areas described in the Symptoms section.

Areas of Concern for RT Assessment

The recreational therapy assessment will vary by setting. The recreational therapist will pay close attention to other treatment team assessments, focusing on immediate safety precautions, presence and relevance of co-occurring conditions, medication side effects that may influence recreational activity, and treatment modalities currently pursued by other treatment team members.

Due to the most common symptoms of MDD, the recreational therapist is likely to find reduced motivation for, participation in, and enjoyment of social, recreational, and leisure pursuits. The recreational therapist should documents deficits discovered using the ICF categories in the Symptoms section.

With a list of areas of concern, the recreational therapist can help the individual with MDD identify reasonable target outcomes for recreational therapy participation and assess current personal and environmental strengths that may aid in the recovery process (Cook et al., 2010). The recreational therapist may also assess information related to a community inclusion and/or reintegration plan if the client is planning to transition from a more to less restrictive living environment. The recreational therapist may also administer instruments and encourage the completion of self-assessments and collaborative assessments designed to facilitate more of a recovery perspective and development of a WRAP.

ICF Core Set

Both a brief and a comprehensive ICF Core Set have been developed for Depression.

Treatment Direction

The recreational therapist can be an integral member of the treatment team when working with a person diagnosed with MDD. Numerous treatment options are available, but with differing results from person to person and dependent on types and severity of symptoms. The treatment team will address acute safety and stabilization needs as a top priority when a person with MDD manifests severe and/or suicidal symptom presentations (APA, 2010; Malhi et al., 2009). Treatment direction is also determined by treatment setting, MDD subtype (if indicated), as well as the client's developmental stage, culture, and co-existing physical and/or psychiatric disorders (APA, 2010).

Whole Team Approach

The quality of services for persons with MDD and other mental illness diagnoses has improved greatly in recent times. These improvements evolved from both the increase in evidence-based practice (EBP) and the development of the recovery movement (Salyers & Tsemberis, 2007). EBP includes well-documented pharmacological, behavioral, and psychotherapeutic interventions that have consistently reduced symptoms across a variety of settings (Drake & Goldman, 2003; Salyers & Tsemberis, 2007). The recovery perspective is more of a self-managed, strengths-based approach endorsed by many advocacy groups and individuals living with mental illness. "Recovery" describes the process by which persons with mental illness participate in their communities as valuable members in the presence or absence of symptoms (Copeland, 1997; Carter Center, 2003). Improvements are seen in the areas of d710 Basic Interpersonal Interactions, d750 Informal Social Relationships, d760 Family Relationships, and d770 Intimate Relationships.

Even though EBP and a recovery perspective may originate from different roots, the two approaches are not mutually exclusive, and a growing research base supports certain recovery approaches as efficacious in the management of severe mental illness (Cook et al., 2010; Copeland, 1997; Ralph, Lambert, & Kidder, 2002; Salyers & Tsemberis, 2007).

A variety of evidence-based tools are available to treat MDD, but the bulk of research still centers around the pharmacological use of antidepressants and psychotherapeutic interventions, such as cognitive behavioral therapy (CBT), behavioral activation strategies (BAS), and interpersonal therapy (IPT) (APA, 2010; Malhi et al., 2009). Setting the stage for effective treatment is important, starting with attention to safety, client education, and the development of a therapeutic alliance with healthcare providers (Malhi et al., 2009). An accurate and complete description of the deficits found during assessment will allow the team to measure the success of treatment with a particular client. These therapies have the potential to bring about improvement in all of the areas described in the Symptoms section. Summaries of some of the most commonly used approaches with persons who have a primary MDD diagnosis are shown below.

Psychological treatment: Several types of therapies are used. Cognitive behavioral therapy (CBT) has a large evidence base and combines cognitive and behavioral techniques. Changes in maladaptive thinking lead to changes in behaviors that feed MDD symptoms. Behavioral approach system (BAS) interventions are regaining popularity and are easier to implement for non-counseling professionals (Hopko et al., 2003). The focus for BAS is on identification of activities that exacerbate symptoms and scheduled participation in positive activities. Interpersonal therapy (IPT) is solutions-focused with attention on adaptive strategies in social contexts. It emphasizes correlations between MDD and the environment. Psychotherapy is an appropriate first line of treatment for mild to moderate MDD with or without antidepressant therapy. Psychotherapies are secondary lines of treatment for persons experiencing atypical features and are often contraindicated for MDD with psychotic or catatonic features (APA, 2010; Craighead et al., 2008; Malhi et al., 2009).

Pharmacological interventions: Medication classes include SSRI, NARI, NaSSA, SNRI, TCA, and MAOIs. Effectiveness of antidepressant class medications varies from person to person; some types are contraindicated due to other co-occurring conditions. Potential side effects are numerous and differ in characteristics and severity between types and individuals. Recreational therapists must be aware of impact that side effects have on recreational activities. SSRIs are generally better tolerated; MAOIs are highly efficacious but, along with TCAs, carry higher risk for serious complications. Due to cost of psychotherapy, antidepressant medications are frequently the sole therapeutic intervention. Antidepressant effectiveness may be enhanced when used in conjunction with psychotherapy. Some individuals experience increased risk of mania or suicide after starting antidepressants. It may take up to four weeks before noticing results (APA, 2010; Malhi et al., 2009).

Electroconvulsive therapy (ECT): Electric shock is conducted to induce a convulsive state while the client is under anesthesia, typically as in-patient care. ECT is considered a safe and effective first-line treatment option in some cases, but is stigmatized by media representations. Short-term memory loss is the most common side effect, but growing evidence indicates risk for long-term memory loss in some cases. It may be indicated for persons with severe cases of MDD that are not sufficiently responsive to other treatment options, where the MDD has catatonic or psychotic features, with persons with unrelenting suicidal ideation, and where there is a history of ECT success (APA, 2010; Malhi et al., 2009).

Assertive community treatment (ACT): This has characteristics of intensive case management models and similar efficacy. It is indicated for persons with a history of severe symptoms and recurrent stays in in-patient mental health facilities, substance abuse treatment facilities, and/or criminal justice settings. Targeted individuals are often non-compliant with traditional treatment. Persons with mild to moderate MDD, or those adequately engaged in and responsive to treatment with severe MDD, would not be appropriate for this level of care. Initiated over 30 years ago, ACT has adapted to shifts and advances in mental health delivery over the years. ACT involves high levels of support from the treatment team with wrap-around services. It takes place in natural community settings or transitional housing settings. ACT has a strong foundation of research to support efficacy in reducing in-patient recidivism, increasing participation in community, and reducing incidence of homelessness by persons with severe mental illness. ACT teams are typically clinician-driven ("clinician as expert") but may also include elements of recovery perspective while maintaining high fidelity to ACT requirements (Salyers & Tsemberis, 2007).

Recovery perspectives: Worldwide, there are multiple recovery-based models of providing mental health services. In the U.S., the Wellness Recovery Action Plan (WRAP) is the most widely embraced (Cook et al., 2010; Ralph et al., 2002). Recovery perspectives focus on self-management and engagement in peer-led services versus clinician-driven treatment in the recovery journey. There is increased focus on the client taking responsibility to build existing personal and environmental strengths, supports, and overall wellness to increase resistance to mental illness symptoms and effects, and a progressively increasing toolbox of skills and strategies (Cook et al., 2010; Ralph et al., 2002).

Complementary and alternative medicine (CAM): CAM therapies are growing in acceptance. They have received scientific study, which has demonstrated their efficacy for MDD, and have been identified as worthy of more rigorous future study. There is a growing trend of integrative approaches to treatment of MDD, combining traditional and non-traditional methods. Some examples are dietary supplements such as folate and St. John's wort, bright light therapy, and exercise. Considerations in using these therapies include evaluating drug interactions between any dietary supplements and prescribed medications. Physical activity and exercise have so much support that they may be prescribed alone, as first-line approaches for persons with mild to moderate depression. These interventions are also recognized as increasing protective properties that promote physical and mental health components that are often impaired directly or indirectly by MDD (APA, 2009).

Recreational Therapy Approach

The recreational therapist may work directly with a person with a MDD diagnosis in a variety of settings, especially considering the frequent co-occurrence with other physical and mental health conditions. A recreational therapist working with someone treated solely for MDD may work in acute mental health at a community hospital, as a treatment team member in a community behavioral health center, or in a long-term mental healthcare facility, such as a state hospital. A recreational therapist may also work as an ACT team member, although often her/his title may be something other than "Recreational Therapist."

The recreational therapy action plan will vary greatly depending on the associated treatment organization's philosophy, approach, and division of practice. Further, the recreational therapist must take into account other co-occurring conditions and contextual factors that influence treatment pathways. The recreational therapy scope of practice may range from a medical model approach concerned with functional intervention to a leisure education and community inclusion approach aimed at health promotion. In all situations an integrated, full-spectrum recreational therapy plan seems most likely to effectively address the holistic needs associated with MDD.

There is a dearth of EBP protocols specific to recreational therapy, resulting from the lack of randomized clinical trials with proven results, but the recreational therapist should develop and build on best practices grounded in available theoretical and research-based evidence in the broader spectrum of literature to guide approaches that are complementary to that of the treatment team and most likely to support recovery in clients with MDD. When possible, the treatment plan creation should be a collaborative process with the client and take the client's goals, aspirations, and preferences into account (Cook et al., 2010; Copeland, 1997; Ralph et al., 2002; Salyers & Tsemberis, 2007).

Recreational Therapy Interventions

The following identifies types of recreational therapy activities and techniques within the recreational therapy scope of practice that potentially hold therapeutic value for a person with MDD in terms of symptom management, functional abilities, social support development, and/or overall quality of life, as derived from current research in behavioral health literature. The recreational therapist may use these techniques in any part of the service continuum, from functional improvement and symptom management to overall health promotion for people experiencing MDD or working to prevent relapse.

Cognitive Behavioral and Behavioral-Action Influences

Recreational therapists are typically not qualified to provide psychotherapy unless they also hold additional credentials. However, a recreational therapist can tap into research and theories related to some of these approaches, and pursue education and training for related skills that may be used in recreational therapy service delivery. Due to the recreational therapy scope of practice, a recreational therapist is well-suited to use CBT and BAS principles to guide recreational therapy delivery, especially in terms of how a person with MDD perceives participation in certain recreation, leisure, and social activities, and how reframing and activity scheduling may help actively address MDD symptoms and improve coping and resilience for the development of quality of life and health promotion.

For example, a behavioral/action approach is currently supported within the nursing home environment, a place where residents are at significantly higher risk for MDD. Positive affect (b152 Emotional Functions), decrease in depression symptoms (b126 Temperament and Personality Functions), and overall quality of life frequently correlate positively with the number of activities engaged in (excluding activities of daily living), and the perception of how pleasant participation was. Some of the highest-rated experiences include receiving social visits, laughing, wearing favorite clothes, attending religious or spiritual services, and being told they were loved (Meeks, Shah, & Ramsey, 2009). Frequency of participation seems to mediate depressive symptoms by the positive influence on overall affect and create feedback to motivate future

engagement (b130 Energy and Drive Functions) (Meeks et al., 2009). Thus, recreational therapists working with nursing home residents should consider their role as important in addressing symptoms regardless of the title they have. The recreational therapist should assess residents on the activities they find enjoyable on an ongoing basis in determining maintenance and changes to options offered and encourage the highest frequency of participation appropriate to each individual resident, in order to establish an enjoyable daily routine (d230 Carrying Out Daily Routine). The recreational therapist should also pursue activities that will encourage humor and laughter and should collaborate with other staff to identify favorite clothing and access to religious services of the resident's preference, if applicable. ICF codes improved by these activities include b126 Temperament and Personality Functions, b130 Energy and Drive Functions, d177 Making Decisions, d710 Basic Interpersonal Interactions, d760 Family Relationships, and d9 Community, Social, and Civic Life.

Recovery Perspective

A recreational therapist grounded in a recovery perspective may work with clients in the development of a personal wellness recovery action plan. There is a significant foundation of support indicating that persons actively pursuing recovery through a WRAP realize higher levels of understandings of self and their status on the personal wellness-illness continuum (b180 Experience of Self and Time Functions), meaningful social supports (d760 Family Relationships, d770 Intimate Relationships), and coping strategies to address active symptoms and mental health crises (d175 Solving Problems, d240 Handling Stress and Other Psychological Demands). Resulting feelings of empowerment may increase overall outlook (b126 Temperament and Personality Functions) and motivation (b130 Energy and Drive Functions), and significant components of developing a wellness toolbox focused on daily routine management (d230 Carrying Out Daily Routine), meaningful community participation (d910 Community Life), developing agency over decision-making in healthcare and other decisions (d177 Making Decisions), health and wellness promotion (d570 Looking After One's Health), and healthy recreation and leisure lifestyle development (d920

Recreation and Leisure) (Cook et al., 2010; Copeland, 1997; Ralph et al., 2002). For more information on WRAP and the general recovery perspective, see "Mental Health Recovery" in the resources for this chapter.

A recreational therapist may incorporate cognitive, behavioral, and/or recovery approaches as foundations for how s/he facilitates any therapeutic intervention, social support development, and specific activity-based approaches.

Social Support Development

The recreational therapist can be a valuable aid in working with the client to develop or renegotiate social skills and or relationships (d350 Conversation, d760 Family Relationships, d770 Intimate Relationships) that are impaired by MDD symptoms or that can act as a protective toolset to buffer and/or decrease MDD symptoms (b126 Temperament and Personality Functions) (Coates & Wortman, 1980; Elliott & Shewchuk, 1995; Malhi et al., 2009, McCormick, 1999; Ralph et al., 2002). In in-patient settings, this may be done through developing therapeutic rapport with the client via one-on-one activities or in group settings, but ideally would take place in the client's natural environment and include existing family and non-kin social supports. Successful implementation of these activities will lead to improvements in d750 Informal Social Relationships, d760 Family Relationships, d770 Intimate Relationships, and d910 Community Life. The recreational therapist may also be charged with facilitating or connecting a client with a mood disorder support group to help provide the client with support and strategies to handle MDD-related stress and demands (d240 Handling Stress and Other Psychological Demands). The role of family-centered treatment is especially beneficial to some clients, with significantly higher efficacy among certain ethnic populations (Almeida et al., 2011).

Specific Activity-Based Modalities

A recreational therapist may utilize almost any recreational activity as part of the overall treatment plan for a person with MDD, but should focus on client preferences to increase self-motivation (b130 Energy and Drive Functions), daily routine (d230 Carrying Out Daily Routine), and development (or redevelopment) of recreation and leisure preferences

(d920 Recreation and Leisure) that are enjoyable and encourage repeated participation. The recreational therapist must also consider safety risks, available resources, and evaluation of how different activities impact MDD symptoms. There is also growing research to indicate additional benefits from certain activities that promote physical activity, combine multiple methods that demonstrate effectiveness, and promote self-managed recovery strategies.

Physical activity and exercise, walking, nature walks: Initiating an exercise program may be difficult for a person experiencing acute MDD symptoms, so in such cases the recreational therapist will help a client set small, achievable goals and then build on them (b126 Temperament and Personality Functions, b130 Energy and Drive Functions). Physical activity has a growing research base that supports therapeutic benefits for MDD treatment and quality of life improvement (APA, 2009; Babyak et al., 2000; Berman et al., 2012), and sedentary behavior is linked with higher rates of depressive episodes (Teychenne, Ball, & Salmon, 2010). Continued exercise routines have also been shown to prevent MDD relapse (Babyak et al., 2000). At the therapeutic dosage, which will vary from person to person, physical activity can promote energy and reduce inertia (b130 Energy and Drive Functions); improve sleep (b134 Sleep Functions), memory (b144 Memory Functions), psychomotor (b147 Psychomotor Functions), and emotional functions (b152 Emotional Functions); reduce sensations of pain (b280 Sensation of Pain); help weight maintenance (b530 Weight Maintenance Functions); increase activity level through daily routine (d230 Carrying Out Daily Routine); and increase ability to manage and cope with stressors (d240 Handling Stress and Other Psychological Demands) (APA, 2009; Babyak et al., 2000; Berman et al., 2012). No special equipment is required as walking is an appropriate method that can be pursued in a variety of environments by those who are ambulatory (Babyak et al., 2000; Berman et al., 2012). However, walking in nature environments seems to provide more benefits than city walking (Berman et al., 2012).

Yoga is another type of physical activity increasingly used to treat depression. Yoga continues to gain popularity as a therapeutic modality for multiple needs based on the potential to simultaneously engage mind, body, and spirit. Evidence is continuing to develop suggesting yoga as an alternative, as well as a complementary addition to traditional MDD treatments (Uebelacker et al., 2010). Hatha yoga emphasizes mindfulness which can be used as a cognitive behavioral tool, and the more obvious benefits of movement, relaxation, and leisure skills development also position yoga as a plausible intervention for MDD. However, more research is needed to fully understand yoga's potential and related implications as a treatment for MDD. ICF codes that may be improved by yoga include b126 Temperament and Personality Functions, b130 Energy and Drive Functions, and b147 Psychomotor Functions.

Animal-assisted interventions: When appropriate for and well tolerated by clients, a recreational therapist may include animal-assisted activities (AAA) and/or animal-assisted therapy (AAT) into an overall recreational therapy plan. A meta-analysis of animal-assisted programs (all with dogs, four programs were AAA and one program was AAT) revealed AAA and/or AAT provided a moderate level of relief to depressive symptoms (Souter & Miller, 2007). In addition to significantly decreasing general depression scores, AAT seems to hold potential to help positively influence cognitive (b117 Intellectual Functions), emotional (b152 Emotional Functions), and motivational (b130 Energy and Drive Functions) functioning, especially with older adults with MDD diagnoses (Moretti et al., 2010). One study on a farm animal-assisted intervention showed some farm work activities presented even higher effectiveness than traditional AAA and AAT, but only when progress in working skills was increased (Pedersen, Martinsen, & Berget, 2011). Some studies examining AAA and AAT impact on depression present conflicting results, and more focused research with methodological rigor is needed in these areas.

Resources

American Academy of Child and Adolescent Psychiatry (AACAP)

www.aacap.org

The AACAP promotes the healthy development of children, adolescents, and families through research, training, prevention, comprehensive diagnosis, and treatment and to meet the professional needs of child and adolescent psychiatrists throughout their careers.

American Association for Geriatric Psychiatry (AAGP)

www.aagponline.org/

A national association providing products, activities, and publications that focus exclusively on the challenges of geriatric psychiatry.

American Foundation for Suicide Prevention (AFSP)

www.afsp.org

The nation's leading organization bringing together people across communities and backgrounds to understand and prevent suicide, and to help heal the pain it causes.

American Psychiatric Association

www.psych.org

The world's largest psychiatric organization. It is a medical specialty society representing more than 33,000 psychiatric physicians from the United States and around the world. Its member physicians work together to ensure humane care and effective treatment for all persons with mental disorders, including intellectual disabilities and substance use disorders.

American Psychological Association

www.apa.org

The American Psychological Association is the largest scientific and professional organization representing psychology in the United States. Its mission is to advance the creation, communication, and application of psychological knowledge to benefit society and improve people's lives.

Centers for Disease Control and Prevention

www.cdc.gov (Search: depression)

As the nation's health protection agency, CDC saves lives and protects people from health threats. To accomplish their mission, the CDC conducts critical science and provides health information that protects the nation against expensive and dangerous health threats and responds when these arise.

Mental Health Recovery

www.mhrecovery.com

Hamilton County, Ohio, Mental Health and Recovery Services Board recovery website.

National Alliance on Mental Illness (NAMI)

www.nami.org

NAMI is the nation's largest grassroots mental health organization dedicated to building better lives for the millions of Americans affected by mental illness. NAMI advocates for access to services, treatment, supports, and research and has a commitment to raise awareness and build a community for hope for all of those in need.

National Coalition for Mental Health Recovery

www.ncmhr.org

Ensures that consumers and survivors have a major voice in the development and implementation of healthcare, mental health, and social policies at the state and national levels, empowering people to recover and lead a full life in the community.

National Institute of Mental Health

www.nimh.nih.gov

The mission of NIMH is to transform the understanding and treatment of mental illnesses through basic and clinical research, paving the way for prevention, recovery, and cure.

National Mental Health Association (NMHA)

www.mentalhealthamerica.net

The National Mental Health Association is a community-based network dedicated to helping all Americans achieve wellness by living mentally healthier lives.

Substance Abuse and Mental Health Services Administration (SAMHSA)

www.samhsa.gov

SAMHSA is the agency within the U.S. Department of Health and Human Services that leads public health efforts to advance the behavioral health of the nation. SAMHSA's mission is to reduce the impact of substance abuse and mental illness on America's communities.

References

Almeida, J., Subramanian, S. V., Kawachi, I., & Molnar, B. E. (2011). Is blood thicker than water? Social support, depression and the modifying role of ethnicity/nativity status. *Journal of Epidemiology and Community Health 65*(1), 51-56.

American Psychiatric Association (APA). (2009). *Complementary and alternative medicine in major depressive disorder: The American Psychiatric Association task force assessment of the evidence, challenges, and recommendations.* Arlington, VA: American Psychiatric Association.

American Psychiatric Association (APA). (2010). *Practice guidelines for the treatment of patients with major depressive disorder.* Arlington, VA: American Psychiatric Association.

American Psychiatric Association (APA). (2013). *Diagnostic and statistical manual of mental disorders* (5th ed.). Arlington, VA: American Psychiatric Association.

Anderson, L. & Heyne, L. (2012). *Therapeutic recreation practice: A strengths approach.* State College, PA: Venture Publishing, Inc.

Babyak, M., Blumenthal, J. A., Herman, S., Khatri, P., Doraiswamy, M., Moore, K., ... & Krishnan, R. (2000). Exercise treatment for major depression: Maintenance of therapeutic benefit at 10 months. *Psychosomatic Medicine, 62*(5), 633-638.

Belmaker, R. H. & Agam, G. (2008). Major depressive disorder. *New England Journal of Medicine, 358*(1), 55-68.

Berman, M. G., Kross, E., Krpan, K. M., Askren, M. K., Burson, A., Deldin, P. J., ... Jonides, J. (2012). Interacting with nature improves cognition and affect for individuals with depression. *Journal of Affective Disorders, 140*(3), 300-305.

Carter Center. (2003). President's new freedom commission on mental health: Transforming the vision. Retrieved from http://www.cartercenter.org/documents/1701.pdf.

Cieza, A., Chatterji, S., Andersen, D., Cantista, P., Herceg, M., Melvin, J., Stucki, G., & de Bie, R. (2004). ICF core sets for depression. *Journal of Rehabilitation Medicine, Suppl. 44*, 128-134.

Coates, D. & Wortman, C. (1980). Depression maintenance and interpersonal control. In A. Baum & J. E. Singer (Eds.), *Advances in environmental psychology* (pp. 149-182). Hillsdale, NJ: Lawrence Erlbaum Associates, Inc.

Cook, J. A., Copeland, M. E., Corey, L., Buffington, E., Jonikas, J. A., Curtis, L. C., ... & Nichols, W. H. (2010). Developing the evidence base for peer-led services: Changes among participants following wellness recovery action planning (WRAP) education in two statewide initiatives. *Psychiatric Rehabilitation Journal, 32*(2), 113-120.

Copeland, M. E. (1997). *Wellness recovery action plan.* Dummerston, VT: Peach Press.

Craighead, W. E., Sheets, E. S., Brosse, A. L., & Ilardi, S. S. (2007). Psychosocial treatments for major depressive disorder. In P.E. Nathan & J. M. Gorman (Eds.), *A guide to treatments that work, third edition* (pp. 289-307). New York: Oxford University Press.

Davidson, L. (2005). Recovery, self management and the expert patient: Changing the culture of mental health from a UK perspective. *Journal of Mental Health, 14*(1), 25-35.

Dehn, D. (1995). *Leisure step up.* Ravensdale, WA: Idyll Arbor.

Drake R. E. & Goldman, H. H. (2003). *Evidence-based practices in mental health care.* Arlington, VA: American Psychiatric Association.

Elliott, T. R. & Shewchuk, R. M. (1995). Social support and leisure activities following severe physical disability: Testing the mediating effects of depression. *Basic and Applied Social Psychology, 16*(4), 471-487.

Holma, K. M., Holma, I. A., Melartin, T. K., Rytsala, H. J., & Isometsa, E. T. (2008). Long-term outcome of major depressive disorder in psychiatric patients is variable. *Journal of Clinical Psychiatry, 69*(2), 196-205.

Hopko, D. R., Lejuez, C. W., Kenneth, J. R., & Eifert, G. H. (2003). Contemporary behavioral activation treatments for depression: Procedures, principles, and progress. *Clinical Psychology Review, 23*(5), 699-717.

Kennedy, S. H., Eisfeld, B. S., Cooke, R. G. (2001). Quality of life: An important dimension in assessing the treatment of depression? *Journal of Psychiatry and Neuroscience, 26*(Suppl.), S23-S28.

Kessler, R. C., Berglund, P., Demler, O., Jin, R., Koretz, D., Merikangas, K. R., ... & Wang, P. S. (2003). The epidemiology of major depressive disorder: Results from the National Comorbidity Survey replication. *Journal of the American Medical Association, 289*(23), 3095-3105.

Koenig, H. G. & Blazer, D. G. (1992). Epidemiology of geriatric affective disorders. *Clinical Geriatric Medicine, 8*, 235-251.

Lorant, V., Deliege, D., Eaton, W., Robert, A., Philippot, P., & Ansseau, M. (2003). Socioeconomic inequalities in depression: A meta-analysis. *American Journal of Public Health, 157*(2), 98-112.

Malhi, G. S., Adams, D., Porter, R., Wignall, A., Lampe, L., O'Connor, N., ... & Mulder, R. T. (2009). Clinical practice recommendations for depression. *Acta Psychiatrica Scandinavia, 119*(Suppl. 439), 8-26.

McCormick, B. (1999). Contributions of social support and recreation companionship to the life satisfaction of people with persistent mental illness. *Therapeutic Recreation Journal, 33*(4), 304-319.

Meeks, S., Shah, S. N., & Ramsey, S. K. (2009). The pleasant events schedule — Nursing home version: A useful tool for behavioral interventions in long-term care. *Aging and Mental Health, 13*(3), 445-455.

Moretti, F., De Ronchi, D., Bernabei, V., Marchetti, L., Ferrari, B., Forlani, C., ... & Atti, A. R. (2010). Pet therapy in elderly patients with mental illness. *Psychogeriatrics, 11*(2), 125-129.

Muntaner, C., Eaton, W. W., Miech, R., & O'Campo, P. (2004). Socioeconomic position and major mental disorders. *Epidemiologic Reviews, 26*(1), 53-62.

Pedersen, I., Martinsen, E. W., & Berget, B. (2011). Farm animal-assisted intervention: Relationship between work and contact with farm animals and change in depression, anxiety, and self-efficacy among persons with clinical depression. *Issues in Mental Health Nursing, 32*(8), 493-500.

Ralph, R. O., Lambert, D., & Kidder, K. A. (2002). *The recovery perspective and evidence-based practice for people with serious mental illness.* Illinois Department of Human Services: Behavioral Health Recovery Management Project.

Roman, M. W. & Callen, B. L. (2008). Screening instruments for older adult depressive disorders: Updating the evidence-based toolbox. *Issues in Mental Health Nursing, 29*(9), 924-941.

Salyers, M. P. & Tsemberis, S. (2007). ACT and recovery: Integrating evidence-based practice and recovery orientation on assertive community treatment teams. *Community Mental Health Journal, 43*(6), 619-641.

Sharp, L. K. & Lipsky, M. S. (2002). Screening for depression across the lifespan: A review of measures for use in primary care settings. *American Family Physician, 66*(6), 1001-1009.

Souter, M. A. & Miller, M. D. (2007). Do animal-assisted activities effectively treat depression? A meta-analysis. *Anthrozoos, 20*(2), 167-180.

Teychenne, M., Ball, K., & Salmon, J. (2010). Sedentary behavior and depression among adults: A review. *International Journal of Behavioral Medicine, 17*(4), 246-254.

Tsuang, M. T., Bar, J. L., Stone, W. S., & Faraone, S. V. (2004). Gene-environment interactions in mental disorders. *World Psychiatry, 3*(2), 73-83.

Uebelacker, L. A., Epstein-Lubow, G., Gaudiano, B. A., Tremont, G., Battle, C. L., & Miller, I. W. (2010). Hatha yoga for depression: Critical review of the evidence for efficacy, plausible mechanisms of action, and directions for future research. *Journal of Psychiatric Practice, 16*(1), 22-33.

Wang, P. S., Simon, G., & Kessler, R. C. (2003). The economic burden of depression and the cost-effectiveness of treatment. *International Journal of Methods in Psychiatric Research, 12*(1), 22-33.

22. Multiple Sclerosis

Marieke Van Puymbroeck, Jasmine Townsend, Karen C. Wenzel, and Jared Allsop

Multiple sclerosis (MS) is an autoimmune disease that causes chronic inflammation of the central nervous system (Fox, 2010). The body's own defense system attacks the fatty substance (myelin) that surrounds and protects the nerve fibers of the brain, optic nerves, and spinal cord. As the damage occurs, the myelin covering of the nerves becomes inflamed, swollen, and detached from the fibers. Eventually, the myelin is destroyed. Scar tissue, also called a lesion or sclerosis, forms over the nerve fibers in place of the myelin (National Multiple Sclerosis Society, 2012).

Nerve impulses do not travel as fast or as accurately across the scarred areas, so impulses are blocked or delayed from traveling to or from the brain. Our bodies rely on the timing and strength of many different nerve impulses to help us interpret the environment. When some of the impulses are sent incorrectly, it can lead to an array of uncomfortable sensations in addition to sensory loss and loss of motor control. Ultimately, the disease process leads to degeneration of the nerves themselves, which accounts for the permanent disabilities that develop in MS (National Multiple Sclerosis Society, 2012).

Multiple sclerosis usually takes one of four disease courses as identified by the National MS Society (2012):

Relapsing-remitting (RRMS): This is the most common type of MS. MS symptoms flare up (exacerbate) and then subside. Exacerbations usually last several days to several weeks. The person may have total or only partial recovery between flare-ups. Around 85% of people with MS initially begin with this course.

Secondary-progressive (SPMS): When exacerbations become steadily progressive and only partial recoveries are achieved with each exacerbation, the course of the disease is described as SPMS. Before disease-modifying drugs became available, more than 50% of those who started with RRMS developed SPMS within 10 years, 90% within 25 years. It still may happen, but the percentages are lower now.

Primary-progressive (PPMS): PPMS is a steady progression of symptoms without signs of remitting, and occurs in about 10% of individuals with MS.

Progressive-relapsing (PRMS): A steady progression of symptoms with obvious acute attacks. Approximately five percent of people with MS appear to have PRMS.

Making a diagnosis of MS is not a simple process. MS symptoms are often attributed to other health problems and consequently misdiagnosed. Often people will wait years after developing symptoms before they are diagnosed with MS. A diagnosis of MS is based on the revised McDonald criteria, established by MS specialists, which focuses on the demonstration of clinical, laboratory, and radiological data of the dissemination of MS lesions in time and space for a non-invasive MS diagnosis (Polman et al., 2005).

Clinical data alone may be sufficient for a diagnosis of MS if an individual has had separate episodes of neurologic symptoms characteristic of MS. The most commonly used diagnostic tools are neuroimaging with magnetic resonance imaging (MRI), analysis of the cerebrospinal fluid, and evoked potentials, which measure how the nervous system responds to stimulation (Northrop & Frankel, 2010). The most helpful test to identify demyelination is magnetic resonance imaging. However, not all lesions can be detected by an MRI, and the presence of lesions does not confirm an MS diagnosis. Lesions can be caused by many other health issues. MRI scans can be helpful in tracking disease progression once a positive MS diagnosis is obtained.

Incidence/Prevalence in U.S.

MS is two to three times more common in women than in men (Northrop & Frankel, 2010); however, among people who develop MS at a later age, the gender ratio is more balanced. Approximately 350,000-400,000 Americans have MS (Fox, 2010; Northrop & Frankel, 2010). Of the various ethnic groups, MS is most common among Caucasians. MS is five times more prevalent in temperate climates — such as those found in the northern United States, Canada, and Europe — than in tropical regions (National Multiple Sclerosis Society, 2012).

Predominant Age

MS generally occurs between the ages of 20 and 30 (early onset), however some individuals do not experience symptoms until after the age of 50 (late onset) (National Multiple Sclerosis Society, 2012). Because MS is more frequent in women, and is most often diagnosed during the ages of 20-30, there is often a concern about bearing children. Having MS does not preclude a woman from having a child, and women typically have a reduction in MS-related symptoms during pregnancy. However, post-pregnancy, 20-40% of women experience an exacerbation in symptoms (National Institute of Neurological Disorders and Stroke, 2010).

Causes

Why the body's defenses attack the myelin sheath is unknown. However, there are several theories about the causes of MS (National Multiple Sclerosis Society, 2012):

Immunologic: MS is an autoimmune process where the body's immune system attacks its own central nervous system destroying the myelin sheath.

Environmental: Epidemiologic studies suggest that early exposure to an environmental agent might be a triggering factor in people who are predisposed by genetic factors to develop MS. The frequency of MS increases for people who live farther away from the equator. MS seems to appear more frequently in states above the 37th parallel. The 37th parallel extends from Newport News, VA, to Santa Cruz, CA, running along the northern border of North Carolina to the northern border of Arizona and including most of California. If a person moves from a higher risk area to a lower risk area, the risk is lowered only if the move occurs prior to adolescence. Certain outbreaks or clusters of MS have been identified, but their significance is unknown. MS is also most prevalent in North America, New Zealand, Australia, and Europe, although the reasons for this are unknown (National Multiple Sclerosis Society, 2012).

Viral: A virus is the triggering agent that causes demyelination and inflammation. Some suggest that mycobacteria, which have some virus-like qualities, might be the cause.

Genetic: Although MS is not hereditary, a genetic marker has been shown to increase the chances of developing MS. If a person has a genetic predisposition to MS and is exposed to a triggering environmental agent, an autoimmune response is more likely to develop.

Systems Affected

MS is a disease of the central nervous system (brain and spinal cord); therefore any system that is directly related to the CNS has the possibility of being affected (s110 Structure of Brain, s120 Spinal Cord and Related Structures). The term "possibility" is used because the course and symptoms of MS vary in severity from person to person, and sometimes from day to day. The primary symptoms are the direct result of demyelination: weakness (b730 Muscle Power Functions); numbness (b840 Sensation Related to the Skin); tingling (b840 Sensation Related to the Skin); tremor (b765 Involuntary Movement Functions); visual problems (double and/or blurry vision) (b210 Seeing Functions); pain (b280 Sensation of Pain); paralysis (b760 Control of Voluntary Movement Functions); poor balance (b755 Involuntary Movement Reaction Functions, d415 Maintaining a Body Position); bowel and bladder dysfunction (b610-b639 Urinary Functions, b525 Defecation Functions); slurred speech (b320 Articulation Functions, b330 Fluency and Rhythm of Speech Functions); decline in cognitive functioning, including reasoning, memory, and processing (b163 Basic Cognitive Functions, b164 Higher-Level Cognitive Functions, b140 Attention Functions, b144 Memory Functions); and dysphagia (b510 Ingestion Functions).

MS symptoms can be aggravated by external variables unrelated to the internal MS disease process. The most common things that aggravate MS symptoms include heat, fatigue, and stress.

Heat: Heat (e225 Climate) from any source, as varied as sunbathing, hot tubs, opening the oven door, a hot shower, or hot weather, worsens MS symptoms. Heat and humidity cause the myelin sheath to conduct electricity less efficiently. Uhthoff's symptom is an increase in blurry vision (b210 Seeing Functions) when the body becomes overheated (Guthrie & Nelson, 1995). This, along with other heat-related symptoms, disappears once the heat is removed and the body's core temperature is brought down. Interestingly, the National MS Society says that the cost of an air conditioner may be tax deductible if a physician writes a prescription. Cold temperatures can also cause problems with spasticity (b765 Involuntary Movement Functions), while cool weather with temperatures in the 60s or 70s seems to provide an optimal environment. In addition, involvement in aquatic programs in a cool pool has been found to help with nerve conduction, thus improving functioning (Kargarfard et al., 2012).

Fatigue: Fatigue (b455 Exercise Tolerance Functions) is one of the major complaints of MS making it both a symptom and something that makes the other symptoms worse. It is not the typical fatigue that a person experiences after a long day. It is an extreme fatigue that affects motivation (b130 Energy and Drive Functions) and the ability to perform daily activities (d230 Carrying Out Daily Routine), not to mention significantly impacting the person's desire and ability to participate in recreation and leisure activities. This type of fatigue seems to be unique to people who have MS. It typically occurs every day and gets worse as the day progresses, despite the activity level of the day. Researchers are still not sure if the fatigue is due to the MS process or another variable such as lack of proper nutrition, lack of adequate sleep, medication, depression, or stress.

Stress: Stressful events and poorly controlled stress levels (d240 Handling Stress and Other Psychological Demands) can lead to exacerbations in MS symptoms (Ackerman et al., 2002; Ackerman et al., 2003).

Secondary Problems

Secondary complications include bowel and bladder dysfunction (b525 Defecation Functions, b610-b639 Urinary Functions), sexual dysfunction (b640 Sexual Functions), muscle atrophy (b730 Muscle Power Functions), poor postural alignment and trunk control (b760 Control of Voluntary Movement Functions), muscle contractures and loss of range of motion (b710 Mobility of Joint Functions), osteoporosis and fractures (s750 Structure of Lower Extremity, s760 Structure of Trunk), respiratory problems (b440-b449 Functions of the Respiratory System), depression (b152 Emotional Functions), decubitus ulcers (b810 Protective Functions of the Skin), deep vein thrombosis (b4303 Clotting Functions), decreased cardiovascular endurance and increase in cardiovascular disease (b455 Exercise Tolerance Functions), orthostatic hypotension (b420 Blood Pressure Functions), pneumonia (b440 Respiration Functions), and spasticity (b735 Muscle Tone Functions).

Common tertiary symptoms in social, vocational, emotional, and psychological areas are caused by the other symptoms. These symptoms include problems with relationships (d7 Interpersonal Interactions and Relationships), driving (d475 Driving), and working (d840-d859 Work and Employment). People also find MS challenges their ability to cope and adjust (d240 Handling Stress and Other Psychological Demands) because of the unpredictable nature of the disease. Emotional and psychological issues that commonly arise include depression (b130 Energy and Drive Functions, b152 Emotional Functions), anxiety (b152 Emotional Functions), and changes in personality (b126 Temperament and Personality Functions), behavior (b125 Dispositions and Intra-Personal Functions), and difficulty solving problems (d175 Solving Problems). These changes may be a direct result of the lesions or from inadequate adaptive coping mechanisms.

Prognosis

The impact that MS has on the individual varies due to the wide range of possible dysfunction, as well as the unpredictability of the disease. Although MS can be defined by four disease courses, it can be difficult to know when exacerbations will occur and how much function will be lost or regained. The prognosis is quite variable and is dependent on the frequency and location of the inflammatory attacks. The site of the inflammatory attack is important because once a certain area of the central nervous system has been attacked, it is more likely to be attacked again. Each subsequent attack leads to more damage to that area. Attacks to critical areas, such as the cervical spine, are more likely to result in physical disability. Because therapies are now available that can effectively stop the inflammatory process, early diagnosis and treatment are important in limiting the impact of MS.

For an individual with MS, the disease makes planning of any kind more difficult, whether that is life planning or day-to-day planning. It is estimated that approximately 95% of people with MS have a normal life expectancy. If a person with MS dies early, it is often due to secondary problems of the disease, such as pneumonia or cardiovascular disease. MS by itself is rarely fatal (National Multiple Sclerosis Society, 2012).

At the present time, MS does not have a cure, although cases of spontaneous remyelination have been seen and medication has helped in slowing down exacerbations or decreasing the duration of the attack. Unpredictable symptoms can have serious effects on the family of a person with MS. People may be unable to work while at the same time accruing high medical bills, as well as additional expenses for home and vehicle modifications, housekeeping, or homecare. The emotional impact on both the person and the family can be overwhelming. Support groups and counseling for people with MS and their families and friends may help in developing appropriate coping skills.

Assessment

Typical Scope of Team Assessment

The first step is to confirm the diagnosis of MS, as described earlier. After that, the treatment team evaluates the course of the disease and the impact of the primary, secondary, and tertiary symptoms on life tasks. The types of assessments vary depending upon observed losses. Some standardized questionnaires that have been utilized with individuals with MS include:

Multiple Sclerosis Functional Composite (MSFC): The MSFC is a commonly used outcome measure used in MS clinical research (Fischer et al., 1999). It is a valid, multidimensional battery that incorporates clinical assessment of ambulation, arm function, and cognition.

Profile of Mood States (POMS): The POMS (McNair, Lorr, & Droppleman, 1992) has 65 items and measures six mood states (tension-anxiety, depression-dejection, anger-hostility, vigor-activity, fatigue-inertia, and confusion-bewilderment) using a scale that ranges from "not at all" to "extremely."

Multiple Sclerosis Impact Scale (MSIS-29): This scale examines the impact that MS has on the individual, both physically (20 questions) and psychosocially (nine questions), and is sensitive to change over time (Hobart et al., 2001).

Fatigue Severity Scale (FSS): The FSS (Krupp et al., 1989) contains nine items and measures the impact of fatigue on the individual's daily function.

Multiple Sclerosis Self-Efficacy (MSSE): The MSSE (Rigby et al., 2003) measures self-efficacy related to overcoming MS-specific challenges for individuals with MS, and has 14 items.

Multiple Sclerosis Neuropsychological Screening Questionnaire (MSNQ): Utilizes a 15-item self-report questionnaire that can be completed by the individual and a family member and does not require a neuropsychologist or rehabilitation professionals to administer or score (Benedict et al., 2003).

Incapacity Status Scale (ISS): The ISS (International Federation of Multiple Sclerosis Societies, 1985) is a 15-item self-administered questionnaire that assesses general functioning in activities of daily living, including bladder control and bowel movements, mobility and transfers, bathing, dressing, grooming, speech, hearing, vision, cognitive and intellectual functions, fatigue, sexual activity and function, and eating.

In order to help an individual maintain a personally meaningful leisure lifestyle, some of the more commonly used recreational therapy assessments may also be used. These tools may help the recreational therapist address the interests and expectations of the individual in light of their limitations (burlingame & Blaschko, 2010). Some recreational therapy-specific assessments that are appropriate to use with individuals with MS include:

Comprehensive Evaluation in Recreational Therapy — Physical Disabilities (CERT-PhysDis): The CERT-PhysDis can be used to establish a starting point for each person's functional skills as they relate to their leisure activities (Parker et al., 1975). It measures functional ability in eight areas (50 items total): (1) gross motor function, (2) fine motor function, (3) locomotion, (4) motor skills, (5) sensory, (6) cognition, (7) communication, and (8) behavior.

Functional Assessment of Characteristics for Therapeutic Recreation — Revised (FACTR-R): The FACTR-R is used to determine the areas where the person has need of improvement in terms of their functional skills and behaviors (Peterson et al., 2002). It measures 11 areas each in three domains (33 items total): physical, cognitive, and social/emotional.

Areas of Concern for RT Assessment

The RT initial evaluation will typically reflect:

Safety concerns: Initiation of and participation in complex community activities may cause safety concerns (d571 Looking After One's Safety), which the person may or may not understand because of cognitive dysfunctions. Furthermore, thermosensitivity (b2700 Sensitivity to Temperature) may cause an exacerbation of symptoms, thus reducing participation in order to avoid over- or under-heating (Thielke et al., 2012).

Patterns of decreased physical activity: As dysfunction and fatigue advance, completing everyday tasks (d230 Carrying Out Daily Routine) requires more time and energy. The person is forced to prioritize activities because of limited energy and function. Consequently, basic self-care, work, and homemaking skills are most often chosen, while recreational pursuits, community tasks, and maintaining relationships are sacrificed (d7 Interpersonal Interactions and Relationships, d9 Community, Social, and Civic Life). Individuals with MS are more likely to be less physically active than individuals without disabilities (Motl, McAuley, & Snook, 2005).

Functional skill impairments: A number of functional skills may be affected by MS (Freeman, 2001). Reduced coordination (b760 Control of Voluntary Movement Functions), ataxic gait (b770 Gait Pattern Functions), and difficulty with balance (b755 Involuntary Movement Reaction Functions, d415 Maintaining a Body Position) are all possible findings, as are tremors of the upper extremity. Upper extremity tremors and spasticity (b765 Involuntary Movement Functions) may significantly impair the person's ability to perform functional tasks of writing (d170 Writing), typing (d360 Using Communication Devices and Techniques), fine crafts (d9203 Crafts), and small object manipulation (d440 Fine Hand Use). Blurry and/or double vision (b210 Seeing Functions) are common visual problems associated with MS.

Therapists typically wait a few days to see if the problem resolves or minimizes before addressing adaptations since it may be transient. If the problem appears to be permanent, an ophthalmologist consult is sought for further evaluation.

Social participation limitations: Participation in life activities (choose specific activity code), leisure and recreation (d920 Recreation and Leisure), and community activities (d910 Community Life) may have been reduced in order to focus on symptom management (Gulick, 1997). This could lead to secondary problems due to limited participation in enjoyable activities.

Fatigue: Fatigue (b455 Exercise Tolerance Functions) is often identified as the most disabling symptom of MS, and occurs in 75-95% of individuals with MS (Kos et al., 2007). Even simple tasks may cause fatigue that greatly impacts the person's ability to participate in life activities (Freal, Kraft, & Coryell, 1984).

Stress: Disease-related stress (d240 Handling Stress and Other Psychological Demands) can be exacerbated by the unpredictable nature of the disease course and loss of ability (Fischer et al., 1994). Since there is a progression of dysfunction, the person constantly has to make adjustments (d230 Carrying Out Daily Routine) to work, family role, self-care, leisure, recreation, and other life tasks. The anticipation of further dysfunction, along with current life stressors, often results in anxiety and depression (b126 Temperament and Personality Functions) expressed through behavior, verbalizations, or physical symptoms. Stress may also exacerbate other MS symptoms (Nisipeanu & Korczyn, 1993).

Cognitive dysfunction: Memory (b144 Memory Functions), word finding and other language issues (b167 Mental Functions of Language), reasoning (b163 Basic Cognitive Functions), and processing information (b163 Basic Cognitive Functions) may be affected (Bobholz & Rao, 2003). This impacts the person's ability to perform instrumental activities of daily living, such as using the telephone (d360 Using Communication Devices and Techniques), balancing a checkbook (b172 Calculation Functions), and using reference materials (b164 Higher-Level Cognitive Functions). Cognitive dysfunction may also impact maintenance of employment (d840-d859 Work and Employment), independence in home and community (d2 General Tasks and Demands, d7

Interpersonal Interactions and Relationships, d8 Major Life Areas, d9 Community, Social, and Civic Life), and education attainment (d810-d839 Education).

Mood issues: Psychosocial challenges associated with MS include clinical depression (b152 Emotional Functions), anxiety (b152 Emotional Functions), sexual dysfunction (d770 Intimate Relationships, b640 Sexual Functions), cognitive changes (b110-b139 Global Mental Functions, b140-b189 Specific Mental Functions), and demoralization (b152 Emotional Functions) associated with MS-related losses. Depression is the most common psychiatric disorder in MS. The depression can be related to the loss of perceived quality of life and impact self-care and adherence to disease modifying therapies. Numerous studies estimate that between 36% and 60% of people with MS will experience an episode of major depression at some point during their lifetime (Group, 2005; Sadovnick et al., 1996; Schiffer et al., 1983; Sullivan et al., 1995).

Resource awareness deficit: Many people might have their first therapy experience after having had MS for a number of years. Therefore, their level of resource awareness (choose specific Environmental Factor code) may be minimal in the area of personal and community resources. Any lack of appropriate adapted equipment should also be documented using the related Environmental Factors code.

ICF Core Set

A brief and comprehensive ICF Core Set for MS is available to help guide the therapist in identifying diagnosis-related ICF codes.

Treatment Direction

Typically people are not admitted to an inpatient stay unless they have moderate to severe loss of function. People with minimal dysfunction are usually seen on an outpatient basis or in adapted recreation settings.

Whole Team Approach

There are several therapies used to treat multiple sclerosis, but so far, there is no cure. Medications are used to modify the disease course, to treat exacerbations, to manage symptoms, and to help improve functional status. Because of the complex nature of the disease and the varying course for each individual comprehensive care is recommended.

The pharmacological agents currently approved to treat MS are known as disease modifying agents (DMAs). These are (National Multiple Sclerosis Society, 2012)

- Aubagio (teriflunomide)
- Avonex (interferon beta-1a)
- Betaseron (interferon beta-1b)
- Copaxone (glatiramer acetate)
- Extavia (interferon beta-1b)
- Gilenya (fingolimod)
- Novantrone (mitoxantrone)
- Rebif (interferon beta-1a)
- Tysabri (natalizumab)

These medications have different efficacy rates and studies are ongoing to determine their long-term effects. All of the first generation of DMAs were injectables (interferons and glatiramer acetate). Of the newer medications, Tysabri is administered by infusion, and Gilenya is the first oral agent. The newest MS medication is Aubagio, a tablet taken daily. Not all people with MS respond to these therapeutic agents, and even with appropriate use of the disease modifying agents, they may continue to experience exacerbations and subsequent disability. Changes caused by the DMAs can be documented using the affected ICF code.

Other recent developments in the treatment of MS include two medications that treat typical problematic symptoms. Ampyra (dalfampridine) was the first medication to treat a symptom of MS and has been shown to improve walking by increasing walking speed (d450 Walking) (Ness, 2011). Nuedexta (dextromethorphan and quinidine) has been shown to treat pseudobulbar affect, which is a neurological disorder that manifests as irregular bouts of anger, crying, laughing, or irritability (b125 Dispositions and Intra-Personal Functions, b126 Temperament and Personality Functions) (Ness, 2011).

An exacerbation of MS, or an acute attack, is generally considered an event that needs treatment. To be considered a true exacerbation, the acute attack must last at least 24 hours and also is separated from a previous exacerbation by at least 30 days. An exacerbation can last from a few days to several weeks, and sometimes lasts for several months.

During acute attacks, people with MS are frequently treated with corticosteroids in order to end the attack sooner and minimize the damage caused by inflammation.

Disease modifying agents are effective in reducing the progression of the disease, but currently do not stop the disease completely. As multiple sclerosis progresses, a person may experience a variety of symptoms. The symptoms of MS vary greatly from person to person, and have a variable course in each individual as well. Most symptoms can be successfully managed with strategies that include pharmaceutical agents, self-care techniques, the use of assistive devices, and therapy with a physical or occupational therapist, speech/language pathologist, recreational therapist, cognitive remediation specialist, and others.

Recreational Therapy Approach

Therapists follow the team approach and address prevention of further secondary and tertiary complications. Given the time constraints often associated with providing treatment and the progressive nature of MS, the therapist often prioritizes adaptation and prevention. During inpatient rehabilitation stays, people typically have a two- to three-week stay and receive a total of six to nine hours of recreational therapy. In outpatient, day treatment, or adapted recreation settings, the length of treatment may be considerably longer. Recreational therapy is also provided in long-term care settings, including adult day programs, assisted living, and skilled nursing facilities.

Recreational Therapy Interventions

Precautions

There are several key safety concerns that recreational therapists should be aware of when programming for and treating individuals with MS.

These precautions typically relate to exercise-based interventions, but are important to know, as many interventions have some type of exercise or physical activity.

Autonomic dysfunction: Precautions about exercise in MS include an autonomic dysfunction in response to exercise, referred to as the pressor response (Anema et al., 1992). Some individuals with MS have a blunted cardiovascular response to isometric handgrip exercises. This suggests that some persons with MS may not be able to sustain adequate perfusion to muscles during exercise, potentially resulting in inability to maintain exercise, as well as the risk of exercise-induced syncope (Pepin et al., 1996).

Thermosensitivity: If thermosensitivity was found during assessment, it requires significant attention from the recreational therapist, as heat and cold can be problematic for individuals with MS (Thielke et al., 2012), and body temperature may rise or fall during RT interventions based on the activity and energy requirements. Individuals with MS should limit temperature rise by lowering core temperature with precooling prior to exercise or intentional cooling during exercise. Methods for precooling or cooling used by individuals with MS include immersion in cold water, cold showers, ice packs, iced drinks, and use of artificial cooling systems (Petajan & White, 2000; White, Davis, & Wilson, 2003; White, Wilson, Davis, & Petajan, 2000).

Interventions

Frequently implemented interventions with people who have MS include the following.

Resistance training: Lack of strength may have significant functional repercussions for mobility in this population and exercise protocols that emphasize strengthening may help offset this. Resistance training has been studied and has shown that it can improve weakness due to inactivity (b730 Muscle Power Functions) (Svensson, Gerdle, & Elert, 1994). Longer-term progressive resistive exercise has demonstrated improvements in functional tasks, such as ambulation and stair climbing, as well as quantitative improvements in muscle strength of the limbs being exercised (Broekmans et al., 2011; Learmonth et al., 2012). In another study, a supervised resistance training program gave MS patients stronger muscles (b730 Muscle Power Functions), better walking ability (d450 Walking), and left them with fewer episodes of fatigue (b455 Exercise Tolerance Functions) and disability (White et al., 2004).

Exercise therapy: Exercise in many forms has demonstrated benefits in improving mobility (d4 Mobility) and upper extremity tremors (b765 Involuntary Movement Functions), as well as numerous other benefits (Beer, Khan, & Kesselring, 2012; Sung et al., 2012). Persons with MS are reported to have reduced strength compared to non-MS controls (Ponichtera et al., 1992).

Exercise can also help with fatigue (b455 Exercise Tolerance Functions) that is prevalent in individuals with MS. Recreational therapy interventions can include exercise and energy conservation techniques to help reduce the effects of fatigue (d230 Carrying Out Daily Routine).

In a 2002 study, researchers compared two groups of MS patients, one who underwent aerobic exercise and a control group. Among other things, the study group had improvements in their health perceptions (b126 Temperament and Personality Functions), increased general daily activity levels (d230 Carrying Out Daily Routine and other codes), and less fatigue (b455 Exercise Tolerance Functions). Additionally, favorable improvements were seen in hip adduction/abduction and internal/external rotation (b710 Mobility of Joint Functions) (Mostert & Kesselring, 2002).

A recent Cochrane review suggests that exercise therapy for people not experiencing an exacerbation can be beneficial in terms of strength (b730 Muscle Power Functions), fitness (b455 Exercise Tolerance Functions), improvements in walking (d450 Walking), and reduced time for transfers (d420 Transferring Oneself), as well as improvements in mood (b126 Temperament and Personality Functions) (Rietberg et al., 2005). However, caution should be taken while exercise training with individuals with MS as heat can exacerbate symptoms. Suggestions to manage heat while exercising include locating a number of movable fans in the temperature-controlled space where exercise is occurring, the use of cooling devices, and wearing light clothing (Petajan et al., 1996).

Aquatic therapy: The use of aquatic therapy (or exercising in water) has been examined as an effective intervention for MS (Kargarfard et al., 2012; Veenstra, Brasile, & Stewart, 2003). The buoyancy of the water decreases the amount of work the person has to perform, thus hypothetically limiting cumulative fatigue, while the coolness of the water limits thermosensitivity (Gehlsen et al., 1986; Kargarfard et al., 2012). The water may also provide a resistive element for ataxia and dysmetria (Apatoff, 1998).

Eastern techniques: Yoga and meditation are often recommended for individuals with MS (Morgante, 2005). Hatha yoga has been shown to significantly improve levels of stress and fatigue for individuals with MS (Oken et al., 2004). Mindfulness-based meditation also has been shown to significantly improve health-related quality of life and reduce depression, stress, and fatigue (Grossman et al., 2010). ICF codes addressed include b126 Temperament and Personality Functions, b455 Exercise Tolerance Functions, and d240 Handling Stress and Other Psychological Demands.

Mobility skills: Mobility skills addressed with this population will vary depending on mobility limitations and activities. Recreational therapists address mobility skills as they specifically relate to participation in life situations. This most commonly includes transfers (d420 Transferring Oneself), lifting and carrying objects (d430 Lifting and Carrying Objects), fine motor skills of the upper and lower extremities (d440 Fine Hand Use, d446 Fine Foot Use), walking (d450 Walking), moving around in different locations (d460 Moving Around in Different Locations), moving around using equipment (d465 Moving Around Using Equipment), and using transportation (d470 Using Transportation). Unresolved visual problems (b210 Seeing Functions) will require adaptations. The therapist helps the person identify, develop, and integrate compensatory strategies for vision as they relate to participation in specifically identified activities. This area of treatment can be related to the assessment of missing adaptation devices noted in the part of the recreational therapy assessment devoted to adequate resource awareness.

Socialization: Social relationships (d730-d779 Particular Interpersonal Relationships) are often sacrificed due to energy limitations and health issues related to MS (Khemthong, 2010; Motl, McAuley, Snook, & Gliottoni, 2009). Social relationships, specifically formation and participation in friendships (d710 Basic Interpersonal Interactions, d720 Complex Interpersonal Interactions), are important for health (Khemthong, 2010; Motl & McAuley, 2009). By identifying the person's interests, compatible social groups can be identified and built upon. Recreational therapists can help foster increased socialization and social relationships by developing interventions around these interests and by including the client's associated social groups in the treatment. Integration training that incorporates learned skills is ideal in many situations to facilitate social engagement. It is important to differentiate between social withdrawal associated with depression and the inability to socialize in one's usual manner due to MS symptoms or impairments.

It has also been demonstrated that improved socialization, through increased quality of life, can be positively impacted by comprehensive outpatient rehabilitation for people with progressive MS (Di Fabio et al., 1997). In one study, outpatient treatment was the sole predictor of positive outcomes for energy and fatigue (b130 Energy and Drive Functions, b455 Exercise Tolerance Functions), change in general health, social function, and social support (d7 Interpersonal Interactions and Relationships).

Adaptive recreation: Adaptive recreation is also a very appropriate health-promoting intervention for individuals with MS. Adaptive recreation is a wide and diverse field ranging from competitive action sports, such as wheelchair tennis and alpine skiing, to more relaxed recreational activities like fly-fishing and swimming. Recreational therapists employed in adaptive recreation settings provide opportunities for engagement, as well as provide interventions and equipment recommendations and training to facilitate healthy recreation activity participation. The role of the therapist is to facilitate the adaptation of the client's leisure interests to ensure the clients safety and to eliminate any possible barriers. Tasks may include identification of appropriate adaptive recreation opportunities, identification of possible barriers and safety issues, assembly and maintenance of required equipment, supervision and facilitation of activity, and leisure education. The primary interventions aimed at community integration are those tailored to the individual's needs and interests. Resource education, adapted activities, and community groups that are important to the individual should be explored. Many facilities that offer adaptive recreation will also offer services for individuals and their families so that the family can recreate together. Changes will usually be noted in ICF codes d910 Community Life, d920 Recreation and Leisure, and solving problems noted in Environmental Factors.

Energy conservation techniques: The use of energy conservation techniques, such as getting adequate sleep, involvement in a cardiovascular exercise program, avoiding heat, eating a healthy

diet, assessing the impact of medications with a physician, and managing stress, may assist with several symptoms of MS including fatigue management (Jalon et al., 2012; Thomas et al., 2010). ICF codes that may be improved include b455 Exercise Tolerance Functions, d230 Carrying Out Daily Routine, d240 Handling Stress and Other Psychological Demands, d570 Looking After One's Health, and d920 Recreation and Leisure.

Stress management: Stress management is especially important, as it has been demonstrated to decrease MS-related symptoms (Artemiadis et al., 2012). Intervention strategies include practicing progressive relaxation, tai chi, and prayer (Freeman, 2001). It is also important to pay attention to emotional health since MS fatigue may be associated with depression and stress (Gold & Irwin, 2009; Grossman et al., 2010; Ziemssen, 2009). Improvements can be documented by looking at changes in ICF codes b152 Emotional Functions and d240 Handling Stress and Other Psychological Demands.

Cognitive interventions: Short-term memory loss is a common problem associated with MS. Recreational therapists seek to improve short-term memory function through neuroplasticity interventions. Short-term memory loss can also be addressed with compensatory strategies. Cognition should be monitored and assessed, as deficits may not always be apparent or reported. Cognitive dysfunction is difficult to detect because language skills and intellectual function are generally preserved (Rao, 1995). Therapeutic interventions designed to restore functions through direct retraining have been developed and studied, with demonstrated improvement in memory (b144 Memory Functions), social behavior (d710-d729 General Interpersonal Interactions), and attention (b140 Attention Functions) (Allen et al., 1998; Benedict et al., 2001; Chiaravalloti, DeLuca, Moore, & Ricker, 2005; Chiaravalloti, Hillary, et al., 2005; Pepping & Ehde, 2005; Rodgers et al., 1996; Solari et al., 2004).

Computer-aided retraining of memory (b144 Memory Functions) and attention (b140 Attention Functions) with MS has also been demonstrated to be effective (Flavia et al., 2010; Solari et al., 2004). Teaching compensatory strategies, such as using intact skills or external aids, have been demonstrated to improve daily functioning (d2 General Tasks and Demands) (Khan & Gray, 2010). Techniques include cognitive restructuring, substitution strategies, scheduling and timelines, use of recording devices, memory strategies, templates for repeated tasks, organizational strategies, assistive technology, structured environments, and using quiet or less stimulating environments (National Clinical Advisory Board of the National Multiple Sclerosis Society, 2006). A study has also correlated premorbid cognitive leisure to cognitive reserve in MS (Sumowski et al., 2010). Individuals who engaged in more cognitive leisure before the development of MS were able to withstand more severe brain atrophy later in life after development of MS. Increased cognitive stimulation can help dampen the negative neurological effects of MS. Premorbid cognitive leisure such as reading and hobbies could be an independent source of cognitive reserve in people with neurodegenerative disease.

Life skills training: Persons living with MS can enhance their development and optimize their health and well-being through life skills training. The achievement of goals in physical, social, emotional, cognitive, and spiritual areas is integral to perceptions of optimal health and well-being. Life domains that are identified as important to achieving and maintaining optimal health and well-being are relationships (d730-d779 Particular Interpersonal Relationships), participating in everyday experiences of home life (d610-d629 Acquisition of Necessities; d630-d649 Household Tasks; d650-d669 Caring for Household Objects and Assisting Others), connections to the community (d910 Community Life) and work (d840-d859 Work and Employment) (Wilhite et al., 2004). The ability to cope emotionally (d240 Handling Stress and Other Psychological Demands) and experience quality of life does not appear to be correlated with severity of disease or disability among people with MS.

Resources

National Multiple Sclerosis Society

733 Third Avenue
New York, NY 10017
800-FIGHT-MS (800-344-4867)
www.nationalmssociety.org
The National Multiple Sclerosis Society provides helpful information on new research, techniques, and resources. The organization provides newsletters, information on a variety of help topics, current research, support groups, and much more. The website has information about living with MS, current research, and links for more information for friends, health professionals, and people with MS.

Multiple Sclerosis Association of America

706 Haddonfield Road
Cherry Hill, NJ 08002
webmaster@msassociation.org
www.mymsaa.org
Tel: 856-488-4500, 800-532-7667
Fax: 856-661-9797
This website has information about living with MS, current research, and links to the MSAA's magazine (*The Motivator*).

Multiple Sclerosis Foundation

6520 North Andrews Avenue
Ft. Lauderdale, FL 33309-2130
support@msfocus.org
www.msfocus.org
Tel: 954-776-6805, 888-MSFOCUS (888-673-6287)
Fax: 954-351-0630
This website is similar to those above, and it has a link to a monthly newsletter about education and information related to MS.

National Institute on Neurological Disease and Stroke

P.O. Box 5801
Bethesda, MD 20824
800-352-9424
www.ninds.nih.gov
This website provides information on current neurological research.

Multiple Sclerosis at the Open Directory Project

www.dmoz.org/Health/Conditions_and_Diseases/Neurological_Disorders/Demyelinating_Diseases/Multiple_Sclerosis/
This website has links to numerous online resources for individuals and healthcare professionals interested in MS.

Database for analysis and comparison of global data on the epidemiology of MS

www.atlasofms.org/
This website has information on the prevalence and incidence of MS, and the availability of resources worldwide for people with MS.

Abstract Index of the Cochrane Library

www.cochrane.org/reviews/en/topics/79.html

This website has a link to all Cochrane reviews related to MS. A great resource for evidence-based practice.

NIH listing of clinical trials related to MS

clinicaltrials.gov/search/term=Multiple+Sclerosis
This website lists all the current and past clinical trials related to MS that are funded by the National Institutes of Health.

Rocky Mountain Multiple Sclerosis Center

www.mscenter.org
This website provides information about the services offered at the Rocky Mountain MS Center, experts in the area of complementary and alternative medicine and MS, as well as extensive information on "Living Well with MS."

References

Ackerman, K. D., Heyman, R., Rabin, B. S., Anderson, B. P., Houck, P. R., Frank, E., & Baum, A. (2002). Stressful life events precede exacerbations of multiple sclerosis. *Psychosomatic Medicine, 64*(6), 916-920.

Ackerman, K. D., Stover, A., Heyman, R., Anderson, B. P., Houck, P. R., Frank, E., ... Baum, A. (2003). Relationship of cardiovascular reactivity, stressful life events, and multiple sclerosis disease activity. *Brain, Behavior, and Immunity, 17*(3), 141-151. doi: S0889159103000473 [pii].

Allen, D. N., Goldstein, G., Heyman, R. A., & Rondinelli, T. (1998). Teaching memory strategies to persons with multiple sclerosis. *Journal of Rehabilitation Research and Development, 35*(4), 405-410.

Anema, J. R., Heijenbrok, M. W., Faes, T. J., Heimans, J. J., Lanting, P., & Polman, C. H. (1992). Cardiovascular autonomic function in multiple sclerosis. *Journal of Neurological Sciences, 104*, 124-134.

Apatoff, B. R. (1998). Multiple sclerosis and exercise. In B. D. Jordan, P. Warren, & P. Tsairis (Eds.), *Sports neurology* (pp. 309-314). Philadelphia: Lippincott, Williams, & Wilkins.

Artemiadis, A. K., Vervainioti, A. A., Alexopoulos, E. C., Rombos, A., Anagnostouli, M. C., & Darviri, C. (2012). Stress management and multiple sclerosis: A randomized controlled trial. *Archives of Clinical Neuropsychology, 27*(4), 406-416.

Beer, S., Khan, F., & Kesselring, J. (2012). Rehabilitation interventions in multiple sclerosis: An overview. *Journal of Neurology, 259*(9), 1994-2008.

Benedict, R. H., Munschauer, F., Linn, R., Miller, C., Murphy, E., Foley, F., & Jacobs, L. (2003). Screening for multiple sclerosis cognitive impairment using a self-administered 15-item questionnaire. *Multiple Sclerosis, 9*(1), 95-101.

Benedict, R. H., Priore, R. L., Miller, C., Munschauer, F., & Jacobs, L. (2001). Personality disorder in multiple sclerosis correlates with cognitive impairment. *The Journal of Neuropsychiatry and Clinical Neurosciences, 13*(1), 70-76.

Bobholz, J. A. & Rao, S. M. (2003). Cognitive dysfunction in multiple sclerosis: A review of recent developments. *Current Opinion in Neurology, 16*(3), 283.

Broekmans, T., Roelants, M., Feys, P., Alders, G., Gijbels, D., Hanssen, I., ... Eijnde, B. O. (2011). Effects of long-term resistance training and simultaneous electro-stimulation on muscle strength and functional mobility in multiple sclerosis. *Multiple Sclerosis Journal, 17*(4), 468-477.

burlingame, j. & Blaschko, T. (2010). *Assessment tools for recreational therapy and related fields* (4th ed.). Ravensdale, WA: Idyll Arbor.

Chiaravalloti, N. D., DeLuca, J., Moore, N. B., & Ricker, J. H. (2005). Treating learning impairments improves memory performance in multiple sclerosis: A randomized clinical trial. *Multiple Sclerosis, 11*(1), 58-68.

Chiaravalloti, N. D., Hillary, F. G., Ricker, J. H., Christodoulou, C., Kalnin, A. J., Liu, W. C., ... DeLuca, J. (2005). Cerebral activation patterns during working memory performance in multiple sclerosis using fMRI. *Journal of Clinical and Experimental Neuropsychology, 27*(1), 33-54.

Di Fabio, R. P., Choi, T., Soderberg, J., & Hansen, C. R. (1997). Health-related quality of life for patients with progressive multiple sclerosis: Influence of rehabilitation. *Physical Therapy, 77*(12), 1704-1716.

Fischer, J., Foley, F., Aikens, J., Ericson, G., Rao, S., & Shindell, S. (1994). What do we really know about cognitive dysfunction, affective disorders, and stress in multiple sclerosis? A practitioner's guide. *Neurorehabilitation and Neural Repair, 8*(3), 151-164.

Fischer, J., Rudick, R., Cutter, G., & Reingold, S. (1999). The Multiple Sclerosis Functional Composite measure (MSFC): An integrated approach to MS clinical outcome assessment. *Multiple Sclerosis, 5*(4), 244-250.

Flavia, M., Stampatori, C., Zanotti, D., Parrinello, G., & Capra, R. (2010). Efficacy and specificity of intensive cognitive rehabilitation of attention and executive functions in multiple sclerosis. *Journal of the Neurological Sciences, 288*(1), 101-105.

Fox, R. J. (2010). Multiple Sclerosis. from http://www.clevelandclinicmeded.com/medicalpubs/disease management/neurology/multiple_sclerosis/.

Freal, J., Kraft, G., & Coryell, J. (1984). Symptomatic fatigue in multiple sclerosis. *Archives of Physical Medicine and Rehabilitation, 65*(3), 135.

Freeman, J. (2001). Improving mobility and functional independence in persons with multiple sclerosis. *Journal of Neurology, 248*(4), 255-259.

Gehlsen, G., Beekman, K., Assmann, N., Winant, D., Seidle, M., & Carter, A. (1986). Gait characteristics in multiple sclerosis: Progressive changes and effects of exercise on parameters. *Archives of Physical Medicine and Rehabilitation, 67*(8), 536-539.

Gold, S. M. & Irwin, M. R. (2009). Depression and immunity: Inflammation and depressive symptoms in multiple sclerosis. *Immunology and Allergy Clinics of North America, 29*(2), 309-320.

Grossman, P., Kappos, L., Gensicke, H., D'Souza, M., Mohr, D. C., Penner, I. K., & Steiner, C. (2010). MS quality of life, depression, and fatigue improve after mindfulness training: A randomized trial. *Neurology, 75*(13), 1141-1149. doi: 10.1212/WNL.0b013e3181f4d80d.

Group, G. C. (2005). The Goldman consensus statement on depression in multiple sclerosis. *Mult Scler., 11*, 328-333.

Gulick, E. E. (1997). Correlates of quality of life among persons with multiple sclerosis. *Nursing Research, 46*(6), 305.

Guthrie, T. C. & Nelson, D. A. (1995). Influence of temperature changes on multiple sclerosis: Critical review of mechanisms and research potential. *Journal of the Neurological Sciences, 129*(1), 1-8.

Hobart, J., Lamping, D., Fitzpatrick, R., Riazi, A., & Thompson, A. (2001). The Multiple Sclerosis Impact Scale (MSIS-29): A new patient-based outcome measure. *Brain, 124*(Pt 5), 962-973.

International Federation of Multiple Sclerosis Societies. (1985). *Incapacity Status Scale: Minimal record of disability for multiple sclerosis.* New York.

Jalon, E. G. G., Lennon, S., Peoples, L., Murphy, S., & Lowe-Strong, A. (2012). Energy conservation for fatigue management in multiple sclerosis: A pilot randomized controlled trial. *Clinical Rehabilitation, 27*(1), 63-74.

Kargarfard, M., Etemadifar, M., Baker, P., Mehrabi, M., & Hayatbakhsh, M. (2012). Effect of aquatic exercise training on fatigue and health-related quality of life in patients with multiple sclerosis. *Archives of Physical Medicine and Rehabilitation, 93*(10), 1701-1708.

Khan, F. & Gray, O. (2010). Disability management and rehabilitation for persons with multiple sclerosis. *Neural Regeneration Research, 5*(4), 301-309.

Khemthong, S. (2010). Influence of fatigue on leisure and quality of life in women with chronic conditions. *Annual in Therapeutic Recreation, 18*, 79-86.

Kos, D., Duportail, M., D'Hooghe, M., Nagels, G., & Kerckhofs, E. (2007). Multidisciplinary fatigue management programme in multiple sclerosis: A randomized clinical trial. *Multiple Sclerosis, 13*(8), 996-1003. doi: 1352458507078392 [pii] 10.1177/1352458507078392.

Krupp, L. B., LaRocca, N. G., Muir-Nash, J., & Steinberg, A. D. (1989). The Fatigue Severity Scale. Application to patients with multiple sclerosis and systemic lupus erythematosus. *Archives of Neurology, 46*(10), 1121-1123.

Learmonth, Y., Paul, L., Miller, L., Mattison, P., & McFadyen, A. (2012). The effects of a 12-week leisure centre-based, group exercise intervention for people moderately affected with multiple sclerosis: A randomized controlled pilot study. *Clinical Rehabilitation, 26*(7), 579-593.

McNair, D. M., Lorr, M., & Droppleman, L. F. (1992). *Manual for the Profile of Mood States.* San Diego: EdITS/Educational and Industrial Testing Service.

Morgante, L. (2005). Healthy living with multiple sclerosis. *MS in Focus 5,* 4-5.

Mostert, S. & Kesselring, J. (2002). Effects of a short-term exercise training program on aerobic fitness, fatigue, health perception and activity level of subjects with multiple sclerosis. *Multiple Sclerosis, 8*(2), 161-168.

Motl, R. W. & McAuley, E. (2009). Pathways between physical activity and quality of life in adults with multiple sclerosis. *Health Psychology, 28*(6), 682.

Motl, R. W., McAuley, E., & Snook, E. M. (2005). Physical activity and multiple sclerosis: A meta-analysis. *Multiple Sclerosis, 11*(4), 459.

Motl, R. W., McAuley, E., Snook, E. M., & Gliottoni, R. C. (2009). Physical activity and quality of life in multiple sclerosis: Intermediary roles of disability, fatigue, mood, pain, self-efficacy and social support. *Psychology Health and Medicine, 14*(1), 111-124.

National Clinical Advisory Board of the National Multiple Sclerosis Society. (2006). *Assessment & management of cognitive impairment in MS.* Professional Resource Center.

National Institute of Neurological Disorders and Stroke. (2010). Multiple sclerosis: Hope through research. Retrieved from http://www.ninds.nih.gov/disorders/multiple_sclerosis/detail_ multiple_sclerosis.htm#159003215.

National Multiple Sclerosis Society. (2012). Multiple sclerosis: About MS. Retrieved from http://www.nationalmssociety.org/about-multiple-sclerosis/what-we-know-about-ms/treatments/index.aspx.

Ness, S. (2011). Significant advances in multiple sclerosis treatment. *Pharmacy Times.* Published online at http://www.pharmacytimes.com/publications/specialty-pt/2011/February-2011/SPT-NPP-0211.

Nisipeanu, P. & Korczyn, A. (1993). Psychological stress as risk factor for exacerbations in multiple sclerosis. *Neurology, 43*(7), 1311-1311.

Northrop, D. E. & Frankel, D. (Eds.). (2010). *Serving individuals with multiple sclerosis in adult day programs: Guidelines and recommendations.* National Multiple Sclerosis Society Professional Resource Center.

Oken, B. S., Kishiyama, S., Zajdel, D., Bourdette, D., Carlsen, J., Haas, M., … Mass, M. (2004). Randomized controlled trial of yoga and exercise in multiple sclerosis. *Neurology, 62*(11), 2058-2064.

Parker, R. A., Ellison, C. H., Kirby, T. F., & Short, M. J. (1975). The comprehensive evaluation in recreational therapy scale: A tool for patient evaluation. *Therapeutic Recreation Journal, 9*(4), 143-152.

Pepin, E. B., Hicks, R. W., Spencer, M. K., Tran, Z. V., & Jackson, C. G. R. (1996). Pressor response to isometric exercise in patients with multiple sclerosis. *Medicine & Science in Sports & Exercise, 28*(6), 656.

Pepping, M. & Ehde, D. M. (2005). Neuropsychological evaluation and treatment of multiple sclerosis: The importance of a neuro-rehabilitation focus. *Physical Medicine and Rehabilitation Clinics of North America, 16*(2), 411-436, viii. doi: 10.1016/j.pmr.2005.01.009.

Petajan, J. H., Gappmaier, E., White, A. T., Spencer, M. K., Mino, L., & Hicks, R. W. (1996). Impact of aerobic training on fitness and quality of life in multiple sclerosis. *Annals of Neurology, 39*(4), 432-441. doi: 10.1002/ana.410390405.

Petajan, J. H. & White, A. T. (2000). Motor-evoked potentials in response to fatiguing grip exercise in multiple sclerosis patients. *Clinical Neurophysiology, 111*(12), 2188-2195.

Peterson, C. A., Dunn, J., Carruthers, C., & burlingame, j. (2002). Functional assessment of characteristics for therapeutic recreation, revised. In j. burlingame & T. M. Blaschko (Eds.), *Assessment tools for recreational therapy and related fields* (4th ed., pp. 364-375). Ravensdale, WA: Idyll Arbor.

Polman, C. H., Reingold, S. C., Edan, G., Filippi, M., Hartung, H. P., Kappos, L., … Wolinsky, J. S. (2005). Diagnostic criteria for multiple sclerosis: 2005 revisions to the "McDonald Criteria". *Annals in Neurology, 58*(6), 840-846. doi: 10.1002/ana.20703.

Ponichtera, J. A., Rodgers, M. M., Glaser, R. M., Mathews, T. A., & Camaione, D. N. (1992). Concentric and eccentric isokinetic lower extremity strength in persons with multiple sclerosis. *The Journal of Orthopaedic and Sports Physical Therapy, 16*(3), 114-122.

Rao, S. M. (1995). Neuropsychology of multiple sclerosis. *Current Opinion in Neurology, 8*(3), 216-220.

Rietberg, M. B., Brooks, D., Uitdehaag, B. M., & Kwakkel, G. (2005). Exercise therapy for multiple sclerosis. *Cochrane Database systematic reviews* (1), CD003980. doi: 10.1002/14651858.CD003980.pub2.

Rigby, S. A., Domenech, C., Thornton, E. W., Tedman, S., & Young, C. A. (2003). Development and validation of a self-efficacy measure for people with multiple sclerosis: The Multiple Sclerosis Self-efficacy Scale. *Multiple Sclerosis, 9*(1), 73-81.

Rodgers, D., Khoo, K., MacEachen, M., Oven, M., & Beatty, W. W. (1996). Cognitive therapy for multiple sclerosis: A preliminary study. *Alternative Therapies in Health and Medicine, 2*(5), 70-74.

Sadovnick, A. D., Remick, R. A., Allen, J., Swartz, E., Yee, I. M., Eisen, K., … Paty, D. W. (1996). Depression and multiple sclerosis. *Neurology, 46*(3), 628-632.

Schiffer, R. B., Caine, E. D., Bamford, K. A., & Levy, S. (1983). Depressive episodes in patients with multiple sclerosis. *The American Journal of Psychiatry, 140*(11), 1498-1500.

Solari, A., Motta, A., Mendozzi, L., Pucci, E., Forni, M., Mancardi, G., & Pozzilli, C. (2004). Computer-aided retraining of memory and attention in people with multiple sclerosis: A randomized, double-blind controlled trial. *Journal of the Neurological Sciences, 222*(1), 99-104.

Sullivan, M. J., Weinshenker, B., Mikail, S., & Bishop, S. R. (1995). Screening for major depression in the early stages of multiple sclerosis. *The Canadian Journal of Neurological Sciences. Le Journal Canadien des Sciences Neurologiques, 22*(3), 228-231.

Sumowski, J. F., Wylie, G. R., Gonnella, A., Chiaravalloti, N., & Deluca, J. (2010). Premorbid cognitive leisure independently contributes to cognitive reserve in multiple sclerosis. *Neurology, 75*(16), 1428-1431. doi: 10.1212/WNL.0b013e3181f881a6.

Sung, C., Chiu, C. Y., Lee, E. J., Bezyak, J., Chan, F., & Muller, V. (2012). Exercise, diet, and stress management as mediators between functional disability and health-related quality of life in multiple sclerosis. *Rehabilitation Counseling Bulletin, 56*(85), 85-95.

Svensson, B., Gerdle, B., & Elert, J. (1994). Endurance training in patients with multiple sclerosis: Five case studies. *Physical Therapy, 74*(11), 1017-1026.

Thielke, S. M., Whitson, H., Diehr, P., O'Hare, A., Kearney, P. M., Chaudhry, S. I., … Sale, J. E. M. (2012). Persistence and remission of musculoskeletal pain in community-dwelling older adults: Results from the cardiovascular health study. *Journal of the American Geriatrics Society, 60*(8), 1393-1400.

Thomas, S., Thomas, P., Nock, A., Slingsby, V., Galvin, K., Baker, R., … Hillier, C. (2010). Development and preliminary evaluation of a cognitive behavioural approach to fatigue management in people with multiple sclerosis. *Patient Education and Counseling. 78*(2), 240-249.

Veenstra, J., Brasile, F., & Stewart, M. (2003). Perceived benefits of aquatic therapy for multiple sclerosis participants. *American Journal of Recreation Therapy, 2*(1), 33-48.

White, A. T., Davis, S. L., & Wilson, T. E. (2003). Metabolic, thermoregulatory, and perceptual responses during exercise after lower vs. whole body precooling. *Journal of Applied Physiology, 94*(3), 1039-1044.

White, A. T., Wilson, T. E., Davis, S. L., & Petajan, J. H. (2000). Effect of precooling on physical performance in multiple sclerosis. *Multiple Sclerosis, 6*(3), 176-180.

White, L. J., McCoy, S. C., Castellano, V., Gutierrez, G., Stevens, J. E., Walter, G. A., & Vandenborne, K. (2004). Resistance training improves strength and functional capacity in persons with multiple sclerosis. *Multiple Sclerosis, 10*(6), 668-674.

Wilhite, B., Keller, M. J., Hodges, J., & Caldwell, L. (2004). Enhancing human development and optimizing health and well-being in persons with multiple sclerosis. *Therapeutic Recreation Journal, 38*, 167-187.

Ziemssen, T. (2009). Multiple sclerosis beyond EDSS: Depression and fatigue. *Journal of the Neurological Sciences, 277*, S37-S41.

23. Neurocognitive Disorders

Juan Tortosa-Martinez and Daniel G. Yoder

Neurocognitive disorders (NCDs) were referred to in the *DSM-IV* as "Dementia, Delirium, and Other Cognitive Disorders." For the *DSM-5* these are all included as neurocognitive disorders. The first *DSM-5* classification in the NCD set is delirium, which is separated out because its onset is rapid, it can be traced to another acute medical condition, and the patient often returns to pre-delirium functioning after the condition is resolved. All the other diagnoses of NCDs are divided into major and mild NCD with descriptions of the underlying cause. These diagnoses usually have a more gradual onset and patients do not return to earlier levels of functioning (APA, 2013).

The *DSM-5* allows for the continued use of the term *dementia* in settings where patients and medical personnel are more familiar with that term, but strongly suggests that the term neurocognitive disorder be used where it is now accepted and replace dementia. The new term more accurately conveys the relationships between all of the possible instances of cognitive deficits. In addition, the ability to classify a mild NCD with a cause was not available in the *DSM-IV* (APA, 2013).

The primary diagnostic feature of each of the NCDs is a cognitive deficit. Other diagnoses may have some cognitive deficits, but the NCD category contains diagnoses that are primarily defined by an acquired cognitive decline — a deficit that was not present from birth or very early life. The other difference between NCDs and all the other *DSM-5* diagnoses is that the underlying pathology and frequently the etiology of the syndromes can potentially be determined. The subtypes included are NCD due to Alzheimer's disease, vascular NCD, NCD with Lewy bodies, NCD due to Parkinson's disease, frontotemporal NCD, NCD due to traumatic brain injury, NCD due to HIV infection, substance/medication induced NCD, NCD due to Huntington's disease, NCD due to prion disease,

NCD due to another medical condition, NCD due to multiple etiologies, and unspecified NCD (APA, 2013). Because recreational therapists are not primarily responsible for treating the underlying diseases, this chapter will focus on the deficits found in all of the NCDs and the RT treatment provided to deal with those deficits.

RTs need first to understand that NCDs are devastating. They progressively steal a person's happiness, relationships, dignity, and any potential contributions to family and community. A review of history shows a deplorable record of ignorance and intolerance that made the conditions even worse. Not too long ago NCDs were considered either a sign of demonic possession or punishment by God for unknown but surely terrible sins. While vestiges of those attitudes remain, NCDs are now largely seen as diseases that can impact people regardless of religion, gender, race, and economic status. The specifics of the deficits that are part of each diagnosis will be discussed in the section on Systems Affected.

Incidence/Prevalence in U.S.

The incidence of neurocognitive disease in older people is rapidly increasing and is creating serious concerns for families, caregivers, professionals, and others in public health systems (Haan & Wallace, 2004). In 2001, there were 24.3 million cases of NCD worldwide (Ferri et al., 2005) and in 2013, 44.4 million (Alzheimer's Disease International, 2013).

To understand the diagnoses, it is important to look at the prevalence of each cause of onset.

The overall prevalence of delirium in the community is just one to two percent. Among those being admitted to a hospital the incidence is 14-24%. The incidence arising during a hospital stay ranges from six percent to as high as 56% (Medscape, 2013d).

An estimated 5.2 million Americans of all ages had Alzheimer's disease in 2013. This included an estimated five million people age 65 and older and approximately 200,000 individuals younger than age 65. The onset of symptoms is most common when people are in their eighties and nineties. The number of Americans with Alzheimer's disease and other NCDs will grow as the U.S. population age 65 and older continues to increase. By 2025, the number of people age 65 and older with Alzheimer's disease is estimated to reach 7.1 million — a 40% increase from the five million age 65 and older currently affected (Alzheimer's Association, 2013a).

Vascular NCD is the second most common cause of NCD in the United States and Europe, but it is the most common form in some parts of Asia. The prevalence rate of vascular NCD is 1.5% in Western countries (affecting about 4.8 million people in the U.S.) and approximately 2.2% in Japan (Alzheimer's Association, 2013a).

Lewy body NCD is an umbrella term for two related diagnoses. It refers to both Parkinson's disease NCD and NCD with Lewy bodies. The earliest symptoms of these two diseases differ, but they reflect the same underlying biological changes in the brain. These NCDs affect an estimated 1.3 million people in the United States (Lewy Body Dementia Association, 2013). Parkinson's disease is estimated to affect nearly two percent of those older than age 65. The National Parkinson Foundation estimates that one million Americans have Parkinson's disease and that 50-80% percent of those with Parkinson's disease eventually experience Parkinson's disease NCD (Alzheimer's Association, 2013b).

Frontotemporal NCD is characterized by severe frontotemporal lobe degeneration. It is distinguished from Alzheimer's disease and Lewy body NCD based on the fact that it does not manifest with amyloid plaques, neurofibrillary tangles, or Lewy bodies (Lynch et al., 1994). In pre-senile (before age 65) cases it is second only to Alzheimer's disease in prevalence, accounting for 20% of the cases (Snowden, Neary, & Mann, 2002).

The incidence of HIV NCD in the Western world prior to the current drug regimen had a cumulative risk of 5-20%. After the treatments changed, the incidence dropped for a while, but is now on the rise again. The estimated number of people with HIV-related NCD is about 77,000 (Medscape, 2013c).

Several epidemiologic studies in the United States, conducted from 1945-1980, show consistent statistics stating that approximately 30,000 people have NCD related to Huntington's disease (Medscape, 2013b).

The other forms of NCD have lower numbers.

Predominant Age

The age of onset of NCD depends on the type of NCD but it is normally late in life, with the highest prevalence at 85 years and older (APA, 2013). Alzheimer's disease is divided into early onset, before 65 years of age, and late onset, after 65 years of age (APA, 2013). Early onset is uncommon. The incidence of Alzheimer's disease doubles every five years after 65 years of age (Querfurth & LaFerla, 2010).

The incidence of vascular NCD is slightly higher among men than among women and appears typically in those between 60 and 75 years of age. The prevalence of vascular NCD rises steeply with age (Alzheimer's Association, 2006). Lewy body and Parkinson's disease NCD also occur most frequently in those over 65.

The other forms of NCD have earlier onsets. Frontotemporal NCD, for example, is seen before age 65 in about 75% of the cases (APA, 2013).

Older adults are the most susceptible to delirium. Infants and children are more susceptible than people who are in early and middle adulthood (APA, 2013).

Causes

Alzheimer's disease is characterized by plaques forming in the brain. These plaques destroy brain cells, creating progressive deterioration of higher cognitive functioning in the areas of memory, problem solving, and thinking. It is characterized by an inability to carry out everyday tasks or perform instrumental activities of daily living (Rimmer & Smith, 2009).

Vascular NCD is caused by disruptions in the supply of blood to the brain (APA, 2013). These disorders may be the result of brain damage from multiple strokes, or infarcts, caused by small clots from heart or neck arteries that clog a branch of a blood vessel in the brain. The relationship between Alzheimer's disease and vascular NCD is complex; however, recent evidence suggests that small strokes may lead to increased clinical presence of Alzheimer's disease (Alzheimer's Association, 2006).

NCDs can also occur from other medical conditions such as Lewy body disease, Parkinson's disease, head trauma, HIV disease, Huntington's disease, Pick's disease, other general medical conditions, substance-induced NCD, and NCD due to multiple etiologies. Each of these conditions follows its own course, but what they all have in common is that brain cells or the connections between neurons are destroyed (APA, 2013).

Developing an NCD may be influenced by genetic, biological, and environmental risk factors. Age may be the most important risk factor for developing NCDs (Querfurth & LaFerla, 2010). Within genetic factors, the APOE e4 lipoprotein of the genetic sequence is associated with a higher risk of developing Alzheimer's disease (Podewils et al., 2005).

Lifestyle factors such as alcohol abuse, smoking, a high fat diet (Gustaw-Rothenberg, 2009), lack of physical activity (Larson et al., 2006; Laurin et al., 2001; Podewils et al., 2005; Rovio et al., 2005; Taaffe et al., 2008), lack of mental stimulation (Akbaraly et al., 2009; Carlson et al., 2008; Verghese et al., 2003; Wilson et al., 2007), and lack of social support and meaningful social networks (Fratiglioni, Paillard-Borg, & Winblad, 2004; Paillard-Borg et el., 2009; Scarmeas et al., 2001; Solfrizzi et al., 2008) through the life span may contribute to development of NCDs. Likewise, stress and depression may also contribute to the development of the disease (Green et al., 2003; Wilson et al., 2007).

For some NCDs, other factors are more important. Huntington's disease is genetic. HIV infections and substance-induced NCDs are usually caused by lifestyle choices.

Systems Affected

Domains

The *DSM-5* (APA, 2013) describes six cognitive domains that are affected by NCDs: complex attention, executive function, learning and memory, language, perceptual-motor abilities, and social cognition. For each of these domains, the *DSM-5* describes the symptoms and observations that mark a mild or major deficit.

Complex attention: In a mild case, the patient takes longer than they used to for tasks. They may need to double check more often, and they find thinking easier when there are fewer other things, such as TV, other conversations, or driving, competing for their attention. Major deficits include being easily distracted by other events in the environment to the extent of not being able to function. Input needs to be simplified to be understood. Even simple information, such as a phone number, may not be remembered. Mental calculations are not possible and all thinking takes longer than usual. The ICF codes that relate to complex attention include b140 Attention Functions, b144 Memory Functions, b156 Perceptual Functions, b160 Thought Functions, b164 Higher-Level Cognitive Functions, b172 Calculation Functions, b176 Mental Functions of Sequencing Complex Movements, d110 Watching, d115 Listening, d160 Focusing Attention, d163 Thinking, d175 Solving Problems, d210 Undertaking a Single Task, d220 Undertaking Multiple Tasks, and d9 Community, Social, and Civic Life.

Executive function: A mild NCD is diagnosed when the person requires increased effort to complete multistage projects; has trouble resuming a task after an interruption; requires extra effort to organize, plan, or make decisions; and/or finds large social gatherings more taxing because of increased effort required to follow shifting conversations. A person has a major NCD when they abandon complex projects, need to focus on one task at a time, and rely on others to plan instrumental activities of daily living or make decisions. The ICF codes that relate to executive function include b130 Energy and Drive Functions, b140 Attention Functions, b144 Memory Functions, b160 Thought Functions, b164 Higher-Level Cognitive Functions, b176 Mental Functions of Sequencing Complex Movements, b180 Experience of Self and Time Functions, d110 Watching, d115 Listening, d160 Focusing Attention, d163 Thinking, d175 Solving Problems, d177 Making Decisions, d210 Undertaking a Single Task, d220 Undertaking Multiple Tasks, d230 Carrying Out Daily Routine, d570 Looking After One's Health, d7 Interpersonal Interactions and Relationships, and d9 Community, Social, and Civic Life.

Learning and memory: In a mild NCD the person will have trouble recalling recent events. There is also increased reliance on list making, trouble keeping track of characters in a movie or novel, and some repetition of stories within a couple of weeks.

In a major NCD the person repeats within the same conversation, cannot keep track of even a short list of items when shopping, and requires frequent reminders to stay with the task at hand. Except in severe forms of NCDs, the person's early memories and implicit memory are preserved, even when recent memories are lost. The ICF codes that relate to learning and memory include b114 Orientation Functions, b117 Intellectual Functions, b140 Attention Functions, b144 Memory Functions, b164 Higher-Level Cognitive Functions, d160 Focusing Attention, d163 Thinking, d166 Reading, d170 Writing, d172 Calculating, and d175 Solving Problems.

Language: In a mild condition there is noticeable word finding difficulty and general terms are substituted for specific terms. The person may not use the names of acquaintances. There are subtle grammatical errors in articles, prepositions, and auxiliary verbs. In a major condition the person has significant difficulties with both expressive and receptive language. General terms are often used ("that thing") and general pronouns are used instead of names. Names of close friends and family are forgotten. Eventually the person may stop speaking altogether. The ICF codes that relate to language include b1142 Orientation to Person, b144 Memory Functions, b160 Thought Functions, b167 Mental Functions of Language, b330 Fluency and Rhythm of Speech Functions, and d3 Communication.

Perceptual-motor abilities: In mild cases the person relies more on maps and directions to get places, especially new places. The person can get lost more easily and has problems with spatial tasks such as carpentry, sewing, and knitting. Major cases present more of the same kind of difficulties to the point where previously familiar activities, such as using tools and going to familiar places, become a problem. Confusion can increase at dusk when the light levels change perceptions. The ICF codes that relate to perceptual-motor abilities include b1141 Orientation to Place, b140 Attention Functions, b147 Psychomotor Functions, b156 Perceptual Functions, b160 Thought Functions, b164 Higher-Level Cognitive Functions, b176 Mental Functions of Sequencing Complex Movements, d110 Watching, d115 Listening, d160 Focusing Attention, d175 Solving Problems, d210 Undertaking a Single Task, and d220 Undertaking Multiple Tasks.

Social cognition: Mild deficits include subtle changes in personality, behaviors, or attitudes. There is less ability to read facial expressions or recognize social cues. There are also changes in the way the person relates to others, often with less inhibition. Major deficits include behavior clearly outside of acceptable range. This can include insensitivity to dress, religious views, or sexual behaviors. There is an inability to react appropriately to cues from others during discussions or when doing things with them. Safety is not a consideration in decisions. The person has little insight into the changes that have taken place. The ICF codes that relate to social cognition include b1142 Orientation to Person, b122 Global Psychosocial Functions, b126 Temperament and Personality Functions, b152 Emotional Functions, b164 Higher-Level Cognitive Functions, b180 Experience of Self and Time Functions, d160 Focusing Attention, d163 Thinking, d3 Communication, d7 Interpersonal Interactions and Relationships, and d9 Community, Social, and Civic Life.

Other ICF consequences: The ICF codes that are affected by NCDs also include b134 Sleep Functions, b176 Mental Functions of Sequencing Complex Movements (which covers the apraxia seen in NCDs), b620 Urination Functions, d240 Handling Stress and Other Psychological Demands (caused by an increasing inability to do tasks), and d6 Domestic Life (because of diminished mental ability). ICF codes d840-d859 Work and Employment and d860-d879 Economic Life represent skills that present significant difficulties for a person with major NCD impairments.

Diagnoses

Different NCDs have different mixes of symptom domains, different onsets, and different courses of the disease. The following information is from the *DSM-5* (APA, 2013).

Delirium: Delirium requires a deficit in attention and an additional deficit in cognition found in any of the other domains described above. It must develop over a short period (hours or days) and fluctuate during the day. There must be evidence that there is some outside cause for the observed deficits, such as intoxication, withdrawal, fever, or other illness. The *ICD-9* and *ICD-10* provide codes for the type of substance in substance-induced delirium.

Major neurocognitive disorder: To diagnose a major NCD there must be evidence of a significant cognitive decline from a previous level of performance in one or more of the domains listed above. The decline can be based on the person's evidence, the reports of others, or an impairment documented by a standardized assessment or clinical observation. The cognitive deficit must interfere with the person's independence in everyday activities and not be associated with delirium or better explained by another mental disorder. Major neurocognitive disorders are then described by specifying what they are caused by, from the list below.

Mild neurocognitive disorder: Mild NCDs require evidence of modest decline from a previous level of performance in one or more of the cognitive areas described above. In this case the cognitive deficits do not stop the person from doing everyday activities, but greater effort, alternate strategies, or some kind of accommodation may be required. As with major NCDs, mild NCDs must not be associated with delirium or better explained by another mental disorder. The disorder is then described by specifying what they are caused by, from the list below.

Causes

Alzheimer's disease: Alzheimer's requires the criteria for a major or mild NCD with an insidious onset and gradual progression in one or more of the cognitive domains. Probable Alzheimer's is diagnosed when there is evidence of a genetic component from genetic testing or family history. Probable Alzheimer's is also diagnosed in a major NCD if there is evidence of a decline in memory, learning, and at least one other cognitive domain, and the decline is steady without extended plateaus. Possible Alzheimer's is diagnosed when the conditions for probable Alzheimer's are not met, but the decline is steady without plateaus.

Frontotemporal NCD: This requires the criteria for a major or mild NCD and an insidious onset and gradual progression. There are two variants. In the behavioral variant the person must have three or more symptoms from behavioral disinhibition, apathy, loss of sympathy or empathy, dietary changes, and behavior that is perseverative or ritualistic. There must also be a decline in social cognition and/or executive function. The language variant has a prominent decline in language abilities.

In either variant there must not be a significant decline in learning, memory, and perceptual-motor function.

Lewy bodies: This requires the criteria for a major or mild NCD and an insidious onset and gradual progression. In addition there is likely to be fluctuating cognition with pronounced variations, recurrent visual hallucinations, spontaneous features of parkinsonism that show up after the onset of cognitive decline, rapid eye movement sleep disorders, and/or severe neuroleptic sensitivity.

Vascular: This requires the criteria for a major or mild NCD. The onset must be consistent with a vascular etiology as demonstrated by being at the same time as a cerebrovascular event or the decline must be most significant in complex attention and executive functioning. There must also be evidence of cerebrovascular disease sufficient to account for the deficits.

Traumatic brain injury: This requires the criteria for a major or mild NCD and must have occurred as the result of a documented TBI.

Substance/medication-induced: This requires the criteria for a major or mild NCD. The impairments must last beyond a period of delirium and it must be reasonable to point to the particular medication or substance as a possible cause with the timing matching up with use of the medication or substance.

HIV infections: This requires the criteria for a major or mild NCD and a documented HIV infection. It must also not be better explained by non-HIV conditions.

Prion disease: This requires the criteria for a major or mild NCD and an insidious onset and rapid progression. Motor features are prominent.

Parkinson's disease: This requires the criteria for a major or mild NCD and an insidious onset and gradual progression. It must also be associated with established Parkinson's disease.

Huntington's disease: This requires the criteria for a major or mild NCD and an insidious onset and gradual progression. It must also be associated with established Huntington's disease or the risk of the disease based on family history or genetic testing.

Other causes: NCDs can also be caused by other medical conditions, multiple etiologies, or unspecified causes. For all of these the NCD must meet the criteria for a major or mild NCD.

Secondary Problems

Secondary problems associated with NCDs are mostly behavioral. Behavioral symptoms contribute significantly to the disability associated with the disease and place great physical and emotional burdens on caregivers (Suhr, Andersen, & Tranel, 1999). Agitation and anxiety (b152 Emotional Functions) are common in individuals with NCDs, which may lead to behaviors such as wandering, screaming, hitting, grabbing, or unwanted sexual advances, such as suggestive comments or touching (Putman & Wang, 2007). It is also common to observe passivity and apathy behaviors, which usually correspond to poor engagement in activities (Heyn, 2003). Other psychological symptoms may occur, such as paranoid delusions (b160 Thought Functions), hallucinations (b160 Thought Functions), or depression (b152 Emotional Functions) (Suhr, Andersen, & Tranel, 1999). Physical fitness is generally lower (b455 Exercise Tolerance Functions). In the later stages of NCDs, the patient will be unable to perform activities of daily living. Providing adequate nutrition is a significant concern.

The hippocampus is a key brain area for memory storage and processing, as well as for spatial orientation (Rothman & Mattson, 2010). Hippocampal atrophy has been shown in individuals with mild cognitive impairment (Lupien et al., 1998) and Alzheimer's disease (Dickerson et al., 2001; Fox et al., 1996).

Prognosis

Delirium is the only one of the NCDs that has the possibility for improved function. The majority of individuals with delirium have a full recovery (APA, 2013). Even so, it is not a hopeful picture for everyone. In patients who are admitted with delirium, mortality rates are 10-26%. Patients who develop delirium during hospitalization have a mortality rate of 22-76% (Medscape, 2013e). As many as 40% of people with delirium die within one year after diagnosis (APA, 2013).

The prognosis of the other NCDs is part of their definition — there is a continuous decline. Different etiologies lead to different rates of decline, but the NCDs do not show improvement. Xie, Brayne, and Matthews (2008) reported a 4.1 years median survival for men and 4.6 years for women diagnosed with NCDs. More recently, Rait et al. (2010)

estimated that people diagnosed with NCDs at age 60-69 had a median survival of 6.7 years, but only 1.9 years for people diagnosed at age 90 or over.

Alzheimer's disease is the sixth leading cause of death in the United States overall and the fifth leading cause of death for those aged 65 and older. It is the only cause of death among the top 10 in America where we haven't found a way to prevent it or cure it. Deaths from Alzheimer's increased 68% between 2000 and 2010, while deaths from other major diseases, including the number one cause of death (heart disease), decreased (Alzheimer's Association, 2013).

In patients with NCDs who have had a stroke, the increase in mortality is significant. The five-year survival rate is 39% for patients with a vascular NCD compared with 75% for age-matched controls (Brodaty et al. 1993). Vascular NCD is associated with a higher mortality rate than Alzheimer's, presumably because of the coexistence of other atherosclerotic diseases.

Assessment

Individuals with NCDs receive a complete physical and cognitive exam to establish the likely cause of the impairment and the stage of the disease.

Typical Scope of Team Assessment

Several classification systems are employed to group individuals with patterns of functional loss. The *DSM-5* divides NCDs into major and mild. The Alzheimer's Association (2009), using the then-appropriate term "dementia" in their classification, developed a more detailed, seven-stage framework to describe how a person's abilities change through time:

1. *No impairment*: The person does not experience memory problems and does not show any other evidence of symptoms of dementia that can be detected by a medical professional.
2. *Very mild decline*: The person starts to experience some memory lapses but symptoms of dementia can't be detected yet.
3. *Mild decline*: Some difficulties start to be noticed by family, friends, or co-workers. Medical professionals may be able to detect some memory or concentration problems. Difficulties in this stage may include problems remembering names, greater difficulties performing tasks in

social or work settings, and problems with planning and organizing.

4. *Moderate decline*: Medical professionals are able to detect several cognitive problems such as forgetfulness of recent events, impaired ability to perform challenging mental arithmetic functions, difficulty performing complex tasks, and mood swings or withdrawal, especially in challenging situations.

5. *Moderately severe decline*: Problems with memory and thinking become evident and the person may need help with daily activities. Difficulties at this stage include remembering their own address or phone number and confusion regarding why and where they are or what day it is. They typically do not require help with eating or using the toilet at this stage.

6. *Severe decline*: The person requires much more help with daily activities. Difficulties include problems remembering the names of spouses and caregivers. They may require help in dressing properly. Persons may also experience major changes in sleep patterns and are likely to experience major personality and behavioral changes.

7. *Very severe decline*: The person loses the ability to interact appropriately with the environment, carry on a conversation, and control movement. At this stage they need help with most daily activities including eating and using the toilet.

Rimmer and Smith (2009, p. 360) have identified and summarized three general progressive phases of the condition:

- *Phase 1*: Forgetting where items are placed, appointments, names, and other daily living and social tasks; having problems with organizing and planning. Forgetfulness usually causes anxiety.

- *Phase 2*: Confusion and intellectual impairment with short-term memory, greater difficulties with performing more complex tasks, problems concentrating, and problems with orientation. Mood disorders often become apparent.

- *Phase 3*: Increased involvement with delusions, agitation, loss of basic abilities, and incontinence. In this phase, individuals need assistance with activities of daily living.

Team assessments consist of several measurement instruments that will help determine individual characteristics of the client. After assessment, therapeutic goals will be determined and a course of action will be designed and implemented. Measurements and instruments researchers have used in the assessment of NCDs and related symptoms are described below. These instruments are relevant to setting goals for any therapeutic program, choosing the appropriate activity, and measuring the efficacy of the treatment. The authors correspond to the articles in which these instruments have been used for assessing patients with NCDs and can be consulted as an example of use in recreational therapy. These are not the authors that originally validated the instruments.

Cognitive function

- *Mini-Mental State Examination* (MMSE) (Onor et al., 2007)
- *Milan Overall Dementia Assessment* (MODA) (Onor et al., 2007)

Behavior

- *Daily Record of Behavior* (DRB) (Woodhead et al., 2005)
- *McCann Instrument* (Schreiner et al., 2005)
- *Need-Driven Dementia-Compromised Behavior* (NDB) model (Fitzsimmons & Buettner, 2002)

Affect

- *Observed Affect Scale* (Williams & Tappen, 2007)
- *Philadelphia Geriatric Center Affect Rating Scale* (Schreiner, Yamamoto, & Shiotani, 2005)

Mood

- *Dementia Mood Assessment Scale* (Williams & Tappen, 2007)
- *Alzheimer's Mood Scale* (Williams & Tappen, 2007)

Depression

- *Geriatric Depression Scale* (GDS) (Buettner and Fitzsimmons, 2002; Onor et al., 2007)
- *Hamilton Depression Rating Scale* (Teri et al., 2003)
- *Cornell Depression Scale for Depression in Dementia* (Teri, et. al., 2003)

Physical function

- *36-item Short Form Health Survey* (SF-36) (Teri et. al., 2003)
- *Sickness Impact Profile* (SIP) (Teri et. al., 2003)
- *Global Deterioration Scale* (GDS) (Fitzsimmons & Buettner, 2002; Buettner, Fitzsimmons & Atav, 2006)

Activities of daily living

- *Katz Index of Activities of Daily Living* (Rolland et al., 2007)
- *Instrumental Activities of Daily Living* (IADL) (Onor et al., 2007)

Past and current interests

- *Farrington Leisure Interest Inventory* (Fitzsimmons & Buettner, 2002; Buettner & Fitzsimmons, 2003; Buettner, Fitzsimmons, & Atav, 2006)

Personality traits

- *NEO-Personality Inventory* (Kolanowski & Richards, 2002)

Areas of Concern for RT Assessment

Recreational therapy assessment will determine therapeutic goals that will direct the RT program. Anticipated findings include the stage of the disease, the cognitive level and deficits (such as memory, attention, aphasia, apraxia, or agnosia) behavioral characteristics (such as agitation, wandering, screaming, aggression, or passivity), physical function level, personality traits, and past and current leisure interests. RTs can use the ICF codes described in the Systems Affected section to document their findings.

Other areas that the recreational therapist can assess include the environmental issues that are affecting the patient. Deficits in the current environment, such as too many stimuli, can be documented using ICF Environmental Factors codes. Areas that are especially relevant include e2 Natural Environment and Human-Made Changes to Environment and e3 Support and Relationships.

ICF Core Set

There are ICF Core Sets for Neurological Conditions during acute care and after acute care, Geriatric Patients, and Traumatic Brain Injury. All of these might provide some guidance for appropriate ICF codes to use when documenting the condition of a patient with an NCD.

Treatment Direction

Whole Team Approach

Pharmacological approaches may be a primary treatment approach for controlling the development of the disease, especially in mild or moderate NCDs, with drugs approved by the U.S. Food and Drug Administration such as donepezil, rivastigmine, or galantamine. These are most helpful early in the course of the disease and have shown some ability to slow the decline. The disease will still continue to progress (Alzheimer's Association, 2009). In order to treat behavior problems, antipsychotic drugs are commonly used, but benefits are controversial and there are potential side effects such as sedation, orthostatic hypotension, and anticholinergic and cardiac side effects (Putman & Wang, 2007).

Non-pharmacological treatment approaches, which help to ameliorate the symptoms of Alzheimer's disease in older adults, may include occupational therapy programs, psychological programs, physical activity programs, and recreational therapy programs. Most of them are interrelated. Recreational therapy strategies include specific programs that aim to increase mental, social, and physical stimulation (Buettner, Fitzsimmons, & Atav, 2006).

Recreational Therapy Approach

In order to achieve desired outcomes, programs are carefully designed while considering therapeutic goals, the person's age and personality style, stage of the disease, cognitive and physical function, behavioral problems, and the individual's leisure interests and skill level. Once the initial assessment is conducted and the therapeutic goals are determined, the program is designed and implemented. Finally, the program must be evaluated to assess the success at reaching the planned outcomes.

Meaningful activities for people with NCDs promote well-being and prevent excess disability. As with most adults, people with NCDs will benefit the most from self-selected activities that promote a sense of personal expression (Kolanowski & Richards, 2002). However, people with NCDs usually have a low rate of participation in activities partially due to their physical and cognitive decline (Buettner & Kolanowski, 2003). Without intervention by a competent recreational therapist, individuals with NCDs are likely to miss out on the benefits of recreation activities.

One possible strategy to increase participation rates is to consider past and current leisure interests. For this purpose, the *Farrington Leisure Interest Inventory* is commonly utilized. The problem with past leisure interests, however, is that physical and cognitive abilities change over time, and activities that were enjoyed years ago may no longer be appropriate and could even lead to frustration and increased inappropriate behavior (Kolanowski et al., 2001). Kolanowski et al. (2001) suggested that personality style influences the type of recreational therapy experiences clients prefer. Planned therapeutic programs that account for personality style may lead to more active physical or social involvements and may enable residents to experience more enjoyment. Among the various types of recreational therapy programs, social and creative experiences may benefit those who are more extroverted. Cooking, gardening, and reading programs may be more attractive to those more introverted.

The Neurodevelopmental Sequencing Program (NDSP) is the conceptual framework chosen by the American Therapeutic Recreation Association to design and implement a program. The NDSP describes the processes of intervention programs for people with NCDs, including the design, the resources needed to deliver it, and the implementation procedures (Buettner & Kolanowski, 2003). The purpose of the NDSP is to improve the quality of life of individuals with NCDs through the enhancement of physical and psychosocial abilities as they relate to recreation participation. Treatment goals are developed based on the person's level of physical and cognitive functioning in an effort to improve engagement and success during recreation activities (Kolanowski et al., 2006).

The results of the treatment need to be measured in order to obtain essential feedback about the effectiveness of the intervention. The measurements and instruments used at the beginning of the program for initial assessment or ICF codes documenting the client's functional abilities should be used to determine the intervention's success.

Recreational Therapy Interventions

Individuals experience significantly higher positive affect (b125 Dispositions and Intra-Personal Functions, b126 Temperament and Personality Functions) during recreation time when compared to non-recreation time (Schreiner, Yamamoto, & Shiotani, 2005). Woodhead et al. (2005) found that positive behaviors increase when people with NCDs participate in activities, and those who engage in more activities have fewer problems with restlessness. Recreational therapy programs for people with NCDs may lead to social, physical, and emotional benefits (Baker et al., 2003; Ballard et al., 2002; Beck et al., 2002; Buettner and Fitzsimmons, 2002; Buettner, Fitzsimmons, & Atav, 2006; Heyn, 2003; Suhr, Andersen, & Tranel, 1999; Rolland et al., 2007; Teri et al., 2003; Williams & Tappen, 2007). Relevant ICF codes include b1142 Orientation to Person, b126 Temperament and Personality Functions, b152 Emotional Functions, b176 Mental Functions of Sequencing Complex Movements, d3 Communication, d7 Interpersonal Interactions and Relationships, and d9 Community, Social, and Civic Life.

Functional Skills

Functional skills will be determined by the person's level of physical, social, and mental functioning according to his/her age and the stage of the disease. Recreational therapy addresses functional skills in all domains. For desired outcomes, it is important to match the functional skill of the person with the challenge of the activity. When a balance of skills and challenge is achieved, the person may enter into "the zone," where optimal activity occurs. According to Csíkszentmihályi (1990) experiencing optimal activities (or being in flow) can lead to long-term benefits. As this relates to NCDs, Jackson and Csíkszentmihályi (1999) maintain that optimal recreation experiences may impose order on mental consciousness. Some relevant ICF codes include b126 Temperament and Personality Functions, b152 Emotional Functions, b176 Mental Functions of Sequencing Complex Movements, d7 Interpersonal Interactions and Relationships, and d9 Community, Social, and Civic Life.

In ordinary life, people typically experience inner conflicts. For example, an office worker might be sitting at his desk and adding up numbers, with part of his attention focused on the job and part of it focused on his wish to be out with his girlfriend. He resents having to sit, to be indoors, and to work on his task. By contrast, in the flow state a person's subjective states are in harmony; the body and mind are working together without internal conflict. "This state of ordered consciousness is one of the main rewards of the flow experience" (Csíkszentmihályi, 1990, p. 165).

Designing the activity according to the person's interests and abilities is a key factor in setting the stage for flow activities (Buettner & Fitzsimmons, 2002). While there is no defined recipe to guarantee flow experiences, it is known that one of the primary conditions of these special times is the reduction of distractions. It may be necessary to limit peripheral activities and noises for a period of time (e2 Natural Environment and Human-Made Changes to Environment).

Education, Training, and Counseling

Teri et al. (2003) proved the effectiveness of a home-based exercise program for persons with NCDs combined with behavioral management training for their caregivers (d7 Interpersonal Interactions and Relationships, e3 Support and Relationships). With the behavioral management group, caregivers were taught to reduce the occurrence of behavioral problems that negatively affected client-caregiver interaction. The participants in the program increased their levels of physical activity, reduced their depression symptoms, and improved their physical health and function. Adherence to the program proved to be quite high. Castro et al. (2002) analyzed retention and adherence to a home-based counseling exercise program for women caring for relatives with NCDs. Women caregivers participating in the program achieved a 74% adherence rate to their prescribed exercise sessions during 12 months. Those who were more depressed had lower adherence. Results show the feasibility of home-based programs for both individuals with NCDs and their caregivers. ICF codes include b126 Temperament and Personality Functions, b130 Energy and Drive Functions, b152 Emotional Functions, d110 Watching, d115 Listening, d160 Focusing Attention, d163 Thinking, d175 Solving Problems, d210 Undertaking a Single Task, d220 Undertaking Multiple Tasks, d230

Carrying Out Daily Routine, d570 Looking After One's Health.

Education programs for people with NCDs have proven effective. For example, Richeson, Boyne, and Brady (2007) showed significant changes in perceived self-efficacy scores and increases in perceived "growth through confidence" by people with NCDs and caregivers after an education program titled Health Promotion for the Body, Mind, and Spirit. Other educational programs target caregivers. For instance, Carbonneau, Caron, and Desrosiers (2011) implemented a leisure education program for caregivers of people with NCDs with a positive impact on these caregivers and their relationships with their patients (d7 Interpersonal Interactions and Relationships, e3 Support and Relationships).

Community Integration

Arkin (2003) involved university students and caregivers in a therapeutic program for individuals with Alzheimer's disease. Participants engaged in 16 to 20 exercise sessions and 10 community activity sessions per semester for two to eight semesters. The physical fitness sessions were performed twice a week for 10 weeks each semester. One weekly session was supervised by a student and combined physical exercise with cognitive and conversation stimulation. The second weekly session was supervised by a family member (caregiver). The compliance of student sessions achieved 100%, but caregivers were less reliable. Participants in the program accomplished significant fitness gains (d570 Looking After One's Health) and improved their moods (b126 Temperament and Personality Functions). Cognitive decline was slowed (b1 Mental Functions). Onor et al. (2007) posited that any therapeutic program should combine treatment for clients and caregivers for best results. Leahey and Singleton (2011) also suggest that involving the caregivers in the programs may assist in transferring skills to caregivers that will help them enable the person with an NCD to be successful in a given activity (d7 Interpersonal Interactions and Relationships, e3 Support and Relationships).

Health Promotion

To promote health in people with NCDs, cognitive, social, and physical stimulation needs to be considered. The combination of these factors increases the possibility of benefits (Fratiglioni & Wang, 2007). Interventions commonly implemented with people who have NCDs include sensory stimulation (b156 Perceptual Functions), leisure time physical activity (d920 Recreation and Leisure), stress reduction techniques (d240 Handling Stress and Other Psychological Demands), animal therapy, or miscellaneous recreation activities based on personal needs.

Sensory stimulation: Different types of sensory stimulation, including multisensory stimulation, aromatherapy, or music, are commonly used for therapy in NCD populations. Multisensory stimulation aims to provide individuals with NCDs with different visual, auditory, olfactory, and tactile stimuli (Baker et al., 2003). In a randomized controlled trial, Baker et al. (2003) tested the effect of standardized multi-sensory stimulation in the Snoezelen room compared to activities such as playing cards, looking at photographs, and taking quizzes over the course of four weeks. The Snoezelen room was originally developed in the Netherlands and is designed to deliver stimuli to different senses. Multi-sensory stimulation was not found to be more effective in changing behavior, mood, or cognition than activities such as playing cards. Further, some individuals with NCDs may be disturbed by the Snoezelen room's random lights, sounds, and shapes (O'Connor et al., 2009).

Individual stimulus: The use of individual stimulus, such as aromatherapy or music therapy, has been successfully used by some researchers. Ballard et al. (2002) proved aromatherapy to be successful in reducing agitation and improving social engagement and constructive activity. Music therapy may result in appropriate behavior, an opportunity to engage in a pleasant creative activity, and a reduction in anxiety (O'Connor et al., 2009). Ragneskog et al., (1996) used three types of music (soft melodious tunes, 1930s jazz, and modern pop) for reducing irritability and depression in individuals with NCDs. While all three types of music successfully reduced irritability and depression, soothing music was most effective. Gerdner (2000) demonstrated that individualized music was more effective than classical relaxation music in reducing the frequency of agitation behaviors in people with Alzheimer's disease and related disorders. ICF codes that can document reduction in agitation and increased engagement include b126

Temperament and Personality Functions, b140 Attention Functions, b144 Memory Functions, d110 Watching, d115 Listening, d160 Focusing Attention, d210 Undertaking a Single Task, d220 Undertaking Multiple Tasks, and d3 Communication.

Combination of stimuli: Other researchers have combined different stimuli. Heyn (2003) evaluated the effects of an exercise program combined with multi-stimulation. The program was composed of a focused attention and warm-up session (storytelling and imagery were used for this component); flexibility and aerobic exercises; a strength training session (imagery and music were used here); and a cool-down session that focused on relaxation and breathing techniques (including thematic music and storytelling). Participants experienced improved resting heart rate, overall mood elevations, and higher engagement in physical activities. ICF codes to document changes include b125 Dispositions and Intra-Personal Functions, b126 Temperament and Personality Functions, b152 Emotional Functions, and b455 Exercise Tolerance Functions.

Stress reduction techniques: Stress increases the risk of developing NCDs and accelerates NCD progression, probably through aberrant levels of cortisol, epinephrine, or glucose and its subsequent effects on memory performance (McEwen, 2008; Wilson et al., 2007). Ironically, NCDs reduce the ability to cope with stress, increasing disturbed behaviors (O'Connor, 2009). Many stress reduction techniques may be used with individuals with NCDs such as yoga, tai chi, progressive muscle relaxation, music, etc. For instance, Suhr, Andersen, and Tranel (1999) successfully used progressive muscle relaxation to decrease psychiatric and behavioral disturbances (d240 Handling Stress and Other Psychological Demands) and improve memory (b144 Memory Functions) and verbal fluency (b167 Mental Functions of Language) in Alzheimer's patients.

Leisure time physical activity: Physical activity is a key component of healthy aging (Taylor et al., 2004). Moderate aerobic exercises such as walking (Friedman & Tappen, 1991; Lautenschlager et al., 2008; Tappen et al., 2000; Williams & Tappen, 2007) seem to be effective for people with NCDs. Strength, flexibility, and balance training have also been used successfully with individuals with NCDs (Teri et al.,

2003; Rolland et al., 2007; Williams & Tappen, 2007). Participating in comprehensive physical activity programs that combine aerobic, strength, balance, and flexibility training may lead to improvements in physical health, physical function, and activities of daily living (Teri et al., 2003; Rolland et al., 2007), mood and affect (Heyn, 2003; Williams & Tappen, 2007) while decreasing symptoms of depression (Teri et al., 2003). The duration of the physical activity training ranges from 30 minutes five times per week to 20 minutes three times per week (Rolland et al., 2008). The physical activity program has to be enjoyable and accessible in order to achieve compliance. Mathews, Clair, and Kosloski (2001) suggested that individual exercises combined with music increase compliance. ICF codes that describe the areas being treated include b125 Dispositions and Intra-Personal Functions, b126 Temperament and Personality Functions, b130 Energy and Drive Functions, b152 Emotional Functions, b455 Exercise Tolerance Functions, d230 Carrying Out Daily Routine, and d415 Maintaining a Body Position.

Animal therapy: Animal-assisted therapy (AAT) is increasing its popularity in nursing and care home settings. AAT involves interactions between clients and trained animals, directed by a trained professional with a specific clinical goal (Buettner, Fitzsimmons, & Barba, 2011). Research indicates that interaction with dogs among people with NCDs reduces aggression and agitation, as well as promoting social interaction. (For more details, see Filan & Llewellyn-Jones, 2006, or Perkins et al., 2008.) The most commonly reported finding is improved social behavior (Buettner, Fitzsimons, and Barba, 2011). For example, Kanamori et al. (2001) used dogs or cats interacting with individuals with NCDs for three months and saw improved NCD-related behavior. Richeson (2003) was able to decrease agitated behaviors and increase social interaction using AAT with a dog. The intervention was conducted for three weeks, five times per week, with a small group approach of three or four participants led by a recreational therapist. However, it is uncertain if the effects of AAT interventions persist over time (Filan & Llewellyn-Jones, 2006). ICF codes to document the therapy include b125 Dispositions and Intra-Personal Functions, b126 Temperament and Personality Functions, and d7 Interpersonal Interactions and Relationships.

Recreation activities individualized according to personal needs: Fitzsimmons and Buettner (2002) suggest recreational therapy is most effective in reducing passivity and agitation when prescribed individually, according to current functioning, past interests, and current needs. Buettner and Fitzsimmons (2003) found small-group recreational therapy experiences that consider individual interests to be successful in engaging individuals in activities 84% of the time. Buettner, Fitzsimmons, and Atav (2006) decreased agitation (b126 Temperament and Personality Functions) in people with NCDs using recreational therapy interventions based on personal needs. Activities were usually offered 30 minutes a day, five days a week and included wheelchair biking, singing, cooking, and exercise. Mahoney (2003) suggests choosing appropriate activities according to the client's age and disease stage, taking into account that those with Alzheimer's disease may actually regress through Piaget's stages of cognitive development. In his research, both age-appropriate and stage-appropriate groups showed significant increases in the expression of positive emotions and a significant reduction in agitation (b126 Temperament and Personality Functions) compared to those in the control groups. Stage-appropriate activities showed significantly more improvements in emotion than age-appropriate activities. Leahey and Singleton (2011), in a case report, found that participating in a Wii bowling activity enabled the client to increase and maintain focus (b130 Energy and Drive Functions, b140 Attention Functions), to engage in a familiar and meaningful activity (d920 Recreation and Leisure), and to learn new skills. A complete recreational therapy assessment was performed in order to choose the most suitable intervention, gathering information from the participant, his wife, and the recreational therapist's observations. The main reason for choosing the activity was the past history of physical activity, bowling, and technology experience of the client.

Miscellaneous

Involving clients in small group activities while keeping individual needs at the forefront has the potential of generating greater positive outcomes, as the social component contributes to the possible benefits. For instance, Phinney and Moody (2011), using a qualitative methodology, demonstrated that participating in a social recreation activity can be a very positive experience for people with mild NCDs. The activity consisted of a group of people with mild NCDs meeting twice a week at a senior center for casual conversation in the morning and a meal together. In the afternoon clients participated in activities such as flexibility exercises, ball games, word games, or dancing. The activities were facilitated by two professional recreational therapists. The program provided participants with enjoyable activities in a comfortable and safe environment. They were happier and more socially engaged (b126 Temperament and Personality Functions, d750 Informal Social Relationships).

The social aspect of the program also helps with compliance and adherence. Group activities promote longer periods of participation and hold individuals' attention for a much longer period than any other activities (Kolanowski & Richards, 2002). Conti, Voelkl, and McGuire (2008) suggested small group formats are preferable for people with NCDs. Group activities are not always the best option. Kolanowski et al. (2001) suggested that because extroverts enjoy interacting with people, group activities could work better. On the other hand, introverts may prefer more individual activities.

Summary

Brookmeyer et al. (2007) estimated that thoughtfully designed interventions that delay disease progression by an average of two years would decrease nearly seven million late stage cases and decrease the global financial, personal, and social burdens of Alzheimer's disease. Because the problem of NCDs is so complex and multifaceted, an integrated approach to intervention is most effective. One component of that multi-pronged effort must be recreational therapy. Recreational therapy must continue to provide well-designed and executed programs for people with NCDs. Such programs, planned and delivered with the individual in mind, have the potential for significant positive results in the fight against these diseases.

Resources

Alzheimer's Association
www.alz.org/

This web site provides information about NCDs and Alzheimer's disease for person's affected, caregivers, and professionals, including definitions, signs, stages, etc.

American Music Therapy Association
www.musictherapy.org/
This web site provides with information about the benefits of musical therapy, programs, training, and certification in the field.

Delta Society
deltasociety.org
This web site provides information about programs, standards of practice, training, and certification in the field of animal-assisted therapy.

Elder Rehab by Students
(Dr. Sharon M. Arkin, University of Arizona)
www.u.arizona.edu/~sarkin/elderrehab.html
This web site provides a description of a student-led home exercise program for people with Alzheimer's disease. It includes a memory and language stimulation protocol and a physical fitness training protocol.

National Center for Physical Activity and Disability
www.ncpad.org/
This web site provides information about physical activity and nutrition for people with NCDs.

Therapet Foundation
www.therapet.com
This web site provides information about programs, standards of practice, training, and certification in the field of animal-assisted therapy.

References

Akbaraly, T. N., Portet, F., Fustinoni, S., Dartigues, J. F., Artero, S., Rouaud, O., Touchon, J., Ritchie, K., & Berr, C. (2009). Leisure activities and the risk of dementia in the elderly. Results from the Three-City Study. *Neurology*, 73(11), 854-861.

Alzheimer's Association. (2013a). Alzheimer's facts and figures. Accessed from http://www.alz.org/alzheimers_disease_facts_and_figures.asp 28-dec-13.

Alzheimer's Association. (2013b). Parkinson's disease dementia. Accessed from http://www.alz.org/dementia/parkinsons-disease-symptoms.asp 28-dec-13.

Alzheimer's Association. (2009). Stages of Alzheimer's. Accessed via website www.alz.org.

Alzheimer's Association. (2006). Vascular dementia. Accessed from https://www.alz.org/cincinnati/documents/vascular.pdf 28-dec-13.

Alzheimer's Disease International. (2013). Dementia statistics. Retrieved from http://www.alz.co.uk/research/statistics.

American Psychiatric Association. (2013). *Diagnostic and statistical manual of mental disorders* (5th ed.) Washington, DC: American Psychiatric Association.

American Psychiatric Association. (2000). *Diagnostic and statistical manual of mental disorders* (IV TR). Washington, DC: American Psychiatric Association.

Arkin, S. M. (2003). Student-led exercise sessions yield significant fitness gains for Alzheimer's patients. *American Journal of Alzheimer's Disease and Other Dementias, 18*(3), 159-170.

Baker, R., Holloway, J., Holtkamp, C. C. M., Larsson, A., Hartman, L. C., Pearce, R., Scherman, B., Johansson, S., Thomas, P. W., Wareing, L. A., & Owens, M. (2003). Effects of multi-sensory stimulation for people with dementia. *Journal of Advanced Nursing, 43*, 465-477.

Ballard, C. J., O'Brian, J. T., Reichelt, K., & Perry, E. K. (2002). Aromatherapy as a safe and effective treatment for the management of agitation in severe dementia: The results of a double blind, placebo controlled trial with Melissa. *Journal of Clinical Psychiatry, 63*, 553-558.

Beck, C. K., Vogelpohl, T. S., Rasin, J. H., Uriri, J. T., O'Sullivan, P., Walls, R., Phillips, R., & Baldwin, B. (2002). Effects of behavioral interventions on disruptive behavior and affect in demented nursing home residents. *Nursing Research, 51*, 219-228.

Brodaty, H., McGilchrist, C., Harris, L., & Peters, K. E. (1993). Time until institutionalization and death in patients with dementia. Role of caregiver training and risk factors. *Arch Neurol, 50*(6), 643-50.

Brookmeyer, R., Johnson, E., Ziegler-Graham, K., & Arrighi, H. M. (2007). Forecasting the global burden of Alzheimer's disease. *Alzheimer's Dementia, 3*, 186-191. Accessed via website http://www.bepress.com/jhubiostat/paper130.

Buettner, L. L. & Fitzsimmons S. (2002). AD-venture program: Therapeutic biking for the treatment of depression in long-term care residents with dementia. *American Journal of Alzheimer's Disease and Other Dementias, 17*, 121-127. doi: 10.1177/153331750201700205.

Buettner, L. L. & Fitzsimmons S. (2003). Activity calendars for older adults with dementia: What you see is not what you get. *American Journal of Alzheimer's Disease and Other Dementias, 18*(4), 215-226. doi: 10.1177/153331750301800405.

Buettner, L. L., Fitzsimmons, S., & Atav, A. S. (2006). Predicting outcomes of therapeutic recreation interventions for older adults with dementia and behavioral symptoms. *Therapeutic Recreation Journal, 40*, 33.

Buettner, L. L., Fitzsimmons, S., & Barba, B. (2011). Animal-assisted therapy for clients with dementia. *Journal of Gerontology Nursing, 37*(5), 10-4. doi: 10.3928/00989134-20110329-05.

Buettner, L. L. & Kolanowski, A. (2003). Practice guidelines for recreation therapy in the care of people with dementia. *Geriatric Nursing, 24*, 18-25. doi: 10.1067/mgn.2003.19.

Carbonneau, H., Caron, C. D., Desrosiers, J. (2011). Effects of an adapted leisure education program as a means of support for caregivers of people with dementia. *Archives of Gerontology and Geriatrics, 53*(1), 31-39. http://dx.doi.org/10.1016/j.archger.2010.06.009.

Carlson, M. C., Helms, M. J., Steffens, D. C., Burke, J. R., Potter, G. G., & Plassman, B. L. (2008). Midlife activity predicts risk of dementia in older male twin pairs. *Alzheimer's and Dementia, 4*(5), 324-331.

Castro, C. M., Wilcox, S., O'Sullivan, P., Baumann, K., & King, A. C. (2002). An exercise program for women who are caring for relatives with dementia. *Psychosomatic Medicine, 64*, 458-468.

Conti, A., Voelkl, J., & McGuire, F. A. (2009). A potential role of leisure in the prevention of dementia. *Annual in Therapeutic Recreation, 17*, 31-45.

Csíkszentmihályi, M. (1990). *Flow: The psychology of optimal experience.* New York: Harper & Row.

Dickerson, B. C., Goncharova, I., Sullivan, M. P., Forchetti, C., Wilson, R. S., Bennett, D. A., Beckett, L. A., & deToledo-Morrell, L. (2001). MRI-derived entorhinal and hippocampal atrophy in incipient and very mild Alzheimer's disease. *Neurobiology of Aging, 22*(5), 747-754.

Ferri, C. P., Prince, M., Brayne, C., Brodaty, H., Fratiglioni, L., Ganguli, M., Hall, K., Hasegawa, K., Hendrie, H., Huang, Y., Jorm, A., Mathers, C., Menezes, P. R., Rimmer, E., & Scazufca, M. (2005). Global prevalence of dementia: A delphi consensus study. *Lancet, 366*, 2112-2117.

Filan, S. L. & Llewellyn-Jones, R. H. (2006). Animal-assisted therapy for dementia: A review of the literature. *International Psychogeriatrics, 18*, 597-611 doi: 10.1017/S1041610206003322.

Fitzsimmons, S. & Buettner, L. L. (2002). Therapeutic recreation interventions for need-driven dementia-compromised behaviors in community-dwelling elders. *American Journal of Alzheimer's Disease and Other Dementias, 17*, 367-381. doi: 10.1177/153331750201700603.

Fox, N. C., Warrington, E. K., Freeborough, P. A., Hartikainen, P., Kennedy, A. M., Stevens, J. M., & Rossor, M. N. (1996). Presymptomatic hippocampal atrophy in Alzheimer's disease: A longitudinal MRI study. *Brain, 119*(6), 2001-2007.

Fratiglioni, L., Paillard-Borg, S., & Winblad, B. (2004). An active and socially integrated lifestyle in late life might protect against dementia. *Lancet Neurology, 3*, 343-53.

Fratiglioni, L. & H. X. Wang. (2007). Brain reserve hypothesis in dementia. *Journal of Alzheimer's Disease, 12*(1), 11-22.

Friedman, R. & Tappen, R. M. (1991). The effect of planned walking on communication in Alzheimer's disease. *Journal of American Geriatric Society, 39*(7), 650-654.

Gerdner, L. (2000). Effects of individualized versus classical "relaxation" music on the frequency of agitation in elderly persons with Alzheimer's disease and related disorders. *International Psychogeriatrics, 12*(1) 49-65.

Green, R. C., Cupples, L. A., Kurz, A., Auerbach, S., Go, R., Sadovnick, D., Duara, R., Kukull, W. A., Chui, H., Edeki, T., Grifith, P. A., Friedland, R. P., Bachman, D., & Farrer, L. (2003). Depression as a risk factor for Alzheimer disease: The MIRAGE study. *Archives of Neurology, 60*, 753-759. Retrieved from www.archneurol.com.

Gustaw-Rothenberg, K. (2009). Dietary patterns associated with Alzheimer's disease: Population based study. *Int J Environ Res Public Health, 6*, 1335-1340. doi: 10.3390/ijerph6041335.

Haan, M. N. & Wallace, R. (2004). Can dementia be prevented? Brain aging in a population-based context. *Annu Rev Public Health 25*, 1-24. doi: 10.1146/annurev.publhealth.25.101802.122951.

Hebert, L. E., Scherr, P. A., Bienias, J. L., Bennett, D. A., & Evans, D. A. (2003). Alzheimer disease in the U.S. population: Prevalence estimates using the 2000 census. *Archives of Neurology, 60*, 1119-1122.

Heyn, P. (2003). The effect of a multisensory exercise program on engagement, behavior, and selected physiological indexes in persons with dementia. *American Journal of Alzheimer's Disease and Other Dementias, 18*, 247-251. doi: 10.1177/153331750301800409.

Jackson, S. & Csíkszentmihályi, M. (1999). *Flow in sports: The keys to optimal experiences and performances.* Champaign, IL: Human Kinetics.

Kanamori, M., Suzuki, M., Yamamoto, K., Kanda, M., Matsui, Y., Kojima, E., Fukawa, H., Sugita, T., & Oshiro, H. (2001). A day care program and evaluation of animal-assisted therapy (AAT) for the elderly with senile dementia. *American Journal of Alzheimer's Disease and Other Dementias, 16*(4), 234-239.

Kolanowski, A. M., Buettner, L., Costa, P. T., Jr., & Litaker, M. S. (2001). Capturing interests: Therapeutic recreation activities for persons with dementia. *Therapeutic Recreation Journal, 35,* 220-235.

Kolanowski, A., Buettner, L., Litaker, M., & Yu, F. (2006). Factors that relate to activity engagement in nursing home residents. *American Journal of Alzheimer's Disease and Other Dementias, 21,* 15-22. doi: 10.1177/153331750602100109.

Kolanowski, A. & Richards, K. (2002). Introverts and extroverts: Leisure activity behavior in persons with dementia. *Activities, Adaptation & Aging, 26,* 1-16. Retrieved from http://www.haworthpressinc.com/store/product.asp?sku=J016.

Larson, E. B., Wang, L., Bowen, J. D., McCormick, W. C., Teri, L., Crane, P., Kukull, W. (2006). Exercise is associated with reduced risk for incident dementia among persons 65 years of age and older. *Ann Intern Med, 144,* 73-81.

Lautenschlager, N. T., Kox, K. L., Flicker, L., Foster, J. K., van Bockxmeer, F. M., Xiao, J., Greenop, K. R., & Almeida, O. P. (2008). Effect of physical activity on cognitive function in older adults at risk for Alzheimer's disease: A randomized controlled trial. *JAMA, 300*(9), 1027-1037. doi: 10.1001/jama.300.9.1027.

Laurin, D., Verreault, R., Lindsay, J., MacPherson, K., & Rockwood, K. (2001). Physical activity and risk of cognitive impairment and dementia in elderly persons. *Archives of Neurology, 58*(3), 498-504.

Leahey, A. & Singleton, J. (2011). Utilizing therapeutic recreation to empower persons with Alzheimer's in a day center. *Journal of Therapeutic Recreation, 45,* 135-146.

Lewy Body Dementia Association. (2013). What is LBD? Retrieved from http://www.lbda.org/node/7 28-dec-13.

Lupien, S. J., de Leon, M., de Santi, S., Convit, A., Tarshish, C., Nair, N. P. V., Thakur, M., McEwen, B. S., Hauger, R. L., & Meaney, M. J. (1998). Cortisol levels during human aging predict hippocampal atrophy and memory deficits. *Nature Neuroscience, 1*(1), 69-73.

Lynch, T., Sano, M., Marder, K. S., Bell, K. L., Foster, N. L., Defendini, R. F., Sima, A. A., Keohane, C., Nygaard, T. G., Fahn, S., Mayeux, R., Rowland, L. P., Wilhelmsen, K. C. (1994). Clinical characteristics of a family with chromosome 17-linked disinhibition-dementia-parkinsonism-amyotrophy complex. *Neurology 44*(10), 1878-1884. doi: 10.1212/WNL.44.10.1878.

Mahoney, A. E. J. (2003). Age-or stage-appropriate? Recreation and the relevance of Piaget's theory in dementia care. *American Journal of Alzheimer's Disease and Other Dementias, 18,* 24-30. doi: 10.1177/153331750301800102.

Mathews, M., Clair, A., & Kosloski, K. (2001). Keeping the beat: Use of rhythmic music during exercise activities for elderly with dementia. *American Journal of Alzheimer's Disease and Other Dementias, 16,* 377-380. doi: 10.1177/153331750101600608.

McEwen, B. S. (2008). Central effects of stress hormones in health and disease: Understanding the protective and damaging effects of stress and stress mediators. *European Journal Pharmacology, 583,* 174-185. doi: 10.1016/j.ejphar.2007.11.071.

Medscape. (2013a). Vascular dementia. Accessed from http://emedicine.medscape.com/article/292105-overview#a0199 28-dec-13.

Medscape. (2013b). Huntington's disease dementia. http://emedicine.medscape.com/article/289706-overview#a0199 28-dec-13.

Medscape. (2013c). HIV Encephalopathy and AIDS Dementia Complex. http://emedicine.medscape.com/article/1166894-overview#aw2aab6b4. 28-dec-13.

Medscape. (2013d). Epidemiology. http://www.medscape.org/viewarticle/590462_2. 28-dec-13.

Medscape. (2013e). Delirium. http://emedicine.medscape.com/article/288890-overview#aw2aab6b2b5aa. 28-dec-13.

O'Connor, D. W., Ames, D., Gardner, B., & King, M. (2009). Psychosocial treatments of behavior symptoms in dementia: A systematic review of reports meeting quality standards. *International Psychogeriatrics, 21,* 225-240. doi: 10.1017/S1041610208007588.

Onor, M. L., Trevisol, M., Negro, C., Alessandra, S., Saina, M., & Aguglia, E. (2007). Impact of a multimodal rehabilitative intervention on demented patients and their caregivers. *American Journal of Alzheimer's Disease and Other Dementias, 22,* 261-272. doi: 10.1177/1533317507302071.

Paillard-Borg, S., Fratiglioni, L., Winblad, B., & Wang, H-X. (2009). Leisure activities in late life in relation to dementia risk: Principal component analysis. *Dement Geriatr Cogn Disord, 28,* 136-144.

Perkins, J., Bartlett, H., Travers, C., & Rand, J. (2008). Dog-assisted therapy for older people with dementia: A review. *Australas J Ageing, 27*(4), 177-82. doi: 10.1111/j.1741-6612.2008.00317.x.

Phinney, A. & Moody, E. M. (2011). Leisure connections: Benefits and challenges of participating in a social recreation group for people with early dementia. *Activities, Adaptation & Aging, 35*(2), 11-130. doi: 10.1080/01924788.2011.572272.

Podewils, L. J., Guallar, E., Kuller, L. H., Fried, L. P., Lopez, O. L., Carlson, M., & Lyketsos, C. G. (2005). Physical activity, APOE genotype, and dementia risk: Findings from the cardiovascular health cognition study. *American Journal of Epidemiology, 161,* 639-651. doi: 10.1093/aje/kwi092.

Putman, L. & Wang, L. T. (2007). The closing group: Therapeutic recreation for nursing home residents with dementia and accompanying agitation and/or anxiety. *American Journal of Alzheimer's Disease and Other Dementias, 22,* 167-175. doi: 10.1177/1533317507300514.

Querfurth, H. W. & LaFerla, F. M. (2010). Mechanisms of disease: Alzheimer's disease. *The New England Journal of Medicine, 362,* 329-344. Retrieved from www.nejm.org.

Ragneskog, H., Bråne, G., Karlsson, I., & Kihlgren, M. (1996). Influence of dinner music on food intake and symptoms common in dementia. *Scandinavian Journal of Caring Sciences, 10,* 11-17.

Rait, G., Walter, K., Bottomley, C., Petersen, I., Illiffe, S., & Nathareth, I. (2010). Survival of people with clinical diagnosis of dementia in primary care: Cohort study. *BMJ, 341,* 1-7.

Richeson, N. E. (2003). Effects of animal-assisted therapy on agitated behaviors and social interactions of older adults with dementia. *American Journal of Alzheimer's Disease and Other Dementias, 18*(6), 353-358.

Richeson, N. E., Boyne, S., & Brady, M. (2007). Education for older adults with early-stage dementia: Health promotion for the mind, body, and spirit. *Educational Gerontology, 33*(9), 723-736.

Rimmer, J. H. & Smith, D. L. (2009). Alzheimer's disease. In Durstine, J. L., Moore, G. E., Painter, P. L. & Roberts, S. D. (Eds.). *ACSM's management for persons with chronic diseases and disabilities* (pp. 368-374). Human Kinetics, Champaign, IL.

Rolland, Y., Pillard, F., Klapouszczak, A., Reynish, E., Thomas, D., Andrieu, S., Rivière, D., & Vellas, B. (2007). Exercise program for nursing home residents with Alzheimer's disease: A 1-year randomized, controlled trial. *Journal of the American Geriatrics Society, 55,* 158-165. doi: 10.1111/j.1532-5415.2007.01035.

Rothman, S. M. & Mattson, M. P. (2010). Adverse stress, hippocampal networks, and Alzheimer's disease. *Neuromolecular Medicine, 12*(1), 56-70. doi: 10.1007/s12017-009-8107-9.

Rovio, S., Kåreholt, I., Helkala, E. L., Viitanen, M., Winblad, B., Tuomilehto, J., Soininen, H., Nissinen, A., & Kivipelto, M. (2005). Leisure-time physical activity at midlife and the risk of dementia and Alzheimer's disease. *Lancet Neurology, 4*(11), 690-691.

Scarmeas, N., Levy, G., Tang, M-X, Manly, J., & Stern, Y. (2001). Influence of leisure activity on the incidence of Alzheimer disease. *Neurology, 57*, 2236-2242.

Schreiner, A. S., Yamamoto, E., & Shiotani, H. (2005). Positive affect among nursing home residents with Alzheimer's dementia: The effect of recreational activity. *Aging & Mental Health, 9*, 129-134.

Snowden, J. S., Neary, D., & Mann, D. M. (2002). Frontotemporal dementia. *Br J Psychiatry, 180*, 140-3. doi: 10.1192/bjp.180.2.14.

Solfrizzi, V., Capurso, C., D'Introno, A., Colacicco, A. M., Santamato, A., Ranieri, M., Fiore, P., Capurso, A., & Panza, F. (2008). Lifestyle-related factors in predementia and dementia syndromes. *Expert Rev Neurother, 8*(1), 133-58.

Suhr, J., Anderson, S., & Tranel, D. (1999). Progressive muscle relaxation in the management of behavioral disturbance in Alzheimer's disease. *Neuropsychological Rehabilitation, 9*, 31-44.

Taaffe, D. R., Irie, F., Masaki, K. H., Abbott, R. D., Petrovitch, H., Ross, G. W., & White, R. L. (2008). Physical activity, physical function, and incident dementia in elderly men: The Honolulu-Asia aging study. *J Gerontol A Biol Sci Med Sci., 63*(5), 529-535.

Tappen, R. M., Roach, K. E., Applegate, E. B., & Stowell, P. (2000). Effect of a combined walking and conversation intervention on functional mobility of nursing home residents with Alzheimer disease. *Alzheimer's Disease and Associated Disorders, 14*(4), 196-201.

Taylor, A. H., Cable, N. T., Faulkner, G., Hillsdon, M., Narici, M., & Van Der Bij, A. K. (2004). Physical activity and older adults: A review of health benefits and the effectiveness of interventions. *Journal of Sports Sciences, 22*(8), 703-725.

Teri, L., Gibbons, L. E., McCurry, S. M., Logsdon, R. G., Buchner, D. M., Barlow, W. E., Kukull, W. A., LaCroix, A. Z., McCormick, W., & Larson, E. B. (2003). Exercise plus behavioral management in patients with Alzheimer disease: A randomized controlled trial. *JAMA, 290*(15), 2015-2022. Retrieved from www.jama.com.

Verghese, J., Lipton, R. B., Katz, M. J., Hall, C. B., Derby, C. A., Kuslansky, G., Ambrose, A. F., Sliwinski, M., & Buschke, H. (2003). Leisure activities and the risk of dementia in the elderly. *New England Journal of Medicine, 348*, 2508-2516.

Williams, C. L. & Tappen, R. M. (2007). Effect of exercise on mood in nursing home residents with Alzheimer's disease. *American Journal of Alzheimer's Disease and Other Dementias, 22*, 389-397. doi: 10.1177/1533317507305588.

Wilson, R. S., Scherr, P. A., Schneider, J. A., Tang, Y., Bennett, D. A. (2007). Relation of cognitive activity to risk of developing Alzheimer disease. *Neurology, 69*, 1911-1920.

Woodhead, E. L., Zarit, S. H., Braungart, E. R., Rovine, M. R., & Femia, E. E. (2005). Behavioral and psychological symptoms of dementia: The effects of physical activity at adult day service centers. *American Journal of Alzheimer's Disease and Other Dementias, 20*, 171. doi: 10.1177/153331750502000314.

Xie, J., Brayne, C., & Matthews, F. (2008). Survival times in people with dementia: Analysis for a population based cohort study with 14 year follow-up. *BMJ, 336*, 258-62.

24. Obesity

Gretchen Snethen, Brenda L. Hart, and Barbara L. Parker

In the United States, obesity is the sixth leading cause of disability (WHO, 2008). More than one-third of Americans are obese (CDC, 2011). Obesity in the general population has elevated to a point where public health officials consider it an epidemic and, as such, a high research priority. In fact, in June 2013, the American Medical Association (AMA, 2013) reclassified obesity as a disease. Research among the general population indicates environmental factors, behavior, and genetics play an important role in obesity (Pi-Sunyer, 2002).

Obesity, defined as excess body fat, is increasingly a concern because it raises the risk of other diseases. Researchers have also examined the risk of metabolic syndrome. Metabolic syndrome is a group of risk factors that increases an individual's risk for diabetes, heart disease, and stroke. The risk factors include a large waistline, high triglyceride levels, low HDL cholesterol, high blood pressure, and high fasting blood sugar (Ford, Giles, & Dietz, 2002). The occurrence of metabolic syndrome increases an individual's risk for diabetes and coronary heart disease.

Individuals are considered obese if their body weight is more than 20% above the appropriate body weight for their age, sex, height, and body build. The most common measure of obesity is the body mass index (BMI). The intersection of an individual's body weight and height indicates an individual's BMI, which is divided into five specific BMI categories: healthy weight (BMI of 18.5-24.9), overweight (BMI of 25-29.9), obesity class 1 (BMI of 30-34.9), obesity class 2 (BMI of 35-39.9), and severe obesity class 3 (BMI of 40 or more).

Despite its common use, the BMI is not a perfect instrument. Individuals who are muscular may have a high BMI due to muscle mass rather than excess fat. Others with low muscle mass and high fat percentage, such as inactive and older adults, may still score low on the BMI (National Institutes of Health, 1998). Although the BMI is still commonly used in individual healthcare, it is a better indicator of disease risk in a population rather than for a specific client (National Institutes of Health, 2008-2009). To better determine an individual's health risks, it is recommended that waist circumference be used in conjunction with the BMI. Waist circumference is determined by wrapping a measuring tape around an individual's waist just above the hipbones and below the rib cage. Women who have a waist circumference of 35" or more and men who have a waist circumference of 40" or more, along with a BMI greater than 25, have a greater risk for developing Type 2 diabetes, hypertension, and cardiovascular disease (The Obesity Society, 2010). Abdominal fat is associated with a higher risk of these conditions than peripheral fat on the legs, buttocks, or hips. If an individual's BMI is in the healthy weight range, but his/her waist circumference is greater than what is recommended, s/he is still at risk due to the high percentage of fat in the abdominal area.

For children, the BMI is measured through a pediatric growth chart. BMI that falls between the 85th and 95th percentile for an age group is considered overweight. A BMI-for-age above the 95th percentile is considered obese (Ogden & Flegal, 2010).

Incidence/Prevalence and Ages in U.S.

Obesity rates have increased in the last 25 years. In 2005-2006, more than one third of the adult population, or over 72 million people, were obese (Ogden, Carroll, Kit, & Flegal, 2012). Currently, less than one-third of the U.S. adult population is at a healthy weight. The 2009-2010 National Health and Nutrition Examination Survey (NHANES) estimated that nearly 70% of U.S. adults are overweight with a BMI greater than 25 and 36% of the population are obese with a BMI greater than 30. Approximately

15% of the population is class 2 obese (BMI ≥ 35) and six percent is class 3 obese (BMI ≥ 40). African-American men and African-American women experience a greater prevalence of obesity than other racial groups (49.5%, 58.6% respectively). Hispanic men and Hispanic women also experience greater prevalence of obesity than the Non-Hispanic white population (Flegal et al., 2012).

Overweight children and teenagers are also a rising concern. The 1999-2008 NHANES found that approximately 19% of children ages 6-19 were overweight. NHANES studies in the 1960s, 1970s, and 1980s indicated that approximately 4-7% of children ages 6-19 were overweight. This number increased to 11% in the late 1980s/early 1990s and has increased again to 19% in the latest survey (Ogden, Carroll, et al., 2010).

Since the 1960s, the number of adults with a healthy weight has significantly decreased. During that time there has been a notable increase in weight. This increase was particularly noticeable between 1980-1991, when the prevalence of overweight increased from 13% to 21% among men and 17% to 26% among women. From 1999 to 2000 there was an increase of overweight to 28% of men and 34% of women (Flegal et al., 2012).

Individuals with disabilities experience greater rates of overweight and obesity than individuals without disabilities (Rimmer & Wang, 2005). In fact, the prevalence of grade 3 obesity (BMI ≥ 40) is four times that of the non-disabled population. Obesity among children without disabilities is approximately 12%, while the prevalence of obesity among children with asthma, learning disabilities, and attention-deficit/hyperactivity disorder is near 20% within each group. Children with autism have a prevalence of obesity exceeding 20% (Chen et. al., 2010). Considering individuals with psychiatric disabilities, obesity is 2.8-3.5 times more likely to occur in those diagnosed with schizophrenia, and 1.2-1.5 times more likely to occur in those diagnosed with bipolar disorder or major depression compared to the general population (De Hert et al., 2011). In a sample of individuals with disabilities from a major city in the Midwest, the percentage of adults with intellectual disabilities who were overweight was 84.8%, and 60% of this population was obese (Rimmer & Wang, 2005).

Causes

Genetic, medical, environmental, psychosocial, and behavioral factors influence obesity (Kopelman, 2000). The following provides information about the causes of obesity. These groups should not be viewed as separate causes, as there is often overlap and influence between the different factors.

Genetics: Children and adolescents are at a greater risk for overweight and obesity if their parents have a history of coronary heart disease (Grotto et al., 2003). Genetics interact with the environment and contribute both to the development of behavioral characteristics associated with weight gain and to the body's processing of energy (Ochoa et al., 2004), which indicates a role for both genetic and environmental factors. Genetics play a role in the development of behavioral tendencies, such as eating patterns and physical activity patterns, that contribute to obesity (Kopelman, 2000).

Medical: Some medical conditions, whether or not they are linked to genetics, are linked to obesity. Further, medications used to treat health conditions may also be associated with excessive weight gain.

Medical conditions that contribute to weight gain, independent of eating and physical activity patterns, include hypothyroidism, Cohen syndrome, Down syndrome, Turner syndrome, Cushing syndrome, Prader-Willi syndrome, Bardet-Biedl syndrome, growth hormone deficiency or resistance, leptin deficiency, precocious puberty, polycystic ovarian syndrome, prolactin-secreting tumors, and Frohlich's syndrome (Kopelman, 2000).

Related to health conditions are the types of medications individuals are prescribed. Certain medications cause individuals to gain weight. These include antipsychotics (e.g., Zyprexa, Clozaril, Seroquel), mood stabilizers (e.g., Eskalith, Depakene, Tegretol), Megace, sulfonylureas, monoamine oxidase inhibitors (MAOIs), oral contraceptives, insulin in excessive doses, thiazolidinediones, risperidone, and clozapine (De Hert et al., 2011).

Environmental: Environmental factors have a direct effect on exercise and dietary behaviors (Swinburn, Egger, & Raza, 1999; Wells et al., 2007) and, as such, a significant impact on weight status. Obesity research defines this as obesogenic environments, that is, micro and macro environments that influence health-related behavior. Macro environments are those at the regional or policy levels that have a direct influence on the more immediate micro level environments in which individuals directly interact. Examples of micro level environments include transportation, service centers, recreational facilities, community groups, local healthcare, and culture. Macro level environments include those overseeing transportation systems, city planning and related municipal departments, national and state health systems, and media (Swinburn et al., 1999). If the environment is felt to be an important part of a patient's obesity problem, it can be documented using an Environmental Factors ICF code, as shown below.

Some of the most prominent macro- and micro-environments that influence body weight include:

- *Recreation and park facilities*: Access to recreation facilities and parks is associated with increased physical activity in adults (e520 Open Space Planning Services, Systems, and Policies) (Sallis et al., 2012).
- *Density/diversity*: Density and diversity of destinations, such as shops and entertainment facilities, are associated with higher levels of incidental physical activity (e565 Economic Services, Systems, and Policies) (Sallis et al., 2012).
- *Public transportation*: People who live near public transportation are more likely to be active and less likely to be overweight (e540 Transportation Services, Systems, and Policies) (Sallis et al., 2012).
- *Food stores*: Access to food stores with more than 50 employees positively impacts eating behavior and reduces obesity risk (e565 Economic Services, Systems, and Policies) (Lopez, 2007).
- *Disadvantaged environments*: In disadvantaged populations, especially those with low socioeconomic status, access to food stores and places to exercise, as well as lack of neighborhood safety correlate with obesity (e520 Open Space Planning Services, Systems, and Policies, e545 Civil Protection Services, Systems, and Policies, e565 Economic Services, Systems, and Policies) (Lopez, 2007; Swinburn et al., 1999).
- *Chronic stress*: The experience of chronic stress, which is often environmentally related, may cause the release of high levels of cortisol, a hormone released by the adrenal cortex. Cortisol is needed for regulating energy and affects fat storage and weight gain. When the body is exposed

to increased levels of cortisol for long periods of time, excessive fat is stored, especially in the abdomen. Stress can be caused by any of e2 Natural Environment and Human-Made Changes to Environment, e3 Support and Relationships, e4 Attitudes, and e5 Services, Systems, and Policies (Daubenmier et al., 2011).

- *Culture*: Cultural and ethnic values can influence an individual's ideal weight. For example, cultures that associate food with pleasure as opposed to health may have different eating patterns. Cultural expectations regarding the role of women may influence levels of physical activity. In Western societies, consumerism has increased the availability of pre-packaged foods, which are often larger in portion size, greater in sodium content, and higher in calories than homemade meals (e135 Products and Technology for Employment) (Ball & Crawford, 2010).
- *Education*: Although being overweight or obese affects people at all levels of education, those with less education have higher rates of overweight and obesity (e585 Education and Training Services, Systems, and Policies) (Kumanyika et al., 2008).

Psychosocial: Psychosocial factors often stem from the physical and cultural environment. Some of the psychosocial factors may include stress and the experience of stigma. While stress is often related to the environment, economic stress, job stress, and social stress may contribute to overweight and obesity. Chronic stress may trigger excess consumption of "comfort foods," which is associated with abdominal obesity (Dallman, Pecoraro, & la Fleur, 2005). The experience of social stigma about weight may increase isolation and decrease physical activity among those who are overweight. Physical educators have a significant anti-fat bias, which may lead to less interaction and encouragement of overweight students (O'Brien, Hunter, & Banks, 2007). Exposure to weight-related stigma is also associated with increased caloric intake (Schvey, Puhl, & Brownell, 2011)

Behavioral: Behavioral patterns are critical factors related to weight status. From a behavioral perspective, weight status is maintained when there is a balance of energy intake (eating) and energy expenditure (physical activity). Thus, weight gain is associated with high energy intake and low energy expenditure (Kumanyika et al., 2008). Eating behaviors that are associated with weight gain include drinking sweetened beverages, eating frequent meals at fast-food restaurants or general eating out, and eating large portions (Kumanyika et al., 2008). Food types associated with weight gain include those that are high in fat and low in fiber (Kumanyika et al., 2008). Physical activity has levels from sedentary activity to vigorous activity. In 1996, the United States released the first Surgeon General's report on physical activity and health, which recommended individuals participate in 30 minutes of moderate to vigorous physical activity (MVPA) daily (USDHHS, 1996). However, the recommended levels of physical activity are related to maintaining cardiovascular health. Recommended levels to prevent weight gain are 60 minutes of moderate to intense physical activity per day (Kumanyika et al., 2008). Sedentary behavior is associated with weight gain (Neville Owen et al., 2010). Sedentary activities are categorized as requiring between 1.0 and 1.5 metabolic equivalent units (METs) and are frequently associated with seated, screen-time activities, such as television viewing and computer use (Owen, Sparling, et al., 2010; Pate, O'Neill, & Lobelo, 2008). Sedentary behavior is also associated with decreased levels of muscle glucose transporter proteins, which affects the metabolism of carbohydrates (Healy, Shaw, et al., 2008; Owen, Healy, et al., 2010).

Systems Affected

The primary issue with obesity is the inability to maintain a healthy weight (b530 Weight Maintenance Functions, d570 Looking After One's Health) but overweight and obesity affect all major bodily systems including the endocrine, cardiovascular, respiratory, muscular, skeletal, and psychosocial systems (Kopelman, 2000).

Endocrine system: One of the most common endocrine diseases related to obesity in the U.S. is Type 2 diabetes (T2D) (Gebel, 2010). T2D is a condition that occurs when the body becomes resistant to the effects of insulin, leading to high levels of blood sugar. The greatest risk factor for developing T2D is being overweight or obese. Over time, T2D causes poor circulation, as blood vessels begin to narrow. This leads to cardiovascular complications, pressure ulcers, reduced kidney functioning, cognitive impairment, and bacterial and/or fungal infections, among other problems (Beers & Berkow, 1999). In both men and women, the risk for diabetes increases significantly with greater BMI. Kopelman (2000) reports that when men with a BMI of 25-27 were compared to men with a BMI of less than 21, they were 2.2 times more likely to develop diabetes. Using the same comparison, men with a BMI of 29-30 were 6.7 times more likely and men with a BMI of greater than 35 were 42 times more likely. For women the risks were much greater. Again compared to a BMI of less than 21, women with a BMI of 25 had a five-fold greater risk. A BMI of 30 had a 28-fold risk, and a BMI of 35 was 93 times more likely to develop diabetes. While the majority of research has examined the risk of diabetes related to obesity in adults, pediatric populations are also at greater risk for both type 1 and type 2 diabetes (Reilly et al., 2003). Endocrine function issues can be documented with ICF code b540 General Metabolic Functions. See the chapter on diabetes for ICF codes to use if diabetes is detected.

Cardiovascular system: Obesity and overweight are associated with greater fat mass and body surface area, which leads to a larger blood volume. The heart has to work harder to accommodate the greater demand, causing an enlargement of the heart's ventricle walls. The structural changes in the heart and the increased blood pressure often lead to the heart's inability to accommodate the needs of the body. When this occurs, sudden death, cardiac failure, stroke, and abnormal heart rhythms may occur (Kopelman, 2000). Risk factors for heart disease include increased diastolic blood pressure, increased systolic blood pressure, increased LDL cholesterol, decreased HDL cholesterol, increased triglycerides, and high fasting insulin concentrations. The risk of coronary heart disease and stroke increases with larger BMI in both adults (Kopelman, 2000) and children (Reilly et al., 2003). Research indicates that over half of obese children (ages 5-10) had at least one cardiovascular risk factor, and one-fourth had two or more risk factors. For adults, the risk becomes even greater with age (Thompson et al., 1999). Cardiovascular problems are documented with ICF codes b410 Heart Functions, b415 Blood Vessel Functions, b420 Blood Pressure Functions, and s410 Structure of Cardiovascular System.

Respiratory system: Dyspnea, or difficulty breathing, is also associated with obesity. This occurs when adipose tissue surrounds the rib cage and abdomen, fills the visceral cavity, and is deposited on the chest wall. The added fat decreases the ability of the diaphragm to move downward. The load on the chest wall reduces the ability of the lungs to expand, while other visceral fat decreases lung capacity even more. All of this leads to inability to take a deep breath and feelings of breathlessness (Salome, King, & Berend, 2009). Respiratory impairment is exacerbated when an individual lies flat, which significantly impacts sleep patterns (Kopelman, 2000). The decreased arterial oxygen saturation contributes to the higher occurrence of sleep apnea in individuals who are obese (Kopelman, 2000). ICF codes related to respiratory functions include b440 Respiration Functions, b445 Respiratory Muscle Functions, b455 Exercise Tolerance Functions, and s430 Structure of Respiratory System. Document sleep apnea with b134 Sleep Functions.

Muscular and skeletal system: Sabharwal & Root (2012) describe many issues related to this system. Obesity has a direct impact on the muscular and skeletal systems. Being obese and carrying increased weight can cause increased stress to lower extremities especially the pelvis, hips, knees, ankles, and feet. In children, there is an increase in back and lower-extremity pain. Depending upon the age of the child when s/he becomes obese, skeletal development can also be impacted, resulting in deformed growth in the lower extremities. Children who are obese also demonstrate a more tentative gait, which may result from the poorer balance experienced by this population. Individuals who are obese also are at greater risk for high velocity related injuries, particularly in the extremities, than their normal-weight counterparts. Among adults, being obese increases the need for both hip and knee arthroplasty. Following knee and/or hip replacement, post-surgery complications are also more likely. While lower extremity injuries are more commonly experienced by individuals who are obese, issues with the upper extremities such as carpal tunnel syndrome and rotator cuff tendonitis are also more likely. There are many ICF codes that may be cited. Most are under b7 Neuromusculoskeletal and Movement-Related Functions, d4 Mobility, and s7 Structures Related to Movement.

Psychosocial system: The physical complications of obesity are well-known; however, obesity is also associated with psychological and social issues. Childhood and adolescent obesity results in an increased risk of developing depression during adulthood (Sanchez-Villegas et al., 2010). Children who are overweight also report greater psychological and weight-related distress than their normal weight peers (Young-Hyman et al., 2006). Weight-related distress is particularly evident in female children and is even higher in white female children (Young-Hyman et al., 2006). In adult populations, the relationship between obesity and major depression is evident, particularly in women; however, the direction of this relationship is unclear (de Wit et al., 2010). Important ICF codes include b125 Dispositions and Intra-Personal Functions, b126 Temperament and Personality Functions, b130 Energy and Drive Functions, and b152 Emotional Functions. Finally, obesity is highly stigmatizing and weight-related discrimination has increased by over 60% between 2000 and 2009. Weight bias exists in employment, healthcare, and educational settings. In addition, weight-related stigma negatively impacts family, friend, and romantic relationships. The experience of weight bias accentuates the impact of weight on psychological and cardiovascular systems (Puhl & Heuer, 2009). Document these issues with d7 Interpersonal Interactions and Relationships and e4 Attitudes.

Secondary Problems

The Systems Affected section provides an overview of the pervasive impact overweight and obesity has on a person's health. However, these issues feed back on one another, meaning the health condition may contribute to weight gain, and obesity contributes to secondary conditions. Overweight and obesity are risk factors for various medical conditions including diabetes, hypertension, osteoarthritis, cerebrovascular accident, heart disease, various cancers, depression, and sleep apnea (Kopelman, 2000; Kumanyika et al., 2008). Obesity can also carry a negative social stigma that affects the development of social relationships, education, and employment (Kumanyika et al., 2008; Puhl & Heuer, 2009; Young-Hyman et al., 2006). Adults who are obese often experience unemployment or underemployment. This may result from obesity-related health conditions, discrimination in the workplace, or a combination of both (McCormick & Stone, 2007). Obesity also negatively impacts performance in work, family, and social settings, which is associated with major disruptions in a person's life (Robard, Fox, & Grandy, 2009). Document these issues with ICF codes d7 Interpersonal Interactions and Relationships, d840-d859 Work and Employment, and e4 Attitudes.

Prognosis

Worldwide, obesity contributes to more than 2.8 million adult deaths (WHO, 2013). In the United States, the effect of obesity on mortality has decreased. However, in 2005, obesity was still associated with over 100,000 excess deaths (Flegal et al., 2005). The increased survival of individuals who are obese is associated with improvements in healthcare and the decrease in deaths related to heart disease (Flegal et al., 2005). In adults over the age of 50, having excess weight was associated with 7.7% of premature deaths in men and 11.7% of premature deaths in women. The association between obesity during midlife and premature deaths was stronger after controlling for smoking (Adams et al., 2006). Research indicates that approximately six percent of total national healthcare costs are associated with obesity (Wolf & Colditz, 1998). Children who are overweight, even at levels that may not be considered obese (50-74 BMI percentiles) are more likely to be overweight as adults (Kumanyika et al., 2008). Adolescents who are obese are up to 20 times as likely to become obese as adults than their non-overweight peers (Kumanyika et al., 2008). Childhood overweight and obesity is associated with poorer adult health outcomes. That is, individuals who were overweight or obese as children are at a greater risk of premature death and physical morbidity. Risks are particularly high for the development of cardiovascular disease (Reilly & Kelly, 2011). Long-term management of obesity class 2 and 3 in adulthood is rarely successful due to the many obstacles that the individual must manage on a daily basis. It is estimated that 90% of individuals who lose a significant amount of weight eventually gain all of it back (Kumanyika et al., 2008).

Obesity also affects the prognosis of individuals being treated for other conditions. Individuals diagnosed with breast cancer who had a BMI of at least 30 were 46% more likely to have distant metastases after 10 years. These women also had an increased chance of dying as a result of breast cancer (Ewertz et al., 2011). In orthopedic patients, individuals who are obese have poorer outcomes post surgery. This is related to increased occurrence of infections and longer recovery time (Sabharwal & Root, 2012).

Because weight loss is difficult to maintain, it is important to examine the personal factors that both contribute to and inhibit the maintenance of weight loss. The following descriptions summarize the relevant factors related to sustained weight loss and relapsed weight gain found in Elfhag and Rossner's (2005) review.

Weight loss patterns: Losing moderate amounts of weight over a longer period of time is associated with sustained weight loss. This likely represents a more sustainable shift in lifestyle characteristics. While significant initial weight loss may seem encouraging, individuals are unlikely to have adopted the lifestyle changes necessary to sustain the weight loss. Weight is more often regained.

Integration of physical activity: Leisure time physical activity that is sustainable, such as walking or cycling that can be integrated into a person's day to replace sedentary behavior, is associated with sustained weight loss. Prescribed physical activity leads to inconsistent results. Many fail to comply with the protocol, which leads to weight gain.

Food intake: Reductions in high-fat foods and increases in fruits and vegetables lead to sustained weight loss. However, individuals who score high on hunger prior to dieting and post dieting are less likely to maintain weight loss that occurred as a result of very low calorie diets or diets that emphasize carbohydrates. Finding the proper diet for each individual is vitally important.

Meal times: Eating breakfast and other meals consistently has aided individuals in making healthier food choices and maintaining weight loss.

Flexible control of diet: Integration of overall healthier eating patterns, but allowing for occasional consumption of less healthy foods, leads to success. Individuals who completely eliminate preferred foods are more likely to feel deprived and do not sustain changed eating patterns or weight loss.

Stressful life events: Loss of a loved one, major illness, and personal or family-related stress often cause weight gain.

Self-monitoring: Recording physical activity, food intake, and regular weighing as a self-directed activity increases weight-loss success and leads to sustainable lifestyle changes.

Social support: Receiving support from friends, believing individuals are available for support, and engaging in weight maintenance support groups all aid in keeping weight off.

Coping style: Active coping styles, such as confronting issues, being active in response to stress, and seeking alternate solutions lead to sustained weight loss. Avoidant coping styles, such as excessive sleeping or ignoring the issues, are associated with weight gain or relapse.

Motivation: Individuals who choose to lose weight or have an internal motivation are more successful in maintaining weight loss. Those with an external motivation often experience weight cycling.

Attribution: Those who attribute weight gain and loss to behavioral choices are more likely to sustain weight loss than those who attribute weight gain to medical or other external factors.

Self-efficacy: Belief that one can be successful in behaviors related to weight loss and weight maintenance is required to be successful.

The literature also supports the notion that the presence of a psychological disorder, distorted eating behaviors, and poor health-related quality of life can significantly impact a person's motivation and response to weight loss interventions (Davin & Taylor, 2009). Due to these obstacles and failure rates, the prevention of obesity in healthy-weight adults and in children at an early age should be the first line of defense in reducing the risk of becoming obese (Kumanyika et al., 2008).

Assessment

Typical Scope of Team Assessment

Underlying medical conditions are treated or ruled out and appropriate referrals are made for psychological evaluations. Height, body weight, and waist circumference are measured and documented to determine a baseline. A diet and physical activity history is taken and evaluated to determine needs. In regards to physical activity participation, it is important to assess the range of activities. This includes assessment of sedentary, light, moderate, and vigorous activity (Hamilton et al., 2008; Healy, Wijndaele, et al., 2008; Pate et al., 2008). Objective physical activity assessments are more accurate than self-report measures. However, the majority of physical activity assessments were developed for individuals without disabilities. Populations that are sedentary or have mobility impairments, abnormal gait patterns, and/or memory impairments may not have assessments that accurately assess physical activity patterns (Warms, 2006). Therefore, it is important to capture as much information as possible regarding the individual's lifestyle, in order to identify factors that may contribute to weight gain. ICF codes identified earlier can be used to record physical problems that are found.

Areas of Concern for RT Assessment

In addition to the team assessment, the recreational therapist conducts a detailed lifestyle assessment to identify areas for change, including but not limited to coping methods, leisure time physical activity, eating habits and patterns, life stressors, time management, holistic self-care, and other personal and psychological traits that might hinder or facilitate success including self-determination, self-efficacy, self-esteem, self-confidence, persistence, optimism, motivation, readiness for change, etc. ICF codes that may be used include b125 Dispositions and Intra-Personal Functions, b126 Temperament and Personality Functions, b130 Energy and Drive Functions, b455 Exercise Tolerance Functions, d240 Handling Stress and Other Psychological Demands, d250 Managing One's Own Behavior, d570 Looking After One's Health, d750 Informal Social Relationships, and d760 Family Relationships.

The recreational therapy assessment will yield information related to the client's lifestyle, emotional status, and environmental supports. The following is a summary of possible findings.

Sedentary lifestyle: Individuals who are overweight or obese (outside of weight gain from medical complications) are likely to have a sedentary lifestyle (Hamilton et al., 2008; Healy, Wijndaele et al., 2008; Pate et al., 2008). Screen time activities are common sedentary activities that may be identified as coping mechanisms or common leisure activities. High rates of sedentary behavior are associated with decreased energy expenditure and screen time activities are also associated with increased caloric intake (Hamilton et al., 2008; Pate et al., 2008). Document the recreational aspects with ICF codes b455 Exercise Tolerance Functions and d920 Recreation and Leisure.

Social isolation: Individuals who are overweight or obese may feel ostracized within their peer group thus limiting the development and maintenance of social relationships (Puhl & Heuer, 2009). Distancing from social interactions may be the choice of the individual due to poor self-esteem or self-confidence and/or the result of others who avoid socializing with the peer who is overweight or obese. The supportive functions of social relationships are a necessary component of health promotion. Document with ICF codes b125 Dispositions and Intra-Personal Functions and d7 Interpersonal Interactions and Relationships.

Poor eating habits: Individuals who are overweight or obese (outside of the effects of a medical condition) typically have poor eating habits that have resulted in increased weight (Kumanyika et al., 2008). Identifying the types of foods and the consumption patterns of individuals will help identify eating habits that contribute to weight gain. Recreational therapists should make note of meal patterns, including frequency and typical content of meals, how food is prepared, and eating location, such as eating in front of the TV, eating in the car, or eating out. Particular eating behaviors are often associated with greater caloric intake and may contribute to weight gain (Ball & Crawford, 2010; Kumanyika et al., 2008). Document with ICF codes d250 Managing One's Own Behavior, d550 Eating, d570 Looking After One's Health, d620 Acquisition of Goods and Services, and d630 Preparing Meals.

Poor cardiovascular endurance: Extra body weight puts more stress on the heart, lungs, and muscles requiring a greater amount of energy for a task (Kopelman, 2000; Reilly et al., 2003). Poor cardiovascular endurance limits an individual's ability to engage in physical activities and often becomes a primary barrier to continued participation in physical activity. Further, some categories of disabilities may impact the individual's heart rate and/or endurance (Warms, 2006). Therefore, it is important to understand the differential impact of the individual's disability and his or her weight status.

Document exercise tolerance with ICF code b455 Exercise Tolerance Functions.

ICF Core Set

A brief and comprehensive ICF Core Set for Obesity is available to help identify diagnosis-related ICF codes.

Treatment Direction

Whole Team Approach

If there is an underlying medical condition that is causing weight gain, appropriate treatment for the condition is recommended and implemented. It is important to note that the focus for an adult who is overweight or obese is to lose weight, while the focus for a child is to slow down the rate of weight gain while achieving normal growth and development (U.S. Department of Health and Human Services, 2010). An initial weight loss goal for individuals who are obese should be no more than 10%, which can reduce many of the health risks associated with obesity (Foster et al., 1997). Typically a last resort to weight loss in markedly obese clients is bariatric surgery where the stomach is made smaller by transecting or stapling one of the stomach curvatures.

The team approach may address sedentary behavior, poor diet, coping skills, and other lifestyle factors. More specific information about these approaches can be found in the recreational therapy interventions. It is important for all members of the treatment team to maintain communication, as lifestyle change is difficult and requires a multifaceted approach.

Outside of the purview of recreational therapy, it is beneficial for the client to meet with a nutritionist to assist with identifying healthy food choices and appropriate portion sizes. Diets that allow for preferred food choices, in moderation, are more likely to yield long-term weight loss (Elfhag & Rossner, 2005). The focus should be on a healthy balance of various foods including fruits, vegetables, whole grains, and lean proteins. Whenever possible, individuals who are overweight or obese should avoid high-risk environments that lead to poor eating habits (Ball & Crawford, 2010).

Recreational Therapy Approach

The recreational therapy approach complements the team approach and focuses on modifications to lifestyle behaviors, coping styles, and identifying social supports. A description of recreational therapy specific interventions related to the team approach follows.

Recreational Therapy Interventions

Often, individuals who are obese, without other diagnostic conditions, are not referred specifically to recreational therapy. However, because there is a high prevalence of overweight and obesity among individuals with disabilities (Rimmer & Wang, 2005), recreational therapists should utilize a holistic approach that addresses both the primary condition, as well as the individual's weight. Often, research examines community-based interventions that may address weight gain or weight loss in large populations. However, characteristics from these interventions can be implemented in individualized intervention programs. Further, it is important to provide interventions based on the individual's "readiness to change" and not where the therapist thinks the client should be. Prochaska and DiClemente's Stages of Change Model is one strategy a therapist might use to determine where the client is in readiness to make the lifestyle changes necessary to improve overall health and well-being (Prochaska & Velicer, 1997). Document the primary goal of weight loss with ICF codes b530 Weight Maintenance Functions and d570 Looking After One's Health.

Functional Skills

Self-monitoring of behavior: Intervention strategies that promote independent behavioral change yield greater weight loss when clients are trained to self-monitor weight, eating behavior, and exercise. Further, computer-generated feedback of individual performance can provide encouragement and help sustain healthy behaviors (Wing et al., 2010). Clients who learn to monitor their own behaviors improve on ICF codes b125 Dispositions and Intra-Personal Functions, d250 Managing One's Own Behavior, d550 Eating, and d570 Looking After One's Health.

Encouraging physical activity: The American College of Sports Medicine (ACSM) has made specific recommendations for interventions that utilize physical activity to lose weight. While the physical activity guidelines recommend at least 150 minutes of MVPA per week, the ACSM recommends at least 250 minutes in order to achieve clinically significant weight loss (Donnelly et al., 2009). Combining reduced energy intake with increased energy expenditure is associated with greater weight loss than dieting alone, when the caloric restriction is modest. Promoting lifestyle physical activity, such as walking for transportation and standing more, is associated with reduced BMI (Donnelly et al., 2009). Finally, aerobic exercise programs lasting greater than six months were associated with a modest decrease in weight and waist circumference. However, the weight loss was minimal, suggesting that these types of interventions should be paired with diet interventions or that there is a need to increase the exercise intensity to maximize weight loss (Thorogood et al., 2011). Increased physical activity may improve ICF codes b130 Energy and Drive Functions, b4 Functions of the Cardiovascular, Hematological, Immunological, and Respiratory Systems, especially b455 Exercise Tolerance Functions, b730 Muscle Power Functions, b735 Muscle Tone Functions, and d4 Mobility.

Reducing television viewing: An intervention aimed at reducing television viewing was effective in reducing the amount of weight gained in children. The six-month intervention consisted of 18 lessons aimed to reduce screen time activity, a 10-day "turn off" period, followed by a weekly budget of seven hours per week of screen time. Families received an electronic TV time manager that could control the power to the TV once budgeted time was used (Robinson, 1999). Given the substantial amount of time adults spend in screen-based activities (Hamer, Stamatakis, & Mishra, 2010), this type of intervention may also be effective with adults. ICF codes that may be affected include b455 Exercise Tolerance Functions, d250 Managing One's Own Behavior, d570 Looking After One's Health, and d920 Recreation and Leisure.

Managing diet: Interventions that address diet are also an important component of weight management. Diet modification is more effective when recipes and training are culturally sensitive (d630 Preparing Meals). For example, participants and family members participated in an intervention that involved a modified version of the Rice Diet, which is a 1000-calorie-per-day diet. The modifications included cost reductions, culturally sensitive recipes, and addressing potential attitudes about weight loss. After the eight-week program, average weight loss was 14.8 pounds (Ard, Rosati, & Oddone, 2000). Regular meal patterns and manageable reductions in caloric intake also help increase and sustain weight loss (Elfhag & Rossner, 2005). The primary ICF code addressed here is d570 Looking After One's Health, but deficits diagnosed in ICF codes d7 Interpersonal Interactions and Relationships and e4 Attitudes are also addressed in this intervention.

Handling stress: Individuals who have active coping styles, and address weight gain systematically are more successful at maintaining weight loss (Elfhag & Rossner, 2005). Avoidant coping patterns like sleeping or eating contribute to weight gain (Elfhag & Rossner, 2005). Stress management techniques (d240 Handling Stress and Other Psychological Demands) should help the client develop skills to confront his or her issues. The recreational therapist can assist the client in recognizing the impact stress has on overall health and well-being and explore non-food related ways to deal with stress. For individuals who experience chronic stress, mindfulness interventions have been effective in reducing cortisol related body fat (Daubenmier et al., 2011).

Confidence: Individuals who gain confidence (b126 Temperament and Personality Functions) in their own skills to maintain healthy behaviors and reduce weight are more likely to lose weight and sustain weight loss (Elfhag & Rossner, 2005). Self-monitoring (Wing et al., 2010) and setting realistic goals (Elfhag & Rossner, 2005) can help increase weight loss self-efficacy.

Community Participation

Leisure-time physical activity: Encouraging clients to integrate enjoyable, leisure-time physical activity into daily life is often more sustainable than strict "exercise" programs. Behaviors might include walking, riding a bicycle, or joining a sports league. These behaviors may be used to replace sedentary behavior (Elfhag & Rossner, 2005). Improvements will be seen in b455 Exercise Tolerance Functions, d570 Looking After One's Health, and d920 Recreation and Leisure.

Social support: Social support is a vital component of maintaining weight-related behavior changes

(Elfhag & Rossner, 2005). Family involvement is a crucial component of weight loss (Ball & Crawford, 2010; Elfhag & Rossner, 2005). Often the entire family needs to change its eating and exercise habits. If the family does not operate as a cohesive unit, one person will find it difficult to change when everyone else in the home is engaging in unhealthy behaviors. This intervention addresses deficits documented with ICF codes d750 Informal Social Relationships, d760 Family Relationships, e310 Immediate Family, and e320 Friends.

Resources

Guidelines on Overweight and Obesity: Electronic Textbook
www.nhlbi.nih.gov/guidelines/obesity/e_txtbk/resources.htm

Physical Activity Guidelines
www.health.gov/paguidelines/default.aspx

Dietary Guidelines
www.health.gov/dietaryguidelines

References

Adams, K. F., Schatzkin, A., Harris, T. B., Kipnis, V., Mouw, T., Ballard-Barbash, R., & Leitzmann, M. F. (2006). Overweight, obesity, and mortality in a large prospective cohort of persons 50-71 years old. *The New England Journal of Medicine, 355*, 763-778.

AMA. (2013). AMA adopts new policies on second day of voting at annual meeting. *AMA News Room,* retrieved from http://www.ama-assn.org/ama/pub/news/news/2013/2013-06-18-new-ama-policies-annual-meeting.page.

Ard, J. D., Rosati, R., & Oddone, E. Z. (2000). Culturally-sensitive weight loss program produces significant reduction in weight, blood pressure, and cholesterol in eight weeks. *Journal of the National Medical Association, 92*(11), 515-523.

Ball, K. & Crawford, D. (2010). The role of socio-cultural factors in the obesity epidemic. In D. Crawford, R. W. Jeffery, K. Ball & J. Brug (Eds.). *Obesity epidemiology: From aetiology to public health* (2nd ed.). New York: Oxford.

Beers, M. H. & Berkow, R. (1999). *The Merck manual of diagnosis and therapy* (17th ed.): Merck and Co, Inc.

CDC. (2011). About the National Health and Nutrition Examination Survey Retrieved 4/13/2012, from http://www.cdc.gov/nchs/nhanes/about_nhanes.htm.

Chen, A. Y., Kim, S. E., Houtrow, A. J., & Newacheck, P. W. (2010). Prevalence of obesity among children with chronic conditions. *Obesity, 18*(1), 210-213.

Dallman, M. F., Pecoraro, N. C., & la Fleur, S. E. (2005). Chronic stress and comfort foods: Self-medication and abdominal obesity. *Brain, Behavior, and Immunity, 19*, 275-280.

Daubenmier, J., Kristeller, J., Hecht, F. M., Maninger, N., Karan, L., & Epel, E. (2011). Mindfulness intervention for stress eating to reduce cortisol and abdominal fat among overweight and obese women: An exploratory randomized controlled study. *Journal of Obesity*. Epub doi: 10.1155/2011/651936.

Davin, S. A. & Taylor, N. M. (2009). Comprehensive review of obesity and psychological considerations for treatment. *Psychology, Health, & Medicine, 14*(6), 716-725.

De Hert, M., Correll, C. U., Bobes, J., Cetkovich-Bakmas, M., Cohen, D., Asai, I., & Leucht, S. (2011). Physical illness in patients with severe mental disorders. I. Prevalence, impact of medications and disparities in health care. *World Psychiatry, 10*(1), 52-77.

de Wit, L., Luppino, F., van Straten, A., Penninx, B., Zitman, F., & Cuijpers, P. (2010). Depression and obesity: A meta-analysis of community-based studies. *Psychiatry Research, 178*(2), 230-235.

Donnelly, J. E., Blair, S. N., Jakicic, J. M., Manore, M. M., Rankin, J. W., & Smith, B. K. (2009). Appropriate physical activity intervention strategies for weight loss and prevention of weight regain for adults. *Medicine and Science in Sports and Exercise, 41*(2), 459-471.

Elfhag, K. & Rossner, S. (2005). Who succeeds in maintaining weight loss? A conceptual review of factors associated with weight loss maintenance and weight regain. *Obesity Review, 6,* 67-85.

Ewertz, M., Jensen, M. B., Gunnarsdottir, K. A., Hojris, I., Jakobsen, E. H., Nielsen, D., & Cold, S. (2011). Effect of obesity on prognosis after early-state breast cancer. *Journal of Clinical Oncology, 29*(1), 25-31.

Flegal, K. M., Carroll, M. D., Kit, B. K., & Ogden, C. L. (2012). Prevalence of obesity and trends in the distribution of body mass index among U.S. adults, 1999-2010. *The Journal of the American Medical Association, 307*(5), 491-497.

Flegal, K. M., Graubard, B. I., Williamson, D. F., & Gail, M. H. (2005). Excess deaths associated with underweight, overweight, and obesity. *The Journal of the American Medical Association, 293*(15), 1861-1867.

Ford, E. S., Giles, W. H., & Dietz, W. H. (2002). Prevalence of the metabolic syndrome among U.S. adults. *The Journal of the American Medical Association, 287*(3), 356-359.

Foster, G. D., Wadden, T. A., Vogt, R. A., & Brewer, G. (1997). What is a reasonable weight loss? Patients' expectations and evaluations of obesity treatment outcome. *Journal of Consulting and Clinical Psychology, 65*(1), 79.

Gebel, E. (2010). Weight-loss surgery and type 2 diabetes: Is bariatric surgery a shortcut to a "cure"? Diabetes Forecast. Retrieved from http://www.diabetesforecast.org/2010/mar/weight-loss-surgery-and-type-2-diabetes.html.

Grotto, I., Huerta, M., Kark, J. D., Shpilberg, O., & Meyerovitch, J. (2003). Relation of parental history of coronary heart disease to obesity in young adults. *International Journal of Obesity, 27,* 362-368.

Hamer, M., Stamatakis, E., & Mishra, G. D. (2010). Television- and screen-based activity and mental well-being in adults. *American Journal of Preventive Medicine, 38*(4), 375-380.

Hamilton, M. T., Healy, G. N., Dunstan, D. W., Zderic, T. W., & Owen, N. (2008). Too little exercise and too much sitting: Inactivity physiology and the need for new recommendations on sedentary behavior. *Current Cardiovascular Risk Reports, 2,* 292-298.

Healy, G. N., Shaw, J. E., Dunstan, D. W., Zimmet, P. Z., Salmon, J., Owen, N., & Cerin, E. (2008). Breaks in sedentary time: Beneficial associations with metabolic risk. *Diabetes Care, 31*(4), 661-666.

Healy, G. N., Wijndaele, K., Dunstan, D. W., Shaw, J. E., Salmon, J., Zimmet, P. Z., & Owen, N. (2008). Objectively measured sedentary time, physical activity, and metabolic risk. *Diabetes Care, 31*(2), 369-371.

Kopelman, P. G. (2000). Obesity as a medical problem. *Nature, 404,* 635-643.

Kumanyika, S. K., Obarzanek, E., Stettler, N., Bell, R., Field, A. E., Fortmann, S. P., & Hong, Y. (2008). Population-based prevention of obesity: The need for comprehensive promotion of healthful eating, physical activity, and energy balance: A scientific statement from American Heart Association Council on Epidemiology and Prevention, Interdisciplinary Committee for Prevention (Formerly the Expert Panel on Population and Prevention Science) *Circulation, 118*(4), 428-464.

Lopez, R. P. (2007). Neighborhood risk factors for obesity. *Obesity Research, 2007*(15), 2111-2119.

Ma, J. & Xiao, L. (2010). Obesity and depression in U.S. women: Results from the 2005-2006 National Health and Nutritional Examination Survey. *Obesity, 18*(2), 347-353.

McCormick, B. & Stone, I. (2007). Economic costs of obesity and the case for government intervention. *Obesity Reviews, 8*(s1), 161-164.

National Institutes of Health. (1998). Clinical guidelines on the identification, evaluation and treatment of overweight and obesity in adults. *The Evidence Report, 57*(4).

National Institutes of Health. (2008-2009). *Review of population indicating specific diseases and increased BMI.*

O'Brien, K. S., Hunter, J. A., & Banks, M. (2007). Implicit anti-fat bias in physical educators: Physical attributes, ideology, and socialization. *International Journal of Obesity, 31*(308-314).

Ochoa, M. C., Marti, A., Axcona, C., Cheueca, M., Oyarzabal, M., Pelach, R., & Martinez, J. A. (2004). Gene — gene interaction between PPAR2 and ADR3 increases obesity risk in children and adolescents. *International Journal of Obesity, 28,* S37-S41.

Ogden, C. L., Carroll, M. D., Curtin, L. R., Lamb, M. M., & Flegal, K. M. (2010). Prevalence of high body mass index in U.S. children and adolescents: 2007-2008. *The Journal of the American Medical Association, 303*(3), 242-249.

Ogden, C. L., Carroll, M. D., Kit, B. K., & Flegal, K. M. (2012). *Prevalence of obesity in the United States, 2009-2010.* Hyattsville, MD: National Center for Health Statistics.

Ogden, C. L. & Flegal, K. M. (2010). *Changes in terminology for childhood overweight and obesity.* Hyattsville, MD: National Center for Health Statistics.

Owen, N., Healy, G. N., Matthews, C. E., & Dunstan, D. W. (2010). Too much sitting: The population health science of sedentary behavior. *Exercise Sport Science Review, 38*(3):105-113.

Owen, N., Sparling, P. B., Healy, G. N., Dunstan, D. W., & Matthews, C. E. (2010). Sedentary behavior: Emerging evidence for a new health risk. *Mayo Clinic Proceedings, 85*(12), 1138-1141.

Pate, R. R., O'Neill, J. R., & Lobelo, F. (2008). The evolving definition of "sedentary." *Exercise Sport Science Review, 36*(4), 173-178.

Pi-Sunyer, F. X. (2002). The obesity epidemic: Pathophysiology and consequences of obesity. *Obesity Research, 10*(s12), 97-104.

Prochaska, J. O. & Velicer, W. F. (1997). The transtheoretical model of health behavior change. *American Journal of Health Promotion, 12*(1), 38-48.

Puhl, R. M. & Heuer, C. A. (2009). The stigma of obesity: A review and update. *Obesity, 17*(5), 941-964.

Reilly, J. J. & Kelly, J. (2011). Long-term impact of overweight and obesity in childhood and adolescence on morbidity and premature mortality in adulthood: Systematic review. *International Journal of Obesity, 35,* 891-898.

Reilly, J. J., Methven, E., McDowell, Z. C., Hacking, B., Alexander, D., Steward, L., & Keinar, C. J. H. (2003). Health consequences of obesity. *Archives of Disease in Childhood, 88*(9), 748-752.

Rimmer, J. H. & Wang, E. (2005). Obesity prevalence among a group of Chicago residents with disabilities. *Archives of Physical Medicine and Rehabilitation, 86*(7), 1461-1464.

Robard, H. W., Fox, K. M., & Grandy, S. (2009). Impact of obesity on work productivity and role disability in individuals with and at risk for diabetes mellitus. *American Journal of Health Promotion, 23*(5), 353-360.

Robinson, T. N. (1999). Reducing children's television viewing to prevent obesity: A randomized controlled trial. *Journal of the American Medical Association, 282*(16), 1561-1567.

Sabharwal, S. & Root, M. Z. (2012). Impact of obesity on orthopaedics. *The Journal of Bone & Joint Surgery, 94*(11), 1045-1052. doi: 10.2106/jbjs.k.00330.

Sallis, J., Floyd, M. F., Rodriguez, D. A., & Saelens, B. E. (2012). Role of built environments in physical activity, obesity, and cardiovascular disease. *Recent Advances in Preventive Cardiology and Lifestyle Medicine, 125*, 729-737.

Salome, C. M., King, G. G., & Berend, N. (2009). Physiology of obesity and effects on lung functioning. *Journal of Applied Physiology, 108*(1), 206-211.

Sanchez-Villegas, A., Pimenta, A. M., Beunza, J. J., Guillen-Grima, F., Toledo, E., & Martinez-Gonzalez, M. A. (2010). Childhood and young adult overweight/obesity and incidence of depression in the SUN project. *Obesity, 18*(7), 1443-1448.

Schvey, N. A., Puhl, R. M., & Brownell, K. D. (2011). The impact of weight stigma on caloric consumption. *Obesity, 19*, 1957-1962.

Swinburn, B., Egger, G., & Raza, F. (1999). Dissecting obesogenic environments: The development and application of a framework for identifying and prioritizing environmental interventions for obesity. *Preventive Medicine, 29*(6), 563-570.

The Obesity Society. (2010). What is obesity? Retrieved from http://www.obesity.org/resources-for/what-is-obesity.htm?qh=YTozOntpOjA7czo1OiJ3YWlzdCI7aToxO3M6MTM6ImNpcmN1bWZlcmVuY2UiO2k6MjtzOjE5OiJ3YWlzdCBjaaXJjdW1mZXJlbmNlIjt9

Thompson, D., Edelsberg, J., Colditz, G. A., Bird, A. P., & Oster. G. (1999). Lifetime health and economic consequences of obesity. *Archives of Internal Medicine, 159*(18), 2177-2183. doi: 10.1001/archinte.159.18.2177.

Thorogood, A., Mottillo, S., Shimony, A., Filion, K. B., Joseph, L., Genest, J., & Eisneberg, M. J. (2011). Isolated aerobic exercise and weight loss: A systematic review and meta-analysis of randomized controlled trials. *The American Journal of Medicine, 124*(8), 747-755.

U.S. Department of Health and Human Services. (2010). Physical activity guidelines for Americans 2008. Retrieved from http://www.health.gov/paguidelines/pdf/paguide.pdf.

USDHHS. (1996). *Physical activity and health: A report of the Surgeon General*. Atlanta, GA: U.S. Department of Health and Human Services, Public Health Service, CDC, National Center for Chronic Disease Prevention and Health Promotion.

Warms, C. (2006). Physical activity measurement in persons with chronic and disabling conditions: Methods, strategies, and issues. *Family and Community Health, 29*(1S), 78S-88S.

Wells, N. M., Ashdown, S. P., Davies, E. H. S., Cowett, F. D., & Yang, Y. (2007). Environment, design, and obesity: Opportunities for interdisciplinary collaborative research. *Environment and Behavior, 39*(6), 6-33.

WHO. (2013). Obesity and overweight. Fact Sheets. Retrieved from http://www.who.int/mediacentre/factsheets/fs311/en/.

Wing, R. R., Crane, M. M., Thomas, J. G., Kumar, R., & Weinberg, B. (2010). Improving weight loss outcomes of community interventions by incorporating behavioral strategies. *American Journal of Public Health, 100*(12), 2513-2519.

Wolf, A. M. & Colditz, G. A. (1998). Current estimates of the economic cost of obesity in the United States. *Obesity Research, 6*(2), 97-106.

Young-Hyman, D., Tanofsky-Kraff, M., Yanovski, S. Z., Keil, M., Cohen, M. L., Peyrot, M., & Yanovski, J. A. (2006). Psychological status and weight-related distress in overweight or at-risk-for-overweight children. *Obesity, 14*(12), 2249-2258.

25. Oppositional Defiant Disorder and Conduct Disorder

Heewon Yang and Margalyn P. Payne

Oppositional defiant disorder (ODD) and conduct disorder (CD) are found in the *Diagnostic and Statistical Manual of Mental Disorders, 5th Edition* (American Psychiatric Association [APA], 2013). ODD and CD are often categorized as externalizing disorders. These disorders are characterized by outward-directed behaviors, such as aggressiveness, noncompliance, over-activity, and impulsivity (Kring et al., 2007).

The *DSM-5* describes ODD as "an ongoing pattern of disobedient, hostile, and defiant behavior toward authority figures which goes beyond the bounds of normal childhood behavior" (APA, 2013). While it may be considered normal to exhibit oppositional defiant behaviors at certain stages of a child's development, if those behaviors are persistent for at least six months and clearly disruptive to the family and home or school, the child's issue may be ODD. Some symptoms that children and adolescents may present are losing their temper, arguing with adults, deliberately annoying others, being angry, negativity, malicious or vindictive behavior, and blaming others for all that goes wrong. Often times, as a result, the child's behavior disrupts his/her daily activities (APA, 2013; Mayo Clinic, 2009).

Conduct disorders (CDs) are behaviors that violate the basic rights of others or major societal roles (APA, 2013). In most cases, these behaviors are illegal, and they are repetitive and destructive enough to go beyond the mischief and pranks common among children and adolescents. Examples of these behaviors identified in the *DSM-5* include aggression and cruelty toward people and animals, damaging property, deceitfulness or theft, and serious violations of rules. The presence of three or more of the above behaviors in the previous 12 months and at least one of them in the previous six months allows for a CD diagnosis (APA, 2013). These behaviors are characterized by cruelty, viciousness, and lack of remorse.

Due to the impact of the child's behavior on people and surroundings, such as parents, peers, and schools, the criminal justice system determines which externalizing behaviors constitute unacceptable conduct. Once adolescents are identified as having conduct problems by legal authority, they may be considered juvenile delinquents (Kring et al., 2007).

Incidence/Prevalence in the U.S.

According to the APA (2013), prevalence rates of ODD, although dependent upon population characteristics and research methods, were reported as two percent to 16% in the U.S. The lifetime prevalence for ODD was found to be 8.5% in a large U.S. epidemiology study conducted by Kessler et al. (2005). The percent of children with ODD is unclear. Steiner and Remsing (2007) found that ODD affects about 20% of school-aged children, while Chandler (2010) found that over five percent of children have ODD. In general, males are diagnosed with ODD more often than females and, as age increases, so does the number of oppositional symptoms (APA, 2013).

In regards to CD, the prevalence estimates range from two percent to more than 10%, with a median of four percent (APA, 2013). In Kessler et al.'s (2005) study, the lifetime prevalence for CD was found to be 9.5%. Like ODD, males are more susceptible to CD than females. Loeber et al. (2000) found CD to be present in four percent to 16% of boys and 1.2% to nine percent of girls. Chandler (2010) also reported similar ranges of prevalence for boys (six to 10 percent) and for girls (two to nine percent). CD appears to occur as early as age three and may persist until late adulthood. It is also more prevalent in urban areas than rural areas (APA, 2013). In addition, social disadvantages such as low socio-economic status and poverty are factors that predispose children to ODD and CD (Carr, 1999). For instance, the longer the child has been living in poverty within the first four years of life, the more prevalent externalizing behavior problems become (Carr, 2006).

Moffitt (1993) theorized that there are two different courses of CD: a life-course-persistent pattern and an adolescence-limited pattern. While the life-course-persistent pattern may begin at age three and serious transgressions continue into late adulthood, the adolescence-limited pattern consists of high levels of antisocial behavior during adolescence only and ceases in adulthood.

Predominant Age

ODD typically begins by age eight, with higher prevalence in late childhood and early teen years. CD typically begins around age 12, peaks sharply around age 17, and drops in young adulthood (Moffitt, 1993). While only a few studies are available, it seems that there are differences regarding gender in relation to the age of onset. For instance, Robins (2006) found that 57% of boys with CD had an onset before the age of 10 years, while for girls with CD the onset was between 14 and 16 years of age.

Causes

Many possible causes are associated with the development of ODD and CD, and some common causes for both disorders are easily found. However, for ODD, since the onset of the disorder is earlier than that of CD, causes of the disorder are less clear than those of CD.

According to Mayo Clinic (2009), the causes may be a combination of inherited and environmental factors. Factors include: (1) a child's natural disposition, (2) limitations or developmental delays in a child's ability to process thoughts and feelings, (3) an imbalance of certain brain chemicals such as a decrease in serotonin, (4) lack of supervision, (5) inconsistent or harsh discipline, and (6) abuse or neglect. In particular, in ODD's case, familial problems, such as harsh parenting styles, lack of structure and guidance, frequent disputes between parents, and lack of emotional and physical availability, including separation or divorce, have been emphasized as main causes of ODD (Encyclopedia of Mental Disorders, 2010).

CD, on the other hand, includes a more comprehensive list of causes that are believed to interact in a complex manner. These include (1) genetic and neurobiological factors, such as inherited aggressive behavior, deficits in communication capability and executive functioning, and neurobiological deficits; (2) cognitive behavioral factors, such as difficulty in understanding and processing information and learned aggression; (3) psychological factors, such as deficiencies in moral awareness and lack of remorse for wrongdoing; and (4) socio-cultural factors, such as peer pressure, ineffective parenting styles, poverty, urban living, living in violent neighborhoods, and poor school achievement (Kring et al., 2007; Hinshaw & Lee, 2003).

Systems Affected

Children with ODD are disobedient and angry much of the time. They start arguments and are usually unable to stop and perceive rational discussion as a continuation of the argument (Encyclopedia of Mental Disorders, 2010). Interestingly, however, they do not perceive themselves as being argumentative or difficult. Rather, they blame their problems on others, provoke others by being annoying, and bully other children (Encyclopedia of Mental Disorders, 2010). Because of these defiant, hostile, and disruptive behaviors, they are more likely to have difficulty interacting with people, particularly with parents and other authority figures such as teachers, coaches, and therapists (Encyclopedia of Mental Disorders, 2010). In addition, the child's academic performance is affected and the child may also develop emotional disturbances such as depression and anxiety (Encyclopedia of Mental Disorders, 2010).

According to Moffitt and Caspi (2001), CD affects many aspects of an individual's life, including academic underachievement and dropping out of school; peer rejection, hostile communication style, and other aspects of social life; and family life, including child abuse and violence. It can also affect physical and emotional aspects of the person's life (Moffitt & Caspi, 2001). Moreover, CD seriously affects society. The financial costs of crimes and corrections for juvenile offenses caused by youth with CD are enormous. Costs may include disruption in classrooms, malfunctioning families, citizen's fear of disordered behavior, damaged public property, and a loss of a sense of safety (Encyclopedia of Mental Disorders, 2010).

Secondary Problems

Common secondary problems associated with ODD include: (1) ADHD, (2) depression, (3) anxiety, and (4) learning and communication disorders (Mayo Clinic, 2010). Researchers believe that in many cases, ODD is a precursor of conduct disorder (CD), or an earlier and milder appearance of CD (Hinshaw & Lee, 2003; Kring et al., 2007).

In CD, it is very rare for a child to have only CD. About 30-50% of children with CD have ADHD, and 25-50% have depression or anxiety (Chandler, 2010). Substance abuse also commonly occurs with CD with the two conditions exacerbating one another. "Children with CD are three times more likely to smoke cigarettes, 2.5 times more likely to drink, and five times more likely to smoke pot" (Chandler, 2010). Other common secondary problems are learning disorders, bipolar disorder, and Tourette syndrome (Chandler, 2010). Adolescents with CD often exhibit altered appetite, irregular sleeping patterns, and signs of hopelessness (Chandler, 2010; Kring et al., 2007).

Prognosis

In *DSM-5*, the diagnosis of CD includes all of the features of ODD, and ODD can be regarded as a precursor to CD (APA, 2013). In the *ICD-10*, ODD is thought to be a milder form of CD and they are considered as unique categories (Kim-Cohen et al., 2003). Thus, the extent to which ODD and CD should be considered as separate or as a single disorder is the subject of some debate (APA, 2013).

At any rate, CD may follow after ODD as children develop into adolescents (Encyclopedia of Mental Disorders, 2010). When ODD is not treated or if treatment is abandoned, the child will have a higher probability of developing CD (Encyclopedia of Mental Disorders, 2010). More specifically, for children who are only mildly defiant, the risk of developing CD is lower. However, the risk of CD becomes higher in children who are more defiant and in children who also have attention-deficit/hyperactive disorder (Encyclopedia of Mental Disorders, 2010). Statistically, about 52% of children with ODD will continue to meet the *DSM-IV-TR* criteria for CD up to three years later and about half of those 52% will progress into CD (Lahey et al., 1994). Longitudinal stability for *DSM-5* criteria is not known yet.

Passive-aggressive behaviors may develop as a result of untreated ODD. Persons with passive-aggressive behaviors typically see themselves as victims and tend to blame others for their problems or wrongdoings (Encyclopedia of Mental Disorders, 2010).

The prognosis for children and adolescents with CD is debatable. While CD in childhood does not necessarily lead to antisocial behavior or antisocial personality disorder (ASD), CD must be a predisposing factor (Kring et al., 2007). As discussed earlier, in the case of adolescence-limited pattern of CD or ASD, individuals engage in high levels of antisocial behavior during adolescence and return to non-problematic lifestyles later in life, while individuals with the life-course-persistent pattern of CD or ASD will continue to exhibit serious behavioral problems throughout the course of their lives (Moffitt, 1993).

Assessment

Typical Scope of Team Assessment

Children exhibiting signs of ODD and/or CD are evaluated by a medical doctor, psychiatrist, and/or psychologist. Tests, such as X-rays and blood tests, are utilized to exclude possible physical illnesses or side effects from medications that mimic ODD or CD symptoms. A behavioral observation, along with a review of reported behaviors and medical history, is conducted. Signs of other mental disorders such as ADHD and depression that often occur along with ODD and CD are additionally evaluated. If there are no suspicious physical origins for the symptoms, the individual is referred to a psychiatrist or psychologist for a mental health assessment to see if the person meets the *DSM-5* criteria for ODD or CD (Chandler, 2010).

The diagnostic criteria for ODD as outlined by the *DSM-5* include the following pattern of behavior (APA, 2013). The behaviors must be present for at least six months and behaviors in the first two categories must occur frequently. There must be at least four of the following behaviors from any of the three categories (Chandler, 2010; American Psychology Association, 2013):

Angry/irritable mood: The person (1) loses his/her temper, (2) is touchy or easily annoyed, or (3) is angry and resentful.

Argumentative/defiant behavior: The person (1) argues with authority figures, (2) actively defies requests from authority figures/rules, or (3) deliberately annoys others and blames others for his/her own mistakes.

Vindictiveness: The person (1) is spiteful.

In addition, to be diagnosed with ODD, a child's behavior: must cause significant problems at work, school, or home; must occur on its own, rather than as part of another mental health problem, such as depression or bipolar disorder; and must not meet the diagnostic criteria for disruptive mood dysregulation disorder.

Diagnostic criteria for CD as outlined by the *DSM-5* include the patterns of behavior listed below (APA, 2013). At least three of the behaviors must be present during the last 12 months and at least one criterion must have been present in the last six months (American Psychology Association, 2013).

Aggression to people and animals: The person (1) is frequently bullying, threatening, or intimidating; (2) frequently starts fights; (3) uses a weapon that can seriously harm others; (4) is physically cruel to people; (5) is physically cruel to animals; (6) steals during a physical confrontation; or (7) forces others into sexual activity.

Destruction of property: The person (1) deliberately sets fires to cause serious damage or (2) deliberately destroys property in ways besides fire setting.

Deceitfulness or theft: The person (1) breaks into someone's house, building, or car; (2) lies to obtain something, or (3) steals without a physical confrontation.

Serious violation of rules: The person (1) frequently stays out at night despite parental prohibitions before age 13; (2) runs away from parental home twice overnight or once for a longer period; or (3) skips school frequently before age 13.

The behaviors must also cause significant impairment in social, academic, and occupational functioning. However, if the individual is age 18 years or older, criteria are not met for antisocial personality disorders (American Psychology Association, 2013).

Beyond the client, the team should also assess the environment the client is in. Changes to the surroundings may be required before treatment can be successful. The primary ICF codes for the environment will be found in e3 Support and Relationships and e4 Attitudes.

Areas of Concern for RT Assessment

The anticipated findings may vary depending on the extent of each disorder, the age of the client, and previous experience with the treatment programs. The primary ICF codes used to document the behavior will probably be found in d7 Interpersonal Interactions and Relationships. ICF codes d710 Basic Interpersonal Interactions and d720 Complex Interpersonal Interactions would be used to document the basic deficits. Other codes in d7 Interpersonal Interactions and Relationships could be used to document deficits with particular groups of people.

The recreational therapist may also anticipate the following (American Psychology Association, 2013; Chandler, 2010):

- Defiant behavior that affects learning and development of appropriate coping mechanisms (b126 Temperament and Personality Functions, d155 Acquiring Skills).
- Argumentative and annoying attitude (b126 Temperament and Personality Functions, b152 Emotional Functions, d250 Managing One's Own Behavior, d910 Community Life).
- Deliberate refusal to participate in the therapy sessions and to comply with requests and rules (d355 Discussion, d720 Complex Interpersonal Interactions).
- Frequent outbursts of anger and resentment (b125 Dispositions and Intra-Personal Functions, b126 Temperament and Personality Functions, b152 Emotional Functions, d250 Managing One's Own Behavior).
- Anxiety and/or depression (b125 Dispositions and Intra-Personal Functions, b152 Emotional Functions).
- Short attention span (b140 Attention Functions, d155 Acquiring Skills).
- Verbal and/or physical aggression toward others, including health professionals (b125 Dispositions and Intra-Personal Functions, b152 Emotional Functions).
- Difficulty in getting along with other participants — social isolation (b126 Temperament and Personality Functions, d240 Handling Stress and Other Psychological Demands, d250

Managing One's Own Behavior, d910 Community Life, d920 Recreation and Leisure)

ICF Core Set

No ICF Core Set has been defined for Oppositional Defiant Disorder or Conduct Disorder.

Treatment Direction

Whole Team Approach

Once ODD or CD has been diagnosed, the treatment team may recommend a combination of therapies (American Academy of Child Adolescent Psychiatry, 2010). While the team treatment approach emphasizes social and psychological methods aimed at particular clients, it would also be important to consider the multiple systems involved in the life of the client, such as family and peers, for the success of treatment efforts documented with ICF codes e3 Support and Relationships and e4 Attitudes (Steiner & Remsing, 2007).

There are many different approaches for the treatment of ODD and CD. The ones that concentrate on the client focus on deficits found in ICF codes b125 Dispositions and Intra-Personal Functions, b126 Temperament and Personality Functions, b152 Emotional Functions, d240 Handling Stress and Other Psychological Demands, d250 Managing One's Own Behavior, d720 Complex Interpersonal Interactions. These approaches include:

Medication: Medication is recommended when ODD and CD are comorbid with other mental disorders such as ADHD, obsessive-compulsive disorder, or anxiety disorder.

Individual psychotherapy: The establishment of a therapeutic relationship between the therapist and the client is the foundation of successful individual therapy. The therapist must provide the client with a forum to explore his/her feelings and behaviors in a non-judgmental environment. The therapist may employ various therapeutic approaches depending on his/her practice philosophy. Examples of individual therapy sessions include anger management, coping skills, problem solving, and conflict resolution.

Cognitive behavioral therapy: Cognitive therapy can teach the client self-control, self-guidance, problem-solving strategies, and other techniques to modify clients' thoughts and belief systems. Behavioral therapy basically utilizes reinforcement techniques and rewards for appropriate behaviors so that the clients can generate positive behaviors.

Social skills training: Social skills training also employs reinforcement strategies and rewards for proper behaviors. Clients learn how to apply one set of social rules to other situations.

Parent and family treatment: The family structure may also contribute to the problem. This intervention tries to improve problems found in e3 Support and Relationships and e4 Attitudes. Parents learn strategies for managing their children's behavior. Parents are taught basic therapy skills such as reinforcement techniques, establishing rapport with their children, and negotiating skills. In family therapy, problems with family interactions are addressed including handling stressful situations and difficulties caused by living with children with ODD and CD.

Programs that incorporate many therapeutic approaches and interventions are proven to be effective in treating disruptive behavior disorders (American Academy of Child Adolescent Psychiatry, 2010; Kring et al., 2007).

Recreational Therapy Approach

Recreational therapy may follow similar approaches as the whole team approach. However, RT focuses more on the development of healthy psychosocial functioning by alleviating the symptoms of ODD and CD in community settings. All of the ICF codes addressed by the treatment team are considered within the primary treatment areas addressed by RTs: d7 Interpersonal Interactions and Relationships and d9 Community, Social, and Civic Life. The therapist provides recreational therapy sessions such as social skills training, leisure education, stress management, and relaxation training by utilizing a primarily cognitive behavioral approach.

Recreational Therapy Interventions

Interventions that are frequently implemented with clients with ODD and CD include:

Functional Skill Development

Changing distorted thinking patterns: The cognitive behavioral approach helps clients with ODD and CD to change their distorted thinking pattern. For example, training of social perspective-taking skills has been proven to be effective in reducing delinquent and antisocial behavior (Chandler, 2010). Cognitive behavioral techniques address diagnosed deficits in ICF codes d250 Managing One's Own Behavior and d720 Complex Interpersonal Interactions.

Communication: While some of the reasons for lack of communication skills are from deficits in body functioning, clients with ODD and CD lack communication skills mainly because of inappropriate thought processes, illogical beliefs, and negative attitudes toward authority figures and other people (Bailey, 2001). Therefore, provision of programs and activities that focus on communication skills are critically important for clients with ODD and CD. These programs and activities can often be facilitated either along with or within the context of the basic social skills and interpersonal relationship activities addressed below. Codes associated with treatment for inappropriate communication styles include b125 Dispositions and Intra-Personal Functions, b126 Temperament and Personality Functions, b152 Emotional Functions, d250 Managing One's Own Behavior, d710 Basic Interpersonal Interactions, d720 Complex Interpersonal Interactions, and d740 Formal Relationships.

Education, Training, and Counseling

Basic social skills: Social skills training is the most important component of the recreational therapy program. Through this training, clients learn how to initiate and develop healthy relationships with other people (Chandler, 2010). Social skills training has an effect as part of a multi-modal package. Direct instruction, discussion, modeling strategies, rehearsal, promoting, feedback, and operant techniques rewarding pro-social behavior and discouraging antisocial behavior are frequently used social skills training methods (Bailey, 2001). For individual codes, look under d7 Interpersonal Interactions and Relationships. Some important codes are d710 Basic Interpersonal Interactions, d720 Complex Interpersonal Interactions, and d740 Formal Relationships.

Interpersonal relationship activities: Along with basic social skills training, the therapist can utilize numerous recreation and leisure activities to develop skills in interpersonal interactions and relationships (d7 Interpersonal Interactions and Relationships).

Anger management: Anger and aggression (b152 Emotional Functions) are common psychological problems that the clients with ODD and CD exhibit. Through an anger management program, the client is provided healthy opportunities to vent feelings of anger through relaxation techniques, journaling, structured recreational sports, and other activities. The client also learns how anger can affect aspects of his/her life (Bailey, 2001). Codes the therapist can consider include b125 Dispositions and Intra-Personal Functions, b126 Temperament and Personality Functions, d240 Handling Stress and Other Psychological Demands, and d250 Managing One's Own Behavior.

Relaxation and stress reduction: There are many different relaxation and stress management techniques that have been proven to be effective in reducing stress and producing relaxation (Hood, 2013). Therapists are addressing deficits documented with the code d240 Handling Stress and Other Psychological Demands.

Leisure education: The recreational therapist educates clients about the benefits of participating in recreational activities. These activities alleviate the symptoms associated with ODD and CD, such as lack of social skills, defiance, anxiety, and aggression. In particular, teaching appropriate leisure activity skills and leisure resources are effective ways to engage the clients in recreational activities (Yang, 2002). Deficits in appropriate recreational activities (d920 Recreation and Leisure) are addressed along with deficits in ICF codes such as b125 Dispositions and Intra-Personal Functions, b126 Temperament and Personality Functions, d240 Handling Stress and Other Psychological Demands, and d250 Managing One's Own Behavior.

Community Integration

Recreation and leisure: Engaging in non-competitive, but expressive and cooperative recreational programs such as arts, crafts, and cultural festivals offered in the community provides the clients with opportunities to express themselves, to explore the differences among people, and to be able to tolerate other people (Yang, 2002). Changes should be documented using d7 Interpersonal Interactions and Relationships.

Miscellaneous

Some general principles apply to the treatment of ODD and CD. In particular, comorbidities and treatable and modifiable risk factors, such as bullying, failure at school, and poor parenting style need to be identified, as they are likely to require treatment in their own right (Quy & Stringaris, 2012). Some of the approaches to treating ODD and CD involve intervening with parents and families of the client. For example, in a program, The Triple P — Positive Parenting Program, parents are taught to enhance parenting skills and improve the parent-child relationship (e3 Support and Relationships). The parents are encouraged to reinforce the pro-social behaviors of their children and to improve the behavior of siblings involved in the program (Bor et al., 2002, Quy & Stringaris, 2012).

A broader treatment approach for ODD and CD is multi-system treatment (MST). The therapist incorporates behavioral, cognitive, family-systems, and case-management techniques and emphasizes the influence of all the factors by involving the individual, family, peers, school, and community. Compared to traditional individual therapy in an office setting, clients who received MST showed fewer behavioral problems and far fewer arrests over the following years (Borduin et al., 1995).

In short, depending on the needs of the individual child and family, there will be a number of treatment options and combinations of those options. While typical treatments for ODD and CD are tailored specifically to the individual child, many other approaches and treatment options can be applied for these diagnoses.

Resources

American Academy of Child and Adolescent Psychiatry

3615 Wisconsin Ave. NW
Washington, DC 20016-3007
Tel: 202-966-7300
Fax: 202-966-2891
www.aacap.org
A medical association that supports children, adolescents, and families with mental, behavior, and developmental disorders.

Mental Health America

2000 N. Beauregard Street, 6th Floor
Alexandria, VA 22311
Phone 703-684-7722, Toll free 800-969-6642
Fax 703-684-5968
www.nmha.org/go/conduct-disorder

An organization that promotes advocacy, education, and empowerment so that we as a community and organization can support mental wellness.

References

American Academy of Child Adolescent Psychiatry. (2010). Your adolescent: Oppositional defiant disorders. Retrieved from http://www.aacap.org/cs/root/publication_store/your_adolescent_oppositional_defiant_disorder.

American Psychiatric Association. (2013). *Diagnostic and statistical manual of mental disorders*, 5th ed. Washington, DC: American Psychiatric Association.

Bailey, V. (2001). Cognitive-behavioural therapies for children and adolescents. *Advances in Psychiatric Treatment, 7*, 224-232.

Bor, W., Sanders, M. R., & Markie-Dadds, C. (2002). The effects of the Triple P-Positive Parenting Program on preschool children with co-occurring disruptive behavior and attentional/hyperactive difficulties. *Journal of Abnormal Child Psychology, 30*, 571-587.

Borduin, C. M., Mann, B. J., Cone, L. T., Henggeler, S. W., Fucci, B. R., Blaske, D. M., & Williams, R. A. (1995). Multisystemic treatment of serious juvenile offenders: Long-term prevention of criminality and violence. *Journal of Consulting and Clinical Psychology, 63*, 569-578.

Burke, J. D., Loeber, R., & Birmaher, B. (2002). Oppositional defiant disorder and conduct disorder: A review of the past ten years, part II. *Journal of the American Academy of Child & Adolescent Psychiatry, 41*(11), p.1275-93.

Carr, A. (2006). *The handbook of child and adolescent clinical psychology: A contextual approach* (2nd Ed.). Abingdon, OX: Routledge, Taylor & Francis Group.

Chandler, J. (2010). Oppositional defiant disorder (ODD) and conduct disorder (CD) in children and adolescents: Diagnosis and treatment. Retrieved from http://www.klis.com/chandler/pamphlet/oddcd/oddcdpamphlet.htm.

Coastal Adolescent Behavioral Health. (2010).Oppositional defiant disorder (ODD). Retrieved from http://www.thecabh.com/odd_signs_treatment.html.

Encyclopedia of Mental Disorders. (2010). Oppositional defiant disorder. Retrieved from http://www.minddisorders.com/Ob-Ps/Oppositional-defiant-disorder.html.

Hinshaw, S. P. & Lee, S. S. (2003). Oppositional defiant and conduct disorder. In E. J. Mash & R. A Barkely (Eds.). *Child Psychopathology* (2nd ed. pp. 144-198). New York: Guilford.

Hood, J. (2013). Monograph: Conduct disorder. Retrieved from http://ed-psych.utah.edu/school-psych/_documents/grants/specific-disabilities/conduct-disorder-monograph.pdf.

Kazdin, A. E. (1985). *Treatment of antisocial behavior in children and adolescents*. Homewood, IL: Dorsey.

Kessler, R. C., Berglund, P., Demler, O., Jin, R., Merikangas, K. R., Walters, E. E. (2005). Lifetime prevalence and age-of-onset distributions of DSM-IV disorders in the national comorbidity survey replication. *Archives of General Psychiatry, 62*(6), 593- 602.

Kim-Cohen, J., Caspi, A., Moffitt, T. E., et al. (2003). Prior juvenile diagnoses in adults with mental disorder: Developmental follow-back of a prospective longitudinal cohort. *Archives of General Psychiatry, 60*, 709-717.

Kring, A. M., Davison, G. C., Neale, J. M., & Johnson, S. J. (2007). *Abnormal psychology* (10th ed). Hoboken, NJ: John Wiley and Sons, Inc.

Lahey, B., Loeber, R., Quay, H., Frick, P., & Grimm, J. (1992). Oppositional defiant and conduct disorders: Issues to be resolved for the DSM-IV. *Journal of the American Academy of Child and Adolescent Psychiatry, 31*, 539-546.

Loeber, R., Burke, J. D., Lahey, B. B., Winters, A., and Zera, M. (2000). Oppositional defiant disorder and conduct disorder: A review of the past 10 years, Part I. *Journal of the American Academy of Child and Adolescent Psychiatry, 39*, 1468-1484.

Mayo Clinic. (2009). Oppositional Defiant Disorder (ODD). Retrieved from http://www.mayoclinic.com/health/oppositional-defiant-disorder/DS00630.

Moffitt, T. E. (1993). Adolescent-limited and life-course persistent antisocial behavior: A developmental taxonomy. *Psychological Review, 100*, 674-701.

Moffitt, T. E. & Caspi, A. (2001). Childhood predictors differentiate life-course persistent and adolescence-limited antisocial pathways among males and females. *Development and Psychopathology, 13*(2), 355-375.

Quy, K. & Stringaris, A. (2012). *International Association for Child and Adolescent Psychiatry and Allied Professions (IACAPAP) text book of child and adolescent mental health.* Retrieved from http://iacapap.org/wp-content/uploads/D.2-ODD-072012.pdf.

Robins, L. N. (2006). Conduct disorder. *The Journal of Child Psychology and Psychiatry, 32*(1), 193-212.

Steiner, H. & Remsing, L. (2007). Practice parameter for the assessment and treatment of children and adolescents with oppositional defiant disorder. *Journal of the American Academy of Child and Adolescent Psychiatry, 46*, 126-141.

Yang, H. (2002). Adolescents with aggressive behavior: Implications for therapeutic recreation. LARNet, the *Cyber Journal of Applied Leisure and Recreation Research* (August 2002). Retrieved from http://larnet.org/2002-2.html.

26. Osteoarthritis

Lei Guo

Osteoarthritis (OA), or degenerative joint disease (DJD), is the most common type of arthritis (Walker, 2011). Unlike other forms of arthritis, it may occur asymmetrically. So, for example, one shoulder may have OA while the other does not. It does not affect internal organs, but slowly wears away the cartilage that cushions the ends of bones in a joint (NIAMS, 2010). When this happens, the bare bone ends begin to rub against each other, causing steady or intermittent pain, swelling, tenderness, and loss of motion in the joint. A crunching feeling or sound may be present (NIAMS, 2010). Bits of bone called osteophytes or damaged cartilage may break off and float inside the joint space causing even greater pain and damage, also resulting in more stiffness of the joint (Arthritis Foundation, 2010).

Incidence/Prevalence in U.S.

Approximately 27 million Americans aged 25 and older have OA. Most persons over the age of 75 are affected with OA in at least one joint, making this condition a leading cause of disability in the U.S. (NIAMS, 2010). OA is predicted to affect one in five adults 65 years and older by 2030 (Farhney et al., 2010). Osteoarthritis is common in all races and backgrounds (Seed, Dunican, & Lynch, 2009).

Predominant Age

OA usually develops after age 45. Men under age 55 are more likely to have OA than women in the same age range. After age 55, however, women are more commonly affected. Overall, more women have osteoarthritis than men. One possible reason is that women's broader hips may put more long-term stress on their knees (Arthritis Foundation, 2010).

Causes

The exact cause is unknown, but a combination of variables is suspected to contribute to the development of OA. These include being overweight, the aging process, joint injury, stresses on joints from certain jobs and sports activities, and genetics (Arthritis Foundation, 2010).

Systems Affected

OA primary affects the musculoskeletal system, such as the thumb, fingers, neck, lumbar section of the spine, and weight-bearing joints (knees and hips). Secondary complications from pain and inactivity may result in hypertension, obesity, and muscle atrophy (Arthritis Foundation, 2010). ICF codes to record the OA symptoms include b280 Sensation of Pain, b710 Mobility of Joint Functions, b730 Muscle Power Functions, s730 Structure of Upper Extremity, s750 Structure of Lower Extremity, and s770 Additional Musculoskeletal Structures Related to Movement. Some of the other ICF codes that may be used to record complications include b130 Energy and Drive Functions, b134 Sleep Functions, d440 Fine Hand Use, d445 Hand and Arm Use, d450 Walking and other codes in d4 Mobility, and d540 Dressing and other codes in d5 Self-Care, and d6 Domestic Life. Other possible codes are discussed in the Secondary Problems section.

Hands: OA in the hands (thumb and fingers) tends to run in families. It affects more women than men. Small, bony knobs called Heberden's nodes may appear on the distal joints of the fingers. Similar knobs, called Bouchard's nodes, can appear on the middle joints of the fingers. Fingers can become enlarged and gnarled, and they may ache or be stiff and numb. The base of the thumb joint is also subject to OA.

Knees: Knees are primary weight-bearing joints and therefore are most commonly affected. They may be stiff, swollen, and painful making daily life tasks, such as walking and climbing stairs, difficult. If not treated, OA in the knees can lead to disability.

Hips: OA of the hip, like OA of the knee, can cause pain, stiffness, and severe disability.

Spine: OA of the spine results in a narrowing of the spaces between the vertebrae, forms bone spurs, and causes pain and numbness in the arms or legs (Mayo Clinic, 2013).

Secondary Problems

Muscle atrophy: Loss of muscle strength is often a consequence of decreased activity levels. Substantial muscle atrophy may manifest in multiple muscle groups along the affected limb, resulting in severe muscle dysfunction and reduced ambulatory capacity of individuals with OA (Rasch et al., 2007). Code with b730 Muscle Power Functions, b735 Muscle Tone Functions, and b740 Muscle Endurance Functions.

Psychological changes: Depression, anxiety, and feelings of helplessness are common in people who live with chronic disease (NIAMS, 2010). Axford et al. (2010) reported that the prevalence of clinically significant anxiety and/or depression was 40.7%. They found that pain correlated with anxiety and depression, and disability was greater in individuals with depression and/or anxiety. Use ICF codes b125 Dispositions and Intra-Personal Functions, b126 Temperament and Personality Functions, and b152 Emotional Functions.

Cardiopulmonary endurance: Decreased involvement in cardiopulmonary conditioning due to primary symptoms such as pain and stiffness and secondary symptoms such as fatigue and depression often results in compromised endurance (Arthritis Foundation, 2010). Studies have found that individuals with OA have lower endurance and aerobic capacities (Patterson et al., 1995) and are physically deconditioned with a decline in cardio-respiratory fitness, exercise tolerance, and functional activity due mainly to pain and musculoskeletal restrictions caused by OA (Philbin et al., 1995). The severity of OA is associated with the severity of cardio-respiratory deconditioning (Ries et al., 1997). People with OA may also develop cardiovascular problems and those undergoing surgery have a higher risk of perioperative complications, such as lower limb phlebitis, deep venous thrombosis, and pulmonary embolism (Ries et al., 1997). Code the endurance issues with ICF codes b410 Heart Functions, b420 Blood Pressure Functions, b440 Respiration Functions, and b455 Exercise Tolerance Functions.

Pain: Painful joints may impact the person's ability to perform life tasks (Arthritis Foundation, 2010). Tsai et al. (2008) suggests that OA of the knee has a significant impact on daily activities such as climbing stairs, walking, dressing, and transferring in and out of a car or chair. Individuals with OA may tend to avoid activity, fearing that it will cause more pain. Unfortunately, this inactivity may contribute to muscle weakness and instability of joints (Steultjens et al., 2001), cause other chronic diseases such as diabetes mellitus and coronary artery disease, and increase the risk of depressive symptoms (Sherman, 2003). Code the impact on life tasks with ICF codes d4 Mobility, d5 Self-Care, and d6 Domestic Life, as appropriate.

Sexual dysfunction: Pain, limited range of motion, limited endurance, and psychological changes can affect ability to participate in physical sexual activity (Wall et al., 2011). Use ICF code d770 Intimate Relationships to document this issue.

Upper and lower extremity weakness and numbness: Upper extremity impairments may occur from OA in the neck, and lower extremity impairments may occur from OA in the lower back. People with OA may experience more pain in the neck and lower back in the morning and evening but feel better during the day as the person's normal movements stir the fluid lubricant of the joints (Ray, 2005). Use the ICF codes for the primary symptoms for these issues.

Sedentary lifestyle: Secondary problems may result due to a sedentary lifestyle including pneumonia, urinary tract infection, decubitus ulcers, deep vein thrombosis, cardiovascular disease, obesity, hypertension, and contractures (Arthritis Foundation, 2010). See separate chapters on these conditions to find appropriate additional ICF codes for these issues.

Prognosis

There are varying degrees of disability and functional compromise depending on the severity of OA. Appropriate exercise and care can often keep symptoms in check and allow the person to live a normal life (NIAMS, 2010). The more invasive approach, joint replacement, is considered when significant pain in weight-bearing joints hinders a person's ability to complete basic life tasks. Significant pain in weight-bearing joints is one of the major causes for joint replacement (NIAMS, 2010). The end stage of hip or knee OA often requires joint replacement surgery (Felson et al., 2000). In the U.S. more than 350,000 knee or hip joint replacement operations are performed each year (Arden & Nevitt, 2006).

Assessment

Total joint replacement (TJR) is the most frequent admitting diagnosis for inpatient physical rehabilitation for those who have OA. Therapists may also see individuals with OA in an inpatient setting as a secondary admitting diagnosis.

Typical Scope of Team Assessment

Although OA is frequently a secondary admitting diagnosis, it still requires attention and treatment. The treatment team assesses the present, as well as the past course and management of the disease. This includes evaluation of activity limitations and participation restrictions that hinder the person's activity performance, functional joint limitations in range of motion and strength, knowledge and skills related to life task adaptations including techniques the has person implemented in the past, knowledge and functional application of joint protection and energy conservation techniques, available resources for assistance, and psychosocial adjustment. In addition to the ICF codes in presented above, the team should record any deficits found in the patient's environment using ICF codes such as e115 Products and Technology for Personal Use in Daily Living, e150 Design, Construction, and Building Products and Technology of Buildings for Public Use, e310 Immediate Family, and e580 Health Services, Systems, and Policies.

Areas of Concern for RT Assessment

There are several issues that the recreational therapist should consider when assessing a patient with OA.

Depression: OA may cause depression (NIAMS, 2010). Sale, Gignac, and Hawker (2008) found that among adults over age 55 with hip or knee OA, 21%

had depressive symptoms but only 14.4% reported being treated for depression. Risk factors associated with depression in persons with OA include perceived pain (Axford et al., 2008; Rosemann et al., 2007), physical disability and few social contacts (Axford et al., 2008; Rosemann et al., 2007), low-education status (Dexter & Brandt, 1994), younger age (Dexter & Brandt, 1994), experiencing greater pain and fatigue, being female, and experiencing stressful life events (Sale, Gignac, & Hawker, 2008). Use ICF codes b126 Temperament and Personality Functions and b130 Energy and Drive Functions to describe emotional issues. Also document the deficits that are caused by depression.

Secondary disability: Conditions that directly relate to a sedentary and inactive lifestyle such as hypertension, obesity, and muscle atrophy (NIAMS, 2010). Using ICF codes discussed earlier document any lifestyle deficits that are found.

Impaired mobility: This can be a result of OA in the hip, knee, or lower back or a secondary complication from a sedentary lifestyle (Sale, Gignac, & Hawker, 2008). Use codes in d4 Mobility as appropriate.

Activity limitations and participation restrictions: Activity limitations are often a result of the primary symptoms of the disease and participation restrictions are often associated with environmental and personal factors, such as transportation, finances, and adaptive devices (NIAMS, 2010). Kjeken et al. (2005) report that people with hand OA have problems in activities requiring considerable grip strength combined with twisting of the hands due to the reduced grip force and joint mobility in the hands. Machado, Gignac, and Badley (2008) suggest that symptom severity of OA does not directly affect older adult's participation in social and leisure activities. Instead it is the effect of pain on their mood and their ability to perform other types of tasks such as getting in and out of a car or using the toilet that may limit their leisure activities. Other than limitations in activities of daily living, more than 20% of individuals with OA reported limitations in sport in a study (Fautrel et al., 2005). Note deficits in activities with ICF codes in d9 Community, Social, and Civic Life. Also document environmental issues with the appropriate Environmental code.

Pain, fear, and anxiety: People often report that fear and anxiety of having pain is a pivotal factor in choosing, initiating, and participating in life tasks (Tsai et al., 2008). The pain is documented elsewhere. Deficits in life tasks can be documented with ICF codes d5 Self-Care, d6 Domestic Life, and d8 Major Life Areas.

Obesity: Being overweight is known to aggravate the development of OA (NIAMS, 2010). There is strong epidemiologic evidence that being overweight or obese, along with knee injury, are associated with increased risk of developing knee OA (Neogi, & Zhang, 2011). See the chapter on Obesity for appropriate ICF codes.

ICF Core Set

A brief and comprehensive ICF core set for Osteoarthritis is available.

Treatment Direction

People with OA often learn to manage the disease via education from their physicians and literature from various organizations. If pain begins to hinder the person's ability to complete basic life tasks, the individual is often referred to outpatient occupational and physical therapy services. Since OA is not reversible, should impairments become disabling, elective joint replacement surgery may be performed.

Primary treatment goals for OA are to improve joint care through rest and exercise, maintain ideal body weight, control pain, and achieve a healthy lifestyle (NIAMS, 2010). Approaches include medication, alternative therapies, surgery, pain relief techniques, rest and joint care, exercise, and weight control (NIAMS, 2010).

Whole Team Approach

Exercise: Research shows that exercise is one of the best treatments for OA. Exercise can improve mood and outlook, decrease pain, increase flexibility, improve the cardiovascular system, maintain a healthy body weight, and promote general physical fitness (Mikesky al., 2006; Penninx et al., 2002). The amount and form of exercise will depend on which joints are involved, how stable the joints are, and whether or not the joint has been replaced with a prosthesis. Strengthening the quadriceps has been found to relieve symptoms of knee OA and prevent more damage (NIAMS, 2010). In addition, individuals with knee OA who are active in a regular exercise program report less pain and improved functioning (Yohannes, & Caton, 2010). ICF codes that are addressed by exercise include b125 Dispositions and Intra-Personal Functions, b126 Temperament and Personality Functions, b130 Energy and Drive Functions, b152 Emotional Functions, b280 Sensation of Pain, b710 Mobility of Joint Functions, b730 Muscle Power Functions, b735 Muscle Tone Functions, and b740 Muscle Endurance Functions. Also record the Activities and Participation codes that are improved with exercise included in d4 Mobility, d5 Self-Care, d6 Domestic Life, d8 Major Life Areas, and d9 Community, Social, and Civic Life.

Psychological health: Developing a positive outlook is vitally important in the management of chronic disease to assist with motivation, initiation, and participation in life tasks that contribute to quality of life (Axford et al., 2010). These interventions address ICF codes b125 Dispositions and Intra-Personal Functions, b126 Temperament and Personality Functions, b130 Energy and Drive Functions, and b152 Emotional Functions.

Rest and joint care: Joints can become painful from excessive activity or prolonged sedentary states (NIAMS, 2010). The person must learn to monitor his/her activity level to manage pain and functioning. Splints may be prescribed, especially for OA in the hands, to minimize pain and allow joints to rest and maintain neutral positions when sleeping. They are not used extensively since stiffness, contracture, and pain can also result from immobilization. Areas addressed include b280 Sensation of Pain and d570 Looking After One's Health.

Stress management and relaxation training: These help to manage pain and relax muscles (Barlow, Turner, & Wright, 2000). This training addresses ICF codes b280 Sensation of Pain and d240 Handling Stress and Other Psychological Demands.

Pain management: Medications can help reduce pain and inflammation (Mayo Clinic, 2013): acetaminophen (such as Tylenol) can relieve pain, but does not reduce inflammation. Nonsteroidal anti-inflammatory drugs (NSAIDs, such as Advil and Motrin) reduce inflammation and relieve pain (b280 Sensation of Pain). In addition to medications, moist heat (warm towels, hot packs, warm showers) may be helpful to reduce pain (NIAMS, 2010).

Weight control: Less weight means less stress on weight-bearing joints. Exercise helps with weight loss. Moreover, individuals who are overweight and who do not have symptomatic OA may reduce their risk of developing symptoms by losing weight (NIAMS, 2010). Weight loss has an immediate effect on **d4 Mobility**.

Surgery: Surgery may be performed to relieve pain and disability of OA. Surgery may be performed to remove loose pieces of bone and cartilage from the joint if they are causing mechanical symptoms of buckling or locking, resurface bones by smoothing them out, or reposition bones. However, joint replacement surgery is the most common, accounting for 80% of all OA surgeries (NIAMS, 2010). Document the reasons for surgery by citing the ICF codes that can be addressed only through surgery.

Recreational Therapy Approach

To manage OA, outside of joint replacement surgery, the recreational therapist focuses on the general treatment directions to manage joint care through rest and exercise (d570 Looking After One's Health), maintain ideal body weight (d570 Looking After One's Health), control pain (b280 Sensation of Pain), and achieve a healthy lifestyle (d570 Looking After One's Health) (NIAMS, 2010). Recreational therapists also address psychological issues that could be impacting participation (Axford et al., 2010).

Recreational Therapy Interventions

OA affects individuals differently. For most people, joint damage develops gradually over years and has a relatively mild impact on ADLs. For some, however, it may cause significant limitations in daily life, including work, leisure, and community activities. Recreational therapists may address the following concerns:

Psychological function: OA may cause depression, anxiety, and/or feelings of helplessness (Yohannes, & Caton, 2010). Studies show that some types of exercises reduce depression and anxiety, such as aerobic exercise (Penninx et al., 2002), strengthening exercise (Diracoglu et al., 2008), aquatic exercise (Belza et al., 2002), and tai chi (Adler, 2007). However, controversy exists regarding the effect of physical exercise on depression. Some studies report that physical exercises have no

significant effect on depression, especially concerning the long-term effect (Yohannes, & Caton, 2010). Therefore, a combination of different types of interventions such as patient education programs, cognitive behavioral therapy, and exercise therapy should be considered for the treatment of depression with OA. In addition, social support has been found to play an important role in moderating the effect of pain and depression in older adults with OA (Blicen & Kippes, 1999). ICF codes that are treated with these interventions include b125 Dispositions and Intra-Personal Functions, b126 Temperament and Personality Functions, b130 Energy and Drive Functions, and b152 Emotional Functions.

Physical exercise: Exercise aids in better sleep (b134 Sleep Functions), reduction of pain (b280 Sensation of Pain), maintenance of a positive attitude (b125 Dispositions and Intra-Personal Functions), and healthy weight control (d570 Looking After One's Health) (NIAMS, 2010). Water exercises are especially beneficial because they provide range of motion (b710 Mobility of Joint Functions), endurance (b455 Exercise Tolerance Functions), and strength building (b730 Muscle Power Functions) with less stress on joints than land-based exercise (Suomi & Lindauer, 1997; Tsae-Jyy et al., 2007). Walking can be an acceptable physical activity for older adults with OA. Farhney et al. (2010) found that a goal-setting intervention is effective in increasing the physical activity levels in walking programs for people with OA. Song et al. (2003) reported that tai chi exercise is effective in improving arthritic symptoms, balance, and physical functioning in older women with OA. Bischoff and Roos (2003) suggest that aerobic and strengthening exercises seem to be equally effective in regards to pain and function in people with OA. Thomas et al. (2002) reported that home-based exercise programs can produce significant reductions in knee pain over two years. In obese individuals with OA, a combination of diet and exercise may be more effective for optimal benefits in health-related quality-of-life and physical function (Bischoff and Roos, 2003). Four types of exercise are important in osteoarthritis management (NIAMS, 2010). Strengthening exercises (b730 Muscle Power Functions) help support and protect joints affected by arthritis (Diracoglu et al., 2008). Aerobic conditioning exercises (b455 Exercise Tolerance Functions) help control weight and improve cardiovascular function (Penninx et al., 2002). Range-of-motion exercises (b710 Mobility of Joint Functions) help reduce stiffness and maintain or increase proper joint movement and flexibility (Aoki et al., 2009). Balance and agility exercises (b235 Vestibular Functions, b755 Involuntary Movement Reaction Functions, d415 Maintaining a Body Position) help prevent falls and improve mobility (Piva et al., 2010).

Recreation and leisure: Recreation and leisure activities may help improve self-efficacy (b126 Temperament and Personality Functions), reduce stress (d240 Handling Stress and Other Psychological Demands), and maintain physical functioning levels (d570 Looking After One's Health) for people with arthritis (Guo, Yang, & Malkin, 2009). Listening to music (McCaffrey, 2008) and making visual art (Reynolds, Vivat, & Prior, 2011) have been found helpful in reducing perceptions of pain among people with OA (b280 Sensation of Pain). Leisure time physical activities such as walking, bicycling, and gardening showed no relationship with incidence of severe knee or hip OA. However, higher leisure time physical activity may have a protective role for the incidence of hip replacement (Ageberg et al., 2012). In addition, providing recreation and leisure activities addresses deficits diagnosed in d920 Recreation and Leisure.

Disease education: People with OA should be educated about the disease. Three kinds of programs could be introduced to help individuals understand osteoarthritis and learn self-care: patient education programs, arthritis self-management programs, and arthritis support groups (NIAMS, 2010). Research shows that patient education and social support are low-cost, effective ways to decrease pain and reduce the use of medication (NIAMS, 2010). Barlow, Turner, and Wright (2000) reported that the Arthritis Self-Management Program significantly reduces depression (b152 Emotional Functions), fatigue (b455 Exercise Tolerance Functions), and anxiety (b152 Emotional Functions), while increasing self-efficacy as shown in the clients' belief that they are capable of managing their own condition (b126 Temperament and Personality Functions). The program also led to a range of health behaviors, often included in d570 Looking After One's Health, that included cognitive symptoms management, communication with physicians, and better dietary habits.

Deficits in e3 Support and Relationships are also addressed here.

Joint care: Individuals are taught joint protection techniques, energy conservation techniques, and proper body mechanics to prevent further joint damage, as well as how to incorporate these techniques in recreation, leisure, play, and community activities. The joint protection techniques help the patient with b280 Sensation of Pain. They also help the client participate in activities that are affected by b7 Neuromusculoskeletal and Movement-Related Functions. Joint care may additionally include prescription and training on adaptive equipment (e1 Products and Technology). If an individual is prescribed a splint, recreational therapists must be sure the individual follows the instructions for when to wear the splint, how to don and doff it correctly, and how to incorporate it into functional activities as appropriate. Document all of these interventions by citing deficits they are addressing from the Activities and Participation codes.

Pain and stress management: Stress management and relaxation training techniques are taught and then monitored for effectiveness in managing pain. Recreational therapists also address negative and distorted thought processes through cognitive behavioral therapy (CBT) interventions that positively correlate with managing stress and pain levels (Yohannes, & Caton, 2010). ICF codes include b280 Sensation of Pain and d240 Handling Stress and Other Psychological Demands.

Healthy lifestyle: The development of a healthy activity pattern that accounts for activity limitations and participation restrictions is a vital component of recreational therapy because the individual needs to learn how to balance exercise and rest. This can address any of the ICF codes found during the assessment (Bijlsma & Knahr, 2007).

Sexual activity: Recreational therapists often include the topic of sexuality (d770 Intimate Relationships) when addressing re-involvement in life tasks since pain, limited range of motion, limited endurance, and psychological changes can affect the person's ability to participate in physical sexual activity (Wall et al., 2011).

Community integration: Carryover of learned skills into a real-life environment is essential to promote follow through with a designed activity pattern. Cite improvements in the specific activity in the real-life setting such as d620 Acquisition of Goods and Services or d920 Recreation and Leisure and/or the specific skills within the integrated setting, e.g., d465 Moving Around Using Equipment. Community integration increases the sense of belonging, which is essential to one's mental health (Mock et al., 2010). ICF codes in d7 Interpersonal Interactions and Relationships are also addressed here.

Caregiver training: Research finds that help from spouses plays an import role in improving physical fitness, coping with pain, and self-efficacy of the person with OA (e310 Immediate Family) (NIAMS, 2010).

Weight reduction: People with OA who are overweight should have weight control programs to reduce stress on weight-bearing joints, limit further injury, and increase mobility (b710 Mobility of Joint Functions). Diet education programs should be included in the weight control program as well as the exercise program (Messier, 2010).

Miscellaneous

Research shows that people with OA who take part in their own care report less pain, make fewer doctor visits, and enjoy a better quality of life (NIH, 2002). There is some evidence to suggest that the intervention of CBT, integrated depression care management, and exercise therapy are associated with reduced depressive symptoms in the short term, while the long-term benefits of depression management in individuals with OA with comorbid depression are unknown (Yohannes, & Caton, 2010).

Resources

Arthritis Foundation

www.arthritis.org

This website has basic information about different types of arthritis, events and programs, current research, and links for more information for caregiver, advocates, and donations.

National Institutes of Health

www.nih.gov

This website has information about health issues, grants and funding, news and events, research and training, and more.

National Institute of Arthritis and Musculoskeletal and Skin Diseases (NIAMS)

www.niams.nih.gov

This website has information related specifically to arthritis and musculoskeletal and skin disease.

References

Adler, P. A. (2007). The effects of Tai Chi on pain and function in older adults with osteoarthritis. Unpublished doctoral dissertation, Case Western Reserve University, Cleveland, OH.

Ageberg, E., Engström, G., de Verdier, M., Rollof, J., Roos, E. M., & Lohmander, L. S. (2012). Effect of leisure time physical activity on severe knee or hip osteoarthritis leading to total joint replacement: A population-based prospective cohort study. *BMC Musculoskeletal Disorders, 13*, 73-79.

Aoki, O., Tsumura, N., Kimura, A., Okuyama, S., Takikawa, S., & Hirata, S. (2009). Home stretching exercise is effective for improving knee range of motion and gait in patients with knee osteoarthritis. *Journal of Physical Therapy Science, 21*(2), 113-119.

Arden, N. & Nevitt, M. C. (2006). Osteoarthritis: Epidemiology. *Best Practice and Research Clinical Rheumatology, 20*(1), 3-25.

Arthritis Foundation (2010). Osteoarthritis. Accessed via website http://www.arthritis.org/disease-center.php?disease_id=32.

Axford, J., Butt, A., Heron, C., Hammond, J., Morgan, J., Alavi, A., et al. (2010). Prevalence of anxiety and depression in osteoarthritis: Use of the Hospital Anxiety and Depression Scale as a screening tool. *Clinical Rheumatology, 29*(11), 1277-1283.

Axford, J., Heron, C., Ross, F., & Victor, C. R. (2008). Management of knee osteoarthritis in primary care: Pain and depression are the major obstacles. *Journal of Psychosomatic Research, 64*, 461-467.

Bijlsma, J. & Knahr, K. (2007). Strategies for the prevention and management of osteoarthritis of the hip and knee. *Clinical Rheumatology, 21*(1), 59-76.

Barlow, J. H., Turner, A. P., & Wright, C. C. (2000). A randomized controlled study of the arthritis self-management programme in the UK. *Health Education and Research, 15*(6), 665-680.

Belza, B., Topolski, T., Kinne, S., Patrick, D. L., & Ramsey, S. D. (2002). Does adherence make a difference? Results from a community-based aquatic exercise program. *Nursing Research, 51*(5), 285-291.

Bischoff, H. A. & Roos, E. M. (2003). Effectiveness and safety of strengthening, aerobic, and coordination exercises for patients with osteoarthritis. *Current Opinion in Rheumatology, 15*, 141-144.

Blicen, C. E. & Kippes, C. (1999). Depression, social support, and quality of life in older adults with osteoarthritis. *Journal of Nursing Scholarship, 31*(3), 221-226.

Dexter, P. & Brandt, K. (1994). Distribution and predictors of depressive symptoms in osteoarthritis. *The Journal of Rheumatology, 21*(2), 279-286.

Diracoglu, D., Baskent, A., Celik, A., Issever, H., & Aydin, R. (2008). Long-term effects of kinesthesia/balance and strengthening exercises on patients with knee osteoarthritis: A one-year follow-up study. *Journal of Back and Musculoskeletal Rehabilitation, 21*(4), 253-262.

Farhney, S., Kelley, C., Dattilo, J., & Rusch, F. (2010). Effects of goal setting on activity level of senior exercisers with osteoarthritis residing in the community. *Therapeutic Recreation Journal, 44*(2), 87-102.

Fautrel, B., Hilliquin, P., Rozenberg, S., Alleart, F., Coste, P., Leclerc, A., et al. (2005). Impact of osteoarthritis: Results of a nationwide survey of 10,000 patients consulting for OA. *Journal of Joint Bone Spine, 72*(3), 235-240.

Felson, D. T., Lawrence, R. C., Dieppe, P. A., Hirsch, R., Helmick, C. G., Jordan, J. M., et al. (2000). Osteoarthritis: New insights. Part 1: The disease and its risk factors. *Annals of Internal Medicine, 133*(8), 635-646.

Guo, L., Yang, H., & Malkin, M. (2009). Self-efficacy and arthritis impact on health: The effect of an Arthritis Foundation aquatic program. *American Journal of Therapeutic Recreation, 8*(4), 9-19.

Kjeken, I., Dagfinrud, H., Slatkowsky-Christensen, B., Mowinckel, P., Uhlig, T., Kvien, T. K., et al. (2005). Activity limitations and participation restrictions in women with hand osteoarthritis: Patients' descriptions and associations between dimensions of functioning. *Annals of the Rheumatic Diseases, 64*, 1633-1638.

Machado, G. M., Gignac, M. M., & Badley, E. M. (2008). Participation restrictions among older adults with osteoarthritis: A mediated model of physical symptoms, activity limitations, and depression. *Arthritis Care & Research, 59*(1), 129-135.

Mayo Clinic. (2013). Arthritis of the spine. Accessed via website http://www.mayoclinic.com/health/medical/IM01682.

McCaffrey, R. (2008). Using music to interrupt the cycle of chronic pain. *Journal of Pain Management, 1*(3), 215–221.

Messier, S. (2010). Diet and exercise for obese adults with knee osteoarthritis. *Clinics in Geriatric Medicine, 26*(3), 461-477.

Mikesky, A. E., Mazzuca, S. A., Brandt, K. D., Perins, S. M., Damush, T., & Lane, K. A. (2006). Effects of strength training on the incidence and progression of knee osteoarthritis. *Arthritis and Rheumatism, 55*(5), 690-699.

Mock, S. E., Fraser, C., Knutson, S., & Prier, A. (2010). Physical leisure participation and the well-being of adults with rheumatoid arthritis: The role of sense of belonging. *Activities, Adaptation & Aging, 34*(4), 292-302.

National Institute of Arthritis and Musculoskeletal and Skin Diseases (NIAMS). (2010). Osteoarthritis. Accessed via website http://www.niams.nih.gov/Health_Info/Osteoarthritis/default.asp#osteoarthritis.

National Institutes of Health. (2002). Handout on health: Osteoarthritis. Accessed via website http://www.niams.nih.gov.

Neogi, T. & Zhang, Y. (2011). Osteoarthritis prevention. *Current Opinion in Rheumatology, 23*(2), 185-191.

Patterson, A. J., Murphy, N. M., Nugent, A. M., Finlay, O. E., Nicholls, D. P., & Boreham, C. A. G., et al. (1995). The effect of minimal exercise on fitness in elderly women after hip surgery. *Ulster Medical Journal, 64*, 118-125.

Penninx, B., Rejeski, W. J., Pandya, J., Miller, M., Bari, M., Applegate, W., et al. (2002). Exercise and depressive symptoms: A comparison of aerobic and resistance exercise effects on emotional and physical function in older persons with high and low depressive symptomatology. *Journal of Gerontology: Psychological Sciences, 57B*(2), 124-132.

Philbin, E. F., Groff, G. D., Ries, M. D., & Miller, T. E. (1995). Cardiovascular fitness and health in patients with end-stage osteoarthritis. *Arthritis & Rheumatism, 38*, 799-805.

Piva, S., Gil, A., Almeida, G., DiGioia, A., Levison, T., & Fitzgerald, G. (2010). A balance exercise program appears to improve function for patients with total knee arthroplasty: A randomized clinical trial. *Physical Therapy, 90*(6), 880-894.

Rasch, A., Bystrom, A. H., Dalen, N., & Berg, H. E. (2007). Reduced muscle radiological density, cross-sectional area, and strength of major hip and knee muscles in 22 patients with hip osteoarthritis. *Acta Orthopaedica, 78*(4), 505-510.

Ray, C. (2005). Osteoarthritis symptoms. Accessed via web http://www.spine-health.com/conditions/arthritis/osteoarthritis-symptoms.

Reynolds, F., Vivat, B., & Prior, S. (2011). Visual art-making as a resource for living positively with arthritis: An interpretative phenomenological analysis of older women's accounts. *Journal of Aging Studies, 25*, 328-337.

Ries, M. D., Philbin, E. F., Groff, G. D., Sheesley, K. A., Richman, J. A., & Lynch, F. (1997). Effect of total hip arthroplasty on cardiovascular fitness. *Journal of Arthroplasty, 12*, 84-90.

Rosemann, T., Backenstrass, M., Joest, K., Rosemann, A., Szecsenyi, J., & Laux, G. (2007). Predictors of depression in a sample of 1021 primary care patients with osteoarthritis. *Arthritis and Rheumatism, 57*(3), 15-22.

Sale, J. E. M., Gignac, M., & Hawker, G. (2008). The relationship between disease symptoms, life events, coping and treatment, and depression among older adults with osteoarthritis. *Journal of Rheumatology, 35*(2), 335-342.

Seed, S., Dunican, K., & Lynch, A. (2009). Osteoarthritis: A review of treatment options. *Geriatrics, 64*(10), 20-29.

Sherman, A. M. (2003). Social relations and depressive symptoms in older adults with knee osteoarthritis. *Social Science & Medicine, 56*, 247-257.

Song, R., Lee, E., Lam, P., & Bae, S. (2003). Effects of tai chi exercise on pain, balance, muscle strength, and perceived difficulties in physical functioning in older women with osteoarthritis: A randomized clinical trial. *The Journal of Rheumatology, 30*(9), 2039-2044.

Steultjens, M. P., Dekker, J., & Bijlsma, J. W. (2001). Coping, pain and disability in osteoarthritis: A longitudinal study. *The Journal of Rheumatology 28*, 1068-1072.

Suomi, R. & Lindauer, S. (1997). Effectiveness of Arthritis Foundation aquatic program on strength and range of motion in women with arthritis. *Journal of Aging and Physical Activity, 5*, 341-351.

Thomas, K., Muir, K., Doherty, M., Jones, A., O'Reilly, S., & Bassey, E. (2002). Home based exercise programme for knee pain and knee osteoarthritis: Randomised controlled trial. *British Medical Journal, 325*, 752-756.

Tsai, Y., Chu, T., Lai, Y., & Chen, W. (2008). Pain experiences, control beliefs and coping strategies in Chinese elders with osteoarthritis. *Journal of Clinical Nursing, 17*(19), 2596-2603.

Tsae-Jyy, W., Belza, B., Elaine-Thompson, F. F., Whitney, J. D., & Bennett, K. (2007). Effects of aquatic exercise on flexibility, strength and aerobic fitness in adults with osteoarthritis of the hip or knee. *Journal of Advanced Nursing, 57*(2), 141-152.

Walker, J. (2011). Effective management strategies for osteoarthritis. *British Journal of Nursing, 20*(2), 81-85.

Wall, P. H., Hossain, M., Ganapathi, M., & Andrew, J. G. (2011). Sexual activity and total hip arthroplasty: A survey of patients' and surgeons' perspectives. *Hip International, 21*(2), 199-205.

Yohannes, A. & Caton, S. (2010). Management of depression in older people with osteoarthritis: A systematic review. *Aging & Mental Health, 14*(6), 637-651.

27. Osteoporosis

Kenneth E. Mobily

Osteoporosis is defined as a decrease in bone strength due to a loss of mineral content, making bones more susceptible to fracture (Marieb & Hoehn, 2010). Osteoporotic bones are more porous, thinner, and lighter than normal (Marieb & Hoehn, 2010). A related malady, osteopenia is a condition where bone mass is below normal but not low enough to be classified as osteoporosis (Martini & Bartholomew, 2003).

Osteoporosis results when bone loss occurs at a faster rate than bone deposition (Marieb & Hoehn, 2010). This dynamic process of deposition (adding minerals to bones) and resorption (taking minerals back out of bones) occurs throughout life in everyone. In the person with osteoporosis, the normal balance between deposition and resorption is disrupted, often by a change in hormone secretion (Marieb & Hoehn, 2010).

Bone density is determined by the actions of several hormones. Calcitonin secreted by the thyroid gland promotes bone growth and storage of calcium and phosphate in bone, leading to strong bones (Marieb & Hoehn, 2010). An antagonistic hormone, parathyroid hormone (PTH), is secreted by the parathyroid gland and causes the breakdown (resorption) of the calcium-phosphate mineral complex in bone (Marieb & Hoehn, 2010). PTH frees minerals, especially calcium, into the blood stream because low levels of calcium in the blood stream are life threatening. Both hormones act by affecting the activity of bone cells, osteoblasts, and osteoclasts (Marieb & Hoehn, 2010).

Sex hormones, testosterone in the male and estrogen in the female, also have significant and favorable effects on bone mineral density (BMD). As people transition into adulthood and age the secretion of sex hormones declines, sharply and precipitously in females during and after menopause (Marieb & Hoehn, 2010). The decrease in the secretion of estrogen with the onset of menopause explains why women are more susceptible to osteoporosis than men. There is no event parallel to menopause for men, though the secretion of testosterone does gradually decline as men age, and the decrease in secretion of testosterone is likewise associated with an increase in the incidence of osteoporosis in men (Marieb & Hoehn, 2010).

The reason a decrease in estrogen secretion leads to increased risk for osteoporosis is that estrogen seems to have a protective effect on bone by blunting the activity of the bone resorbing osteoclast (Marieb & Hoehn, 2010). With the decrease in estrogen secretion during menopause, the balance of osteoblast and osteoclast activity is disrupted, resulting in the net loss of minerals in bones (Marieb & Hoehn, 2010).

Incidence/Prevalence in U.S.

An estimated ten million people in the United States have osteoporosis, and as many as four times that number are at risk for developing the affliction (National Osteoporosis Foundation, 2012a). Osteoporosis is as prevalent among women as breast, uterine, and ovarian cancers combined (National Osteoporosis Foundation, 2012a).

Race is also a risk factor; non-Hispanic, Caucasian, and Asian women are at greatest risk (National Osteoporosis Foundation, 2012b). Hispanic women have the next highest risk of developing osteoporosis (National Osteoporosis Foundation, 2012b). Although black women have the lowest risk of developing osteoporosis, it is under-treated among all racial groups (National Osteoporosis Foundation, 2012b).

Predominant Age

About 50% of women and 25% of men over the age of 50 can expect to develop osteoporosis in their lifetimes (National Osteoporosis Foundation, 2012b). The percentage at risk is even more sobering, with 55% of those aged 50 and over at risk (National Osteoporosis Foundation, 2012b). Older age is strongly and positively correlated with osteoporosis and older women are four times more likely to develop the condition than men (National Osteoporosis Foundation, 2012b). A staggering 70% of American women have osteoporosis by the age of 80, compared to only 30% who have it between the ages of 60 and 70 (Marieb & Hoehn, 2010).

Causes

The leading predictor of bone health in old age is bone health in youth. Specifically, the greater the bone mass acquired during the developmental years of puberty, the greater the bone mass reserve available for later years. In particular, women acquire almost all of their bone mass by about the age of 20 (National Osteoporosis Foundation, 2012b).

Unfortunately, osteoporosis is often a latent disorder until the individual sustains a fracture. Some may experience pain, especially if the spine is affected, but many report no pain in advance of an associated injury (National Osteoporosis Foundation, 2012b).

Like heart disease, osteoporosis is associated with identifiable risk factors, both modifiable and non-modifiable. Non-modifiable risk factors include being older and female, post-menopausal, either non-Hispanic or Asian, and genetic predisposition, often shown by a family history of fractures (National Osteoporosis Foundation, 2012b).

There are many more modifiable risk factors that can be corrected by behavioral changes. Smoking and excess alcohol consumption contribute to osteoporosis. Alcohol is thought to interfere with mineral absorption in the digestive system, while smoking is thought to inhibit estrogen secretion (Marieb & Hoehn, 2010). Light body weight is a risk factor as well. Although one should not encourage excessive weight gain because of the obesity epidemic in the United States, higher body weight puts more favorable stress on the skeleton and stimulates the deposition of more minerals in response (Marieb & Hoehn, 2010). Adequate dietary intake of calcium and phosphorus is key, as these minerals cannot be manufactured by the body (Marieb & Hoehn, 2010). A sedentary lifestyle, especially the absence of weight-bearing exercise, is another risk factor. Some exercise is better than none, as long as the precautions discussed in the Treatment section are followed, and weight-bearing exercise is better yet. When it comes to osteoporosis, walking, because it puts more stress on the bones, is better than swimming (Marieb, Wilhelm, & Mallatt, 2011). Like body weight, weight-bearing exercise stresses the skeleton in an optimal manner, causing it to add bone-strengthening minerals (Marieb, Wilhelm, & Mallatt, 2011).

Less frequent risk factors the practitioner may encounter are secondary to eating disorders and rheumatoid arthritis. Eating disorders may cause amenorrhea in association with decreased estrogen secretion, which is correlated with bone loss (Marieb & Hoehn, 2010). Persons with rheumatoid arthritis often receive anti-inflammatory steroids which cause bone loss (Surgeon General, 2004).

Systems Affected

The skeletal system is the focal point of osteoporosis. Bones consist of organic and inorganic components. The organic components include several bone cell types, an inter-cellular matrix, called osteoid, and collagen fibers (Marieb & Hoehn, 2010). Important cells for the purpose of understanding osteoporosis are osteoblasts and osteoclasts. The osteoblasts are responsible for producing new bone tissue, while osteoclasts are responsible for breaking down bone tissue and freeing minerals into the bloodstream (Marieb & Hoehn, 2010). The balance of osteoblast and osteoclast activities ultimately determine the bone mass of the skeleton (Marieb & Hoehn, 2010).

The inorganic component of the skeleton is represented by its mineral content, primarily calcium and phosphorus (Marieb & Hoehn, 2010). It is the mineral portion of bone that gives it strength and determines bone mass (Marieb & Hoehn, 2010). The mineral part of bone is likewise the target of osteoporosis, with significant loss of the mineral content leading to a positive diagnosis of osteoporosis (Marieb & Hoehn, 2010).

Osteoporosis is an exaggeration of a normal process that occurs in everyone. Bone is dynamic tissue, with osteoblasts producing new bone matrix throughout life and osteoclasts resorbing old, worn out bone tissue at the same rate (Marieb & Hoehn, 2010). When bone resorption outpaces bone deposition, osteoporosis is more likely (Marieb & Hoehn, 2010).

The primary observation of reduced bone mass is documented with ICF codes in s7 Structures Related to Movement, most often s750 Structure of Lower Extremity and s760 Structure of Trunk.

Secondary Problems

Loss of bone mass is associated with an increased risk for fractures, particularly among older adults (National Osteoporosis Foundation, 2012a 2012b). Joints and skeletal components most at risk for fracture are hip (femur), spine (vertebrae), and wrist (radius) (National Osteoporosis Foundation, 2012b). Microscopic fractures in the thoracic region of the spine may lead to an exaggeration of the normal thoracic curvature. In its most severe form it may result in an excess concavity on the spine's anterior presentation, called a "dowager's hump" (Marieb & Hoehn, 2010). The excessive curvature may lead to all manner of functional difficulty, from abnormal ambulation to so much compression of the chest that it reduces vital capacity during respiration (Marieb & Hoehn, 2010). Other distortions of the spine are possible, including scoliosis and other posture alignment deformities (Marieb, Wilhelm, & Mallatt, 2011). Functional issues can be coded with ICF codes that include b280 Sensation of Pain, b440 Respiration Functions, b455 Exercise Tolerance Functions, b710 Mobility of Joint Functions, b720 Mobility of Bone Functions, b770 Gait Pattern Functions, and relevant codes in d4 Mobility.

A concern for recreational therapy in some severe cases is cosmetic disfigurement, which can alert others to differences when the person participates in usual activities. There are good data supporting the negative effects of cosmetic differences and attempts on the part of the impaired person to fit in (e.g., Hoenk & Mobily, 1987). Reactive depression is one psychosocial consequence that may develop secondary to osteoporosis (Mobily & Ostiguy, 2004). This condition is defined as the depression and helplessness that are a result of a significant and negative life event, such as a traumatic injury or significant chronic condition (Mobily & Ostiguy, 2004). The

ICF code b152 Emotional Functions can be used to document these issues.

Prognosis

Osteoporosis is a treatable chronic condition. Similar to diabetes, it can be managed to improve the person's quality of life, but no currently available treatment can cure it (Marieb & Hoehn, 2010). Fractures are the most serious consequences of osteoporosis. Furthermore, fractures among older adults, especially hip fractures, not only decrease quality of life but are associated with death; 24% of people who sustain a hip fracture die within one year of their injury (National Osteoporosis Foundation, 2012b).

Assessment

Typical Scope of Team Assessment

One or more tests of bone mineral density (BMD) initiate the treatment process, with the dual energy x-ray absorptiometry (DXA) assessment the most common. Osteoporosis is formally diagnosed by a test of BMD. The DXA test can also diagnose osteopenia. A risk assessment for fractures and identification of osteoporosis risk factors in combination with densitometric measurement by DXA is necessary before any therapy. This is especially important in cases of younger women at high risk for osteoporotic driven fractures (Tremollieres, 2012). Osteoporotic compression fractures in (usually thoracic) vertebra may present with or without pain. Hence, back pain among patients at risk for osteoporosis represents a secondary assessment criterion for the detection of osteoporosis (Lee et al., 2012). Deficits can be recorded in ICF codes under s7 Structures Related to Movement.

Areas of Concern for RT Assessment

Assessments chosen and anticipated results for recreational therapy relate primarily to quality of life, both in terms of independent functioning and the client's emotional response to diagnosis and lifestyle afterward (Shephard, Thomas, & Weller, 1991). The *Physical Activity Readiness Questionnaire* and functional fitness tests for older adults inform the judicious implementation of an exercise program (Mobily, 2009). Lifestyle assessments that reveal the social-psychological impact of the disorder on quality of life supplement functional data. In combination with the fact that osteoporosis is primarily a disease of later life, any of the following are good assessments of the individual's quality of life: life satisfaction and any of a number of assessments of leisure attitudes, including those that measure perceived freedom in leisure, leisure satisfaction, leisure attitude, and leisure motivation.

Invariably, the primary result of an overall assessment of the patient with osteoporosis will yield a finding of significantly reduced BMD. As indicated below in the treatment section, steps can be taken by all members of the treatment team to address various aspects of reduced BMD.

In addition, specific to recreational therapy intervention, and as with many chronic conditions, osteoporosis is associated with a number of comorbid, psychological symptoms. Psychological markers, including self-esteem, body image, and general mood are negatively associated with osteoporosis (Surgeon General, 2004). These can be coded with b126 Temperament and Personality Functions, b180 Experience of Self and Time Functions. These symptoms are above those of depression and anxiety, customarily expected of someone who has little control over the onset of a chronic condition (Surgeon General, 2004). Further, osteoporosis exacerbates a person's handicap because of its association with the fear of falling and the risk of a resulting fracture (Surgeon General, 2004). Fear of falling tends to have a restrictive effect, with even those who remain independent reporting a significantly reduced quality of life (de Oliveira et. al., 2009), leading to a decrease in engagement in meaningful activities (Surgeon General, 2004). In fact, when given a choice between death and a hip fracture resulting in nursing home placement, 80% of women older than 75 indicated a preference for death (NIH, 2002). Restrictions in lifestyle choices may be found in any of the codes under d2 General Tasks and Demands, d4 Mobility, d5 Self-Care, d6 Domestic Life, d8 Major Life Areas, and d9 Community, Social, and Civic Life.

ICF Core Set

A brief and comprehensive ICF Core Set for Osteoporosis is available.

Treatment Direction

Drug treatments are designed to slow the rate of mineral loss from the skeleton. Drugs designed to promote accumulation of bone mass and minerals in the skeleton have had mixed success. Some have even proven to be contraindicated because they can result in other detrimental effects. For example, hormone replacement drugs have been related to an increased incidence of cancer and heart disease (Marieb & Hoehn, 2010). Otherwise, most treatments address either risk factor exposure and/or secondary conditions or symptoms.

Some treatments have variable effectiveness. For instance, calcitonin is not an appropriate treatment for osteoporosis. Calcium and vitamin D effectiveness varies depending on circumstance. Calcium was found to be effective in reducing the risk of hip fractures, but not vertebral fractures. There is some evidence that vitamin D is effective at reducing overall fracture risk. Calcium and vitamin D in combination reduce the fracture risk in elderly women but not in elderly men (Levis & Theodore, 2012). These treatments are specifically directed at ICF codes in s7 Structures Related to Movement.

Whole Team Approach

Exercise is a typical recommendation for persons with osteoporosis or osteopenia (Surgeon General, 2004). Direct treatment here means that the client is guided, coached, or otherwise directed through an exercise program. With individuals who have advanced osteoporosis and are at especially high risk for a fall and fracture (Reginster, 2011), the intervention is more likely to be delivered under the close supervision of the attending physician (National Osteoporosis Foundation, 2012a, b). ICF codes being addressed include b280 Sensation of Pain, b440 Respiration Functions, b455 Exercise Tolerance Functions, b710 Mobility of Joint Functions, b720 Mobility of Bone Functions, b770 Gait Pattern Functions, and relevant codes in d4 Mobility.

For those with osteoporosis, but otherwise in good health or those at the level of osteopenia, other allied therapies, including recreational therapy, may be involved in exercise interventions. Furthermore, at the less advanced level of the disease the objective is more one of patient education instead of direct exercise treatment delivery. If preventive efforts fall within the practitioner's scope of service, it is worth noting that BMD acquisition during puberty is enhanced through appropriate diet and weight-bearing exercise. As a corollary, BMD acquired during youth postpones the onset of osteoporosis in the later years (Ohta, 2012). Hence, youth programs pertaining to exercise and nutrition, perhaps within a health promotion initiative for at-risk youth, may present an opportunity to impact the onset of osteoporosis and osteopenia in later life.

Regardless of the level of exercise program delivery and which profession is delivering the exercise, the therapist must monitor the amount of weight bearing that is intrinsic to the exercise. This is the case because weight-bearing exercise is known to produce the best results with respect to bone health (Roghani et al., 2013; Surgeon General, 2004). Regular weight bearing loads the skeleton and causes it to adapt to that stress by depositing more minerals in the skeleton. However, this is a case where the "cure" may be hazardous if the exercise intervention is not carefully monitored. Weight bearing may load the weakened osteoporotic skeleton to the point of failure depending on the severity of the condition (National Osteoporosis Foundation, 2012a, b).

Exercise is often a large part of fall prevention programs for frail older adults, many of whom have osteoporosis (Surgeon General, 2004). Lower extremity weakness is among the leading predictors of falls in older adults (Clemson et al., 2012, Lacour, Kostka, & Bonnefoy, 2002). To exercise interventions, one may deliberately add balance practice exercises (b235 Vestibular Functions, b755 Involuntary Movement Reaction Functions, d415 Maintaining a Body Position), usually at the beginning or end of the program (Surgeon General, 2004; National Osteoporosis Foundation, 2012a, b).

Prevention of secondary disorders is frequently addressed. In some cases osteoporosis may lead to other preventable disorders, including scoliosis, kyphosis (dowager's hump), and frailty (National Osteoporosis Foundation, 2012a, b). Scoliosis and kyphosis are deformities of the spine that may be prevented through good posture and regular exercise (National Osteoporosis Foundation, 2012a. b). In addition, patients with osteoporosis are at risk for reactive depression (Surgeon General, 2004), as are others who experience an abrupt recognition of a health condition. Because the person with osteoporosis knows s/he is at greater risk for a fracture if a fall

occurs, s/he may significantly decrease motor activity. This not only leads to de-conditioning of the cardio-respiratory complex, but also low muscle fitness and frailty. Frailty, of course, is an important risk factor for a fall (Lord & Clark, 1996). If problems have been noted with ICF codes b410 Heart Functions, b440 Respiration Functions, b735 Muscle Tone Functions, or b730 Muscle Power Functions, the need for an exercise program is indicated.

Pain management (b280 Sensation of Pain) is a frequent concern (National Osteoporosis Foundation, 2012a, b) in the intervention plan for individuals with osteoporosis. The team physician may prescribe analgesics to treat pain; and physical therapy may use thermal techniques and massage to relieve pain.

Patient education is ubiquitous in rehabilitation and healthcare today because of managed care. Treatment and management of osteoporosis is no exception. The general goal of patient education is to promote compliance with lifestyle changes conducive to successfully managing osteoporosis, including a sound diet, regular exercise habit, smoking cessation, etc. (Surgeon General, 2004). ICF codes that are improved with education can be cited as the reason for the education.

Recreational Therapy Approach

When working as a member of the treatment team, recreational therapists have the same treatment goals as the whole team, indicated above. In community and outpatient service programs, prevention and a broader definition of quality of life programming may be embraced by recreational therapy. Best practice suggests that the recreational therapist should do some preliminary screening before initiating an exercise program with a patient. One field-tested questionnaire that has proven valid and reliable is the *Physical Activity Readiness Questionnaire* (PARQ, Shephard, 1988), which has been widely used in Canada. The PARQ consists of seven yes/no screening questions; an affirmative answer to any question should alert the therapist to clear exercise with the client's primary care physician before beginning the program.

Recreational Therapy Interventions

Exercise

When recreational therapy is involved in the delivery of exercise programs to persons with osteoporosis and osteopenia, caution is warranted. Fortunately, several methods for managing the amount of load on the skeleton exist. For those with less advanced conditions, programs that are a reasonably safe choice include dancing, walking outside, including hiking over uneven terrain, and group exercise programs that include some low impact exercises such as marching and stair climbing. For those with more advanced osteoporosis, the practitioner should look to the physician for precautions that should be operative during the intervention. Likely, lower impact exercise will be safe. These include activities such as step machines, elliptical machines, walking on treadmill machines, and group exercise programs that do not include any lifting of the foot leading to impact (Surgeon General, 2004).

For almost any but the most severe cases of osteoporosis, resistance training with weights, resistance bands, or medicine balls is useful (Surgeon General, 2004). Although not always weight bearing, resistance training also loads the skeleton but in a manner slightly different from weight bearing. Because muscles attach to bones to produce movement by way of tendons, when resistance opposes any given movement, the tendon and muscle must pull more forcefully on the bone being moved. The thinking is that the pulling of the tendon stimulates the bone remodeling physiology (Frost, 2001) to produce bone tissue. In sum, a well-rounded program of exercise is recommended because skeletal adaptation to load is specific to the site loaded (Surgeon General, 2004; Suominen, 2006). Hence, all parts of the body and, by association, the entire skeleton must be stressed or loaded. The Centers for Disease Control publish general exercise recommendations and recommendations for resistance training for older adults that are prudent to apply to older adults with osteoporosis and osteopenia.

Overload and progression are the two principles that guide resistance training (Mobily & MacNeil, 2002). Overload means that a muscle must work harder than normal to become stronger, and this principle applies to the skeleton, too. That is why load-bearing exercise is positively associated with gains in bone mass. The companion notion of progression means that once the muscle system and skeletal system adapt to the increased load, subsequent increases in load are needed to assure that muscles and bones will continue to improve.

Another method for getting exercise with different weight-bearing options is aquatic exercise. The benefits of exercising in water are several. First, the water provides natural resistance to movement when the body part is moved under water, resulting in the same sorts of localized load bearing as resistance training (Mobily & MacNeil, 2002). Second, by adjusting the depth of the water, the person may bear more or less of his or her own weight (Mobily & MacNeil, 2002). A rough estimate of weight bearing in the water is about 75% of the body weight is borne at knee depth, 50% at waist level, 25% at chest level, and 10% at neck level. Third, if the participant does lose his/her balance, water cushions the fall (Mobily & MacNeil, 2002).

Aquatic exercise leadership certification is an appealing skill to add to the recreational therapist's resume, with certification available through a one-day workshop with the Arthritis Foundation. This skill set is attractive because it does not require that the therapist have exceptional aquatic skills, such as lifeguard certification or water safety instructor training.

The exercise programs described above are all directed at issues documented with ICF codes b440 Respiration Functions, b455 Exercise Tolerance Functions, b710 Mobility of Joint Functions, b720 Mobility of Bone Functions, b730 Muscle Power Functions, b740 Muscle Endurance Functions, b770 Gait Pattern Functions, s7 Structures Related to Movement, and relevant codes in d4 Mobility.

Balance training (Surgeon General, 2004) may be delivered as a separate program, as part of a group exercise program, or it may be intrinsic to an exercise program — such as tai chi or yoga. These sorts of programs are within the recreational therapist's scope of practice and reasonably safe. Balance practice may also be a component within a larger exercise group or, even better, an aquatic exercise group (Arthritis Foundation, 2012a, b). Improved balance (b755 Involuntary Movement Reaction Functions, b765 Involuntary Movement Functions, d415 Maintaining a Body Position) may assist in avoiding falls among persons with susceptible bones (Kemmier &

Stengel, 2010), as in osteoporosis, and is recommended as part of a complete exercise program for older adults in general (Centers for Disease Control and Prevention, 2008) and older adults with osteoporosis in particular (Surgeon General, 2004). Improved balance has also been associated with improved quality of life in older women with osteoporosis (Madureira et al., 2010).

Depression may also result from chronic experience with osteoporosis (Surgeon General, 2004). But a little exercise goes a long way because some research shows that older adults who walk daily are significantly less likely to report depression, and those who adopt exercise subsequent to reporting depression are much less likely to report depression at follow-up (Mobily, et. al, 1996). More generally, regardless of the lifestyle management techniques adopted by the patient, compliance adds to perceptions of control and effectance, which in turn promote reductions in depressive symptoms (Mobily & Ostiguy, 2004). In this case exercise is addressing ICF codes b126 Temperament and Personality Functions, b152 Emotional Functions, and b180 Experience of Self and Time Functions.

Pain Management

Pain management is a common concern for persons with osteoporosis (Mobily & MacNeil, 2002; National Osteoporosis Foundation, 2012a). Various techniques are available to alleviate pain. Relaxation techniques of various types, including progressive relaxation, meditation, and biofeedback, contribute to easing the body's response to pain, and may result in perceptions of psychological control (b126 Temperament and Personality Functions, b280 Sensation of Pain) (Mobily & MacNeil, 2002).

Direct massage is another technique that is useful, though it should be administered with caution (Uhlemann & Lange, 2006). The aim of massage and other sensory stimulation techniques, such as TENS units, is to stimulate heavily myelinated touch nerve fibers that transmit impulses more rapidly than lightly myelinated pain nerve fibers (Marieb & Hoehn, 2010). Somewhere in the nervous system exists a "gate" that limits the flow of incoming sensory information (Melzack and Wall, 1965). Some have maintained its existence in the spinal cord, while others assert its location in the thalamus. When the heavily myelinated fibers transmitting touch infor-

mation reach the gate, they interfere with and block the pain transmitted by the smaller diameter fibers. Casual and daily experiences with bumps verify that if we rub an injured area it does feel better, so long as we keep rubbing.

If the therapist is not qualified to administer direct massage, immersion of the individual in the water is a good substitute. While no direct aquatic interventions were identified with osteoporotic patients, Mobily and Verburg (2001) were able to use aquatics effectively in reducing pain in fibromyalgia. Like touch sensations, thermal sensations are transmitted by heavily myelinated fibers (Marieb & Hoehn, 2010) and will also yield the same short-term relief. However, do use a warm water pool if the subject is not moving or exercising very much because hypothermic conditions will aggravate pain instead of producing relief. In addition, the buoyancy attribute of the water relieves the load on the skeleton thus easing pain (Arthritis Foundation, 2012).

Exercise, if administered with the precautions indicated above, may also promote pain relief. Two types of mechanisms for pain relief have been suggested. First, exercise is associated with the secretion of natural analgesics which will help reduce pain (Thoren et al., 1990). Second, stronger muscles will stabilize joints and skeletal structures, also reducing pain (Arthritis Foundation, 2012).

In addition, the Arthritis Foundation teaches joint protection (b710 Mobility of Joint Functions) in all its consumer education programs. Joint protection is useful to the person with osteoporosis as well as arthritis.

Massage, warm water experiences, and exercise all can address ICF code b280 Sensation of Pain.

Recreation Activities

Secondary conditions may well develop in response to a diagnosis of osteoporosis. Although their research was not specific to osteoporosis, Smith and Yoshioka (1992) investigated the lifestyle impact of a related impairment (arthritis). Their findings may have implications for practitioners working with persons with osteoporosis. They found that arthritis caused subjects to make significant changes in their leisure pursuits, often abandoning their favorite activities, leading to deficits in d920 Recreation and Leisure. The authors suggested that increasing the subject's leisure repertoire through teaching leisure skills would help with adaptation to the disorder. The same likely applies to persons with osteoporosis. Adaptation can address issues with b126 Temperament and Personality Functions, b152 Emotional Functions, and b180 Experience of Self and Time Functions.

Nutrition

The patient education component of the team approach that recreational therapists, among others, may be responsible for pertains to teaching the person exercises they can do at home and cooking and nutrition support for osteoporosis (Dishman, 1994; Simone et. al, 2011; Marcelli, 2010). Cooking groups that specialize in augmenting calcium and other minerals in the diet are useful if the program teaches the person to recognize food rich in minerals and vitamin D, and how to cook foods so they do not deplete the minerals and vitamins they contain (Marieb & Hoehn, 2010). Proper nutrition addresses ICF codes in s7 Structures Related to Movement.

Community Integration

Because of the demographics associated with osteoporosis, senior center exercise programs are most apt to have participants with osteoporosis, both manifest and latent. Hence, the recreational therapist working in situations where the most members are older adults acts prudently when s/he assumes that everyone has osteoporosis. Further, despite the general mantra of inclusion and integration, older adults more often prefer to exercise alone or in segregated settings with their peers (Dishman, 1994). The reason may be that older adults are self-conscious about their appearance and ability to be competent in exercise when in the company of younger cohorts. If true, this means that exercise programs customized for older adults may be more effective if restricted to only older adults, especially when trying to encourage adoption of a regular exercise habit. These exercise programs address d9 Community, Social, and Civic Life.

Life Activities

Transitioning and adjusting to limitations may take considerable emotional energy because of lifestyle changes that come with orthopedic impairments such as osteoporosis. As mentioned above, a study of persons with arthritis reported by Smith and Yoshioka (1992) found that subjects typically had to surrender their favorite leisure pursuits following diagnosis. Because of the overlap in symptoms, these findings likely apply to persons with osteoporosis as well as those with arthritis. Clearly, professionals need to assist the subject in identifying alternative leisure activities and adapting favored leisure activities to continue meaningful participation. Beyond that, therapists can look at the whole range of activities covered by ICF codes d2 General Tasks and Demands, d4 Mobility, d5 Self-Care, d6 Domestic Life, d8 Major Life Areas, and d9 Community, Social, and Civic Life to address areas where the client is not functioning as well as possible because of concerns about osteoporosis and help the client find adaptations that make these activities possible again.

Health Promotion

Prevention programs for persons with disabilities who are at greater risk for osteoporosis (e.g., spinal cord injuries, rheumatoid arthritis, immobility impairments, kidney dialysis, etc.) and for the general community-dwelling population may be planned and implemented by the community-based recreational therapist. Research shows that past and present exercise habits independently predict risk for hip fracture (Surgeon General, 2004). What this means is that if prevention programs for young women can be introduced early, they may give the participant a head start on maintaining bone health in later life. In addition, the recreational therapist in a community setting should be alert to those at risk for osteoporosis and fractures secondary to another condition when programming in general. For example, for persons with rheumatoid arthritis an aquatic exercise program is preferred over a weight-bearing exercise program, such as walking (Arthritis Foundation, 2012).

Resources

National Osteoporosis Foundation
1150 17th St NW, Suite 850
Washington, DC 20036
www.nof.org.

References

Arthritis Foundation. (2012). The many benefits of exercise. Accessed via website www.arthritis.org.

Arthritis Foundation. (2009). *Arthritis Foundation instructors manual*. Atlanta, GA: Arthritis Foundation.

burlingame, j. & Blaschko, T. M. (2010). *Assessment tools for recreational therapy and related fields* (4th edition). Ravensdale, WA: Idyll Arbor.

Centers for Disease Control and Prevention. (2008). Facts about physical activity. Accessed via website www.cdc.gov.

Clemson, L., Fiatarone, S., Bundy, A., Cumming, R. G., Manollaras, K., O'Loughlin, P., & Black, D. (2012). Integration of balance and strength training into daily life activity to reduce rate of falls in older people (the LIFE study): Randomised parallel trial, *BMJ (Clinical Research), 345*, 1-15.

de Oliveira, F. N., Arthuso, M., da Silva, R., Pedro, A. O., Neto, A. M., & Costa-Pavia, L. (2009). Quality of life in women with postmenopausal osteoporosis: Correlation between QUALEFFO 41 and SF-36. *Maturitas, 62*, 85-90.

Dishman, R. K. (1994). Motivating older adults to exercise. *Southern Medical Journal, 87*, S79-S82.

Frost, H. M. (2001). From Wolff's law to the Utah paradigm: Insights about bone physiology and its clinical applications. *The Anatomical Record, 262*, 398-419.

Hoenk, A. H. & Mobily, K. E. (1987). Mainstreaming the play environment: Effects of previous exposure and salience of disability. *Therapeutic Recreation Journal, 21*(4), 233-31.

Kemmier, W. & Stengel, S. (2011). Exercise and osteoporosis-related fractures: Perspectives and recommendations of the sports and exercise scientists. *The Physician and Sportsmedicine, 39*, 142-157.

Lacour, J. R., Kostka, T., & Bonnefoy, M. (2002). Physical activity to delay effects of aging on mobility. *Presse Medicale, 31*, 1185-1192.

Lee, H. M., Park, S. Y., Lee, S. H., Suh, S. W., & Hong, J. Y. (2012). Comparative analysis of clinical outcomes in patients with osteoporotic vertebral compression fractures (OVCFs): Conservative treatment versus balloon kyphoplasty. *The Spine Journal, 12*(11), 998-1005.

Levis, S. & Theodore, G. (2012). Summary of AHRQ's comparative effectiveness review of treatment to prevent fractures in men and women with low bone density or osteoporosis: Update of the 2007 report. *Journal of Managed Care Pharmacy, 18*, S1-15.

Lord, S. R. & Clark, R. D. (1996). Simple physiological and clinical tests for accurate prediction of falling in the elderly. *Gerontology, 42*, 199-203.

Madureira, M. M., Bonfá, E., Takayama, L., & Pereira, R. M. (2010). A 12-month randomized control trail of balance training in elderly women with osteoporosis: Improvement of quality of life. *Maturitas, 66*, 206-211.

Melzack, R. & Wall, P. (1965). Pain mechanisms: A new theory. *Science, 150*, 971-979.

Marcelli, C. (2010). Role of nonphysician healthcare providers in improving treatment adherence among patients with severe osteoporosis. *Joint, Bone, Spine, 77*(Suppl. 2), S117-S119.

Marieb, E. N. & Hoehn, K. (2010). *Human anatomy and physiology* (8th edition). San Francisco: Benjamin Cummings.

Marieb, E. N., Wilhelm, P. B., & Mallatt, J. (2011). *Human anatomy* (6th edition). Boston: Benjamin Cummings.

Martini, F. H. & Bartholomew, E. F. (2003). *Essentials of anatomy and physiology* (3rd edition). Upper Saddle River, NJ: Prentice-Hall.

Mobily, K. E. (2009). Role of exercise and physical activity in therapeutic recreation services. *Therapeutic Recreation Journal, 43*, 9-26.

Mobily, K. E. & MacNeil, R. D. (2002). *Therapeutic recreation and the nature of disabilities.* State College, PA: Venture.

Mobily, K. E. & Ostiguy, L. J. (2004). *Introduction to therapeutic recreation: U.S. and Canadian perspectives.* State College, PA: Venture Publishing.

Mobily, K. E., Rubenstein, L. M., Lemke, J. H., O'Hara, M. W., & Wallace, R. B. (1996). Walking and depression in a cohort of older adults: The Iowa 65+ rural health study. *Journal of Aging and Physical Activity, 4*, 119-135.

Mobily, K. E. & Verburg, M. D. (2001). Aquatic therapy in community-based therapeutic recreation: Pain management in a case of fibromyalgia. *Therapeutic Recreation Journal, 35*, 57-69.

NIH. (2002). National Institutes of Health Consensus Statements. Bethesda, MD: National Institutes of Health.

National Osteoporosis Foundation. (2012a). Bone health basics, Retrieved from http://www.nof.org/aboutosteoporosis/bonebasics/whyboneh ealth.www.nof.org.

National Osteoporosis Foundation. (2012b). Prevalence report. Retrieved from http://www.nof.org/advocacy/resources/prevalencereport.

Ohta, H. (2012). Prevention of osteoporosis. *Clinical Calcium, 22*, 825-831.

Osness, W. H., Adrian, M., Clark, B., Hoeger, W., Raab, D., & Wisnell, R. (1990). *Functional fitness assessment for adults over 60 years (a field based assessment).* Reston, VA: American Alliance for Health. Physical Education Recreation and Dance.

Reginster, J. Y. (2011). Antifracture efficacy of currently available therapies for postmenopausal osteoporosis. *Drugs, 71*, 65-78.

Roghani, T., Torkaman, G., Movasseghe, S., Hedayati, M., Goosheh, B., & Bayat, N. (2013). Effects of short-term aerobic exercise with and without external loading on bone metabolism and balance in postmenopausal women with osteoporosis. *Rheumatology International, 33*(2), 291-8. doi: 10.1007/s00296-012-2388-2.

Shephard, R. J. (1988). Canadian Home Fitness Test and exercise screening alternatives. *Sports Medicine, 5*, 185-195.

Shephard, R. J., Thomas, S., and Weller, I. (1991). The Canadian Home Fitness Test: 1991 Update. *Sports Medicine, 1*, 359.

Simone, M. J., Roberts, D. H., Irish, J. T., Neeman, N., Schulze, J. E., Lipsitz, L. A., Schwartzstein, R., Aronson, M. D., & Tan, Z. S. (2011). An educational intervention for providers to promote bone health in high risk older adults. *Journal of the American Geriatric Society, 59*, 291-296.

Smith, S. A. & Yoshioka, C. F. (1992). Recreation functioning and depression in people with arthritis. *Therapeutic Recreation Journal, 26*, 21-30.

Suominen, H. (2006). Muscle training for bone strength. *Aging Clinical and Experimental Research, 18*, 85-93.

Surgeon General. (2004). *Bone health and osteoporosis.* Rockville, MD: Office of the Surgeon General.

Thoren, P., Floras, J. S., Hoffmann, P., & Seals, D. R. (1990). Endorphins and exercise: Physiological mechanisms and clinical implications. *Medicine and Science in Sports and Exercise, 22*, 417-428.

Tremollieres, F. (2012). What patients need to know about the risk of bone fracture and its prevention. *Journal of Obstetrics and Biological Reproduction, 12*, 220-227.

Uhlemann, C. & Lange, U. (2006). Physiotherapy strategies in osteoporosis — recommendations for daily practice. *Zeitschrift Fur Rhematologie, 65*, 407-410, 412-416.

28. Parkinson's Disease

Heather R. Porter, Brenda P. Wiggins, and Natalie Haynes

Parkinson's disease (PD) is a progressive, degenerative neurological disorder of the basal ganglia in the brain. It is the second most common neurodegenerative disorder after Alzheimer's disease (de Lau & Breteler, 2006). The neurons located at the base of the brain die, or are damaged, causing a slow degeneration of the nervous system. When the brain sends a message to a muscle for movement, the message passes through the basal ganglia. The basal ganglia are located deep in the brain at the base of the cerebrum. This collection of neurons helps to smooth out and coordinate muscle movements. As an impulse travels through the basal ganglia, the neurons release a neurotransmitter called dopamine. Dopamine allows the neurons in the basal ganglia to communicate with each other. PD impairs those nerve impulses. The result is a depressed production of dopamine and poor connections among neurons in the basal ganglia. When approximately 60-80% of the dopamine-producing cells in the brain are damaged and do not produce enough dopamine, the motor symptoms of PD appear (National Parkinson Foundation, 2013).

Incidence/Prevalence in U.S.

It is estimated that four to six million people worldwide have PD (National Parkinson Foundation, 2010). In the United States alone, 50,000-60,000 new cases of PD are diagnosed each year, adding to the over one million people who currently have PD (National Parkinson Foundation, 2008).

Predominant Age

Age of PD onset predominately occurs between 55 and 75 years of age (Jankovic, 2008); and is 1.5-2 times more common in men than women (Haaxma et al., 2007).

Causes

Although there is no identified cause, researchers tend to agree that genes, as well as environment, play a large role in the onset of PD. Non-genetic risk factors for PD include expose to pesticides, herbicides, and heavy metals; and tobacco, coffee, and alcohol use (de Lau & Breteler, 2006).

Systems Affected

PD affects the neuromuscular system. The primary structural deficits are in the basal ganglia (s1103 Basal Ganglia and Related Structures).

Motor Symptoms

There is no definitive test to diagnose PD; therefore, it is diagnosed based on the clinical presentation of the individual (Jankovic, 2008). A person must have two out of three motor cardinal features to be diagnosed with PD. These include an asymmetric resting tremor (tremor when the limb is not being used), rigidity of muscles (determined by resistance to passive range of motion of a joint), and bradykinesia (slowed, reduced movement) (National Parkinson Foundation, 2013; Jankovic, 2008). A fourth cardinal sign, postural instability with loss of balance typically emerges eight or more years into the disease process (Hauser, 2010).

Asymmetric tremors: Tremors (b765 Involuntary Movement Functions) usually begin in one upper extremity and initially may be intermittent. As with most tremors, the amplitude increases with stress and resolves during sleep. After several months or years, the tremors may affect the extremities on the other side, but asymmetry is usually maintained. PD tremors may also involve the lower extremities, tongue, lips, or chin (Hauser, 2010).

Rigidity of muscles: Increased muscle tone (rigidity) is caused by excessive and continuous contraction of muscles (Jankovic, 2008). During the early stages of PD, rigidity tends to be asymmetrical, often starting in the shoulder and neck. Record this with ICF codes b710 Mobility of Joint Functions and b780 Sensations Related to Muscles and Movement Functions. As the disease progresses, rigidity in the individual's muscles and facial expressions become evident (O'Sullivan et al., 2007). The face becomes rigid and expressions are compromised (Hemmesch et al., 2009). Eye blinking is also decreased and gives the impression of staring. The flat facial expression causes a depressive look or mask-like appearance where facial expressions seldom change. Difficulties with showing facial emotion, such as smiling at a joke or frowning when sad, can affect social relationships, so successful interaction with others diminishes over time (Hemmesch et al., 2009). Record social issues with ICF codes in d7 Interpersonal Interactions and Relationships.

Bradykinesia: Slowed movement (bradykinesia) is the reduction of movement speed. The individual's movements become increasingly slow and over time the muscles may randomly freeze (National Parkinson Foundation, 2013). Use ICF codes b760 Control of Voluntary Movement Functions and b765 Involuntary Movement Functions.

Postural instability: Impaired balance negatively affects functional independence and activities of daily living (ADLs) for individuals with PD. The decline of balance and mobility associated with PD leads to a tremendous decrease in the ability to perform even the simplest daily activities, while increasing the risk of falls (Gobbi et al., 2009), impairing the quality of life for individuals with PD (Varanese et al., 2010; Plotnik, 2011). Record the physical condition with b755 Involuntary Movement Reaction Functions, b770 Gait Pattern Functions, and d415 Maintaining a Body Position. Activity issues are addressed by many ICF codes in d2 General Tasks and Demands, d4 Mobility, d5 Self-Care, d6 Domestic Life, d8 Major Life Areas, and d9 Community, Social, and Civic Life.

Non-Motor Symptoms

Although motor dysfunction, as described above, typically represents the chief symptoms of individuals with PD, non-motor symptoms of the condition are often equally disabling (Breen & Drutyte, 2012). Non-motor symptoms include:

Mood: Depression can be a primary symptom of PD due to changes in brain chemicals or a consequence of coping with a chronic, progressive disability. With depression, other symptoms such as anxiety, loss of internal locus of control, and frustration can co-occur (Becker et al., 2011; Foster et al., 2011). Use ICF codes b125 Dispositions and Intra-Personal Functions and b126 Temperament and Personality Functions.

Cognitive changes including neurocognitive disorders: It is estimated that 30-40% of individuals with PD develop cognitive impairments that interfere with daily functioning including executive function, memory, bradyphrenia (slowed mental processing which can further impair problem solving and memory), language, attention, particularly for complex situations that require divided or shared attention, and visual-spatial abilities (Poletti et al., 2012; Johns Hopkins Medicine, 2011). Personality changes, psychosis, and hallucinations might also occur (National Parkinson Foundation, 2013). Cognitive impairments in PD are due to the depletion of dopamine in the striatum causing disruption in the frontal lobes (Kudlicka et al., 2013). The *DSM-5* (APA, 2013) includes Parkinson's as one of the causes of neurocognitive disorder. All of the ICF codes in b1 Mental Functions may need to be used, depending on the particular individual. Also consider ICF codes in d2 General Tasks and Demands.

Orthostatic hypotension: Lightheadedness and low blood pressure upon standing (b110 Consciousness Functions, b420 Blood Pressure Functions) (National Parkinson Foundation, 2013).

Constipation and early satiety: A feeling of fullness after eating small amounts (b515 Digestive Functions, b525 Defecation Functions) (National Parkinson Foundation, 2013).

Hyperhidrosis: Excessive sweating, especially of the hands and feet (b270 Sensory Functions Related to Temperature and Other Stimuli) (National Parkinson Foundation, 2013).

Seborrhea dermatitis: Dry skin, dandruff (b8 Functions of the Skin and Related Structures) (National Parkinson Foundation, 2013).

Urinary problems: Urgency, frequency and incontinence (b620 Urination Functions) (National Parkinson Foundation, 2013).

Loss of sense of smell (anosmia): A compromised sense of smell (b255 Smell Function) is a complaint in approximately 80% of individuals with PD (Shah et al., 2009). This olfactory dysfunction may be caused by difficulty breathing in enough air required for sniffing or it may be caused by degeneration of neurons and striatal dopamine transporters (Berendse et al., 2001). Lack of smell can impair appetite and increase risk for malnutrition, as well as raise safety concerns because the client is unable to smell gas or rancid food.

Sleep disorders: These can include insomnia, excessive daytime sleepiness, rapid eye movement behavioral disorder or active dreaming, dream enactment, involuntary movements and vocalizations during sleep, restless legs syndrome, or periodic leg movements disorder (b134 Sleep Functions, b765 Involuntary Movement Functions) (National Parkinson Foundation, 2013).

Sensory problems: Including pain, tingling, or burning (b280 Sensation of Pain), or tightness (b780 Sensations Related to Muscles and Movement Functions) (National Parkinson Foundation, 2013).

Mixed Motor and Non-Motor Symptoms

Sialorrhea: Drooling due to slowed swallowing (b510 Ingestion Functions) (National Parkinson Foundation, 2013)

Speech problems: Muffled speech (hypokinetic dysarthria) initially begins with sounding breathy or hoarse; which eventually leads to reduced speech volume and inability to articulate consonants (Howell et al., 2009). The mouth, lips, and lingual gestures also become difficult to decipher, specifically when producing "u" characters (Weismer et al., 2003). Individuals with PD often stutter due to muscular problems forming words; and speech becomes soft and takes on a monotonous tone (National Parkinson Foundation, 2010). These can be documented with b3 Voice and Speech Functions.

Swallowing problems: Due to muscle rigidity in the face, swallowing becomes difficult causing drooling and choking (b510 Ingestion Functions) (Nobrega et al., 2008). As a result of the swallowing dysfunction, both malnutrition and dehydration can occur if the individual does not consume enough nourishment (Nobrega et al., 2008).

Secondary Problems

Individuals with PD are at risk for numerous secondary conditions.

Falls: Individuals with PD report frequent falls, at a rate 60-70% higher than that of the general geriatric population (Plotnick et al., 2011). There are a variety of factors that increase risk of falls in this population. First, individuals with PD have difficulty initiating a first step, called "start-hesitation." With start-hesitation, walking halts without any warning because the individual's foot doesn't advance. The feet feel as if they are glued to the floor, complicating functional ambulation, including turning and maneuvering around obstacles (Factor et al., 2011). This freezing, in combination with postural instability, accounts for approximately 80% of all falls by individuals with PD (Factor et al., 2011). Other impairments caused by PD also further increase the risk of falls and subsequent injury, including a short, shuffling gait with a hanging head and shoulders and limited arm swing. ICF codes b760 Control of Voluntary Movement Functions, b770 Gait Pattern Functions, and d4 Mobility can be used to document mobility issues.

Sexual dysfunction: Sexual dysfunction (b640 Sexual Functions) can occur in individuals with PD due to low dopamine levels in the brain, decreased ability to move, and medication (National Parkinson Foundation, 2010).

Decreased activity: Movement dysfunction from PD decreases activity. Complications from inactivity among individuals with PD can include cardiac deconditioning, skin breakdown, and pneumonia (Archer et al., 2011). General deconditioning and reduced exercise capacity can cause early fatigue and decreased isotonic strength and endurance (Archer et al., 2011; Kluding et al., 2006). Inactivity or decreased activity can also cause neurodegeneration (see "Exercise" in the RT Interventions later in the chapter). ICF codes that describe the problems of reduced activity include d7 Interpersonal Interactions and Relationships, d8 Major Life Areas, and d9 Community, Social, and Civic Life. Document the consequences of decreased activity, too, with codes such as b455 Exercise Tolerance Functions, b730 Muscle Power Functions, b740 Muscle Endurance Functions, and s810 Structure of Areas of Skin.

Quality of life: Health-related quality of life (HRQoL) is significantly impaired for individuals with PD. In a four-year longitudinal study, participants with PD reflected a decrease in HRQoL in the dimensions of physical mobility, emotional reactions, pain, and social isolation (Karlsen et al., 2000). ICF codes described earlier can be used to document specifics about quality of life issues.

Prognosis

About 25-40% of people with PD eventually develop dementia, which is largely responsible for decreased life expectancy (de Lau & Breteler, 2006). Predictors for more rapid motor progression, nursing home placement, and short survival time include older age at onset of PD, associated comorbidities, presentation with rigidity and bradykinesia, and decreased dopamine responsiveness (Suchowersky et al., 2006).

Assessment

Typical Scope of Team Assessment

Diagnosis of PD is problematic even for specialists (Macphee & Stewart, 2012). Consequently, practitioners may typically see individuals who deny the PD diagnosis. They may consult several health professionals before accepting the diagnosis (Leritz et al., 2004). The progression of PD can take twenty years or more; however, for some individuals, the disease can progress rapidly (Hobson et al., 2010). There is no way to predict the course of the disease, but there are assessment instruments that classify the progression of the disease.

Hoehn and Yahr Scale: Classifies PD into five stages (1, 2, 3, 4, 5). There is also a Modified Hoehn and Yahr Scale that begins with 0 and includes half-stages (0, 1, 1.5, 2, 2.5, 3, 4, and 5) (Movement Disorder Virtual University, n.d.).

- Stage 0: No signs of disease.
- Stage 1: Unilateral disease; symptoms on one side of the body only.
- Stage 1.5: Unilateral plus axial involvement.
- Stage 2: Bilateral disease; symptoms on both sides of the body, no balance impairment.
- Stage 2.5: Mild bilateral disease, with recovery on pull test.
- Stage 3: Mild to moderate bilateral disease; some postural instability; physically independent.
- Stage 4: Severe disability, but still able to walk or stand unassisted.

- Stage 5: Wheelchair-bound or bedridden unless assisted.

Schwab and England Activities of Daily Living Scale: A 0-100 scale that rates the person's level of independence (0 = vegetative functions such as swallowing, bladder, and bowel function are not functioning; 100 = completely independent, able to do chores without slowness, difficult, or impairment) (Movement Disorder Virtual University, n.d.).

Unified Parkinson Disease Rating Scale (UPDRS) (Movement Disorder Virtual University, n.d.): The UPDRS is a six-part scale that classifies level of impairment, which includes (1) mentation, behavior, and mood (includes intellectual impairment, thought disorder, depression, and motivation/initiative), (2) activities of daily living (includes speech, salivation, swallowing, handwriting, handling utensils, cutting food, dressing, hygiene, turning in bed and adjusting bed clothes, falling, freezing when walking, walking, tremor, and sensory complaints), (3) motor examination (including speech, facial expression, tremor at rest, action or postural tremor of hands, rigidity, finger taps, hand movements, rapid alternating movements of hands, leg agility, arising from chair, posture, gait, postural stability, and body bradykinesia and hypokinesia), (4) complications of therapy in the past week (related to dyskinesia, clinical fluctuations, and other complications), (5) Modified Hoehn and Yahr stages, and (6) *Schwab and England Activities of Daily Living Scale* complex scale.

Other scales and assessment tools recommended by the National Parkinson Foundation (2013) include:

- *Abnormal Involuntary Movement Scale (AIMS)*: Used to assess the severity of levodopa-induced dyskinesia.
- *PDQ39*: PD-specific measure of subjective health status (self-report).
- *Mini-Mental State Examination (MMSE)*: Screening for cognitive impairment.
- *Montreal Cognitive Assessment (MoCA)*: Detects mild cognitive impairment.
- *Dementia Rating Scale*: Assesses dementia in individuals with neuropsychological conditions.
- *Epworth Sleep Scale*: Measures daytime sleepiness.

- *PD Sleep Scale (PDSS)*: Measures sleep disturbances.
- *Geriatric Depression Scale*: Assesses depressive symptoms in elderly population.
- *Beck Depression Inventory (BDI)*: Measures severity of depression.
- *Hamilton Depression Rating Scale*: Assesses primary depression.
- *Parkinson Disease Fatigue Scale (PFS)*: Assesses physical aspects of fatigue and impact on daily function.
- *Neuropsychiatric Inventory (NPI)*: Evaluates behavioral abnormalities that occur in individuals with dementia.
- *Brief Psychiatric Rating Scale*: Used to measure psychosis in medication trials.
- *Patient diaries*: Individual documents motor state when not being observed.

Quality of life: Den Oudsten and colleagues (2011) note that "the assessment of medical intervention outcomes has moved from the traditional focus (e.g., mortality and morbidity) to more comprehensive assessment that incorporates individuals' own perspectives and beliefs regarding their health and well-being" (p. 2490). Consequently, the authors conducted focus group sessions with 54 individuals with PD and their caregivers to identify themes related to quality of life. The authors found the following themes: overall quality of life, pain and discomfort, energy and fatigue, sleep and rest, mobility, activities of daily living, dependence on medication or treatments, working capacity, positive feelings, thinking/learning/memory, self-esteem, negative feelings, religion/personal beliefs, personal relationships, social support, sexual activity, physical safety, home environment, financial resources, health and social care, opportunities for learning, leisure activities, physical environment, and transport (all of which are reflected in *World Health Organization Quality of Life* assessment [*WHOQoL*]). The additional themes of autonomy, physical adaptations to disability, personal adaptations to disability, communication ability, communication supports, social acceptance, social network and interaction, social inclusion and contribution, and barriers to access were also identified in the study and are currently not part of the *WHOQoL*. The authors note that "the results of this study pointed out that the impact of PD on QoL goes beyond the physical,

social, and emotional domains of Health Related Quality of Life [HRQoL]" (p. 2506). Consequently, recreational therapists should conduct a multi-faceted evaluation of quality of life to identify themes of concern for a particular client so they can implement interventions for those concerns to improve subjective QoL. Appropriate ICF codes for recording these issues were discussed in the System Affected and Secondary Problems sections.

Cognitive function: Mitchell and colleagues (2010) conducted a systematic search and review of the literature on quality of life and cognitive complications of neurological disorders including PD. The authors noted that common cognitive impairments associated with PD negatively impact HRQoL including executive performance, visuospatial function, memory, and language. The authors note that cognitive impairments cause difficulties with life tasks and roles, including, social interactions, ADLs, and mobility, which impact HRQoL. Consequently, the authors recommend "that a thorough cognitive examination should be part of routine clinical practice in those caring for neurological patients" (p. 8). Cognitive issues are typically recorded with ICF codes in b1 Mental Functions. Codes to record the impacts have been discussed earlier.

Other areas of assessment: In addition to the above assessment tools, a 12-week study by Cieza and colleagues (2013) assessed 741 patients with brain disorders (including PD). They identified a set of psychosocial difficulties that impact health outcomes including energy and drive, sleep, emotional functions, problem solving, conversation, areas of mobility and self-care, relationships, community life, and recreation and leisure. All of these were significant predictors of health outcomes. Many, as previously described, are issues for individuals with PD. Consequently, the authors advocate for the addition of these items to health assessments "to adequately describe the experience of general health for persons with brain disorders, and thereby to gain the advantages for intervention planning and other applications of a more extensive understanding of this experience" (p. 8). ICF codes for recording these issues have been discussed earlier.

Areas of Concern for RT Assessment

In addition to the previously reviewed PD symptoms and secondary complications, common findings from the RT assessment include:

Decreased recreation, leisure, and community activity: Studies have shown that PD has a significant negative effect on engagement in recreation, leisure, and community activities affecting health, quality of life, and functional skills (Trail et al., 2012; Foster & Hershey, 2011; McCabe et al., 2008). Record these deficits in engagement with d9 Community, Social, and Civic Life.

Changes in life roles: Role changes that may occur as the disease progresses may or may not be well accepted by the individual (Leritz et al., 2004). Relationship issues can be documented with d7 Interpersonal Interactions and Relationships.

Difficulty coping: Individuals with PD who have poor cognition use less problem-focus coping, which includes facing the problem head-on and developing strategies to solve the problem. They use more emotional-focused coping, such as anger, withdrawal, and isolation, which leads to higher depression and anxiety and lower quality of life (Hurt et al., 2012). ICF codes b125 Dispositions and Intra-Personal Functions and b126 Temperament and Personality Functions address these issues.

ICF Core Set

A brief and comprehensive ICF Core Set for Neurological Conditions is available. It covers a wider range of diagnoses than just Parkinson's disease so some of the codes listed may not be appropriate for Parkinson's and some codes may be missing.

Treatment Direction

Whole Team Approach

The treatment goals for individuals with PD are prioritized based on management of symptoms, involvement in life tasks specific to the individual, and activities that promote health and optimize quality of life (Hanna & Cronin-Golomb, 2011). The treatment team works toward restoration or maintenance of functioning when deconditioning occurs. Medication is prescribed or adjusted to restore dopamine receptor function and secondarily to inhibit muscarinic cholinergic receptors, a type of protein

receptor in the brain (Brotchie, 2008). Antiparkinsonian medications may cause side effects like involuntary movements and, as a result, precautionary measures must be taken to remove obstacles and protect against falls (Carter & Van Andel, 2011).

Recreational Therapy Approach

Recreational therapy addresses gross motor movement, maintenance of muscle tone, range of motion, endurance, strength, balance, relaxation techniques, fostering social interaction and support, use of assistive devices when necessary, affect, self-esteem, well-being, involvement, and independence (Robertson & Long, 2008).

Recreational Therapy Interventions

Exercise

Regular engagement in exercise might hold the key to prevent brain degeneration in conditions such as Alzheimer's and PD. Based on the following studies, s1103 Basal Ganglia and Related Structures or any ICF code under b1 Mental Functions can be cited as the reason for treatment. ICF codes in b4 Functions of the Cardiovascular, Hematological, Immunological, and Respiratory Systems, b7 Neuromusculoskeletal and Movement-Related Functions, and d4 Mobility are also improved according to this research.

A review of the literature by Marques-Aleixo and colleagues (2012) found that "physical exercise modulates several physiological mechanisms that may increase brain resistance to aging and neurodegeneration" (p. 158). The authors note that exercise triggers neuroprotective mechanisms that "represent an important strategy against many cerebral pathophysiological conditions… [and] may have preventive and/or therapeutic potential" (p. 158). An earlier review of the literature by Farley and colleagues (2008) also found support for the neurological value of exercise, finding that "[r]esearch in the area of exercise neurobiology has shown that exercise may interfere with multiple mechanisms involved in cell death, stimulate the proliferation of new neurons, alter metabolic and immune system responses, increase blood supply, and protect again the erosive neural events of aging, neurodegeneration, and brain injury" (p. 101).

Exercise intervention studies have also shown support for the value of exercise in treating PD. For example, Combs and colleagues (2013) conducted a study of 31 adults with PD. The participants were randomly assigned to boxing training (stretching, lateral footwork, punching bags, resistance exercises, aerobic training, and balance activities) or traditional exercise (stretching, resistance exercises, aerobic training, and balance activities) for 24-36 sessions, each lasting 90 minutes over 12 weeks. The traditional exercise group had significantly greater gains in balance confidence, and the boxing group had significantly greater gains in gait velocity and endurance. Both groups had significant improvements in balance, mobility, and quality of life. The authors state that "supporting options for long-term community-based group exercise for persons with PD will be an important future consideration for rehabilitation professionals" (p. 117).

A study by Poliakoff and colleagues (2013) also had similar findings. Thirty-two adults with PD, who were not regularly exercising, participated in a community gym training program at a local recreation center. Following the interventions, participants had significant improvement in reaction time and reported feelings of enjoyment, additional social benefits, and increased confidence.

As a result of the research boom in exercise as a disease-modifying agent, researchers are beginning to explore how best to apply exercise interventions in the PD population. Farley and colleagues (2008) advocate that therapists working with individuals with PD should not be quick to implement compensatory strategy training that bypasses the basal ganglia pathology, but instead adopt a neuroplasticity model, such as is used in stroke rehabilitation, where clients repeat complex, high-effort tasks within novel environments, force limb use within everyday activities, or have general, whole-body progressive locomotion training. Within their literature review, they found that the timing of exercise is critical. The timings they found are

Prior to diagnosis of PD: Depending on baseline fitness level and how early exercise is started, exercise may protect dopamine neurons.

After diagnosis of PD (injury): Regular engagement in exercise may be required to maintain the growth and survival of the remaining viable dopamine neurons. Inactivity or failure to engage damaged systems, either impairment-related or self-imposed, may contribute to further degradation of brain function.

Advanced PD: Exercise has been shown to produce changes in the damaged basal ganglia pathways, but progressively higher intensity, velocity, longer duration practice, and task-specific exercises may be required.

Given the above findings, engagement in leisure time physical activity (LTPA) is a vital component of recreational therapy treatment to prevent neurodegeneration and promote neuron growth. Therapists can cite the ICF codes listed at the beginning of this topic and any deficits noted in d920 Recreation and Leisure as justification for implementing the following treatment modalities:

- exploring leisure interests, motivation, satisfaction, and needs to identify forms of LTPA best suited to the client.
- assessing barriers and facilitators to engagement in LTPA at the intrapersonal, interpersonal, and structural levels with the goal of minimizing barriers and strengthening or maintaining facilitators. For example, Ellis and colleagues (2013) studied 260 adults with PD and found that expectations from exercise, lack of time to exercise, and fear of falling were primary barriers to exercise engagement.
- assessing functional skill baselines for LTPA participation to determine skill and ability needs and implementing treatment services to maximize LTPA performance and independence.
- obtaining precautions and parameters from the treating physician to guide LTPA choices and engagement, as well as for monitoring.
- determining and implementing education, training, and counseling needs related to LTPA benefits, resources, adaptation, etc.
- assessing and addressing challenges or needs related to LTPA participation in community settings to promote social connectedness.

Recreation, Leisure, and Community Engagement

As previously reviewed, engagement in recreation, leisure, and community activities is significantly affected by PD. Individuals give up previously enjoyed activities, activity becomes more passive, and social isolation commonly ensues. Decreased activity can hasten neurodegeneration and further contribute to the advance of the disease. Interventions to foster engagement in active recreation, leisure, and community activities is necessary, as well as forms of passive recreation, leisure, and community activities that foster cognitive, psychological, and social well-being. The studies listed below demonstrate that deficits in ICF codes b125 Dispositions and Intra-Personal Functions, b126 Temperament and Personality Functions, d230 Carrying Out Daily Routine, d4 Mobility, d7 Interpersonal Interactions and Relationships, and d9 Community, Social, and Civic Life can be improved with these activities.

Several recent studies further highlight the need for increased activity. For example, McCabe, Roberts, and Firth (2008) conducted individual interviews with 110 adults with neurological illnesses (of which 31 had PD). In regards to recreation, only 13% indicated positive recreational outcomes from the development of their illness. They cited increased leisure time, more time to spend pursuing hobbies, and spending time with family. The majority of clients, caregivers, and healthcare professionals indicated that the illness negatively affected recreational activities leading to reduction in social and physical activities, curtailment of hobbies, and difficulties in holiday travel. The authors note that the negative change in recreational activities is a major concern because if "these enjoyable activities are no longer accessible, there may be a deterioration in the well-being of both patients and carers" (p. 609). The authors advocate for the organization of activities to keep people active outside their homes and that "engagement and ensuring social contact is likely to lead to an enhanced sense of well-being" (p. 609).

Engagement in recreation, leisure, and community activities, however, is not as simple as offering opportunities. A study by Meligrana and colleagues (2011) of 55 adults with PD found that executive efficiency, independence in performing complex activities of everyday life, and neurobehavioral symptoms were the most significant predictors of social and community functioning. In another study, Trail et al. (2012) studied 100 veterans with PD and found that fatigue, physical and cognitive limitations, and psychosocial reasons such as being too busy, not having enough money, lack of motivation, depression, and memory problems kept participants from participating in their favorite activities. As a final example, Foster and Hershey (2011) found that

individuals with PD participated in fewer activities compared to matched controls that did not have PD; that they had lower cognition; and that everyday executive function after controlling for motor dysfunction and depressive symptoms was associated with reduced activity participation.

Given the outcomes from the above studies, functional skill development, compensatory training, adjustment to disability and coping, leisure exploration, leisure education and counseling, reduction of barriers and strengthening of facilitators, and community integration training focused on engagement or re-engagement in healthy forms of recreation, leisure, and community activities should be key rehabilitation components of recreational therapy for individuals with PD. Recreational therapists working in residential and community settings should include the provision of healthy forms of activity that promote holistic health.

Activity Specific Interventions

Cycling: Ridgel and colleagues (2012) found that cycling, in the PD population, improved tremors and bradykinesia (b765 Involuntary Movement Functions). The participants were between 45 and 74 years of age with Hoehn and Yahr stages of 1 to 3. They utilized a motorized bike for forty minutes of active-assisted cycling. The researchers noted that the sessions were well tolerated by the participants after monitoring heart rate, pedaling power, and perceived exertion. When looking at pre- and post-assessments during resting, postural and kinetic tremor showed improvements in both tremors and bradykinesia after one session. In an earlier study, Buettner and Fitzsimmons (2002) utilized wheelchair bikes in a two week recreational therapy protocol combined with small group activity therapy for adults with dementia in long-term residential care, of which 4.7% had PD. Depression scores significantly improved following the protocol and were maintained at a 10-week follow-up assessment (b126 Temperament and Personality Functions). Sleep (b134 Sleep Functions) and levels of activity engagement (b130 Energy and Drive Functions) also improved.

Nordic pole walking: In a study by Reuter and colleagues (2011), participants with PD participated in Nordic walking three times per week for six months, with each session lasting 70 minutes. Each session consisted of a warm up including flexibility and strength exercises, with and without the poles, and a cool down. One session each week was devoted to Nordic walking technique and the other two sessions focused on endurance training. Training sessions took place in a local park or forest. Video-taping was used to assess technical skills, along with a checklist for technical skill assessment, including diagonal sequence, opening of the hands, and planting of the poles. Pain, balance, quality of life, stride length, gait pattern and variability, maximum walking speed, exercise capacity, postural stability, and PD-specific disability on the *UPDRS* all improved. All of the participants continued Nordic walking after the completion of the study. Relevant ICF codes include b280 Sensation of Pain, b740 Muscle Endurance Functions, b770 Gait Pattern Functions, d410 Changing Basic Body Position, d415 Maintaining a Body Position, d450 Walking, and d465 Moving Around Using Equipment.

Yoga: Lee (2006) conducted a study of 17 adults with mild to moderate PD who participated in a 10-week Iyengar Yoga program of two, one-hour classes per week and daily 30-minute home exercises. Following the program, participants demonstrated improved gait efficiency, lower extremity function, and balance, as well as decreased fear of falling. ICF codes include b740 Muscle Endurance Functions, b770 Gait Pattern Functions, d410 Changing Basic Body Position, d415 Maintaining a Body Position, and d450 Walking.

Tai chi (d920 Recreation and Leisure, d570 Looking After One's Health): A randomized controlled trial and blinded outcome study by Li and colleagues (2012) consisted of 185 adults with PD (Hoehn and Yahr Stages 1-4). Participants were randomized into a tai chi group, resistance group, or stretching group. All three groups trained for 24 weeks, twice a week, for 60-minute sessions. At the end of the 24 weeks, the tai chi group (compared to both the resistance group and the stretching group) had significantly better maximum excursion, direction control, stride length, and functional reach. The tai chi group also had significantly better knee flexion and extension, timed up and go, and URPDS scores then the stretching group, but not the resistance group; and lower falls incidents compared to the stretching group. ICF codes include b710 Mobility of Joint Functions, b770 Gait Pattern

Functions, d410 Changing Basic Body Position, and d450 Walking.

Dance: A randomized controlled trial with base-line assessments was undertaken with 52 adults with PD (Hoehn and Yahr 1-4) (Foster et al., 2013). Participants were randomly assigned to participate in a community Argentine tango group dance class (one-hour dance classes, two times per week for 12 months; dance partners did not have PD) or a control group (asked to continue with normal life routine). Participants in the tango group reported "increased participation in complex daily activities, recovery of activities lost since the onset of PD, and engagement in new activities," indicating that the incorporation of "dance into the clinical management of PD may benefit participation and subsequently quality of life for this population" (p. 240). Rabbia (2010) conducted a review of the literature on community-based dance for older adults and found that "[d]ance for individuals with PD… provides external cues through music and incorporates functional movement strategies, specifically moving sideways and backwards; movements that often are related to falls." In a mixed method study by Houston and McGill (2013), 24 adults with PD participated in a 12-week ballet class with 1.5 hour session, one time a week, which included other events such as watching rehearsals of the company, going to ballet perform-ances at the theatre, behind-the-scenes talks, live music during the dance sessions, and refreshments after each dance class. All of the participants had 100% adherence to the program and valued the classes as an important part of their lives. They also demonstrated improved balance and stability. The authors note that "[d]ancing may offer benefits to people with PD through its intellectual, artistic, social, and physical aspects" (p. 103). The improve-ments in balance, movement, and stability address needs found in ICF codes b710 Mobility of Joint Functions, b760 Control of Voluntary Movement Functions, and d4 Mobility.

Nintendo Wii: The use of Nintendo Wii is be-coming a popular therapy tool for the treatment of PD, and the Wii balance board has been identified as "a valid tool for the quantification of postural stability among individuals with Parkinson's" (Holmes et al., 2012, p. 361). In a study of 10 subjects with PD (Hoehn and Yahr Stages 2.5 or 3), participants engaged in Wii balance board game sessions with a therapist three times a week for eight weeks. Each session was 30 minutes long, consisting of participation in three ten-minute games including marble tracking, skiing, and bubble rafting. The participants demonstrated improved balance and gait (Mhatre et al., 2013). In a longitudinal study by Mendes and colleagues (2012), 16 adults with early stage PD were taught 10 Wii Fit games over 14 sessions. Sixty 60 days later they retained cognitive and motor abilities. The authors found that "motor difficulty can impair the performance of patients with PD on the majority of games, but they do not affect the ability to improve performance with practice or to retain these benefits after training. However, impairment in some cognitive functions, particularly quick decision making and management of attention and/or working memory, may have hampered learning on some games" (p. 222). The authors found that the following games had the greatest indication for therapeutic use: (1) Single Leg Extension — balance on one leg while moving arms and leg contralaterally while remaining stable, sustain attention to mimic movements shown by avatar, self-awareness (2) Torso Twists — perform torso twists, moving arms and keeping feet still while remaining stable, sustain attention to mimic movements shown by avatar, self-awareness, (3) Rhythm Parade — perform stationary walk to auditory and visual rhythm provided by game, while performing flex-extension of elbows in different rhythm to walk, divide attention between gait and task of hitting random targets with one or both arms, (4) Table Tilt — shift center of gravity slowly in all directions with feet in a fixed position, plan movements in order to hit targets, (5) Basic Step — alternate steps mounting and dismounting the Wii Balance Board according to the rhythm determined by the game, sustain attention to follow visual and auditory cues that direct foot movements, and (6) Obstacle Course — perform stationary walk as fast as possible, halt and resume walking, decide on best walking speed, when to halt and resume, response inhibition. The use of Nintendo Wii at home has also shown positive outcomes. For example, a study of 10 subjects with moderate PD who participated in a six-week, home-based balance-training program using the Nintendo Wii Fit and Balance Board showed significant gains in dynamic balance, mobility, and functional abilities (Esculier et

al., 2012). Most of these Wii interventions address deficits in d4 Mobility.

Compensatory Training and Environmental Design for Functional Mobility

Although the current push is to utilize a neuroplasticity approach in PD, compensatory training continues to have a place in helping individuals with PD manage mobility problems (d4 Mobility). Project RESCUE developed 15 evidence-based guidelines to help therapists identify compensatory strategies to help with motor difficulties, such as freezing, getting stuck in a chair, and involuntary movements. All are available online at http://hces-online.net/websites/rescue/pubs/info_sheets.htm.

Overall, the project recommends therapists help clients by teaching them to use visual cues, rhythmical cues, and attentional strategies to improve mobility:

Visual cues: When experiencing freezing, imagine a line on the floor that you need to step over or on, or look at lines or patterns on the floor or carpet when walking. Helps keep size of steps uniform and fosters attention on stepping.

Rhythmical cues: Play a song in your head or listen to music that has a comfortable, steady stepping beat. Advance your step in time with the beat.

Attentional strategies: Rehearse movements in your mind or count a rhythm in your head. As you walk, focus on the visualized movement or stepping beat.

Making changes to the person's environment to decrease risk of falls can also be helpful (e115 Products and Technology for Personal Use in Daily Living). A review of the literature by Lord, Menz, and Sherrington (2006) found that the interaction between an older person's physical abilities, cognition, and their exposure to environmental stressors increases falls risk. Environmental modifications made in the studies reviewed included: fixing unsafe stairs, adding handrails, removing throw rugs and floor mats, removing cords strung across rooms, removing unsafe chairs, making clear pathways through the home, installing well-designed lighting, etc.

Cognitive Retraining

As reviewed earlier, level of cognition affects leisure, recreation, and community participation. It can also impair functional performance, independence, and quality of life. Consequently, cognitive evaluations are recommended with subsequent interventions (Foster & Hershey, 2011). Cognitive retraining for remediation, compensatory strategies, and/or environmental design are common interventions for neurological impairments, however research related to PD specifically is lacking.

In regards to cognitive retraining for improving deficits in ICF codes b1 Mental Functions and d1 Learning and Applying Knowledge, a review of the literature prior to July 2011 by Calleo and colleagues (2012) only turned up four studies (two pilot studies, two small randomized controlled trials). All showed positive outcomes. Two of the studies utilized computerized cognitive programs, and two utilized in-person sessions. One of the in-person studies consisted of practice exercises, worksheets on attention tasks, and homework that improved executive functioning; while the other in-person study used search tasks, matrices, puzzles, speech production, picture completion, and storytelling that improved executive function and maintained working memory. The authors conclude that more research is needed, but that "[p]ersonalized approaches to tailor treatment to individual strengths and deficits are recommended" (p. 5).

Compensatory strategy training might also be addressed as part of cognitive retraining. Compensatory strategy training assists clients in identifying and implementing external and internal strategies to compensate for lost cognitive functions.

External strategies: Paper calendars, lists, sticky notes, planners, technology items such as iPhone and iPad apps or electronic calendars that send reminders to phone, diaries, tape recorders, flow charts for making decisions and solving problems, pill boxes, key finders, bulletin boards and dry erase boards, watches with alarms, and organizational strategies such as things kept in consistent places all can lead to better functioning.

Internal strategies: Acronyms, visualization, mnemonics, associations, chunking, and rhymes can be used.

Psychological Adjustment

Depression and anxiety (b126 Temperament and Personality Functions, d240 Handling Stress and Other Psychological Demands) may be separate and distinct conditions, a result of coping or adjustment to functional loss and lifestyle changes, a part of the pathophysiological process of PD, or some combination. They are estimated to be prevalent in 33% of the PD population. Pharmacological interventions for treating depression and anxiety can exacerbate PD symptoms, resulting in a "critical need for alternative treatment approaches" (Yang et al., 2012, p. 113). Consequently, Yang and colleagues (2012) conducted a review of the literature prior to April 2011 related to psychosocial interventions and found support (although not generalizable) for the following interventions: cognitive behavioral therapy; psychodrama; group sessions focused on psychosocial issues; strategy training for motor behavior; relaxation techniques; social skills training; and multi-disciplinary education programs that focused on activities of daily living, speech therapy, mobility, group relaxation training, and expert presentations on disease, diet, and medication. The authors concluded that in "spite of the methodological limitations…it appears that psychosocial interventions have the potential for improving depressive and anxiety outcomes among people with PD" (p. 118).

Pain Management

Sophie and Ford (2012) conducted a review of the literature on pain management in PD (b280 Sensation of Pain). They found that up to 80% of individuals with PD have significant pain that impacts functioning; and that musculoskeletal pain was the most frequent, resulting from rigidity, lack of mobility, posture deformities, and awkward gait mechanics. Recommendations for treating such pain include a combination of medication, physical therapy, and exercise programs, along with recommendations for passive range of motion exercises to prevent contractures in clients with limited mobility. For extreme musculoskeletal pain, other interventions may be considered including corticosteroid injections, nerve blocks, or surgery. The authors recommend that clinicians conduct routine screenings for depression, as this is a frequent comorbidity that can contribute to chronic pain. Recreational therapy interventions aimed at engagement in physical activity and reduction of depressive symptoms are key to assist with pain management. However, other common recreational therapy pain management interventions such as relaxation training, positive mood, coping, and stress management are not currently reflected in the literature, offering opportunities for research.

Resources

National Parkinson Foundation, Inc.

www.parkinson.org

A national organization whose mission is to improve the lives of people with Parkinson's disease through research, education, and outreach.

Offers a download of the Hoehn and Yahr scale (www.parkinson.org/Professionals/Professional-Resources/Screening-Instruments), as well as other scales reviewed in this chapter.

American Parkinson Disease Association

www.apdaparkinson.org

A grassroots organization serving Americans with Parkinson's (news, research, treatments).

References

American Psychiatric Association. (2013). *Diagnostic and statistical manual of mental disorders* (5th ed.). Arlington, VA: American Psychiatric Publishing.

Archer, T., Fredriksson, A., & Johansson B. (2011). Exercise alleviates Parkinsonism: Clinical and laboratory exercise. *Acta Neurological Scandinavica, 123,* 73-84.

Becker, C., Robert, G. P., Johansson, S., Jick. S. S., & Meier, C. R. (2011). Risk of incident depression in patients with Parkinson disease in the UK. *European Journal of Neurology, 18,* 448-453.

Berendse, H., Booij, J., Francot, C., Bergmans, P., Hijman, R., Stoof, J., & Wolters, E. (2001). Subclinical dopaminergic dysfunction in asymptomatic Parkinson's disease patients' relatives with a decreased sense of smell. *Annals of Neurology, 50*(1). 34-41.

Breen, K. C. & Drutyte, G. (2013). Non-motor symptoms of Parkinson's disease: The patient's perspective. *Journal of Neural Transmission, 120*(4), 531-535.

Brotchie, J. M. (2008). Pharmacology of Parkinson's disease, in *Therapeutics of Parkinson's Disease and Other Movement Disorders* (eds. M. Hialett and W. Poewe), John Wiley & Sons, Ltd, Chichester, UK. doi: 10.1002/9780470713990.ch3.

Buettner, L. L. & Fitzsimmons, S. (2002). AD-venture program: Therapeutic biking for the treatment of depression in long term care residents with dementia. *American Journal of Alzheimer's Disease and Other Dementias, 17*(2), 121-7.

Calleo, J., Burrows, C., Levin, H. Marsh, L., Lai, E., & York, M. K. (2012). Cognitive rehabilitation for executive dysfunction in Parkinson's disease: Application and current directions. *Parkinson's Disease, 2012,* 512892, 1-6.

Carter, M. J. & Van Andel, G. E. (2011). *Therapeutic recreation.* Long Grove, IL: Waveland Press, Inc.

Cieza, A., Bostan, C., Ayuso-Mateos, J. L., Oberhauser, C., Bickenbach, J., Raggi, A., Leonardi, M., Vieta, E., & Chatterji, S. (2013). The psychosocial difficulties in brain disorders that explain short term changes in health outcomes. *BMC Psychiatry, 12*(78), 1-12.

Combs, S., Diehl, M. D., Chrzastowski, C., Didrick, N., Mccoin, B., Mox, N., Staples, W., & Wayman, J. (2013). Community-based group exercise for persons with Parkinson disease: A randomized controlled trial. *NeuroRehabilitation, 32*(1), 117-124.

de Lau, L. & Breteler, M. (2006). Epidemiology of Parkinson's disease. *Lancet Neurology, 5,* 525-35.

Den Oudsten, B. L., Lucas-Carrasco, R., Green, A. M., & The WHOQoL-DIS Group. (2011). Perceptions of persons with Parkinson's disease, family and professionals on quality of life: An international focus group study. *Disability and Rehabilitation, 33*(25-26), 2490-2508.

Ellis, T., Boudreau, J. K., DeAngelis, T. R., Brown, L. E., Cavanaught, J. T., Earhart, G. M., Ford, M. P., Foreman, K. B., & Dibble, L. E. (2013). Barriers to exercise in people with Parkinson disease. *Physical Therapy, 93*(5), 628-636.

Esculier, J. F., Vaudrin, J., Beriault, P., Gangnon, K., & Tremblay, L. E. (2012). Home-based balance training programme using Wii Fit with balance board for Parkinson's disease: A pilot study. *Journal of Rehabilitation Medicine, 44*(2), 144-50.

Factor, S. A., Steenland, N. K, Higgins, D. S., Molho, E. S., Kay, D. M., Montimurro, J., Rosen, A. R., Zabetian, C. P., & Payami, H. (2011). Postural instability/gait disturbance in Parkinson's disease has distinct subtypes: An exploratory analysis. *Journal of Neurology, Neurosurgery & Psychiatry, 82*(5), 564-568.

Farley, B. G., Fox, C. M., Ramig, L. O., & McFarland, D. H. (2008). Intensive amplitude-specific therapeutic approaches for Parkinson's disease: Toward a neuroplasticity-principled rehabilitation model. *Topics in Geriatric Rehabilitation. 24*(2), 99-114.

Foster, E. R., Golden, L., Duncan, R. P., & Earhart, G. M. (2013). Community-based Argentine tango dance program is associated with increased activity participation among individuals with Parkinson's disease. *Archives of Physical Medicine and Rehabilitation, 94,* 240-9.

Foster, E. & Hershey, T. (2011). Everyday executive function is associated with activity participation in Parkinson disease without dementia. *OTH: Occupation, Participation and Health, 31,* 16-22.

Foster, P. S., Drago, V., Crucian, G. P., Sullivan, W. K., Rhodes, R. D., Shenal, B. V., Skoblar, B., Skidmore, F. M., & Heilman, K. M. (2011). Anxiety and depression severity are related to right but not left onset Parkinson's disease duration. *Journal of Neurological Sciences, 305,* 131-135.

Gobbi, L., Oliveira-Ferreira, M., Caetano, M., Lirani-Silva, E., Barbieri, F., Florindo, S., & Gobbi, S. (2009). Exercise programs improve mobility and balance in people with Parkinson's disease. *Parkinsonism and Related Disorders, 15*(S3), 49-52.

Haaxma, C. A., Bloem, B. R., Borm, G. F., Oyen, W., Leenders, K., Eshuis, S., Booij, J. Dluzen, D. E., & Horstink. M. (2007). Gender differences in Parkinson's disease. *Journal of Neurology and Neurosurgery Psychiatry, 78*(8), 819-824.

Hauser, R. (2010). Parkinson disease. Retrieved from www.emedicine.com.

Hanna, K. K. & Cronin-Golomb, A. (2012). Impact of anxiety on quality of life in Parkinson's disease, *Parkinson's Disease, 2012,* 1-8.

Hemmesch, A. R., Tickle-Degnen, L., & Zebrowitz, L. (2009). The influence of facial masking and sex on the older adult's impressions of individuals with Parkinson's disease. *Psychology and Aging, 24*(3), 542-549.

Hobson, P., Meara, J., & Ishihara-Paul, L. (2010). The estimated life expectancy in a community cohort of Parkinson's disease patients with and without dementia, compared with the UK population. *Journal of Neurology, Neurosurgery & Psychiatry, 81*(10), 1093-1098.

Holmes, J. D., Jenkins, M. E., Johnson, A. M., Hunt, M. A., & Clark, R. A. (2012). Validity of the Nintendo Wii balance board for the assessment of standing balance in Parkinson's disease. *Clinical Rehabilitation, 27*(4), 361-366.

Houston, S. & McGill, A. (2013). A mixed-methods study into ballet for people living with Parkinson's. *Arts and Health, 5*(2), 103-119.

Howell, S., Tripoliti, E., & Pring, T. (2009). Delivering the Lee Silverman Voice Treatment (LSVT) by web camera: A feasibility study. *International Journal of Language and Communication Disorders, 44*, 287-300.

Hurt, C. S., Landau, S., Burn, D. J., Hindle, J. V., Samuel, M., Wilson, K., & Brown, R. G. (2012). Cognition, coping, and outcome in Parkinson's disease. *International Psychogeriatrics, 24*(10), 1656-1663.

Jankovic, J. (2008). Parkinson's disease: Clinical features and diagnosis. *Journal of Neurology, Neurosurgery and Psychiatry, 79*(4), 368-76.

Johns Hopkins Medicine. (2011). Six signs of cognitive impairment in Parkinson's patients. Accessed via website http://www.johnshopkinshealthalerts.com/alerts/memory/cognitive-impairment-Parkinsons_5902-1.html.

Karlsen, K. H., Tandberg, E., Arsland, D., & Larsen, J. P. (2000). Health related quality of life in Parkinson's disease: A prospective longitudinal study. *Journal of Neurology & Neurosurgery Psychiatry, 69*, 584-589.

Kluding, P. & McGinnis, P. Q. (2006). Multidimensional exercise for people with Parkinson's disease: A case report. *Physiotherapy Therapy and Practice, 22*(3), 153-162.

Kudlicka, A., Clare, L., & Hindle, J. V. (2013). Awareness of executive deficits in people with Parkinson's disease. *Journal of the International Neuropsychological Society, 19*, 559-570.

Lee, L. (2006). Poster Board S33: Enhancing balance, lower extremity function, and gait in people with Parkinson's disease. *American Journal of Physical Medicine and Rehabilitation, 85*(3), 284.

Leritz, E., Loftis, C., Crucian, G., Friedman, W., & Bowers, D. (2004). Self-awareness of deficits in Parkinson disease. *The Clinical Neuropsychologist, 18*(3), 352-361.

Levy, R., Lang, A., Dostrovsky, J. O., Pahapill, P., Romas, J., Saint-Cyr, J., Hutchinson, W. D., & Lozano, A. M. (2001). Lidocaine and muscimol microinjections in subthalamic nucleus reverse Parkinsonian symptoms. *Brain, 124*, 2105-2118.

Li, F., Harmer, P., Fitzgerald, K., Eckstrom, E., Stock, R., Galver, J., Maddalozzo, G., & Batya, S. S. (2012). Tai chi and postural stability in patients with Parkinson's disease. *New England Journal of Medicine, 366*, 511-519.

Lord, S. R., Menz, H. B., & Sherrington, C. (2006). Home environment risk factors for falls in older people and the efficacy of home modifications. *Age and Aging, 25*(S2), ii55-ii59.

Macphee, G. J. A. & Stewart, D. A. (2012). Parkinson's disease — Pathology, etiology and diagnosis. *Reviews in Clinical Gerontology, 22*(3), 165-178.

Marques-Aleixo, I., Oliveira, P. J., Moreira, P. I., Magalhaes, J., & Ascensao, A. (2012). Physical exercise as a possible strategy for brain protection: Evidence from mitochondrial-mediated mechanisms. *Progress in Neurobiology, 99*, 149-162.

McCabe, M. P., Roberts, C., & Firth, L. (2008). Work and recreational changes among people with neurological illness and their caregivers. *Disability and Rehabilitation, 30*(8), 600-610.

Meligrana, L., Sgaramella, T., Bartolomei, L., Carrieri, L., Perini, F., Cracco, A., & Soresi, S. (2011). The role of cognitive, functional and neuropsychiatric symptoms on community integration in Parkinson's disease. *International Journal of Child Health and Human Development, 4*(3), 323-330.

Mendes, F. A., Pompeu, J. E., Lobo, A. M., da Silva, K. G., Oliveira, T., Zomignani, A. P., & Piemonte, M. E. (2012). Motor learning, retention and transfer after virtual-reality based training in Parkinson's disease — effect of motor and cognitive demands of games: A longitudinal, controlled clinical study. *Physiotherapy, 98*, 217-223.

Mhatre, P. V., Vilares, I., Stibb, S. M., Albert, M. V., Pickering, L., Marciniak, C. M., Kording, K., & Toledo, S. (2013). Wii fit balance board improves balance and gait in Parkinson Disease. *PM & R: The Journal of Injury, Function, and Rehabilitation, 5*(9), 769-770.

Mitchell, A. J., Kemp, S., Benito-Leon, J., & Reuber, M. (2010). The influence of cognitive impairment on health-related quality of life in neurological disease. *Acta Neuropsychiatrica, 22*, 2-13.

Movement Disorder Virtual University. (n.d.). Unified Parkinson's disease rating scale. Accessed via website http://www.mdvu.org/library/ratingscales/pd/updrs.pdf.

National Parkinson Foundation. (2013). About Parkinson disease. Retrieved from www.parkinson.org.

Nobrega, A. C., Rodrigues, B., Torres, A. C., Scarpel, R., Neves, C. A., & Melo, A. (2008). Is drooling secondary to a swallowing disorder in patients with Parkinson's disease? *Parkinsonism and Related Disorders, 14*, 243-245.

O'Sullivan, S., Schmitz B., & Thomas J. (2007). Parkinson's disease. *Physical Rehabilitation* (5th Ed.) pp. 856-857. Philadelphia: F. A. Davis.

Plotnik, M., Giladi, N., Dagan, Y., & Hausdorff, J. M. (2011). Postural instability and fall risk in Parkinson's disease: Impaired dual tasking, pacing, and bilateral coordination of gait during the "on" medication state. *Exploratory Brain Research, 210*, 529-538.

Poliakoff, E., Galpin, A., McDonald, K., Kellett, M., Dick, J. P., Hayes, S., & Wearden, A. J. (2013). The effect of gym training on multiple outcomes in Parkinson's disease: A pilot randomized waiting-list controlled trial. *NeuroRehabiltiation, 32*(1), 125-134.

Poletti, M., DeRosa, A., & Bonuccelli, U. (2012). Affective symptoms and cognitive functions in Parkinson's disease. *Journal of Neurological Sciences, 317*, 97-102.

Rabbia, J. (2010). Dance as a community-based exercise in older adults. *Topics in Geriatric Rehabilitation, 26*(4), 353-360.

Reuter, I., Mehnert, S., Leone, P., Kaps, M., Oeschsner, M., & Engelhardt, M. (2011). Effects of a flexibility and relaxation programme, walking, and Nordic walking on Parkinson's disease. *Journal of Aging Research, 2011*, 232473, 1-18.

Ridgel, A. L., Peacock, C. A., Fickes, E. J., & Kum, C. H. (2012). Active-assisted cycling improves tremor and bradykinesia in Parkinson's disease. *Archives of Physical Medicine and Rehabilitation, 93*(11), 2049-2054.

Robertson, T. & Long, T. (2008). *Foundations of therapeutic recreation*, Champaign, IL: Human Kinetics.

Shah, M., Deeb, J., Fernando, M., Noyce, A., Visentin, E., Findley, L., & Hawkes, C. (2009). Abnormality of taste and smell in Parkinson's disease. *Parkinsonism and Related Disorders, 15*, 232-237.

Sophie, M. & Ford, B. (2012). Management of pain in Parkinson's disease. *CNS Drugs, 26*, 937-948.

Suchowersky, O., Reich, S., Perlmutter, J., Zesiewicz, T., Gronseth, G., & Weiner, W. (2006). Practice parameter: Diagnosis and prognosis of new onset Parkinson disease: An evidence-based review. *American Academy of Neurology, 66*, 968-975.

Trail, M., Petersen, N. J., Nelson, N., & Lai, E. C. (2012). An exploratory study of activity in veterans with Parkinson's disease. *Journal of Neurology, 259*(8), 1686-93.

Varanese, S., Birnbaum, Z., Rossi, R., & DiRocco, A. (2010). Treatment of advanced Parkinson's disease. *Parkinson's' Disease, 2010*, 1-9. 480260.

Weismer, G., Yunusova, Y., & Westbury, J. (2003). Interarticulator coordination in dysarthria: An x-ray microbeam study. *Journal of Speech, Language, and Hearing Research, 46*, 1247-1261.

Yang, S., Sajatovic, M., & Walter, B. L. (2012). Psychosocial interventions for depression and anxiety in Parkinson's disease. *Journal of Geriatric Psychiatry and Neurology, 25*(2), 113-121.

29. Post-Traumatic Stress Disorder

Kathy Neely, Dean Parker, and John Campbell

Post-traumatic stress disorder (PTSD) was once considered a condition that resulted from being in combat. Now it is seen as a disorder that also affects people after traumatic events outside of combat situations, including events that were only witnessed (National Institute of Mental Health, 2010).

PTSD was classified as an anxiety disorder in the *Diagnostic and Statistical Manual of Mental Disorders IV-TR* (American Psychiatric Association, 2000a; American Psychiatric Association, 2000b). The *DSM-5* (American Psychiatric Association, 2013) classifies PTSD in a separate area entitled "Trauma- and Stressor-Related Disorders." "The essential feature of post-traumatic stress disorder (PTSD) is the development of characteristic symptoms following exposure to one or more traumatic events" (American Psychiatric Association, 2013, p. 274).

Those events may include rape, abuse, natural disaster, being in a war zone, or exposure to a terrorist attack (Friedman, Keane, & Resick, 2007). Other traumatic events that may trigger the onset of symptoms of PTSD include "threatened or actual physical assault (e.g., physical attack, robbery, mugging, childhood physical abuse), threatened or actual sexual violence (e.g., forced sexual penetration, alcohol/drug facilitated sexual penetration, abusive sexual contact, noncontact sexual abuse, sexual trafficking)" (American Psychiatric Association, 2013, p. 274). Individuals who are kidnapped, taken hostage, experience a terrorist attack, "torture, incarceration as a prisoner of war, natural or human-made disasters, and severe motor vehicle accidents" are also considered to have experienced traumas. Additionally, traumatic medical incidents which can precipitate PTSD "involve sudden, catastrophic events (e.g., waking during surgery, anaphylactic shock)" (2013, p. 274). In the *DSM-5*, a greater emphasis is now being placed on how a person experienced events which are considered to be traumatic, such as first responders.

Characteristic symptoms develop following the exposure to an extreme traumatic stressor. After the traumatic event, if PTSD develops, the person may avoid anything associated with the trauma (Kahn and Fawcett, 2001). A person who has developed PTSD may feel emotionally numb or may easily become hyper-aroused. An individual with PTSD symptoms may re-experience the traumatic events through flashbacks, nightmares, and frightening thoughts. Other symptoms may be anhedonia, dissociation, or a combination of various symptoms (American Psychiatric Association, 2013). Some "co-occurring areas may include binge-eating, gambling, over-spending, sexual addiction and other impulse control problems" (Najavits, 2002, p. 337), and there may simultaneously be "a lack of healthy pleasures, such as hobbies, sports or outdoor activities" (p. 337).

To be diagnosed with PTSD, symptoms that impair important life functions need to be present for a duration exceeding one month (American Psychiatric Association, 2013). Symptoms for children with PTSD also include bedwetting, excessive forgetting, difficulties with verbal expression, nightmares, agitated behavior, acting out the traumatic event during playtime, and enmeshment with parental figures (National Institute of Mental Health, 2010). Responses and behaviors that develop are often attempts to reduce stress.

Incidence/Prevalence in U.S.

PTSD is a frequently occurring condition. Recent estimates vary due to the occurrence of PTSD with multiple comorbidities. Even though PTSD has been studied for decades, varying viewpoints regarding measures of prevalence persist.

Estimates reported by the Anxiety Disorders Association of America (n.d.) indicate that of those individuals exposed to some type of mass violence, 67% develop PTSD. Those who are exposed to natural disasters or other types of traumatic events have lower rates of PTSD than those exposed to mass violence. The Anxiety Disorders Association of America estimates that "7.7 million Americans age 18 and older have PTSD" (p.1). In a differing view, Friedman, Keane, and Resick (2007) indicate that 10-20% of those exposed to trauma actually develop PTSD. PTSD appears to be more common among persons "with chronic pain, anxiety disorders, and both major and other depression" (Liebschutz et al., 2007, p. 72).

Other sources with estimates on prevalence include Riggs (2010), who reports that one to three percent of the civilian population has PTSD. The proportions are higher for military populations and especially those returning from combat zones. Newhouse (2008) cites numbers from the Department of Defense and the Office of Mental Health Disaster Preparedness that suggest between 30% and 57% of returning veterans could be diagnosed with PTSD. Therapists working with service members returning from deployments should note co-occurring problems that cluster with PTSD. These often include substance abuse, depression, suicide, anxiety, panic, physical health problems, and traumatic brain injury, as well as relationship problems (Riggs, 2010).

The American Psychiatric Association (2013) reports that prevalence for PTSD among adults in the United States over a 12-month period is 3.5%, which is similar to the three percent prevalence reported by Riggs (2010). "In the United States, projected lifetime risk for PTSD using *DSM-IV* criteria at age 75 years is 8.7%" (p. 276). Europe and most Asian, African, and Latin American countries have lower numbers clustering around 0.5-1.0% (American Psychiatric Association, 2013).

Also addressed in the *DSM-5* is the higher risk of traumatic exposure among first responders and veterans and the increased attention given to PTSD in children. Although preschool children, children, and adolescents are reported to have a lower prevalence of PTSD, there is a possibility that this may be because "previous criteria were insufficiently developmentally informed" (American Psychiatric Association, 2013, p. 276.) The highest rates of PTSD "are found among survivors of rape, military combat and captivity, and ethnically or politically

motivated internment and genocide." Fully "one-third to more than one-half of those exposed" to these specific types of trauma develop PTSD (p. 276).

Since most people who experience trauma do not develop PTSD, more data are reported on trauma and trauma risk than on the actual diagnosis of PTSD. There are at least one to two times as many persons in the current population with severe subsyndromal PTSD, or indicators of PTSD, without an actual diagnosis of PTSD as there are persons with PTSD (Friedman et al., 2007).

One challenge with obtaining current, consistent national incidence data on the general or civilian population regarding PTSD is that most people with PTSD initially present to their primary care providers. Slone (2006, p. 1) indicated that "a patient's trauma history is often undetected during routine medical visits unless the patient mentions trauma as the main reason for the visit." Samson et al. (1999) supported the belief that undiagnosed PTSD in primary care settings has been an on-going problem, and that persons with PTSD present with more somatic complaints than other patients. Of critical importance is that these patients may not connect the experience of trauma to their physical health problems (Samson et al., 1999).

Since PTSD is often undiagnosed, both patients and providers often experience a disconnect between presenting problems and a diagnosis of PTSD. Jankowski (2007) identified this as a significant issue because PTSD has been associated with cardiovascular diseases, and recommends greater collaboration between primary care and specialty medical care personnel. The diagnosis of PTSD is often not made until some time after a person has experienced a significant trauma. It is less likely that providers without specialized training or experience in PTSD will review five months or more of a patient's life history to identify the original trauma and to connect symptom clusters, therefore, the diagnosis of PTSD is often not made initially. Slone (2006) concurs that PTSD is prevalent in primary care settings.

Persons with lower incomes and those who already have other health problems are more likely to be in the group of those who are undiagnosed, even though they have had PTSD for a considerable period of time (Davis et al., 2008). Income levels and access to resources are variables that also influence the diagnosis of PTSD. This would seem to be especially true for non-veteran populations with less access to healthcare.

For detailed findings which estimate prevalence and differences by gender, age, and ethnicity, see Friedman et al. (2007) and the *DSM-5* (American Psychiatric Association, 2013).

Predominant Age

Since trauma precipitates PTSD and traumatic events can occur at any time in a person's life, PTSD can occur at any age, including childhood. The *DSM-5* indicates that PTSD can be experienced by young children (American Psychiatric Association, 2013).

Though currently accepted, Dyregrov and Yule (2006) reported that prior to 1980 children were not believed to experience PTSD. These authors also indicated that there is less agreement about preschool children, regarding the "range and severity of their stress reactions" (p. 176). Incidence rates vary and in selected samples of children in special groups, such as child refugees from war-torn countries, they reported that rates ranged from 25-70%. As might be expected, when serving children, the focus has been primarily on trauma and not PTSD, due to the passage of time before symptoms were noticed (Fairbank, 2008).

The *DSM-5* includes diagnostic information which clearly indicates a shift in thinking regarding children and PTSD. The diagnostic criteria presented now include a separate section specifically for use with children six years old and younger. Noteworthy for the recreational therapist is that prior to the age of six, "young children are more likely to express re-experiencing symptoms through play that refers directly or symbolically to the trauma" (American Psychiatric Association, 2013, p. 277). This would seem to support intuitive and anecdotal observations from therapists who work with children. For those therapists who discerned that they were observing PTSD symptoms in young children but did not find sufficient support for those observations in the literature on children and PTSD, current information may be particularly useful.

Grasso et al. (2009) found that even in children considered to be maltreated, PTSD "is frequently underdiagnosed" (p. 157) and that "PTSD is one of the most frequent diagnoses associated with a history of abuse" (p. 158).

When older adults were studied for trauma and PTSD, a concern regarding trauma-related research was that some researchers have not "recruited sufficient numbers of older adults to examine age effects or have failed to include older adults at all" (Cook & Niederehe, 2006, p. 255). They also reported that a number of older adults are considered to have sub-threshold PTSD symptoms and that this warrants both research and clinical attention.

There has been concern about the existence of subsyndromal PTSD (Cook & Niederehe, 2006; Friedman et al., 2007). However, with regard to older adults, "the prevalence of full-threshold PTSD also appears to be lower among older adults compared with the general population; there is evidence that subthreshold presentations are more common than full PTSD in later life and that these symptoms are associated with substantial clinical impairment" (American Psychiatric Association, 2013, p. 276).

Causes

PTSD has many causes. These can include surviving a traumatic event or injury, witnessing other persons being injured or killed, the sudden unexpected death of a loved one (Smith & Segal, 2013), as well as the loss of a job or home, terrorist incidents, rape, or some other life-threatening event (Anxiety Disorders Association of America, n.d.). The *DSM-5* includes an extensive description of the precursory events which can result in the development of PTSD (American Psychiatric Association, 2013).

Certain resilience factors are believed to reduce the risk of PTSD. Individuals who seek support from friends and family, involve themselves in a support group, develop a coping strategy, and who can respond effectively even though they experience fear are considered to be resilient. Persons in this category are less likely to develop PTSD (National Institute of Mental Health, 2010).

Persons at higher risk for developing PTSD include those who have experienced repeated exposure to trauma and those who experience trauma but who do not receive social support after the trauma (Friedman et al., 2007). This would also include persons without the adequate or well-developed coping skills required to effectively deal with stress. Additionally, "social support prior to event exposure is protective" (American Psychiatric Association, 2013, p. 277).

Systems Affected

PTSD affects a person's mood and ability to cope effectively with ongoing stressful events, even events that most people would not experience as stressful. Symptoms include a diminished interest in significant activities, recurring distressing recollections and/or dreams of the event, feeling separate from others, and negative beliefs concerning the future (Kahn & Fawcett, 2001). ICF codes that cover the mood and stress symptoms include b125 Dispositions and Intra-Personal Functions, b126 Temperament and Personality Functions, b130 Energy and Drive Functions, b134 Sleep Functions, b152 Emotional Functions, b160 Thought Functions, and d240 Handling Stress and Other Psychological Demands

PTSD can affect a person's social functioning as a result of the detachment they feel from others and as a result of their avoidance of people, places, and activities that remind them of the trauma (American Psychiatric Association, 2000). ICF codes can include d230 Carrying Out Daily Routine, d240 Handling Stress and Other Psychological Demands, d250 Managing One's Own Behavior, d7 Interpersonal Interactions and Relationships, d910 Community Life, and d930 Religion and Spirituality. Also important related to social functioning is that the client has people in his/her community who are capable of providing appropriate social support. This aspect can be documented with ICF codes under e3 Support and Relationships.

Cognitive difficulties as a result of PTSD can present as poor concentration and focus (Mobily & MacNeil, 2002). PTSD can affect the brain structure known as the limbic system (Mahan & Ressler, 2012). It has been suggested that changes in the limbic system may account for difficulties concerning emotional learning (Quirk & Mueller, 2008) as well as the emotional dysregulation symptoms often associated with PTSD (Etkin & Wager, 2007). ICF codes that may be used to note cognitive difficulties include b164 Higher-Level Cognitive Functions.

Secondary Problems

According to the *DSM-IV-TR* (American Psychiatric Association, 2000a), there may be an increased risk for an individual with PTSD for agoraphobia, obsessive-compulsive disorder, social phobia, specific phobia, major depressive disorder, somatization disorder, and substance-related disorders. The *DSM-5* (p. 280) notes that "individuals with PTSD are 80% more likely than those without PTSD to have symptoms that meet diagnostic criteria for at least one other mental disorder (e.g., depressive, bipolar, anxiety, or substance use disorders)" (American Psychiatric Association, 2013). An individual with PTSD can also be at risk for panic disorder and suicidal feelings and thoughts (National Institute of Mental Health, 2010). Researchers suggest there is a significant overlap between fibromyalgia and PTSD (Cohen et al., 2002; Raphael, Janal, & Nayak, 2004). PTSD commonly occurs with other disorders. The co-occurrence of PTSD with mild traumatic brain injury is 48%. See chapters in this book that discuss the specific comorbidities for information about ICF codes to use to describe those findings. One related effect of PTSD that should be assessed is the client's ability to continue his/her education and find employment (d810-d839 Education, d845 Acquiring, Keeping, and Terminating a Job).

Comorbidity issues related to children exhibit different patterns than those of adults. For example, young children are more likely to display comorbidity with separation anxiety and oppositional defiant disorder.

Prognosis

One of the challenges of addressing the issue of prognosis for persons with PTSD is that, not unlike trauma, specific prognostic indicators are affected by the prevalence, intensity, and duration of multiple comorbidities. Keane et al. (2007) report that comorbidity is a significant issue in PTSD. One other issue that appears to affect prognosis is the degree to which PTSD is initially addressed as a specific diagnosis (Liebschutz et al., 2007). If a person with PTSD is treated only for its symptoms with the PTSD remaining undiagnosed, the prognosis is much worse.

One complicating issue in the treatment of PTSD is that there is not one standard screening for PTSD and especially so with the existence of comorbidities. There are also barriers to treatment for some individuals, especially those with few financial resources, even though they may desire treatment.

Some of those barriers include "transportation and finances, family disapproval and unfamiliarity with accessing treatment" (Davis et al., 2008, p. 218). For military members or veterans, fears that talking about PTSD may hinder one's career, cause a loss of confidence in leadership ability, or result in a person being seen as "weak" are also barriers to treatment (National Center for PTSD, 2012, p.1).

Taylor (2006) found that studies regarding prognosis differed in their findings. He attributed these inconsistencies to small sample sizes with lower predictive power. He suggested that subtle predictors of PTSD would be identified in studies with larger sample sizes. PTSD was also found to be "comorbid with chronic pain in survivors of road traffic collisions, industrial accidents and other causes of traumatic injury" (p. 78). Regardless of the use of interventions otherwise considered successful, such as pain management techniques and relaxation training, poorer prognosis for persons diagnosed with PTSD and severe pain due to soft tissue injuries was noted by Taylor (2006).

Again, prognosis is influenced by the number and severity of comorbidities. For extensive treatment of comorbidities and their effect on outcomes see Keane et al., 2007, or Taylor, 2006.

Assessment

Typical Scope of Team Assessment

The specific indicators for the assessment of PTSD are clearly delineated in the diagnostic criteria of the *DSM-5* (American Psychiatric Association, 2013, pp. 271-272). In summary, the primary focus is on identifying whether a person has symptoms related to:

A. "Exposure to actual or threatened death, serious injury, or sexual violence" (p. 271). This includes the experience of a traumatic event (or events) either directly, as a witness, as others experienced the event, or learning that significant others experienced the event(s). An individual can also be traumatized by repeated or extreme exposure to the traumatic event(s). The latter category would include people watching news reports.

B. Presence of one (or more) of five identified intrusion symptoms resulting from the traumatic event(s). These symptoms include distressing trauma-related memories, dreams, dissociative reactions, psychological distress, and physiological reactions that involve internal or external trauma-related cues.

C. Persistent avoidance of stimuli associated with the traumatic event(s). This includes the avoidance of "distressing memories, thoughts, or feelings" about trauma-related experiences or avoiding people, places, conversations, activities, objects, and situations that arouse distressing memories. These symptoms can be considered a quick screen for PTSD, as they represent core behavioral areas common to the experience of and response to trauma.

D. Negative alterations in cognitions and mood associated with the traumatic event(s), as evidenced by two problems that include memory-related factors that are unrelated to other issues like alcohol, drugs, or head injuries. Other criteria include exaggerated beliefs that persist, detachment and estrangement-related feelings, as well as a "persistent inability to experience positive emotions" (p. 272).

E. Marked alterations in arousal and reactivity associated with the traumatic event(s) that meet at least two of six criteria. Those criteria include hypervigilance, irritable behavior coupled with angry outbursts, an exaggerated startle response, sleep disturbance, and problems with concentration.

F. Criteria B, C, D, and E need to have lasted more than one month.

G. The symptoms must cause clinically significant distress or impairment in social, occupational, or other important areas of functioning.

H. The disturbance cannot be attributed to the physiological effects of a substance (e.g., medication, alcohol) or other medical condition.

Because treatment for PTSD is more successful when a diagnosis of PTSD is made (Liebschutz et al., 2007), it is important for the person doing the assessment to note both the *DSM-5* diagnosis and the ICF codes that identify specific deficits noted during the assessment process.

When conducting assessments, some significant considerations include therapist and interviewer training, the administration time required for the assessment, cost, and the need for items which include both severity and frequency measures of symptoms (National Center for PTSD, 2013).

Medical and psychological assessments are central to the delivery of services to persons with PTSD, due to the nature of prevalent comorbidities. Many individuals who experience traumatic brain injury develop PTSD. There are some symptoms that overlap. Symptoms can include problems with sleeping and memory loss as well as depression and anxiety (National Center for PTSD, n.d.).

One complicating issue in the treatment of PTSD is that healthcare providers have not settled on one standard of practice for screening for PTSD. Especially with the existence of comorbidities, PTSD is often undiagnosed or diagnosed after the person has experienced a significant number of PTSD-related problems, even in individuals who present for treatment later in life (Keane et al., 2007).

Areas of Concern for RT Assessment

The following may be found as part of the RT assessment:

Limited leisure activities: These may be the result of an avoidance of people, places, and activities perceived as stressful, or isolation from others as a way of numbing oneself (Selz, Agcaoili, & Mason, 1995/1996; Whealin, Decarvalho, & Vega, 2008). When assessing leisure involvement, the assessment should consist of more than just an inventory and allow for differentiation between healthy and unhealthy coping (d240 Handling Stress and Other Psychological Demands, d570 Looking After One's Health) and leisure patterns (d920 Recreation and Leisure). For example, it would benefit the treatment process for the person to be aware of whether or not the choice of leisure is motivated by attempts to engage in avoidance, isolation, or self-harm (Griffin, 2005).

Traumatic reenactment: This describes a potential to react to current experiences as though these were past, trauma-associated experiences (Griffin, 2005). This can include variety of outcomes associated with an avoidance of people, places, and activities that remind the individual of the traumatic event (American Psychiatric Association, 2013). ICF codes include b160 Thought Functions and d240 Handling Stress and Other Psychological Demands.

Positive-emotion deficits: This may include limited pleasure derived from activities; lack of desire or diminished interest to participate in activities (Najavits, 2002; American Psychiatric Association, 2000b). The American Psychiatric Association (2013) describes this as "A persistent inability to feel positive emotions (especially happiness, joy,

satisfaction, or emotions associated with intimacy, tenderness, and sexuality)" (p. 275). There may also be difficulty engaging in healthy "self-nurturing" activities, which are done to comfort and soothe oneself (Griffin, 2005; Najavits, 2002). Most of these observations can be documented with ICF code b126 Temperament and Personality Functions. ICF codes b152 Emotional Functions and d570 Looking After One's Health may also be used.

Negative emotions: These include poor self-efficacy and feelings of helplessness (Bloom, 1997), emotional disconnection and deficits in self-awareness (Griffin, 2005), and an increased stress level and possible deficits in stress management (Mobily & MacNeil, 2002). ICF codes include b125 Dispositions and Intra-Personal Functions, b126 Temperament and Personality Functions, b180 Experience of Self and Time Functions, and d240 Handling Stress and Other Psychological Demands.

ICF Core Set

No ICF Core Set has been defined for Post-Traumatic Stress Disorder.

Treatment Direction

Whole Team Approach

A variety of approaches are utilized in the treatment of PTSD. The treatment approaches and interventions can include cognitive processing therapy, therapeutic exposure, and relaxation techniques. Cognitive processing therapy combines a key element of exposure therapy with an approach that addresses conflicts and provides information that may help correct distorted thoughts and beliefs (Resick & Calhoun, 2001). During therapeutic exposure clients safely confront stressors by imagining themselves in fear-producing situations or recalling their particular traumas. Time frames for therapeutic exposure may vary but generally involve forty-five minute sessions that last for at least four weeks (Resick & Calhoun, 2001). Relaxation techniques such as progressive muscle relaxation, guided imagery, and breathing control are coping skills that are often utilized to help the client develop feelings of mastery and control concerning fears and anxiety (Mobily and MacNeil, 2002).

A holistic (or biopsychosocial and spiritual) approach is critical to address the varied needs of the person seeking treatment, including all of the individual's medical issues. The person seeking treatment has likely had past experiences that have resulted in some degree of fragmentation of his or her life experiences, including symptoms and some type of treatment prior to a diagnosis of PTSD. Slone (2006) describes the challenges health practitioners experience in primary care settings as they deliver health services and attempt to screen for mental health problems as well. The concern is that the treatment not be fragmented, but consider all relevant issues. "Treating the whole person is a particularly appropriate charge for therapeutic recreation professionals" (Dustin et al., 2011, p. 330).

The treatment team needs to be prepared to address issues related to TBI, depression, chronic pain, and substance use in a holistic manner, as symptoms and problems often cluster (Najavits, 2002). Additionally, some veterans who served in the military during Operation Enduring Freedom or Operation Iraqi Freedom (OEF/OIF) have experienced a type of brain injury identified as blast-induced neurotrauma (BINT). Due to the nature of BINT, additional considerations are suggested when developing treatment approaches. One significant ICF code to consider is b7 Neuromusculoskeletal and Movement-Related Functions. For additional detail regarding BINT, see the *Life Skills* section of *Recreational Therapy Basics, Techniques, and Interventions* and Schneider et al., 2009.

Veterans who struggle with what they perceive to be a "transgression of moral, spiritual, or religious beliefs" (Maguen & Litz, 2012, p. 1) are believed to also experience other issues such as shame, guilt, and self-condemnation. These feelings are related to difficulties in experiencing forgiveness. The linkages between these feelings, PTSD, and suicide are nascent areas of research which are expected to become increasingly valuable. The identification of specific linkages will likely result in the development of more clearly targeted interventions that include persons in community settings who provide services to veterans, as well as leaders from faith-based and spiritual communities. Some early attempts are described in Newhouse (2008).

Treating children can bring up a different set of issues. A history of abuse in children who were maltreated was most frequently associated with a diagnosis of PTSD (Grasso et al., 2009). Rape, childhood sexual abuse, and other traumas were observed as precursors or precipitating events for persons diagnosed with PTSD and substance abuse (Najavits, 2002; American Psychiatric Association, 2013).

When working with some persons, it is common for those who present with PTSD symptoms to experience difficulty relating to or trusting other people (Najavits, 2002). This is described as "emotional numbing" and is not limited to veterans, but considered to be a common reaction to extreme stressors in both adults and children (Whealin, Decarvalho & Vega, 2008).

Recreational Therapy Approach

Recreational therapists provide therapy to achieve the goals in the whole team approach. Recreational therapists should take special effort to consider situations and activities that may trigger traumatic memories.

Recreational Therapy Interventions

Recreational therapy interventions include the application of the following approaches during leisure experiences. The focus is on maximizing the client's emotional adjustment (b125 Dispositions and Intra-Personal Functions, b126 Temperament and Personality Functions, b130 Energy and Drive Functions, b152 Emotional Functions) and coping skills (d240 Handling Stress and Other Psychological Demands) in leisure and other life situations. For example, activities and experiences that increase a person's involvement in leisure while having the person engage in an enjoyable activity that involves other people or people who are part of the person's social network has the potential to increase positive moods and reduce negative moods like anger, depression, and tension (Lundberg et. al, 2011).

Leisure education group: Outcomes of recreational therapy interventions should benefit the group members by enabling them to identify specific ways in which people engage in avoidance behaviors and how they isolate themselves through their leisure (d920 Recreation and Leisure) (Griffin, 2005). For example, after participating in the group, each person should be able to identify one healthy and one unhealthy leisure choice. Each group member should also be able to identify at least one leisure experience that might trigger a trauma-related response as well as a healthy response if an unpleasant memory is triggered. Additionally, teaching individuals how to plan and implement leisure experiences in which they find pleasure and feel safe would likely reduce stress (d240 Handling Stress and Other Psychological Demands) and subsequently reduce hyperarousal (Selz et al., 1995/1996; Griffin, 2005).

Social activities: Some clinicians have used activities that help to decrease stress (d240 Handling Stress and Other Psychological Demands) and increase positive moods (b126 Temperament and Personality Functions) (Whealin et al., 2008). Walking, bicycling, swimming, weight training, and cleaning house are activities that increase physical activity and can also be done with others (Najavits, 2002). Activities that can be engaged in with others provide opportunities for social interaction (d710 Basic Interpersonal Interactions), which is important in community reintegration and increasing involvement in leisure (d920 Recreation and Leisure). The therapist's approach is to specifically address trauma-related actions (Najavits, 2002; Griffin, 2005). Having a person with PTSD identify potential triggers for selected activities and develop a plan in advance to manage the accompanying emotions (d240 Handling Stress and Other Psychological Demands) could be done through role-playing (Najavits, 2002). Lundberg, Bennett, and Smith (2011) reported that participation in adaptive sports and recreation activities, which included water skiing, kayaking, river rafting, canoeing, fly-fishing, or skiing, snowboarding, ice skating, and Nordic skiing, over a period of five days decreased mood disturbances including anger, depression, and tension (b152 Emotional Functions) (Mowatt & Bennett, 2011). In addition to reducing mood disturbances, a general sense of vigor (b130 Energy and Drive Functions) and perceived competence (b126 Temperament and Personality Functions) were reported to increase (Lundberg et al., 2011). Significant others were included in these activities, which were conducted with veterans returning from combat with acquired disabilities. Dustin et al. (2011) used nature-based activities, which included paddle boating, kayaking, camping, day hiking, shared meals, campfire experiences, and journaling about these experiences, with veterans. Positive outcomes reported by Dustin et al. (2011) included an increased ability of participants to accept the diagnosis of

PTSD and the related symptoms. Understanding the on-going nature of PTSD-related issues and changing leisure lifestyles to adjust to the PTSD diagnosis were also observed. Other positive outcomes were the reported experience of joy (b152 Emotional Functions) and awareness of triggers (d240 Handling Stress and Other Psychological Demands).

Social skills training: The focus here is to reduce issues of isolation and family problems, which tend to cluster with a diagnosis of PTSD. The person experiencing PTSD may not be aware of the social skill deficits that impact interpersonal relationships (d7 Interpersonal Interactions and Relationships). Whealin et al. (2008) identified issues that affect social functioning and leisure, such as the avoidance of social contact, working for extended hours as an avoidance behavior, and "dropping out of recreational activities" (p.53). These are crucial areas, and especially so for the veteran returning from war, because the individual must express social skills to exist cohesively with others and reintegrate. With children, early intervention which focuses on family communication about traumatic events, clarifying misunderstandings, preventing family secrets, and providing an environment where children experience feelings of safety is recommended (d760 Family Relationships) (Dyregrov & Yule, 2006). Individuals with social skills deficits would find these actions challenging and would benefit from training. Selz, Agcaoili, and Mason (1995/1996) also identified social problems that co-exist with PTSD.

Physical exercise: Physical exercise (d920 Recreation and Leisure, d570 Looking After One's Health) is important, and whenever possible should include the building of "social networks through recreation opportunities" (Kelley & Loy, 2008, p. 116). Lundberg et al. (2011) and Dustin et al. (2011) both reported that physical activity had a positive effect on veterans. For example, walking and aquatic therapy (Kelly & Loy, 2008) have been found to be helpful in the reduction of chronic pain associated with fibromyalgia. Fibromyalgia is mentioned because fibromyalgia is often a comorbid condition with PTSD or related diagnoses like anxiety and depression (Harvard Mental Health Letter, 2009; Raphael et. al, 2004). See the chapter on Fibromyalgia for information about ICF codes used in treatment of fibromyalgia.

Social support: This is a critical area, consistent across the literature and especially so for persons with multiple traumas. With children who have been maltreated, "the availability of a caring and stable parent or alternate guardian" was one of the most important factors that distinguished between good outcomes and "more deleterious outcomes" (Grasso et al., 2009). In selecting activity interventions, especially with children, the RT needs to create opportunities for positive and reliable connections to peers, adults, and the community (d7 Interpersonal Interactions and Relationships, d910 Community Life) and make sure appropriate social support is available (e310 Immediate Family, e315 Extended Family) (Kinniburgh, Blaustein, & Spinazzola, 2005).

Life skills: This area will be increasingly important as individuals who have been in war zones (Schneider et al., 2009) return with blast-induced neurotrauma (BINT) and who also have PTSD. Due to the explosive weapons used in the current wars, clinicians have reported an increase in the numbers of veterans who return with a BINT, which is a blast-induced brain injury that produces symptoms similar to mild traumatic brain injury. However, due to the nature of these types of injuries, the affected veteran's level of functioning is not immediately apparent, but changes over a period of time. Interventions used should have value for the veteran whether the veteran will be reassigned, medically discharged, or enter the civilian workforce. They should assist the veteran in reintegrating into the community. In addition to identifying and resolving barriers to leisure, therapists can have individuals focus on improving management of symptoms of stress (d240 Handling Stress and Other Psychological Demands) and arousal (b152 Emotional Functions) (Selz et al., 1995/1996). For military members returning from combat zones with BINT and PTSD, an interdisciplinary approach is recommended due to the complexity of the comorbidities the person faces (Schneider et al., 2009).

Functional Skills

Some specific areas of concern include:

Physical: Due to the common comorbidities of chronic pain, depression, and the stress of reliving traumatic events, physical activity can be used to help manage pain (b280 Sensation of Pain), decrease stress (d240 Handling Stress and Other Psychological Demands), and improve well-being (b126 Temperament and Personality Functions). Physical interventions can be used to specifically address a person's level of hyperarousal or avoidance (b125 Dispositions and Intra-Personal Functions) and are best initiated at a lower or moderate level to avoid aggravating other health conditions. Recreational therapists also address physical impairments related to presenting comorbid conditions, such as those associated with BINT. These impairments often include balance and strength issues and can be coded using b7 Neuromusculoskeletal and Movement-Related Functions.

Cognitive: Any involvement in RT should consider the tendency of persons to relive past traumas by focusing on those painful thoughts and dwelling on faulty thoughts (b160 Thought Functions) (Griffin, 2005; Selz et al., 1995/1996). Recreational therapists additionally address impairments related to comorbid conditions, such as memory and problem solving issues (b144 Memory Functions, d175 Solving Problems) noted as part of the BINT comorbidity.

Emotional: Comorbidities that commonly occur with PTSD affect the emotional domain. They include depression, chronic pain, and often substance use disorders. ICF codes addressed in treatment will be found in the chapters describing those comorbid disorders. Interventions which include increasing the person's awareness of his/her emotions and which elevate mood are useful (Najavits, 2002).

Spiritual: Individuals report that prayer, participating in church-related activities, and meditation are helpful in the healing process. These activities can address any deficits noted in d930 Religion and Spirituality. These types of experiences are related to self-nurturing, which is a concept addressed by Najavits (2002) and Griffin (2005).

Education, Training, and Counseling

Recreational therapists have the training to provide education, training, and counseling in the context of activities. Some of the topics that are important to address can be taught through:

- Activities and counsel that promote spontaneity and playfulness (b126 Temperament and Personality Functions) (Bloom, 1997).

- Relaxation techniques — formal and informal techniques (d240 Handling Stress and Other Psychological Demands).
- Reducing anxiety provoking thoughts (b152 Emotional Functions) and changing thinking patterns that have become distorted as a result of trauma (b160 Thought Functions).
- Teaching coping strategies — strategies that decrease focus on anxiety and focus on mastery and internal locus of control (b152 Emotional Functions, d240 Handling Stress and Other Psychological Demands, b126 Temperament and Personality Functions).
- Spirituality and values clarification — learning to make meaning in the face of challenges to belief systems as the result of trauma (d930 Religion and Spirituality) (Kahn and Fawcett, 2001).
- Appropriate activities that promote abdominal breathing for handling stress and are cooperative in nature (d240 Handling Stress and Other Psychological Demands, d920 Recreation and Leisure).
- Identification and development of social supports (d7 Interpersonal Interactions and Relationships, e3 Support and Relationships).
- Activities and counsel that promote self-esteem and improve self-concept (b126 Temperament and Personality Functions).

Community Integration

Current challenges in community reintegration include the lack of "a consensual definition of successful community reintegration" (Resnik et al., 2012, p. 97). Key dimensions of participation that are important to veterans include leisure (d920 Recreation and Leisure); social interactions (d7 Interpersonal Interactions and Relationships), especially with spouses and significant others (d770 Intimate Relationships); education and returning to work (d810-d839 Education, d845 Acquiring, Keeping, and Terminating a Job); spiritual and religious experience (d930 Religion and Spirituality); and self-care (d5 Self-Care) (Resnik et al., 2012). Recreational therapists can be involved in each of these areas to assist in the community reintegration process. Recreational therapists need to "connect with various community resources and ensure that veterans and other clients have the necessary skills to utilize community resources independently, which may include advocating for appropriate transportation and funding" (Lundberg et al., 2011, p. 116). Therapists can also assist the individual to overcome alienation (Smith & Segal, 2013), in part by seeking support from others and finding a support group (National Institute of Mental Health, 2010).

Health Promotion

Individuals with PTSD can seek treatment provided by mental health counselors or specialists, hospitals, behavioral health centers, outpatient clinics, members of the clergy, employee assistance programs, and peer support groups (Smith & Segal, 2013; Kahn & Fawcett, 2001). Other sources of health promotion currently being tested for survivors of mass trauma events include telephone-assisted therapy and internet-based self-help therapy (Smith & Segal, 2013). Ruzek and Hamblin (n.d.) identified specific examples of health promotion resources which include telephone applications, such as the PTSD Coach mobile phone application for persons with PTSD. The application can be used to obtain educational information, as a self-assessment tool, or to supplement face-to-face contact with a healthcare provider. Williams and Poijula (2002) recommend that individuals with PTSD engage in ongoing self-care (d570 Looking After One's Health) including eating regular meals, exercising regularly, getting adequate sleep, meditating, setting healthy boundaries, spending time with family and friends, and maintaining health through prayer, joining a church, or nature appreciation. These activities can also affect ICF codes b134 Sleep Functions, d7 Interpersonal Interactions and Relationships, and d930 Religion and Spirituality.

Resources

National Center for PTSD
U.S. Department of Veteran Affairs
810 Vermont Avenue NW
Washington DC 20420
802-296-6300
www.ptsd.va.gov
This resource provides information pertaining to research, education, prevention, understanding, and treatment of PTSD in order to help and assist American veterans.

National Panic and Anxiety News

editor@npadnews.com

www.npadnews.com

Free articles and information for individuals who have panic or anxiety disorders and PTSD.

Anxiety Disorder Association of America

8701 Georgia Ave., Ste. 412

Silver Spring, MD 20910

240-485-1001

www.adaa.org

This resource provides information pertaining to the prevention, treatment, and cure of anxiety, depression, and stress-related disorders, as well as quick links to a variety of anxiety disorders.

Gift from Within

16 Cobb Hill Road

Camden, Maine 04843

Voice: 207-236-8858

Fax: 207-236-2818

www.giftfromwithin.org

This resource provides educational webcasts on PTSD for survivors and therapists. The web site also provides the opportunity to join a network of willing peer support participants.

CTU-Online: Clinician's Trauma Update

www.ptsd.va.gov/professional/publications/ctu-online.asp

Defense Centers of Excellence for Psychological Health and Traumatic Brain Injury

www.dcoe.mil/

Faces of Combat

facesofcombat.us

Resources for veterans with PTSD and a blog about current news for veterans and providers.

References

American Psychiatric Association. (2013). *Diagnostic and statistical manual of mental disorders* (5th ed.). Arlington, VA: American Psychiatric Association.

American Psychiatric Association. (2000a). *Diagnostic and statistical manual of mental disorders* (IV-TR). Washington DC: American Psychiatric Association.

American Psychiatric Association. (2000b). *Quick reference to the diagnostic criteria from DSM-IV-TR*. Washington, DC: American Psychiatric Association.

Anxiety Disorders Association of America. (n.d.). Treatment. http://www.adaa.org/understand-anxiety/post traumatic-stress-disorder-ptsd/treatment, accessed December 6, 2010.

Bloom, S. (1997). *Creating sanctuary: Toward the evolution of sane societies*. New York, NY: Routledge.

Cohen, H., Neumann, L., Haiman, Y., Matar, M., Press, J., & Buskila, D. (2002). Prevalence of post traumatic stress disorder in fibromyalgia patients: Overlapping syndromes or post-traumatic fibromyalgia syndrome? *Seminars in Arthritis and Rheumatism, 32*(1), 38-50.

Cook, J. M. & Niederehe, G. (2007). Trauma in older adults. In Friedman, M. J., Keane, T. M. & Resick, P. A. (Eds.), *Handbook of PTSD: Science and practice*. New York, NY: Guilford Press.

Davis, R. G., Ressler, K. J., Schwartz, A. C., Stephens, K. J., & Bradley, R. G. (2008). Treatment barriers for low-income urban African Americans with undiagnosed posttraumatic stress disorder. *Journal of Traumatic Stress, 21*(2), 218-222.

Dyregrov, A. & Yule, W. (2006). A review of PTSD in children. *Child and Adolescent Mental Health, 11*(4), 176-184.

Dustin, D., Bricker, N., Arave, J. Wall, W., & Wendt, G. (2011). The promise of river running as a therapeutic medium for veterans coping with post-traumatic stress disorder. *Therapeutic Recreation Journal, XLV*(4), 326-340.

Etkin, A. & Wager, T. D. (2007). Functional neuroimaging of anxiety: A meta-analysis of emotional processing in PTSD, social anxiety disorder, and specific phobia. *American Journal of Psychiatry. 167*, 1476-1488.

Fairbank, J. (2008). The epidemiology of trauma and trauma related disorders in children and youth. *PTSD Research Quarterly, 19*(1), 1-7.

Friedman, M., Keane, T., & Resick, P. (2007). *Handbook of PTSD science and practice*. New York: Guilford Press.

Grasso, D., Boonsiri, J., Lispschitz, D., Guyer, A., Houshyar, S., Douglas-Palumberi, H., Massey, J., & Kaufman, J. (2009). Posttraumatic stress disorder: The missed diagnosis. *Child Welfare, 80*(4), 157-176.

Griffin, J. (2005). Recreation therapy for adult survivors of childhood abuse: Challenges to professional perspectives and the evolution of a leisure education group. *Therapeutic Recreation Journal, 39*, 207-228.

Harvard Mental Health Letter. (2009). Treating fibromyalgia in the mental health setting. *Harvard Mental Health Letter*, July 2009 issue.

Jankowski, K. (2007). PTSD and physical health. National Center for PTSD. Retrieved from http://www.ptsd.va.gov/professional/pages/ptsd-physical-health.asp.

Kahn, A. P. & Fawcett, J. (2001). *The encyclopedia of mental health*. New York, NY: Facts on File.

Keane, T., Brief, D., Pratt, E., & Miller, M. (2007). Assessment of PTSD and its comorbidities in adults. In Friedman, M., Keane, T., and Resick, P. *Handbook of PTSD science and practice*. New York: Guilford Press.

Kelley, C. & Loy, D. P. (2008). Comparing the effects of aquatic and land-based exercise on the physiological stress response of women with fibromyalgia. *Therapeutic Recreation Journal, XLII*(2), 103-118.

Kinniburgh, K. J., Blaustein, M., & Spinazzolla, J. (2005). Attachment, self-regulation, and competency: A comprehensive framework for children with complex trauma. *Psychiatric Annals, 35*(5), 424-430.

Liebschutz, J., Saitz, R., Brower, V., Keane, T., Averbuch, T., Lloyd-Travaglini, C., & Samet, J. (2007). PTSD in urban primary care: High prevalence and low physician recognition. *Society of General Internal Medicine, 22*, 719-726.

Lundberg, N., Bennett, J., & Smith, S. (2011). Outcomes of adaptive sports and recreation participation among veterans returning from combat with acquired disability. *Therapeutic Recreation Journal, XLV*(2), 105-120.

Maguen, S. & Litz, B. (2012). Moral injury in veterans of war. *PTSD Research Quarterly, 23*(1), 1-6.

Mahan, A. L. & Ressler, K. J. (2012). Fear conditioning, synaptic plasticity and the amygdala: Implications for posttraumatic stress disorder. *Trends in Neurosciences. 35*, 24-35.

Mobily, K. & MacNeil, R. (2002). *Therapeutic recreation and the nature of disabilities*. State College, PA: Venture Publishing.

Mowatt, R. & Bennett, J. (2011). War narratives: Veteran stories, PTSD effects and therapeutic fly-fishing. *Therapeutic Recreation Journal, XLV*(4), 286-308.

Najavits, L. M. (2002). *Seeking safety: A treatment manual for PTSD and substance abuse*. New York: Guilford Press.

National Center for PTSD. (2013, November 4-Last Reviewed/Updated). FAQs about PTSD assessment: For professionals. (Originally published in 2007). Retrieved from http://www.ptsd.va.gov/professional/pages/faq-ptsd-professionals.asp.

National Center for PTSD. (2012, September). What's stopping you? Overcoming barriers to care. Retrieved from http://www.ptsd.va.gov/public/pages/faq-ptsd-professionals.asp.

National Center for PTSD. (n.d.). Understanding PTSD. Retrieved from http://www.ptsd.va.gov/public/understanding_ptsd/booklet.pdf.

National Institute of Mental Health. (2010, August 31). Post-traumatic stress disorder (PTSD). Retrieved October 17, 2010, from http://www.nimh.nih.gov/health/publications/post-traumatic-stress-disorder-ptsd/complete-index.shtml.

National Institute of Mental Health. (2007, July). Fact sheet post-traumatic stress disorder (PTSD). Retrieved October 17, 2010, from http://www.nimh.nih.gov.

Newhouse, E. (2008). *Faces of Combat, PTSD & TBI*. Enumclaw, WA: Issues Press.

Quirk, G. J. & Mueller, D. (2008). Neural mechanisms of extinction learning and retrieval. *Neuropsychopharmachology. 33*(1), 56-72.

Raphael, K. G., Janal, M. N., & Nayak, S. (2004). Comorbidity of fibromyalgia and posttraumatic stress disorder symptoms in a community sample of women. *Pain Medicine, 5*(1), 33-41.

Resick, P. A. & Calhoun, K. S. (2001). Posttraumatic stress disorder. In David H. Barlow (Ed.), *Clinical handbook of psychological disorders: A step-by-step treatment manual* (3rd ed., Rev., pp. 60-114). New York: Guilford Press.

Resnick, L., Bradford, D. W., Glynn, S. M., Jette, A. M., Hernandez, C. J., Wills, S. (2012). Issues in defining and measuring veteran community reintegration: Proceedings of the working group on community reintegration, VA Rehabilitation Outcomes Conference, Miami, Florida. *Journal of Rehabilitation Research & Development, 49*(1), 87-100.

Riggs, D. (2010). Impact of deployment on the health of service members and their families — why clinicians should ask. Power Point presentation. Centers for Disease Control (CDC).

Ruzek, J. & Hamblen, J. (n.d.) Improving care for veterans with PTSD. National Center for PTSD, VA Palo Alto Health Care System.

Samson, A. Y., Bensen, S., Beck, A. Price, D., & Nimmer, C. (1999, March). Posttraumatic stress disorder in primary care. *The Journal of Family Practice, 48*(3), 222-227.

Schneider, S., Haak, L., Owens, J., Herrington, D., & Zelek, A. (2009). An interdisciplinary treatment approach for soldiers with TBI/PTSD: Issues and outcomes. *Perspectives on Neurophysiology and Neurogenic Speech and Language Disorders, 19*(2), 36-46.

Selz, L., Agcaoili, G., & Mason, R. (1995/1996). A framework for recreational therapy interventions in the treatment of post traumatic stress disorder. *Annual in Therapeutic Recreation, 6*, 1-13.

Slone, L. (2006) Prevalence of PTSD in primary care settings. The National Center for Post Traumatic Stress Disorder, *PTSD Research Quarterly, 17*(2).

Smith, M. & Segal, J. (2013). Post traumatic stress disorder. Retrieved from http://www.helpguide.org/mental/post_traumatic_stress_disorder_symptoms_treatment.htm.

Taylor, S. (2006). *Clinician's guide to PTSD: A cognitive-behavioral approach*. New York: Guilford Press.

Whealin, J. M., Decarvalho, L. T., & Vega, E. M. (2008). *Clinician's guide to treating stress after war: Education and coping interventions for veterans*. Hoboken, NJ: John Wiley & Sons, Inc.

Williams, M. B. & Poijula, S. (2002). *The PTSD workbook: Simple, effective techniques for overcoming traumatic stress symptoms*. Oakland, CA: New Harbinger Publications.

30. Pressure Ulcers

Heather R. Porter

When a client stays in one body position for a prolonged period of time, increased pressure occurs on the skin that covers boney processes — areas that have little fat and muscle over boney prominences such as the buttocks, elbows, and heels. When pressure over a boney process is not relieved, blood circulation to the skin and its underlying body tissue is cut off due to the pressure. Without a supply of fresh, oxygenated blood to the skin and underlying tissues, the cells become damaged and the skin begins to break down and die. Pressure ulcers, also known as decubitus ulcers or skin breakdowns, occur from the inside out and can develop in as little as two to six hours (Hughes, 2008).

The increased pressure begins with the tissue pressing against the boney process. Cells at the innermost area begin to break down, eventually reaching the outside surface of the skin if the pressure is not relieved. There are four stages of pressure ulcers:

Stage One: Intact skin with nonblanchable redness of a localized area. This can be difficult to detect on dark skin.

Stage Two: Partial-thickness loss of dermis presenting as a shallow, open ulcer with a red-pink wound bed OR open/ruptured serum-filled blister OR a shiny or dry shallow ulcer.

Stage Three: Full-thickness tissue loss, where subcutaneous fat may be visible but bone, tendon, and/or muscle are not exposed.

Stage Four: Full-thickness tissue loss with exposed bone, tendon, and/or muscle (see Figure 1) (Weiss & Weiss, 2010).

The depth and size of the ulcer will vary depending on the length of time that the pressure continues and other reasons including other trauma that has occurred, shear injuries, fever, amount of moisture, and infection. The longer the breakdown goes untreated, the worse it gets.

The specific areas affected will depend on the body position that the client has been in for a prolonged period of time. For example, a client who has been in a sitting position for a long period of time is at an increased risk of developing decubitus ulcers on the shoulder blades from leaning against the back of the chair; spine from leaning against the back of the chair; hips from pressing against the side of the chair; buttocks from sitting on the hip bones without adequate padding; back of the upper arm and lower arm from leaning against the back of the chair and leaning on armrests; hand, wrist, and elbow all from leaning on armrests; and feet, especially the heels and toes from leaning against the wheelchair foot pedals. For a client who has been in a supine position for a prolonged period of time, decubitus ulcers are most likely to appear on the back of the head, shoulder blades, hip bones, elbows, spine, between the knees (especially when lying on the side), hip, and anywhere the leg touches the bed, especially the heels.

Devices such as casts, splints, braces, and prostheses can also cause skin breakdowns. Decubitus ulcers might also be seen in uncommon areas due to engagement in particular activities. For example, it is not uncommon for clients who have complete paraplegia from a spinal cord injury to pick up and rest the heel of one foot on the opposite knee to change their appearance. They may also carry heavy items on their lap for prolonged periods of time in order to use both hands to propel the wheelchair. In both of these situations, decubitus ulcers could occur on the tops of the knees.

Incidence/Prevalence

Pressure ulcers affect 1.3 to three million adults in the U.S. (Chou et al., 2013). It is estimated that 3-10% of the hospitalized populations experience a pressure ulcer; 5-8% of young patients with neurologic impairments experience a pressure ulcer during the course of a year; 25-85% of these patients will develop a pressure ulcer sometime during their lifetime; and 8-29% of older adults who are house-bound will develop a pressure ulcer (Elsevier, 2012). The majority of pressure ulcers occur in the hip and buttock region (67%) and lower extremities (25%) (Elsevier, 2012).

Predominant Age

Two-thirds of pressure ulcers occur in individuals over 70 years of age; however any individual with a medical condition that leads to long periods of uninterrupted pressure is at risk for pressure ulcer development (Elsevier, 2012).

Causes

There is no single factor that causes pressure ulcer risk; rather it is an interplay of many factors that increase the probability of pressure ulcer development (Coleman et al., 2013). In general, clients who are unable to change body positions or who are unaware that body position needs to be changed are at an increased risk for developing skin breakdowns. Other risk factors include individuals who use a manual wheelchair and have had previous pressure ulcers (Taule et al., 2013); cognitive impairments; physical impairments; comorbid conditions that affect soft tissue integrity and healing such as urinary incontinence, edema, impaired microcirculation, hypoalbuminemia, and malnutrition; reduced mobility or activity; pressure ulcer status; skin moisture; age; hematological measures; and deficits in nutrition, perfusion, and general health status (Chou et al., 2013; Coleman et al., 2013). Other contributory factors include aging with increased fragility of blood vessels and connective tissue and loss of fat and muscle that previously helped to dissipate pressure, conditions that affect wound healing (e.g., diabetes, peripheral vascular disease), conditions associated with low tissue oxygen tension (e.g., atrial fibrillation, myocardial infarction, chronic obstructive pulmonary disease), conditions that cause sensory loss, such as spinal cord injury, and conditions that result in paralysis and insensibility, which causes atrophy of the skin leading to thinning and more susceptibility to friction and shear forces (Elsevier, 2012).

Stage One: Skin is unbroken, but red or discolored. Redness does not fade within 30 minutes after pressure is removed.

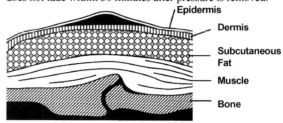

Stage Two: The epidermis is broken, creating a shallow open sore. Drainage may or may not be present.

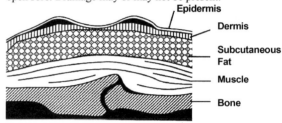

Stage Three: The break in the skin extends through the dermis into the subcutaneous fat tissue.

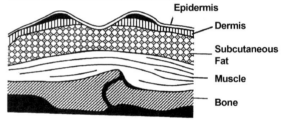

Stage Four: The breakdown extends into the muscle. Dead tissue and drainage are usually present.

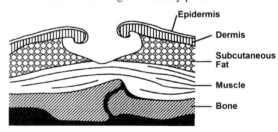

Stage Four: The breakdown may extend to the bone.

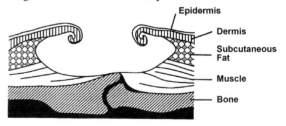

Systems Affected

Pressure ulcers affect the skin (b810-b849 Functions of the Skin, s810 Structure of Areas of Skin), as well as underlying tissue, muscle, and bone. If other systems are affected, code the appropriate part of the Body Functions codes and Body Structures codes. If infection occurs and becomes systemic, other body systems can be subsequently affected. Code Body Functions and Body Systems as appropriate.

Secondary Problems

Pressure ulcers are associated with decreased quality of life; impaired function; complications, such as infection; poorer prognosis; and increased costs of care (Chou et al., 2013).

Prognosis

There are many factors that contribute to the healing process; therefore it is difficult to determine a prognosis. As a general rule, pressure ulcers that do not reduce in size between 30% and 50% in a two- to four-week period of time are less likely to heal than ulcers that do reduce by these amounts (Sussman & Bates-Jensen, 2007).

Assessment

Typical Scope of Team Assessment

The *Braden Scale for Predicting Pressure Sore Risk* is the most widely used tool for predicting the development of pressure ulcers (Ayello, 2012). The client is rated in six areas and a numeric score is given for each (Braden & Maklebust, 2005):

Sensory perception: Completely limited (1), very limited (2), slightly limited (3), no impairment (4)

Moisture: Constantly moist (1), very moist (2), occasionally moist (3), rarely moist (4)

Activity: Bedfast (1), chairfast (2), walks occasionally (3), walks frequently (4)

Mobility: Completely immobile (1), very limited (2), slightly limited (3), no limitation (4)

Nutrition: very poor (1), probably inadequate (2), adequate (3), excellent (4)

Friction and shear: problem (1), potential problem (2), no apparent problem (3)

The total score indicates the client's pressure ulcer risk: ≤ 9 is severe risk, 10-12 is high risk, 13-14 is moderate risk, 15-18 is mild risk, and 19-23 is no risk.

Areas of Concern for RT Assessment

Recreational therapists further explore the six areas on the Braden Scale to determine underlying issues that could be affecting the Braden Scale scores. ICF codes can be used to provide details of the risk areas. For example, the client might have memory deficits that interfere with ability to remember to perform regular weight shifts (b144 Memory Functions); have decreased activity level due to psychosocial issues (b125 Dispositions and Intra-Personal Functions, b130 Energy and Drive Functions); have inadequate nutrition due to inability to get to the grocery store (d470 Using Transportation, d620 Acquisition of Goods and Services); or have an injury or illness that causes decreased mobility by confining the client to bed or a wheelchair (d410 Changing Basic Body Position).

One deficit that is almost certain to be found is d5200 Caring for Skin, although it may be better documented for treatment as a lack of support from others to provide skin care, e340 Personal Care Providers and Personal Assistants and e355 Health Professionals. RTs should also document if a lack of recreational activities (d920 Recreation and Leisure) is also putting the client at greater risk.

ICF Core Set

No ICF Core Set for Pressure Ulcers is available, although looking at core sets for conditions that increase the risk of pressure ulcers, such as Spinal Cord Injuries, may be helpful.

Treatment Direction

Whole Team Approach

Levine and colleagues (2013) reviewed the literature for best practices related to treatment of pressure ulcers and identified the following: Immediately transfer client to a specialized air mattress, optimize nutrition, and initiate parenteral ascorbic acid (500 mg twice daily); turning every two hours; at Stage One, continue to observe; at Stage Two, utilize wound cleansers; at Stage Three and Four, undergo debridement. Skin flap surgery is a last resort to promote healing of deep ulcers. This part addresses ICF codes b810-b849 Functions of the

Skin, s810 Structure of Areas of Skin. In addition, the six areas on the Braden Scale are incorporated into pressure ulcer protocols to prevent, as well as care for, pressure ulcers (Ribeiro & Cruz, 2013). This part addresses ICF codes e340 Personal Care Providers and Personal Assistants and e355 Health Professionals.

Recreational Therapy Approach

Recreational therapists employ an educational approach to teach clients and caregivers how to reduce the risk of pressure ulcer development (d5200 Caring for Skin e340 Personal Care Providers and Personal Assistants and e355 Health Professionals), as well as employ therapeutic interventions to help promote the healing process (b810-b849 Functions of the Skin, s810 Structure of Areas of Skin).

Recreational Therapy Interventions

Identifying pressure ulcers: Nursing regularly assesses skin integrity as part of the nursing evaluation. However, identifying pressure ulcers is also the entire team's responsibility, as they can occur quickly. Recreational therapists who work with clients who are at risk for pressure ulcers regularly evaluate exposed skin areas during therapy sessions and alert nursing staff if pressure ulcers are seen.

Monitoring pressure ulcers: Once a client is identified as having a pressure ulcer, recreational therapists monitor pressure ulcers that are not covered with dressings during therapy sessions. For example, if a client has a Stage One pressure ulcer on her elbow, the therapist evaluates the ulcer during therapy sessions to make sure it hasn't progressed and positions the client during the session to alleviate pressure on that particular area (e355 Health Professionals).

Healing and preventing pressure ulcers: The following interventions can be utilized to promote healing, as well as prevent pressure ulcers in those who do not have pressure ulcers:

- Provide recreational therapy sessions focused on leisure skill development and community integration, perhaps addressing d410 Changing Basic Body Position or another mobility issue defined during assessment. In the SCIRehab Project, these two areas of intervention resulted in less rehospitalization and less pressure ulcer development after discharge (Cahow et al., 2012).

- Promote an active and healthy lifestyle, as sedentary behavior increases risk of pressure ulcers, addressing deficits noted in d920 Recreation and Leisure (Dobbins et al., 2013).

- Address underlying issues that affect the Braden Scale, such as increasing opportunities for mobility, social eating to promote better nutritional intake, and following proper technique when performing a transfer so not to shear skin.

- Educate clients about pressure ulcers including weight shift techniques, as described next, and graphic pictures of stages of pressure ulcers, which can be very motivating.

Weight shift techniques: Teach clients how to perform regular weight shifts to alleviate pressure on boney areas and address deficits noted in d410 Changing Basic Body Position and d5200 Caring for Skin. Weight shifts should be performed every 20-30 minutes. This relieves pressure from boney areas and allows fresh, oxygenated blood to reach and nourish the area. Weight shifts can be very difficult for clients to remember, especially when engaged in activities. A watch that is set to beep every 30 minutes can be a helpful external reminder. The initiation and correct performance of weight shifts during activity is a common recreational therapy objective when working with clients who have a spinal cord injury (e.g., "Perform effective weight shifts every 30 minutes during activity in clinic without prompting"). The type of weight shifts performed by the client will vary depending on the abilities and limitations of the client.

- *Push up*: Lock the brakes if sitting in a wheelchair. Place both hands on the armrests. Push up with the arms so that the elbows are extended and the buttocks are lifted off the chair seat. Hold for 30 seconds.

- *Side lean*: Sit upright in the chair. Hang one arm over the side of the chair and reach toward the floor until the opposite buttock is lifted off the chair. Hold for 30 seconds.

- *Forward lean*: Lock brakes if sitting in a wheelchair. Lean forward by moving the chest toward the knees until the back of buttocks is lifted off the chair. Hold for 30 seconds.

- *Tilt*: This can be performed in three ways. For the client who is using a manual wheelchair and can independently perform a wheelie, a wheelie position is initiated and maintained for 30 seconds. For the client who has a manual wheelchair and is unable to independently perform a wheelie, another person tips the wheelchair backwards and maintains the balance point position for 30 seconds. For the client who is using a tilt-n-space power wheelchair, the client presses a button or moves the joystick or performs a sip-n-puff sequence so that the wheelchair moves into a tilt position. The position is held for at least 30 seconds.

Education

Clients need to understand why it is important to prevent pressure ulcers and the techniques they can use to minimize their risks (d5200 Caring for Skin). Here are some suggested education topics that RTs can use in educational sessions with their clients. (1) Teach clients how to evaluate the impact of activities on the development of pressure ulcers and problem solve on how to reduce risks. Some examples include using a backpack on the back of wheelchair to carry heavy items instead of placing heavy items on the lap and techniques for performing weight shifts in the community. (2) Remind clients to perform regular daily skin checks with a long-handled mirror to see all body areas to increase awareness of a skin breakdown. (3) Remind clients to keep skin dry at all times, as moisture increases the fragility of the skin, quickening skin breakdown. (4) Remind clients to alert healthcare professionals immediately of any signs of skin breakdown. If skin breakdown is treated during the beginning stages through the removal of pressure, the body can begin to heal. If the skin breakdown is allowed to continue, the client's health, level of independence, and functioning in life tasks can be severely affected.

References

Ayello, E. (2012). Predicting pressure ulcer risk. *Best Practices in Nursing Care to Older Adults, 5*, Accessed via website http://consultgerirn.org/uploads/File/trythis/try_this_5.pdf.

Braden, B. J. & Maklebust, J. (2005). Preventing pressure ulcers with the Braden Scale: An update on this easy-to-use tool that assesses a patient's risk. *Wound Wise*. Accessed via website http://www.fchs.ac.ae/fchs/uploads/Files/Semester%201%20-%202010-2011/3971/Article%20(Preventing%20Presssure%20Ulcers%20with%20the%20Braden%20Scale).pdf.

Cahow, C., Gassaway, J., Rider, C., Joyce, J. P., Bogenshutz, A., Edens, K., Kreider, S. E., & Whiteneck, G. (2012). Relationship of therapeutic recreation inpatient rehabilitation interventions and patient characteristics to outcomes following spinal cord injury: The SCIRehab project. *The Journal of Spinal Cord Medicine, 35*(6), 547-64.

Chou, R., Dana, T., Bougatsos, C., Blazina, I., Starmer, A. J., Reitel, K., & Buckley, D. I. (2013). Pressure ulcer risk assessment and prevention: A systemic comparative effectiveness review. *Annals of Internal Medicine, 159*, 28-38.

Coleman, S., Gorecki, C., Nelson, A., Closs, S. J., Defloor, T., Halfens, R., Farrin, A., Brown, J., Schoonhoven, L., & Nixon, J. (2013). Patient risk factors for pressure ulcer development: Systematic review. *International Journal of Nursing Studies, 50*, 974-1003.

Dobbins, C., Stratton, G., Rosenberg, M., & Merabti, M. (2013). Monitoring and reducing sedentary behavior in the elderly with the aid of human digital memories. *Telemedicine and E-Health, 19*(3), 173-185.

Elsevier. (2012). Pressure ulcer. Accessed via website https://www.clinicalkey.com/topics/infectious-disease/pressure-ulcer.html.

Hughes, R. G. (2008). *Patient safety and quality: An evidence-based handbook for nurses*. Rockville, MD: Agency for Healthcare Research and Quality.

Levine, S., Sinno, S., Levine, J. P., & Saadeh, P. B. (2013). Current thoughts for the prevention and treatment of pressure ulcers. *Annals of Surgery, 257*(4), 603-608.

Ribeiro, A. P. & Cruz, I. (2013). How effective is the development of skin care in critically ill patients using the Braden Scale scores aiming to prevent the incidence of pressure ulcers? Systematic literature review. *Journal of Specialized Nursing Care, 6*(1).

Sussman, C. & Bates-Jensen, B. (2007). *Wound care: A collaborative practice manual*. Lippincott Williams & Wilkins.

Taule, T., Bergfjord, K., Holsvik, E. E., Lunde, T., Stokke, B. H., Storlid, H., Sorheim, M. S., & Rekand, T. (2013) Factors influencing optimal seating pressure after spinal cord injury. *Spinal Cord, 51*(4), 273-7.

Weiss, L. & Weiss, J. (2010). *Oxford American handbook of physical medicine and rehabilitation*. Oxford University Press.

31. Rheumatoid Arthritis

Lei Guo

Rheumatoid arthritis (RA) is a chronic disease that involves inflammation of the lining (synovium) of the joints, causing joint damage, chronic pain, loss of function, and possibly permanent disability (Arthritis Foundation, 2010). RA is considered an autoimmune disorder, which occurs when the immune system attacks the body's own tissues. In addition to joint problems, RA can also cause fevers and fatigue (Mayo Clinic, 2013).

RA develops in three stages (Arthritis Foundation, 2010). The first stage is the swelling of the synovial lining, causing pain, warmth, stiffness, redness, and swelling around the joint. Second is the rapid division and growth of cells, which causes the synovium to thicken. In the third stage, the inflamed cells release enzymes that may digest bone and cartilage, often causing the involved joint to lose its shape and alignment leading to increased pain and loss of movement.

Incidence/Prevalence in U.S.

RA affects approximately 1.3 million Americans, or about 0.6% of the U.S. adult population (NIAMS, 2010). Approximately 294,000 children under the age of 18 are affected by juvenile arthritis (Arthritis Foundation, 2010).

Predominant Age

RA can affect anyone, including children, though onset usually occurs between 30 and 50 years of age. Women make up 70% of people with RA (Arthritis Foundation, 2010).

Causes

Scientists still do not know exactly what causes the immune system to turn against itself in RA, but research over the last few years has identified the following factors (NIAMS, 2010):

Genetic factors: Specific genes may play a role in whether a person develops RA and how severe the disease will become. However, some clients possess these genes and don't develop RA, while others don't have these genes and develop RA. Therefore, one's genetic make-up is believed to be one of many variables in the development of RA.

Environmental factors: It is believed that an environmental factor, such as a virus, bacterium, or mycobacterium may trigger the disease process. The exact agent is unknown.

Hormones: Deficiencies or changes in certain hormones may promote the development of RA in genetically susceptible clients who have been exposed to an environmental triggering agent.

Systems Affected

RA predominantly affects the musculoskeletal system, though sensory changes, involvement of other organs, lower energy levels, and psychological issues may also be present (Arthritis Foundation, 2010).

RA primarily affects wrist joints and finger joints closest to the hand; however it can also affect the neck, shoulders, elbows, hips, knees, ankles, and feet. It presents in a symmetrical pattern, meaning that it affects the same joints on the right and left sides. Clients typically complain of feeling pain and stiffness that lasts for more than 30 minutes upon awakening in the morning or after a long rest. Joints become swollen, reddened, and painful during and after excessive use. The primary ICF codes to document this include b280 Sensation of Pain, b710 Mobility of Joint Functions, b730 Muscle Power Functions, b780 Sensations Related to Muscles and Movement Functions, s710 Structure of Head and Neck Region, s720 Structure of Shoulder Region, s730 Structure of Upper Extremity, s750 Structure of Lower Extremity, d440 Fine Hand Use, d445 Hand and Arm Use, and d450 Walking.

Some additional symptoms and problems that a client may experience with RA include (NIH, 2010):

Anemia: A decrease in the normal number of red blood cells. Proteins released from the inflamed tissues may impact the body's ability to use iron and produce red blood cells, leading to low red blood cell counts. Medications commonly used to treat RA, including non-steroidal anti-inflammatory drugs (NSAIDs) and steroids, may also cause anemia (Sullivan, 2008). Use ICF code b430 Hematological System Functions.

Depression: Most people with RA experience some degree of depression, anxiety, and/or feelings of hopelessness (Tak, 2006). ICF codes b125 Dispositions and Intra-Personal Functions and b126 Temperament and Personality Functions.

Fatigue: Fatigue is sometimes the first sign of inflammation of the joints and one of the most common symptoms of RA. In part it is caused because of the increased time and effort required to complete life tasks (Arthritis Foundation, 2010). Fatigue can make it harder for people to concentrate or deal with pain thus possibly leading them to feel helpless. ICF codes b455 Exercise Tolerance Functions, b730 Muscle Power Functions, and b740 Muscle Endurance Functions.

Functional limitations: Functional limitations in activities of daily living are common among adults with arthritis; 40% report it is "very difficult" or they "cannot do" at least one of nine important daily functional activities. Almost eight million adults with limitations due to their arthritis report severe limitation in their ability to stoop, bend, or kneel. Six million cannot walk a quarter mile (Centers for Disease Control and Prevention, 2010). ICF codes d410 Changing Basic Body Position and d450 Walking.

Impaired range of motion: The joints most commonly affected in RA include hands, wrists, feet, ankles, knees, shoulders, and elbows. ICF codes b710 Mobility of Joint Functions, d440 Fine Hand Use, and d445 Hand and Arm Use.

Inflammation: One of the main problems in RA is joint inflammation. Each joint has a capsule around it for protection. The lining of the capsule is called the synovium, which is only a few cells thick. In affected joints, the synovium grows thicker. The joint swells and the cartilage protecting the ends of the bones in the joints get damaged, along with the ends of the bones themselves (Metcalf, 2008). ICF codes b710 Mobility of Joint Functions, b715 Stability of Joint Functions, and s7 Structures Related to Movement.

Joint deformity: Commonly seen in fingers, impacting grip strength and hand function. ICF codes b710 Mobility of Joint Functions, b730 Muscle Power Functions, and d440 Fine Hand Use.

Malaise: Malaise, a feeling of illness, is a non-specific symptom associated with nearly all infectious, metabolic, or systemic diseases. Malaise is often accompanied by fatigue. ICF code b130 Energy and Drive Functions.

Neck pain: RA may cause neck pain and neck stiffness. Pain may radiate into the arms, causing numbness and weakness in the arms and hands. ICF codes b280 Sensation of Pain and b780 Sensations Related to Muscles and Movement Functions.

Rheumatoid nodules: Bumps under the skin that often form close to the joints affect about one fourth of people with RA. While many people with RA have no pain with the nodules, some find the nodules painful. Sometimes rheumatoid nodules may interfere with daily activities, put pressure on nerves, limit movement, or affect organ function if rheumatoid nodules grow in areas such as the heart and lungs. ICF codes b280 Sensation of Pain, b710 Mobility of Joint Functions, b730 Muscle Power Functions, d440 Fine Hand Use, and other codes for organs as needed.

Fever: Occasionally (b550 Thermoregulatory Functions).

Dry eyes and mouth: A less common symptom (b215 Functions of Structures Adjoining the Eye, b510 Ingestion Functions).

Secondary Problems

Bone loss: Women with RA are at an increased risk of bone loss and fracture in the areas immediately surrounding the affected joints due to the development of osteoporosis for several reasons (NIH, 2010). Medications (especially corticosteroids) prescribed for the treatment of RA can trigger significant bone loss. Pain and loss of joint function caused by the disease can result in inactivity, further increasing osteoporosis risk. Bone loss in RA may occur as a direct result of the disease. Women, a group already at increased osteoporosis risk, are two to three times more likely than men to have RA. See the chapter on Osteoporosis if this is a co-occurring issue.

Cardiopulmonary endurance: Decreased involvement in cardiopulmonary conditioning due to the primary symptoms (pain, stiffness, limited range of motion) and secondary symptoms (fatigue, depression) often results in compromised endurance (Arthritis Foundation, 2010). Document with ICF code b455 Exercise Tolerance Functions.

Muscle atrophy: Loss of muscle strength is often a consequence of decreased activity levels (NIH, 2010). ICF codes b455 Exercise Tolerance Functions, b730 Muscle Power Functions, and b740 Muscle Endurance Functions.

Life tasks: Joints become tender and painful during and after excessive use, impacting the client's ability to perform life tasks (Arthritis Foundation, 2010). ICF codes b280 Sensation of Pain, b780 Sensations Related to Muscles and Movement Functions, d230 Carrying Out Daily Routine, and d850 Remunerative Employment.

Psychological changes: Depression, anxiety, and feelings of helplessness are common in clients who live with any chronic disease (NIASM, 2010). ICF codes b125 Dispositions and Intra-Personal Functions and b126 Temperament and Personality Functions.

Sexual dysfunction: Pain, limited range of motion, resultant inflammation from activity, limited endurance, and psychological changes can affect the client's desire to participate in sexual activity (Hill, Bird, & Thorpe, 2003). ICF code b640 Sexual Functions.

Prognosis

As many as 75% of clients improve somewhat with conservative treatment, such as physical therapy, recreational therapy, diet, and vitamin supplements, during the first year of disease. Ten percent are eventually disabled despite full treatment (Berkow, 1992). Studies have shown that people who are well-informed and participate actively in their own care experience less pain and make fewer visits to the doctor than other people with RA (NIH, 2010).

RA varies from person to person. For some people the symptoms may last from months to years, but then disappear without causing any noticeable damage. Others may experience periods of worsening symptoms (called flares) and periods when they feel better (called remissions). Still others may have serious joint damage and disability (NIAMS, 2010).

RA can interfere with every area of a person's life from family life to work life. For example, a study reported that more than a quarter of the women with RA stopped working within four years after being diagnosed (NIAMS, 2010). RA can also affect the normal family life, including the decision to have children (NIH, 2010).

Women with RA may feel better during pregnancy. The reason is not clear. It may be related to differences in certain proteins that are transferred between a mother and her unborn child. These proteins help the immune system distinguish between the body's own cells and foreign cells. Such differences may change the activity of the mother's immune system during pregnancy and relieve pain caused by RA (NIH, 2010).

Assessment

Typical Scope of Team Assessment

A person with RA often learns to manage the disease through education from his/her physician and literature from various organizations. If joint deformity, inflammation, and pain begin to hinder the ability to complete basic life tasks, the client is often referred to outpatient therapy services. A person is only admitted to an inpatient physical rehabilitation center if the RA has substantially affected his/her ability to complete life tasks and a more comprehensive approach to treatment is needed. Therapists may also see people with RA in an inpatient setting as a secondary admitting diagnosis.

Since most people with RA have adopted techniques for managing the disease prior to their inpatient rehab admission, the treatment team assesses both the present and the past course and management of the disease. This includes evaluation of activity limitations and restrictions that hinder the client's participation in life situations. Specific areas of assessment include the extent of joint deformity (Johnsson & Eberhardt, 2009); the process of the disease, including intervals between flares and remissions; functional joint limitations in range of motion, strength, and coordination (Aletaha, Smolen, & Ward, 2006); ability to perform life tasks and skills; knowledge and skills related to life task adaptations, including techniques the client has implemented in the past; knowledge and functional applications of joint protection and energy conservation techniques; available resources for assistance (Niedermann et al., 2011); and psychosocial adjustment (Sterba et al., 2008). In addition to the ICF codes discussed in the Systems Affected section, it is important to document significant deficits noted in d5 Self-Care, d6 Domestic Life, d7 Interpersonal Interactions and Relationships, d8 Major Life Areas, and d9 Community, Social, and Civic Life. Environmental Factors codes can be used, where appropriate, to document adaptations for the disease. The codes suggested in the ICF Core Set include e115 Products and Technology for Personal Use in Daily Living, e310 Immediate Family, e355 Health Professionals, e570 Social Security Services, Systems, and Policies, and e580 Health Services, Systems, and Policies.

Areas of Concern for RT Assessment

Depression: Depression is a common psychological issue for clients with RA. A change from premorbid recreational activities, lack of control over lifestyle, and unpredictable pain and/or unexpected functional limitations may affect the client's ability to cope with the disease and lead to depressive symptoms (Guo & Lee, 2010; Smith & Yoshioka, 1992). Note the depression with ICF code b126 Temperament and Personality Functions and also document the cause of the depression.

Impaired mobility: This can be a result of RA in the hip, knee, or ankle joints or a secondary complication, such as hip contractures, from a sedentary lifestyle (NIH, 2010). Use ICF code in d4 Mobility.

Pain, fear, and anxiety: Clients often report that fear and anxiety of having or causing inflammation and the resultant pain is a pivotal factor in choosing, initiating, and participating in life tasks (Arthritis Foundation, 2010). Use ICF codes b125 Dispositions and Intra-Personal Functions and b126 Temperament and Personality Functions.

Changes in physical activity participation: Research has confirmed that most individuals with RA experienced changes in their favorite activities because of RA and most of them discontinued relatively physical activities such as bowling, running, or dancing and replaced them with more sedentary activities, such as reading and crafting

(Smith & Yoshioka, 1992). Due to fatigue and pain, people with arthritis tend to spend less time on physical activities than those without arthritis (LaPlante, 1997). Document deficits in recreation with ICF code d920 Recreation and Leisure

Secondary disabilities: People with arthritis are more likely to be inactive and overweight or obese than people without arthritis (Greene et al., 2006). One study found that only 24% of people with arthritis report engaging in physical activities at the recommended level, which requires 30 minutes of moderately intense physical activity on most days of the week (Hootman et al., 2003). In addition, lack of exercise may increase the risk of cardiovascular disease. Some of the drugs used to treat RA may be a factor for the increased risk of developing infections (NIH, 2010). Document these observations with the codes discussed in the Secondary Problems section.

ICF Core Set

A brief and comprehensive ICF Core Set for Rheumatoid Arthritis is available.

Treatment Direction

Whole Team Approach

Focus is on management of symptoms and prevention of secondary disability. The goals of treatment are to relieve pain, reduce inflammation, slow down or stop joint damage, and improve the client's sense of well-being and ability to function (NIAMS, 2010). ICF codes that are addressed by these treatments include b280 Sensation of Pain, b455 Exercise Tolerance Functions, b710 Mobility of Joint Functions, b730 Muscle Power Functions, b780 Sensations Related to Muscles and Movement Functions, s710 Structure of Head and Neck Region, s720 Structure of Shoulder Region, s730 Structure of Upper Extremity, s750 Structure of Lower Extremity, d230 Carrying Out Daily Routine, d410 Changing Basic Body Position, d440 Fine Hand Use, d445 Hand and Arm Use, and d450 Walking. Medical interventions to address these issues include (NIAMS, 2010):

Medication: To control pain, decrease inflammation, and/or slow down the course of the disease.

Surgery: To reduce pain, improve joint function, and improve functional performance in life tasks.

Joint replacement: To remove a damaged joint and replace it with a prosthetic joint.

Tendon reconstruction: Tendons are reconstructed by attaching an intact tendon to the damaged tendon. This is most frequently done to the hand to increase hand function.

Synovectomy: This is the removal of the inflamed synovial tissue as part of tendon reconstructive surgery. Synovectomy is seldom performed by itself anymore because not all the tissue can be removed, and it eventually grows back.

Recreational Therapy Approach

Mobily and MacNeil (2002) suggest that recreational therapists seek to intervene with RA by managing pain and decreasing depression while increasing self-esteem and preventing secondary disabilities. In addition to the ICF codes used by the medical team, recreational therapists are providing treatment to address concerns with b126 Temperament and Personality Functions and b130 Energy and Drive Functions. Learning strategies to cope with the disease (d230 Carrying Out Daily Routine) is an area where RT is especially important. These suggestions can easily be absorbed into the three stages of the disease. Trombly (1989) recommends specific goals that can be adopted by allied health professionals. Clients are taught the rationale for stages of treatment prior to discharge and are educated on the importance of maintaining mobility and protecting joints throughout their lives.

Acute Stage: Synovial Inflammation and Proliferation

The overall approach is to prevent joint deformity and pain by resting the affected joints through the use of splints and positioning, assisting the client to cope with the unpredictable nature of the disease, and beginning energy conservation education. Recreational therapists follow prescriptive splint-wearing schedules as established by the occupational therapist and physician. The recreational therapist may need to assist the client in donning and doffing the splint. The therapist can monitor the inflammation process by asking the client to rate his/her pain level prior to, during, and after activity. During the acute stage, activity should be minimized. The recreational therapist can look for activities that do not aggravate inflammation. Passive or very gentle active-assisted motion is done by the occupational or physical therapist to each joint daily to maintain mobility (Christie et al., 2007).

Subacute Stage: Post-Inflammation

The general approach in this stage is to maintain or increase mobility, strength, and endurance; maintain or increase functional abilities; prevent deformity by using splinting and joint protection techniques; develop problem-solving skills relative to energy conservation and joint protection (Niedermann et al., 2011); and assist in psychosocial adjustment to chronic pain and disability.

Chronic Stage: Burn Out of Disease

At this stage, inflammation has fully subsided and resultant deformity is evident. The therapist's approach at this stage is a continuation of the subacute stage approach with a stronger focus on preparation for discharge and long-term health promotion. Premorbid leisure activities may need to be replaced if they cause pain, are incompatible with joint protection techniques, or if the client does not desire to participate in an adaptive form of the activity (Guo & Lee, 2010). Prescription and training on the use of adaptive equipment is a common need. The development of healthy activity patterns that account for activity limitations and participation restrictions is a vital component of therapy at this stage, as the client needs to learn how to balance exercise and rest. The more involved a patient is in planning and controlling his/her own care, the greater the chance of successful compliance (Brus et al., 1997). Frequent short rests are recommended over long rests due to the increased risk of secondary complications from prolonged sedentary activity.

Since depression is a common psychological issue experienced by clients with RA, the activity pattern should have activities that help manage the symptoms of depression and energy conservation techniques to avoid fatigue and resulting frustration. Social opportunities with activities that reflect strengths of the client can promote self-esteem and confidence.

Therapists should be careful to include the topic of sexuality (b640 Sexual Functions, d770 Intimate Relationships) when addressing re-involvement in life tasks since pain, limited range of motion, resultant inflammation from activity, limited endurance, and psychological changes may have affected the client's ability to participate in sexual activity (Guo, Yang, & Malkin, 2007). Carryover of learned skills into a real-life environment is essential to promote follow through with activity patterns (Smith & Yoshioka, 1992).

Recreational Therapy Interventions

The overall goal is to prevent joint deformity and pain by resting the affected joints, assist the client to cope with the unpredictable nature of the disease, and begin energy conservation education (Christie et al., 2007).

Adaptations to function: People with RA may have problems in d430 Lifting and Carrying Objects, d440 Fine Hand Use, d450 Walking, d470 Using Transportation, d475 Driving, and d540 Dressing. If these are noted during the assessment, treatment provides adaptation techniques to participate in activities that promote health and quality of life.

Exercise and mobility: Exercise is important for maintaining strong, healthy muscles, preserving joint mobility, and maintaining flexibility. Rall and Roubenoff (2000) reported that after three months of resistance strength training, patients with RA demonstrated improvement in strength, reported less pain and fatigue, and achieved better performance in walking and maintaining balance. Exercise can also help people sleep well, reduce pain, maintain a positive attitude, and lose weight (NIH, 2010). ICF codes that are addressed include b126 Temperament and Personality Functions, b134 Sleep Functions, b280 Sensation of Pain, b455 Exercise Tolerance Functions, b710 Mobility of Joint Functions, d410 Changing Basic Body Position, d415 Maintaining a Body Position, and d450 Walking. Exercise programs for individuals with RA should take into account the person's physical abilities, limitations, and changing needs (NIASM, 2010). Recreational therapy focuses not only on the specific form of exercise, such as walking, swimming, and tai chi, but also on the systemic issues, such as pain management and stress coping, that surround the client's ability to continue involvement in exercise after discharge (Guo & Lee, 2010).

Rest: People with RA need a good balance between rest and exercise (d570 Looking After One's Health, d230 Carrying Out Daily Routine), with more rest when the disease is active and more exercise

when it is not (Rall & Roubenoff, 2000). Rest helps to reduce active joint inflammation and pain and to fight fatigue (NIH, 2010). The length of time for rest will vary from person to person, but in general, shorter rest breaks every now and then are more helpful than long times spent in bed (NIAMS, 2010).

Leisure education: In addition to teaching individuals with RA about the important role of leisure in coping with RA (d240 Handling Stress and Other Psychological Demands), recreational therapists teach people with RA how to adapt to the leisure activities they did before or choose new activities that are more suitable for their current conditions (d920 Recreation and Leisure) (Guo & Lee, 2010). Wikström, Jacobsson, and Arvidsson (2005) reported that even though people with RA experienced constraints in leisure participation like needing more time and being dependent, they still attempted to find solutions to carry out leisure participation by choosing, planning, and adapting.

Joint care: Some people with RA find using a splint for a short time around a painful joint reduces pain and swelling by supporting the joint and letting it rest (NIASM, 2010). Splints are used mostly on wrists and hands, but also on the ankles and feet. Other ways to reduce stress on joints include self-help devices, such as zipper pullers and long-handled shoe horns (e1 Products and Technology); devices to help with getting on and off chairs, toilet seats, and beds; and changes in the ways that a person carries out daily activities. The assistive devices can promote independence and increased engagement in recreational and community activities (d9 Community, Social, and Civic Life) (Brichford, 2009).

Community integration: Mock et al. (2010) suggested that sense of belonging is an important mediator to help explain the significant association between physical leisure activity and well-being among people with RA. Community integration may increase a person's sense of belonging, compared to staying in a hospital or institution. Community integration provides an opportunity for increased frequency of physical leisure participation, which is associated with higher ratings of mental and physical health (Mock et al., 2010). Assessed deficits in community integration can be coded with ICF code d910 Community Life. If other issues are the reason for community integration, for example better mental health (b126 Temperament and Personality Functions), use the code for the issue being addressed.

Identification and engagement in activities: Recreational therapists help people with RA identify and engage in programs in the community that are beneficial to maintain health (d570 Looking After One's Health), reduce pain and stress (b280 Sensation of Pain, d240 Handling Stress and Other Psychological Demands), and improve quality of life (Guo, Yang, & Malkin, 2007). Programs such as yoga, tai chi, walking clubs, and aquatic exercises are possible choices for people with RA (Guo & Lee, 2010). Yoga and tai chi are gentle exercises that are suitable for those who have RA to reduce pain and increase range of motion (Guo, 2011). The Arthritis Foundation recommends walking as a daily exercise for people with RA. The buoyancy of water facilitates pain-free range of motion, making water exercise ideal for people with RA (Roller et al., 2008). Gusi et al. (2006) reported that exercise in waist-high warm water decreases pain and improves health-related quality of life and strength in the lower extremities in women with RA.

Sexuality: Pain and depression could be the principle factors contributing to sexual dysfunction for people with RA (b640 Sexual Functions). The treatment of sexual dysfunction will be dependent upon each person's symptoms. However, recreational therapists should know some general recommendations, such as exploring different positions; using analgesics, heat, and muscle relaxants before sexual activity; and exploring alternative methods of sexual expression (Tristano, 2009).

Stress reduction: People with RA encounter both physical and emotional challenges, which may increase their stress level (d240 Handling Stress and Other Psychological Demands). The negative emotions they may feel because of RA could be fear, anger, dissatisfaction, and frustration (Guo & Lee, 2010). Some techniques for coping with stress include frequent short rest breaks, relaxation, distraction, visualization exercises, participation in support groups, and good communication with the healthcare team (NIASM, 2010). Guo and Lee (2010) reported that leisure activities serve important roles in releasing stress through escaping, expressing negative emotions, relaxing, enhancing moods, and being with friends and others.

Healthful diet: There is no scientific evidence that any specific food or nutrient helps or harms people with RA (NIAMS, 2010). However, an overall nutritious diet with enough — but not an excess of — calories, protein, and calcium is important for the joints (d570 Looking After One's Health). Alcoholic beverages may need to be avoided because of the medications used for RA. For example, those taking methotrexate should not drink alcohol because it may cause liver damage (NIAMS, 2010). Research shows that special diets and vitamin supplements (for example, fish oil supplements) may help reduce arthritis inflammation. For most diets and supplements, controlled scientific studies have not found definite benefits (NIAMS, 2010).

Resources

Arthritis Foundation

www.arthritis.org

This website has basic information about different types of arthritis, events and programs, current research, and links for more information for caregivers and advocates.

National Institutes of Health

www.nih.gov

This website has information about health issues, grants and funding, news and events, research and training, and more.

National Institute of Arthritis and Musculoskeletal and Skin Diseases (NIAMS)

www.niams.nih.gov

This website has information related specifically to arthritis and musculoskeletal and skin disease.

References

Aletaha, D., Smolen, J., & Ward, M. M. (2006). Measuring function in rheumatoid arthritis: Identifying reversible and irreversible components. *Arthritis & Rheumatism, 54*, 2784-2792.

Arthritis Foundation. (2010). Osteoarthritis. Accessed via website http://www.arthritis.org/disease-center.php?disease_id=32.

Berkow, R. (1992). *The Merck manual of diagnosis and therapy.* Rahway, NJ: Merck & Co, Inc.

Brichford, C. (2009). Assistive devices for rheumatoid arthritis. Accessed via website http://www.everydayhealth.com/rheumatoid-arthritis/assistive-devices-for-rheumatoid-arthritis.aspx.

Brus, H., van de Laar, M., Taal, E., Rasker, J., & Wiegman, O. (1997). Compliance in rheumatoid arthritis and the role of formal patient education. *Seminars in Arthritis and Rheumatism, 26*(4), 702-710.

Centers for Disease Control and Prevention. (2010). NHIS arthritis surveillance. Accessed via website http://www.cdc.gov/arthritis/data_statistics/national_nhis.htm .

Christie, A., Jarmtvedt, G., Dahm, K. T., Moe, R., Haavardsholm, E., & Hagen, K. B. (2007). Effectiveness of nonpharmacological and nonsurgical interventions for patients with rheumatoid arthritis: An overview of systematic reviews. *Physical Therapy, 87*(12), 1697-1715.

Greene, B. L., Haldeman, G. F., Kaminski, A., Neal, K., Lim, S. S., & Conn, D. L. (2006). Factors affecting physical activity behavior in urban adults with arthritis who are predominantly African-American and female. *Physical Therapy, 86*(4), 510-519.

Guo, L. (2011). Examining the impact of rheumatoid arthritis on the discontinuity, continuity, and development patterns of physical activities. *American Journal of Recreation Therapy, 9*(4), 9-18.

Guo, L. & Lee, Y. (2010). Examining the role of leisure in the process of coping with stress in adult women with rheumatoid arthritis. *Annual in Therapeutic Recreation, 18*, 100-113.

Guo, L., Yang, H., & Malkin, M. (2007). Learning to cope: Leisure and recreation can improve the life of people with rheumatoid arthritis. *Parks and Recreation Magazine, 42*(7), 26-29.

Gusi, N., Tomas-Carus, P., Hakkinen, A., Hakkinen, K., & Ortega-Alonso, A. (2006). Exercise in waist-high warm water decreases pain and improves health-related quality of life and strength in the lower extremities in women with fibromyalgia. *Arthritis & Rheumatism: Arthritis Care & Research, 55*(1), 66-73.

Hill, J., Bird, H., & Thorpe R. (2003), Effects of rheumatoid arthritis on sexual activity and relationships. *Rheumatology, 42*, 280-286.

Hootman, J. M., Marcera, C. A., Ham, S. A., Helmick, C. G., & Sniezek, J. E. (2003). Physical activity levels among the general U.S. adult population and in adults with and without arthritis. *Arthritis Care & Research, 49*(1), 129-135.

LaPlante, M. P. (1997). Prevalence of leisure-time physical activity among persons with arthritis and other rheumatic conditions. *Morbidity & Mortality Weekly Report, 46*, 389-393.

Johnsson, P. M. & Eberhardt, K. (2009). Hand deformities are important signs of disease severity in patients with early rheumatoid arthritis. *Rheumatology, 48*(11), 1398-1401.

Mayo Clinic. (2013). Rheumatoid arthritis. Accessed via website http://www.mayoclinic.com/health/rheumatoid-arthritis/DS00020.

Metcalf, E. (2008). The facts on inflammation. Accessed via website http://www.everydayhealth.com/rheumatoid-arthritis/rheumatoid-arthritis-inflammation.aspx.

Mobily, K. & MacNeil, R. (2002). *Therapeutic recreation and the nature of disabilities*. State College, PA: Venture Publishing, Inc.

Mock, S. E., Fraser, C., Knutson, S., & Prier, A. (2010). Physical leisure participation and the well-being of adults with rheumatoid arthritis: The role of sense of belonging. *Activities, Adaptation & Aging, 34*(4), 292-302.

National Institute of Arthritis and Musculoskeletal and Skin Diseases (NIAMS). (2010). Rheumatoid arthritis. Accessed via website http://www.niams.nih.gov/Health_Info/Rheumatic_Disease/default.asp.

National Institutes of Health. (2010). Rheumatoid arthritis. Accessed via website http://www.niams.nih.gov/hi/topics/arthritis/ rahandout.htm.

Niedermann, K., de Bie, R. A., Kubli, R., Ciurea, A., Steurer-Stey, C., & Villiger, P. M., et al. (2011). Effectiveness of individual resource-oriented joint protection education in people with rheumatoid arthritis. A randomized controlled trial. *Patient Education and Counseling, 82*(1), 42-48.

Rall, L. C. & Roubenoff, R. (2000). Benefits of exercise for patients with rheumatoid arthritis. *Nutrition in Clinical Care, 3*, 209-215.

Roller, J., Johnson, M., Jones, E., Hunt, H., & Kirkwood, N. (2008). Effectiveness of a water-based exercise program on Berg Balance Test scores in community-living older women. *Journal of Aquatic Physical Therapy, 16*(1), 1-5.

Smith, S. & Yoshioka, C. (1992). Recreation functioning and depression in people with arthritis. *Therapeutic Recreation Journal, 26*(4), 21-30.

Sterba, K. R., DeVellis, R. F., Lewis, M. A., DeVellis, B. M., Jordan, J. M., & Baucom, D. H. (2008). Effect of couple illness perception congruence on psychological adjustment in women with rheumatoid arthritis. *Health Psychology, 27*(2), 221-229.

Sullivan, S. L. (2008). Rheumatoid arthritis and anemia. Accessed via Website http://www.everydayhealth.com/rheumatoid-arthritis/rheumatoid-arthritis-and-anemia.aspx.

Tak, S. H. (2006). An insider perspective of daily stress and coping in elders with arthritis. *Orthopaedic Nursing Journal, 25*(2), 127-132.

Tristano, A. G. (2009). The impact of rheumatic diseases on sexual function. *Rheumatology International, 29*(8), 853-860.

Trombly, C. (1989). *Occupational therapy for physical dysfunction* (3rd ed.). Baltimore, MD: Williams & Wilkins.

Wikström, I., Jacobsson, L. T. H., & Arvidsson, B. (2005). How people with rheumatoid arthritis perceive leisure activities: A qualitative study. *Musculoskeletal Care, 3*(2), 74-84.

32. Schizophrenia Spectrum and Other Psychotic Disorders

Gretchen Snethen

Schizophrenia spectrum and other psychotic disorders (SSD) are complex in nature. The diagnoses covered in the *DSM-5* include schizophrenia; schizophreniform disorder; schizoaffective disorder; delusional disorder; brief psychotic disorder; and psychotic disorder caused by substances, medications, or other medical conditions. Schizotypal disorder is considered to be in the schizophrenia spectrum, but it is also classified as a personality disorder and described in that section of the *DSM-5*. The presence of catatonia is also included as part of SSD (APA, 2013). The *DSM-IV-TR* included subtypes of paranoid, disorganized, catatonic, undifferentiated, and residual. The *DSM-5* removed separate diagnoses due to changes in symptomology across the course of the diagnosis (APA, 2013).

Symptoms

Each diagnosis has a specific set of symptoms found in one or more of five categories: delusions, hallucinations, disordered thinking or speech, grossly disorganized or abnormal motor behavior (including catatonia), and negative symptoms (APA, 2013). In the *DSM-IV-TR* the first four categories were called positive symptoms, as these are characteristics added to the individual (APA, 2000).

Delusions: Delusions are beliefs that the client will not change even though they are contradicted by evidence in the current situation. The *DSM-5* (APA, 2013) lists several types of delusions: Persecution is the belief that someone or some organization intends harm the client. Referential delusions happen when the client believes that certain gestures or environmental cues are directed at the client; this would include the belief that secret messages are being given to the client by a character in a television program. Grandiose delusions happen when the client

inaccurately believes s/he has exceptional abilities. Erotomanic delusions are the incorrect belief that someone is in love with him/her. Nihilistic delusions refer to a belief in impending destruction. Somatic delusions are inaccurate beliefs about health. Delusions are classified as bizarre when they seem clearly implausible. Some examples are thoughts being inserted into or removed from the client's mind and the idea that someone else is in control of the client's actions.

Hallucinations: Hallucinations seem to the client to be vivid perceptions of something that is occurring in the real world, even though nothing in the environment is causing the perception. Auditory hallucinations are the most common type in SSD. Hallucinations that occur when falling asleep or waking are considered normal. Hallucinations may also be considered normal in some religious contexts (APA, 2013).

Disordered thinking and speech: Disordered thinking is usually determined by observations of disordered speech. To be considered disordered the speech must be disordered enough to substantially impair communication. Some possible aspects of disordered speech are switching topics in ways that the listener can't follow and giving answers that are not related to the questions that are being asked. Disordered speech can be inaccurately diagnosed when the clinician and the client come from different linguistic backgrounds (APA, 2013). Other aspects of disordered thinking that have been discussed in the past include memory deficits, delayed recall, difficulty accessing vocabulary, difficulty or inability to plan, impairments in organizing information, and problems attending to single or multiple tasks (Badcock, Michie, & Rock, 2005; Lysaker, Lancaster, Nees, & Davis, 2004; Todman et al., 2009).

335

While these cognitive issues are still prevalent within individuals with this diagnosis, these aspects are no longer included as part of disordered thinking in the *DSM-5*.

Motor behavior: Problems with motor behavior are diagnosed when the behavior interferes with activities of daily living or other goal-directed behaviors. Catatonia is included in this category and includes behaviors such as resistance to instructions, rigid or bizarre postures, and lack of response. Catatonia can also include purposeless and stereotyped movements, grimacing, staring, and echoing of speech (APA, 2013).

Negative symptoms: These indicators are called negative symptoms because they are cited when something seems to be missing from the person with SSD. In schizophrenia there is a great likelihood that the therapist will see diminished emotional expression and avolition. Diminished emotional expression is demonstrated when the client puts less emotion than normal into interactions with others. The diminished emotional expression is also referred to as flattened affect. It can include fewer or less emphatic facial expressions, lack of intonation in speech, less eye contact, and fewer physical movements while communicating. Avolition refers to a decrease in or a lack of motivation, particularly in initiating behavior. This may be evident in social or work activities and may also impact activities of daily living. At times, avolition is mistaken for laziness. It is important for clinicians to recognize this as a symptom of schizophrenia. Other negative symptoms include alogia (poverty of speech), asociality (decreased desire to interact with others), and anhedonia (inability to experience pleasure (Kirkpatrick et al., 2006). Negative symptoms substantially contribute to the functional impairments experienced by individuals with schizophrenia, more so than the other psychotic disorders included in SSD (APA, 2013).

Diagnoses

All of the disorders in SSD are diagnosed based on the symptoms described. Decisions about which disorder to diagnose are based on the relative prevalence and types of the symptoms and the length of time the symptoms have been present. At any given time the severity of the condition may be calculated by grading the severity of the five symptoms on a zero-to-four scale called the Clinician-Rated Dimensions of Psychosis Symptom Severity (APA, 2013).

Schizophreniform disorder: This is diagnosed when two or more of the five symptoms of SSD are present. At least one of them must be delusions, hallucinations, or disorganized speech. The episode must last at least one month and less than six months (APA, 2013).

Schizophrenia: This is diagnosed when two or more of the five symptoms of SSD are present. At least one of them must be delusions, hallucinations, or disorganized speech. The symptoms must have lasted at least six months and there must have been a marked decrease in the ability to work, interact with others, perform self-care, or perform in other major life areas. The diagnosis includes the number of episodes the client has experienced and whether there are catatonic features (APA, 2013).

Schizoaffective disorder: Schizoaffective disorder is diagnosed when schizophrenia criteria are met and there is a co-occurring mood disorder. There must also be at least two weeks where there are delusions or hallucinations without a major mood disorder. During a substantial portion of rest of the duration of the illness the mood disorder must be present. The diagnosis includes the number of episodes the client has experienced and whether there are catatonic features (APA, 2013). Hospital discharge data suggests schizoaffective disorder is the most commonly diagnosed form of SSD (Weber et al., 2009).

Delusional disorder: This is diagnosed when there have been one or more delusions that have lasted at least a month. All of the other symptoms must be missing or minor aspects of the condition for a diagnosis of delusional disorder. The type of delusion is specified (APA, 2013).

Brief psychotic disorder: This is diagnosed when one or more symptoms from delusions, hallucinations, disorganized speech, and grossly disorganized or catatonic behavior have been observed. If there is only one symptom, it must be one of the first three. The duration of the symptoms must be between one day and one month and may not be attributable to other causes such as drugs or another medical condition. The diagnosis includes information about whether stressors are present and whether it has occurred postpartum (APA, 2013).

Psychotic disorders (induced): In the *DSM-5* there are categories for psychotic disorders induced by substances, medications, and other medical conditions. These are diagnosed when there are prominent hallucinations and/or delusions that can be attributed to another cause (APA, 2013).

Schizotypal personality disorder: Schizotypal disorder is considered a personality disorder that is part of the schizophrenia spectrum. It is used when there is a pervasive pattern of deficits described in the symptoms of SSD, which are not severe enough to be classified as psychotic. The diagnosis requires five or more of the following nine behaviors: ideas of reference not severe enough to be classified as delusions, odd beliefs or magical thinking, unusual perceptual experiences that are not hallucinations, odd thinking as demonstrated by odd speech patterns, suspiciousness not reaching paranoia, abnormal affect, odd or eccentric behavior, lack of close friends, and excessive social anxiety associated with paranoid fears rather than a negative self-image (APA, 2013).

Incidence/Prevalence in U.S.

Lifetime prevalence indicates that approximately seven individuals in 1,000 will be affected by an SSD (McGrath et al., 2008). SSD affects approximately one percent of the U.S. population (Narrow et al., 2002). The male to female incidence ratio is 1.4, which suggests that, on average, for every three men diagnosed with SSD, two women will be affected (McGrath et al., 2008). There is a greater incidence of SSD among individuals with immigrant status (McGrath et al., 2008). The U.S. hospital discharge survey found there were a greater percentage of blacks (1.8%) than whites (0.9%) discharged with a diagnosis of SSD between 1979 and 2003. Individuals admitted to the hospital with an SSD diagnosis, regardless of primary admitting diagnosis, were hospitalized an average of 6.5 days longer than individuals without a SSD diagnosis (Weber et al., 2009).

Predominant Age

Onset of SSD usually occurs between the ages of 15 and 30. Onset is broken down into four age categories: adolescent onset (10-17 years of age), early adult onset (18-30 years of age), middle-age onset (30-45 years of age), and late onset (Versola-

Russo, 2006). After the age of 45, the risk of developing this illness sharply decreases. Although the incidence of SSD in both men and women is similar, there is a significant difference in the age of onset and prognosis. Men are often diagnosed earlier, and have a poorer prognosis (Nolen-Hoeksema, 2004). The peak age of onset for men is 10 to 25 years old, while women peak between the ages of 25 and 35 years old. About 90% of clients in treatment for SSD are between age 15 and 55.

Causes

There is not a known cause for SSD; however, genetics appear to play a role in the development. A close genetic relationship to an individual with SSD increases the risk (Versola-Russo, 2006).

Structure and chemical composition of the brain are also contributing factors. More specifically, research has determined that individuals with SSD are more likely to have enlarged ventricles, possibly related to tissue deterioration, and less activity in the frontal cortex when compared to the general population (Versola-Russo, 2006). Chemical imbalances, specifically dopamine, in different areas of the brain correlate with SSD occurrence.

Environmental factors also contribute to the onset of SSD. Individuals with the same genetic predisposition are more likely to develop SSD if they also live in environmentally stressful settings (Versola-Russo, 2006). These often include urban settings, particularly those in impoverished neighborhoods (Dragt et al., 2011). Individuals in lower socioeconomic groups have higher incidence rates of SSD (Dragt et al., 2011; Versola-Russo, 2006). Immigrants also have higher incidence rates of SSD, suggesting abrupt cultural change is a stressor that may contribute to the onset of SSD (Versola-Russo, 2006). Among individuals without a familial diagnosis, earlier onset is predicted by birth complications and cannabis abuse (Scherr et al., 2012).

Psychosocial factors also contribute to the onset of SSD. Contemporary psychodynamic theory suggests individuals with SSD have a biological condition that prevents them from developing an integrated sense of self (Versola-Russo, 2006). However, families with deviant styles of communication, such as using words inappropriately or combining words together in an odd sequence, and who frequently express emotion are more likely to have children who develop SSD. This is particularly true in families who also have a genetic predisposition to SSD. Stressful situations often trigger a psychotic relapse (Todman, 2003). In fact, the diathesis-stress model of schizophrenia suggests that when individuals with poor information processing, attention, coping mechanisms, and social skills experience stress, their inability to handle the stress may lead to a psychotic episode. This, in turn, causes more stress, which perpetuates the cycle (Nolen-Hoeksema, 2004). However, individuals with a stress-induced onset of SSD have a better prognosis than individuals who develop SSD independent of external stressors.

Systems Affected

SSD can directly affect multiple areas of functioning (Tenorio-Martinez, del Carmen Lara-Munoz, & Medina-Mora, 2009). Cognitive, emotional, and social systems are all affected by SSD.

Cognitive functioning: The symptoms of delusion and disordered thinking and speech are cognitive issues (b160 Thought Functions).

Perceptual functioning (b156 Perceptual Functions) is the most commonly known area of functional impairment. Positive symptoms, specifically sensory hallucinations, represent impairment in perceptual functioning. While auditory hallucinations are the most common, hallucinations may be experienced in all five sensory areas and may also involve the misinterpretation of external stimuli (Basavanthappa, 2007).

Individuals with SSD often experience impairments in receiving, processing, and initiating conversation (d350 Conversation, d710 Basic Interpersonal Interactions); planning (b164 Higher-Level Cognitive Functions), problem solving (b164 Higher-Level Cognitive Functions, d175 Solving Problems), initiating tasks (d210 Undertaking a Single Task, d220 Undertaking Multiple Tasks), managing multiple tasks (d220 Undertaking Multiple Tasks), and organizing information (b164 Higher-Level Cognitive Functions); and fine motor skills (d440 Fine Hand Use) (Tenorio-Martinez et al., 2009).

The structural composition of the brain, specifically the decreased activity in the frontal lobe, contributes to these impairments. The frontal lobe is responsible for speech fluency (b330 Fluency and Rhythm of Speech Functions), understanding (d310-d329 Communicating — Receiving, b167 Mental Functions of Language), and using language (d330-d349 Communicating — Producing, b167 Mental Functions of Language). It is also responsible for executive functioning (d155 Acquiring Skills, b164 Higher-Level Cognitive Functions, d210 Undertaking a Single Task, d220 Undertaking Multiple Tasks, and d130-d159 Basic Learning). Additionally, the frontal cortex has a role in processing information and emotion regulation (b152 Emotional Functions) (Basavanthappa, 2007).

Emotional functioning: An individual's emotional functioning is also impacted by SSD. Negative symptoms often involve blunted or flattened affect (b152 Emotional Functions) (Kirkpatrick et al., 2006). Individuals with SSD may also experience anhedonia, which is the inability to experience pleasure (b152 Emotional Functions) (Kirkpatrick et al., 2006).

Social functioning: Asociality is also a negative symptom of SSD and affects the individual's ability to empathize with others (d710 Basic Interpersonal Interactions, d720 Complex Interpersonal Interactions). This has a significant impact on social functioning, including communication (Kirkpatrick et al., 2006; Lysaker & Davis, 2004; Lysaker, Lancaster, Nees, & Davis, 2004). Amotivation in social situations affects an individual's motivation (b130 Energy and Drive Functions) and ability to initiate behavior (d210 Undertaking a Single Task, d220 Undertaking Multiple Tasks) (Kirkpatrick et al., 2006).

Secondary Problems

Individuals with SSD have poor physical health and, on average, die 25 years earlier than the general population (Everett et al., 2008). When considering the leading causes of death in the United States (heart disease, cancer, stroke, chronic lower respiratory diseases, accidents, Alzheimer's disease, diabetes, influenza and pneumonia, nephritis, and septicemia), individuals with SSD have higher death rates for all of them except cancer and Alzheimer's. Cancer and Alzheimer's are probably the exceptions because people with SSD are likely to die before onset occurs (Everett et al., 2008).

Comorbid anxiety disorders as well as substance abuse diagnoses are more likely in individuals with

SSD, and those with dual diagnoses have a poorer prognosis. Those with anxiety disorders may also experience higher rates of hospitalization, as anxiety can trigger positive symptoms (Pokos & Castle, 2006). Depression is also common for individuals with SSD, and suicide is the leading cause of premature death, with nearly 50% of individuals with SSD attempting suicide (Cohen, Test, & Brown, 1990). See the chapters on Anxiety and Depression for appropriate ICF codes to use with these comorbid conditions.

Prognosis

Individuals with SSD who receive recreational therapy services are often individuals who experience more chronic symptoms and greater functional impairment, leading to a poorer prognosis.

Approximately one-third of individuals with SSD will have one psychotic episode and show no further symptoms of SSD, one-third show functional improvements but require occasional hospitalization, and one-third have permanent functional impairments (Ascher-Svanum & Krause, 1991). The majority of functional decline will likely occur within the first five years of diagnosis. Those with worsening negative symptoms may continue to experience functional decline. While early definitions of recovery focused on recovery as an outcome, this section, as well as the broader mental health field, approaches recovery as an individual process. In this orientation, mental health professionals are concerned with the overall functioning of the individual, rather than the elimination of symptoms (Harvey & Bellack, 2009).

Specific characteristics are thought to be indicators of a good or poor prognosis in schizophrenia (Nolen-Hoeksema, 2004). A client is more likely to have a good prognosis if s/he has: (1) a late onset of schizophrenia; (2) stressful precipitating life events prior to the onset of schizophrenia; (3) a current acute onset of symptoms; (4) a healthy social, sexual, and work history; (5) symptoms of a depressive mood disorder and a family history of mood disorders; and (6) a marriage that includes a good support system (Nolen-Hoeksema, 2004).

A client is more likely to have a poor prognosis if s/he has: (1) early onset; (2) no obvious precipitating life stressors; (3) an insidious onset (slow and subtle development so a beginning date is hard to identify); (4) not in a marriage and a poor support system; (5) an unhealthy social, sexual, and work history; (6) withdrawn and autistic behavior; (7) a family history of schizophrenia; (8) neurological signs and symptoms; (9) a history of perinatal trauma; (10) no remissions within a three-year period or many relapses; (11) severe negative symptoms; and (12) a history of assault (Nolen-Hoeksema, 2004).

Assessment

Typical Scope of Team Assessment

The team assessments should focus on a client's underlying symptoms, cognitive functioning, current levels of community participation, and capacity to participate within the community. Given the frequency of physical health problems in this population, it is also important to assess physical health in individuals with SSD.

Assessment tools typically focus on symptoms related to SSD. The *Global Assessment of Functioning* (GAF) is one of the most common assessment tools for individuals with SSD (Hall, 1995). While the GAF assesses functioning, criticism suggests it is too closely tied to symptoms to truly measure functional impairments (Bellack et al., 2007). The *Clinician-Rated Dimensions of Psychosis Symptom Severity* (CRDPSS) can be used to calculate the current condition by grading the severity of each of the five symptom categories on a zero-to-four scale (APA, 2013). The CRDPSS requires special training, but may be used by other members of the treatment team. Having an understanding of the relative symptom severity and how symptoms impact functioning will help therapists evaluate the effectiveness of overall treatment.

The treatment team may also use the ICF codes described earlier to document to condition of the client.

Areas of Concern for RT Assessment

Recreational therapists should focus on assessments that address functional impairments in the following areas: social, communication, emotional, and executive functioning. Many ICF codes that can be used to document findings were discussed earlier. Additional codes that might be useful will be found in d5 Self-Care, d7 Interpersonal Interactions and

Relationships, and d8 Major Life Areas. When determining functional impairments, it is important to understand both the individual's capacity to function and his/her normal participation in life settings. This is particularly important with individuals who have SSD, as their capacity to function is frequently not predictive of actual participation (Bellack et al., 2007).

Given the relationship between stress and psychotic episodes, RTs should also assess stress levels and coping skills (d240 Handling Stress and Other Psychological Demands). Hutchinson, Bland, and Kleiber (2008) suggest a hierarchy of informal questions to assess perceived stress, perceived usefulness, and access to leisure-related resources.

All assessments should attend to the resources available to the individual by citing appropriate Environmental Factors codes because individuals with SSD often have limited financial and social resources. Prior to assessing clients, the RT should conduct an assessment of resources in the community. When integrating specific leisure activities into treatment, RT professionals should also focus on the assessment of functional skills related to the specific goals and requirements of participation in the activity (Rudnick, 2005). Furthermore, recommendations for assessing interest-based activities include focusing on activities that are available in the specific community. RT professionals working towards independent community participation should assess both the individual's interest and perceived barriers to participation (Snethen, McCormick, Smith, & Van Puymbroeck, 2011)

ICF Core Set

No ICF Core Set has been defined for Schizophrenia Spectrum and Other Psychotic Disorders.

Treatment Direction

Individuals with SSD receive treatment in multiple settings. These include both ambulatory and inpatient care. Ambulatory services include outpatient clinics based out of psychiatric hospitals, mental health centers, general hospitals, the Veterans Administration (VA), alcohol/drug treatment centers, mental health specialists, mental health crisis centers, as well as general hospital emergency rooms and general practitioners. Inpatient treatment facilities include state and county mental hospitals, general

hospitals, community and private mental health centers, the VA psychiatric unit, inpatient substance abuse units, and nursing homes. In relation to ambulatory care, individuals with severe and persistent SSD, on average, visit alcohol/drug outpatient clinics 40 times per year, and other settings averaged about 15 visits per year (Narrow et al., 2000).

Whole Team Approach

Within the overall treatment direction, practitioners should facilitate interventions that incorporate the elements of process-oriented recovery to address issues documented with ICF codes including b152 Emotional Functions, b160 Thought Functions, b156 Perceptual Functions, b164 Higher-Level Cognitive Functions, b167 Mental Functions of Language, d210 Undertaking a Single Task, and d220 Undertaking Multiple Tasks. These interventions may include support from professionals and peers and plans to increase participation in personally meaningful activities (Mancini, 2007).

Psychopharmacology is the primary form of treatment for SSD. Early treatment with antipsychotics often is predictive of better outcomes and a shorter duration of acute symptoms. However, antipsychotic medication does little to address negative symptoms and problems in functioning (Buchanan, 2007). All therapists should help address medication compliance, as it is a critical focus of any mental health treatment. Employment is not always feasible, nor does it meet the preferences of all individuals diagnosed with SSD; therefore, participation in meaningful activities outside of remunerative employment is important to the recovery process (Harvey & Bellack, 2009). Overall treatment targets include medication management (d5 Self-Care), development of coping skills, social skills, functional skills, and increased independent community participation (d710 Basic Interpersonal Interactions, d720 Complex Interpersonal Interactions) (Kreyenbuhl et al., 2010).

The 2009 Schizophrenia Patient Outcomes Research Team (PORT) (Dixon et al., 2010; Kreyenbuhl et al., 2010), which reviews the most current evidence-based practice, made recommendations for the psychosocial treatment of individuals with SSD. Recommendations for treatment are described below.

Assertive community treatment (ACT): A community-based treatment program having a multidisciplinary team with a low client-to-staff ratio, which provides frequent services in the community. ACT services are beneficial for reducing hospitalization and homelessness.

Supported employment: Individuals with SSD who desire employment should receive services targeted at obtaining and maintaining a job placement. Essential factors of supported employment include individualized job skills development, rapid search and placement, ongoing support, and the integration of vocational services with mental health services. Outcomes include increased competitive employment, higher wages, and more working hours than those who did not receive supported employment services.

Skills training: Services should also target the development of skills that will benefit the individual with SSD in social situations, participation in activities of daily living, and other skills that have a direct impact on participation in the community. Skills development should utilize positive feedback, behavioral modeling, rehearsal, and constructive feedback. Because of the difficulty individuals with SSD have in transferring skills into different environments, skills training should also target participation in day-to-day activities and training to transfer skills from one setting to another.

Cognitive behavioral therapy (CBT): CBT attempts to change the way individuals cognitively assess a situation, and, as such, how they react to it behaviorally. Through cognitive retraining, individuals are challenged to assess their reaction to stressors and, in the case of schizophrenia, to positive symptoms. Through modeling and the development of self-managing techniques, individuals are taught to deal with daily stressors and situations directly related to their conditions (d240 Handling Stress and Other Psychological Demands). Individual or group-based CBT that lasts at least four to nine months should be provided to individuals with SSD. These services should complement psychiatric medication and should target both cognitive and behavioral strategies to manage stress and reduce symptoms. Outcomes of CBT include reduced positive and negative symptoms and improved social functioning.

Functional cognitive behavioral therapy (FCBT): Another type of CBT that has been proposed is functional cognitive behavioral therapy (Penn et al., 2004). FCBT proposes the use of CBT and supportive therapy to increase an individual's functioning. Modeling is strongly encouraged in this type of CBT, using supervised social and recreational activities as a place to learn and practice behaviors. These learned behaviors can then transfer to independent situations, improving functioning. FCBT is a specific 16-session intervention. Readers should refer to the referenced article for information on these sessions. Specifics of FCBT include focusing on the individual's functioning as opposed to his or her symptoms. The primary areas FCBT addresses are increasing social relationships, developing hobbies, and finding daily activities in which to participate.

Token economy interventions: Service providers in residential or long-term inpatient settings should use token economy interventions that are based in Bandura's (1999) social learning theory. These interventions use consistent positive reinforcement for predefined behaviors and have been successful in improving personal hygiene habits (d5 Self-Care), social skills (d710 Basic Interpersonal Interactions), and adaptive behaviors (d250 Managing One's Own Behavior).

Family-based services: Clients who have ongoing contact and support from family members and significant others and receive family-based services that last from six to nine months have lower rates of rehospitalization. These services should include illness education, crisis intervention, emotional support, and coping skills training. Outcomes include higher medication adherence, reduction of psychiatric symptoms, and lower stress levels for family members.

Psychosocial interventions for weight management: Individuals with SSD have higher rates of obesity and diabetes than the general population. Therefore, in an effort to address person-centered care, individuals who are overweight or obese should receive interventions of at least three months duration that target weight loss. These interventions should be comprehensive and include nutrition counseling and behavioral self-management that includes portion control, goal setting, weigh-ins, self-monitoring of diet and physical activity, and physical activity modifications.

Recreational Therapy Approach

RT professionals should attend to the same treatment recommendations as the whole team, particularly those that are theoretically based, such as CBT and token economy interventions. While RT professionals are often employed in inpatient settings, there is also a clear role for RT in community-based mental health programs. This need will only increase as community-based mental health shifts more towards functional outcomes and community integration.

Recreational Therapy Interventions

Because the mental health field is still in the early stages of studying evidence-based practices (EBP), a comprehensive list of EBP interventions is not currently possible. However, practitioners should consider the applicability of the treatment recommendations put forth by the schizophrenia PORT study (Kreyenbuhl et al., 2010), as these recommendations have application for all service providers. The following is a short list of EBP interventions that may be used by recreational therapists.

Functional Skills and Symptom Reduction

Cognitive social skills training: Cognitive social skills training through recreational activities is a manualized intervention that uses recreational activities for the improvement of neurocognition (b160 Thought Functions), social skills (d7 Interpersonal Interactions and Relationships), and well-being (b126 Temperament and Personality Functions). The development of recreational skills was also correlated with treatment motivation and general social functioning (Mueller & Roder, 2005).

Body-oriented psychotherapy: Participation in a body-oriented psychotherapy group, which involves sharing, stretching and exercise, structured tasks (e.g., interacting with props, mirroring others, and exploring space), creative movement, and a closing circle was associated with reduced negative symptoms (b130 Energy and Drive Functions, d210 Undertaking a Single Task, d220 Undertaking Multiple Tasks) (Rohricht & Priebe, 2006).

Adventure therapy: Adventure therapy programs are associated with improved global functioning and self-esteem (b126 Temperament and Personality Functions) (Voruganti et al., 2006)

Video games: Participation in an internet video game intervention over an eight-week period was related to a significant decrease in positive symptoms and involuntary movement (b156 Perceptual Functions, b160 Thought Functions) (Han et al., 2007).

Progressive muscle relaxation: Progressive muscle relaxation training has been shown to significantly reduce anxiety in adults with SSD (d240 Handling Stress and Other Psychological Demands) (Chen et al., 2009).

Yoga: Individuals with SSD were randomly assigned either to a yoga treatment group or to an exercise group. After four months of participation, those in the yoga treatment group experienced significant reductions in psychopathology, as well as significant improvements in social (d7 Interpersonal Interactions and Relationships) and occupational (d8 Major Life Areas) functioning as well as overall quality of life (b126 Temperament and Personality Functions) (Duraiswamy et al., 2007).

Community Integration

Community integration continues to be an ongoing need for this population. However, limited research exists that demonstrates effective interventions. Research does encourage practitioners to provide services in the community, so that clients have a higher likelihood to generalize behavior from treatment to everyday living (Kreyenbuhl et al., 2010). Community-peer interventions that pair individuals with SSD with community volunteers for intentional friendships have been successful in increasing peer support (e320 Friends). Individuals who responded to the intervention also saw an increase in subjective well-being as well as a decrease in psychiatric symptoms (McCorkle et al., 2008). The Independence through Community Access and Navigation (ICAN) (Snethen, McCormick, Smith, & Van Puymbroeck, 2011; Snethen, McCormick, & Van Puymbroeck, 2011) is an RT-specific intervention that focuses on the development of functional skills related to independent, community-based recreation participation.

Health Promotion

Advocacy: RT professionals, particularly those who target community integration, will likely meet attitudes that are not accepting of individuals with

SSD. Working with other mental health providers to reduce stigmatizing attitudes in the community can help reduce the attitudinal barriers that are prevalent in the community (e460 Societal Attitudes).

Accessibility: Given the limited resources available to individuals with SSD, RT professionals should work with community agencies to promote the availability of need-based scholarships (e575 General Social Support Services, Systems, and Policies).

Miscellaneous

Case examples related to RT and SSD can be found in the following references: Snethen, McCormick, Smith, & Van Puymbroeck, 2011 and Rudnick, 2005.

Resources

National Alliance on Mental Illness (NAMI)
nami.org/
Local NAMI branches are a resource to practitioners, individuals with SSD, and family members.

Mental Health America
www.nmha.org/
Dedicated to public policy and advocacy initiatives.

References

American Psychiatric Association. (2013). *Diagnostic and statistical manual of mental disorders* (5th ed.). Arlington, VA: American Psychiatric Publishing.

American Psychiatric Association. (2000). *Diagnostic and statistical manual of mental disorders* (IV-TR). Washington, DC: American Psychiatric Association.

Ascher-Svanum, H. & Krause, A. (1991). *Psychoeducational groups for patients with schizophrenia: A guide for practitioners*. Gaithersburg, MD: Aspen Publications.

Badcock, J. C., Michie, P. T., & Rock, D. (2005). Spatial working memory and planning ability: Contrasts between schizophrenia and bipolar I disorder. *Cortex, 41*, 753-763.

Bandura, A. (1999). Social cognitive theory: An agentic perspective. *Asian Journal of Social Psychology, 2*(1), 21-41.

Basavanthappa, B. T. (2007). *Psychiatric mental health nursing*. New Deli, India: Jaypee Brothers Medical Publishers Ltd.

Bellack, A. S., Green, M. F., Cook, J. A., Fenton, W., Harvey, P. D., Heaton, R. K., et al. (2007). Assessment of community functioning in people with schizophrenia and other severe mental illnesses: A white paper based on an NIMH-sponsored workshop. *Schizophrenia Bulletin, 33*(3), 805-822.

Buchanan, R. W. (2007). Persistent negative symptoms in schizophrenia: An overview. *Schizophrenia Bulletin, 33*(4), 1013-1022.

Chen, W., Chu, H., Lu, R., Chou, Y., Chen, C., Cang, Y., et al. (2009). Efficacy of progressive muscle relaxation training in reducing anxiety in patients with acute schizophrenia. *Journal of Clinical Nursing, 18*(15), 2187-2196.

Cohen, L. J., Test, M. A., & Brown, R. L. (1990). Suicide and schizophrenia: Data from a prospective community treatment study. *American Journal of Psychiatry, 147*, 602-607.

Dixon, L. B., Dickson, F., Bellack, A. S., Bennett, M., Dickinson, D., Goldberg, R. W., et al. (2010). The 2009 schizophrenia PORT psychosocial treatment recommendations and summary statements. *Schizophrenia Bulletin, 36*(1), 48-70.

Dragt, S., Nieman, D. H., Veltman, D., Becker, H. E., van de Fliert, R., de Haan, L., et al. (2011). Environmental factors and social adjustment as predictors of a first psychosis in subjects at ultra high risk. *Schizophrenia Research, 125*(1), 69-76.

Duraiswamy, G., Thirthalli, J., Nagendra, H. R., & Gangadhar, B. N. (2007). Yoga therapy as an add-on treatment in the management of patients with schizophrenia — a randomized controlled trial. *Acta Psychiatrica Scandinavica, 116*(3), 226-232.

Everett, A., Mahler, J., Biblin, J., Ganguli, R., & Mauer, B. (2008). Improving the health of mental health consumers: Effective policies and practices. *International Journal of Mental Health, 37*(2), 8-48.

Hall, R. C. W. (1995). Global Assessment of Functioning: A modified scale. *Psychosomatics, 36*, 267-275.

Han, D. H., Renshaw, P. F., Sim, M. E., Kim, J. I., Arenella, L. S., & Lyoo, K. (2007). Letter to the editor: The effect of internet video game play on clinical and extrapyramidal symptoms in patients with schizophrenia. *Schizophrenia Research, 103*, 338-340.

Harvey, P. D. & Bellack, A. S. (2009). Toward a terminology for functional recovery in schizophrenia: Is functional remission a viable concept? *Schizophrenia Bulletin, 35*(2), 300-306.

Hutchinson, S. L., Bland, A. D., & Kleiber, D. A. (2008). Leisure and stress-coping: Implications for therapeutic recreation practice. *Therapeutic Recreation Journal, 42*(1), 9-23.

Kirkpatrick, B., Fenton, W. S., Carpenter, W. T., Jr., & Marder, S. R. (2006). The NIMH-MATRICS consensus statement on negative symptoms. *Schizophrenia Bulletin, 32*(2), 214-219.

Kreyenbuhl, J., Buchanan, R. W., Dickerson, F. B., & Dixon, L. B. (2010). The schizophrenia Patient Outcomes Research Team (PORT): Updated treatment recommendations 2009. *Schizophrenia Bulletin, 36*(1), 94-103.

Lysaker, P. & Davis, L. (2004). Social function in schizophrenia and schizoaffective disorder: Associations with personality, symptoms and neurocognition. *Health and Quality of Life Outcomes, 2*(1), 15.

Lysaker, P. H., Lancaster, R. S., Nees, M. A., & Davis, L. W. (2004). Attributional style and symptoms as predictors of social function in schizophrenia. *Journal of Rehabilitation Research & Development, 41*(2), 225-232.

Mancini, M. A. (2007). The role of self-efficacy in recovery from serious psychiatric disabilities: A qualitative study with fifteen psychiatric survivors. *Qualitative Social Work, 6*, 49-74.

McCorkle, B. H., Rogers, E. S., Dunn, E. C., Lyass, A., & Wan, Y. M. (2008). Increasing social support for individuals with serious mental illness: Evaluating the Compeer model of intentional friendship. *Community Mental Health Journal, 44*, 359-366.

McGrath, J., Saha, S., Chant, D., & Welham, J. (2008). Schizophrenia: A concise overview of incidence, prevalence, and mortality. *Epidemiologic Reviews, 30*, 67-76.

Mueller, D. R. & Roder, V. (2005). Social skills training in recreational rehabilitation of schizophrenia patients. *American Journal of Recreational Therapy, 4*(3), 11-19.

Narrow, W. E., Rae, D. S., Robins, L. N., & Regier, D. A. (2002). Revised prevalence estimates of mental disorders in the United States: Using a clinical significance criterion to reconcile two surveys' estimates. *Archives of General Psychiatry 59*, 115-123.

Nolen-Hoeksema, S. (2004). *Abnormal Psychology* (3rd ed.). New York: McGraw-Hill.

Penn, D. L., Mueser, K. T., Tarrier, N., Gloege, A., Cather, C., Serrano, D., & Otto, M. W. (2004). Supportive therapy for schizophrenia: Possible mechanisms and implications for adjunctive psychosocial treatments. *Schizophrenia Bulletin, 30*(1), 101-112.

Pokos, V. & Castle, D. J. (2006). Prevalence of comorbid anxiety disorders in schizophrenia spectrum disorders: A literature review. *Current Psychiatry Review, 2*(3), 285-307.

Rohricht, F. & Priebe, S. (2006). Effect of body-oriented psychological therapy on negative symptoms in schizophrenia: A randomized controlled trial. *Psychological Medicine, 36*(5), 669-678.

Rudnick, A. (2005). Psychiatric leisure rehabilitation: Conceptualization and illustration. *Psychiatric Rehabilitation Journal, 29*(1), 63-65.

Scherr, M., Hamann, M., Schwethoffer, D., Frobose, T., Vukovich, R., Pitschel-Walz, G., et al. (2012). Environmental risk factors and their impact on the age of onset of schizophrenia: Comparing familial to non-familial schizophrenia. *Nordic Journal of Psychiatry, 66*(2), 107-114.

Snethen, G., McCormick, B. P., Smith, R. L., & Van Puymbroeck, M. (2011). Independence through Community Access and Navigation (I-CAN) in adults with schizophrenia spectrum disorders: Treatment planning & implementation [Part II] *American Journal of Recreational Therapy, 10*(1), 35-46.

Snethen, G., McCormick, B. P., & Van Puymbroeck, M. (2011). Independence through Community Access and Navigation (I-CAN) in adults with schizophrenia spectrum disorders: Theoretical & practical foundations [Part I] *American Journal of Recreational Therapy, 10*(1), 25-34.

Tenorio-Martinez, R., del Carmen Lara-Munoz, M., & Medina-Mora, M. E. (2009). Measurement of problems in activities and participation in patients with anxiety, depression and schizophrenia using the ICF checklist. *Social Psychiatry & Psychiatric Epidemiology, 44*, 377-384.

Todman, M. (2003). Boredom and psychotic disorders: Cognitive and motivational issues. *Psychiatry, 66*(2), 146-167.

Todman, M., Sheypuk, D., Nelson, K., Evans, J., Goldberg, R., & Lehr, E. (2009). Boredom, hallucination-proneness and hypohedonia in schizophrenia and schizoaffective disorder. In K.-s. Yip (Ed.), *Schizoaffective Disorders: International perspectives on understanding, intervention and rehabilitation* (pp. 153-157). New York: Nova Science Publishers, Inc.

Versola-Russo, J. (2006). Cultural and demographic factors of schizophrenia. *International Journal of Psychosocial Rehabilitation, 10*(2), 89-103.

Voruganti, L. N. P., Whatham, J., Bard, E., Parker, G., & MacCrimmon, D. J. (2006). Going beyond: An adventure- and recreation-based group intervention promotes well-being and weight loss in schizophrenia. *Canadian Journal of Psychiatry, 51*(9), 575-580.

Weber, N. S., Cowan, D. N., Millikan, A. M., & Niebuhr, D. W. (2009). Psychiatric and general medical conditions comorbid with schizophrenia in the national hospital discharge survey. *Psychiatric Services, 60*(8), 1059-1067.

33. Sickle Cell Disease

Julie Hoehl and Karen Smith

Sickle cell disease (SCD) is an inherited blood disorder that affects red blood cells (also called erythrocytes). SCD is caused by a mutated form of hemoglobin, which results in red blood cell (RBC) rigidity during low oxygen states. A normal RBC's lifespan is approximately 100-120 days. In SCD the cell's lifespan is closer to 10-20 days creating chronic anemia, which leads to other pathological conditions. In addition to the anemia, the defective hemoglobin becomes stiff and rod-like or sickle-shaped when it gives up its oxygen. The shape does not go through small blood vessels as easily as normal RBCs causing vessel occlusions when a cluster of cells blocks a blood vessel. This leads to tissue micro-infarctions.

The RBC membrane is also affected, which allows it to become attached to vessel walls as well as cluster with other affected red blood cells. Recent studies reveal that the defective hemoglobin fails to actuate the biosensor responsible for opening vessels to allow appropriate blood flow (Kato, Gladwin, & Steinberg, 2007; Miller & Gladwin, 2012). All of these defective processes lead to recurrent vaso-occlusive crises that cause disabling pain and damage to the tissues not receiving an adequate blood supply.

The most common types of SCD are sickle cell anemia (Hb SS), sickle cell hemoglobin C (Hb SC), and sickle beta thalassemia (Hb SB).

The events that drive an individual with SCD to medical care fall into three major categories (Ballas et al., 2012): anemia, pain, and infection. At baseline, clients with SCD typically report pain, disturbed sleep, reduced daytime functioning, and absence from work or school, all of which can be exacerbated during a vaso-occlusive crisis (Anie et al., 2012).

Incidence/Prevalence in U.S.

According to the National Heart, Lung, and Blood Institute (2011), SCD affects millions throughout the world. It is particularly common among people whose ancestors come from sub-Saharan Africa; South America; Cuba; Central America; Saudi Arabia; India; and Mediterranean countries such as Turkey, Greece, and Italy.

In the United States, it affects around 72,000 people, most with ancestors who come from Africa (Smith, 1999). The disease occurs in about one in every 500 African-American births and once in every 1000 to 1400 Hispanic-American births (NHLBI, 2011). About two million Americans, or one in 12 African Americans, carry the sickle cell trait (NHLBI, 2011).

Current prevalence information focuses on the frequency of pain resulting in emergency department use and the number of hospitalizations due to pain crisis in SCD, however few studies focus on these pain manifestations outside the typical healthcare delivery system or how individuals manage their pain outside of accessing their physician. Furthermore, it is unclear the percentage of individuals who are able to self-manage their crises at home without accessing healthcare professionals (Smith et al., 2005).

Predominant Age

Since sickle cell disease is a chronic, hereditary disorder, it is found in all ages of clients (Howard, Thomas, & Rawle, 2009). The first symptoms usually develop after six months of age (CDC, 2011).

Causes

SCD is an inherited condition. Two copies of the sickle cell gene are needed for the body to make the abnormal hemoglobin found in sickle cell anemia. Sickle cell disease goes through vaso-occlusive events (VOE), cycles of remission, and acute crises that are brought on by the environment and the individual's activity choices, including overexertion, exposure to cold temperatures, exposure to infections, increased body temperature, significant emotional stress, and dehydration (Wright & Ahmedzai, 2010).

Systems Affected

SCD affects the entire body throughout the lifespan of the client. Depending on the severity and type of the disease, the number of crises will determine the effect on the body. The underlying cause of the disease is documented with ICF codes in b430 Hematological System Functions.

The premature death of affected red blood cells exceeds the body's ability to produce new red blood cells. The resulting anemia leaves everything in the body in a low-oxygen state producing symptoms of tiredness and subnormal functioning in every activity (b130 Energy and Drive Functions). In addition to the anemia there are crises when the hemoglobin has lost enough oxygen that it becomes stiff and sickle shaped. During a crisis, tissue ischemia (a reduction in the supply of oxygenated blood to cells) causes pain (b280 Sensation of Pain) and decreased function of the affected tissue or organ. If the lack of blood supply lasts long enough, it causes necrosis (death of body tissue). The effects on some of the important body systems include:

Brain: Strokes and silent cerebral infarct (SCI) are major complications of SCD. About 10-15% of children with SCD will have a stroke (Adams, Ohene-Frempong, & Wang, 2001; King, DeBaun, & White, 2008). SCI occurs in 27% of this population before they turn six and 37% by their 14th birthday (DeBaun et al., 2012). See the chapter on Cerebrovascular Accident for information on ICF codes to use.

Bones: Through multiple crises, the bones are weakened with the potential of bone rarefaction (decrease in the density) and osteoporosis. This increases the client's potential for fracturing bones. Other skeletal deformities may also develop including lordosis (a spinal deformity that causes the lumbar spine to have an excessive curve backwards) and kyphosis (a spinal deformity that causes the thoracic portion of the spine to curve forward causing rounded shoulders and impairing lung capacity). Individuals with SCD are often treated with high doses of steroids, which cause necrosis in bone and joint tissues. This can require joint replacement (Arya & Agarwal, 2012; Osunkwo et al., 2012; Pack-

Mabien & Haynes, 2009). The chapters on Osteoporosis and Total Joint Replacement provide information on relevant ICF codes. Spinal deformities should be noted with ICF code s760 Structure of Trunk and codes in d4 Mobility that describe particular issues.

Central nervous system: Because of the potential for blockage of the vascular system, clients have an increased risk of a cerebrovascular accident. For example, research shows that children with sickle cell anemia scored one standard deviation lower than their siblings on cognitive tests. The assumption is that this difference is due to brain damage from ischemia, specifically strokes and SCIs, and the resulting necrosis (Feliu et al., 2011; Hijmans et al., 2011; King et al., 2008). See the chapter on Cerebrovascular Accident for information on ICF codes to use.

Heart: Cardiac exam findings are rarely normal in SCD. Clients with sickle cell anemia often have an enlarged or damage heart due to ischemia and necrosis (Claster & Vichinsky, 2003; Miller & Gladwin, 2012; Voskaridou, Christoulas, & Terpos, 2012). A lack of appropriate levels of physical activity and the emotional stress associated with sickle cell disease may also play a factor (Waltz et al., 2012; Wendel-Vos et al., 2004). The specific findings for the heart can be documented with ICF code s410 Structure of Cardiovascular System. Resulting functional problems may be noted with codes such as b410 Heart Functions and b455 Exercise Tolerance Functions.

Kidney: Tissue ischemia and necrosis of the kidney causes inability to concentrate urine, which leads to enuresis (bedwetting) (Daniel et al., 2010; Lehmann et al., 2012; Portocarrero et al., 2012), hematuria (blood in the urine) (Kryvenko & Epstein, 2012), and nephritic syndrome (inflammation of the kidneys) (Osei-Yeboah & Rodrigues, 2011; Pham et al., 2000). ICF codes b610 Urinary Excretory Functions, b620 Urination Functions, and d530 Toileting describe these issues.

Liver: Multiple crises may cause necrosis of liver tissue, which means healthy liver tissue is replaced with fibrotic (scar) tissues (Berry et al., 2007). The liver produces bile that helps the body digest fats in the small intestine; balances the body's level of bilirubin (if not balanced, jaundice results that produces yellow discoloration of the skin and eyes); secretes fats, glucose, proteins, and vitamins (all necessary for feeding the cells in the body); processes hemoglobin to allow the body to use its iron; and converts poisonous ammonia produced as a by-product of cell function into urine. ICF codes include b430 Hematological System Functions, b515 Digestive Functions, and b610 Urinary Excretory Functions.

Lungs: Lungs are a major target organ for acute and chronic complications of SCD. Asthma is thought to be a significant comorbidity for individuals with SCD. Acute chest syndrome (ACS) and pulmonary hypertension have the highest associated mortality rates in this population and are second to pain for causes of hospitalizations (Miller & Gladwin, 2012). Although the methods of diagnosing pulmonary hypertension are controversial, it has been reported to occur in as many as 30% of the people with SCD (Parent et al., 2011; Ristow & Schiller). ICF codes include b440 Respiration Functions.

Physical stature and maturation: Clients with sickle cell anemia tend to reach physical maturity one to two years later than their peers. Height and weight were about 84% of normal in a study of 148 subjects with SCD (Zemel et al., 2007). Anemia and more difficulty getting adequate nutrition appear to be significant causes of the delayed maturity and smaller size (Dekker et al., 2012; Zemel et al., 2007). This difference compared to peers causes additional stress for adolescents, who, as a group, already have a lot to cope with. Due to ongoing pain, even at times when their body is not in crisis, and frequent hospitalizations, clients are not inclined to participate in activities as much as their peers. A loss of appetite and anorexia due to treatment and medications may also be a problem, further compounding body image issues. One ICF code to use to document this issue is b560 Growth Maintenance Functions.

Spleen: The spleen becomes enlarged with sickle cells during a crisis, as it tries to remove what appear to be damaged red blood cells from the circulatory system (Ebert, Nagar, & Hagspiel, 2010). At all times the spleen is overworked trying to remove cells that are sickled. One of complications of the spleen being overworked is that it is less efficient at removing antibody-coated bacteria, which can result in increased susceptibility to infection. ICF codes that can be used to document these issues include b430 Hematological System Functions and b435 Immunological System Functions

Skin: Clients with SCD are at an increased risk of developing skin ulcers on their lower extremities (b810-b849 Functions of the Skin) due to poor circulation caused by sickled hemoglobin. In the United States, 2.5% of individuals with SCD are likely to have reoccurring problems with ulcers (Koshy et al., 1989).

Secondary Problems

Common secondary problems include acute chest syndrome; pulmonary hypertension; anemia; blindness or vision impairment; disease of the kidney, liver, and lung; narcotic drug abuse; gallstones; hemolytic crisis; pneumonia; gallbladder inflammation; osteomyelitis (bone infection); urinary tract infection; joint destruction; leg sores; parvovirus B19 infection, leading to low red blood cell production and an aplastic crisis; splenic sequestration syndrome; and tissue death in the kidney (MedlinePlus, 2012).

Prognosis

In the past, individual with SCD often died from acute chest syndrome (ACS), pulmonary hypertension, organ failure, and/or infections. Due to better understanding and management of the disease, individuals with SCD can now live into their 50s or beyond (McKerrell, Cohen, & Billett, 2004). The average life expectancy for males and females with SCD has been determined to be 42 and 48 years, respectively (Platt et al., 1994). Some people with the disease experience minor, brief, infrequent episodes. Others experience severe, long-term, frequent episodes with many complications.

The only cure for SCD at this time is a stem cell transplant. Transplants have been most successful with a related, matched donor. In selected clients who are disease free, the overall survival rate is greater than 80% (Bolanos-Meade & Brodsky, 2009). As the risk of the disease increases, the need to try cord blood and hematopoietic transplants increases. Allowing clients to be able to weigh the symptoms with the risks of the transplant is important (Kamani et al., 2012; Shenoy, 2011).

Assessment

Typical Scope of Team Assessment

During a crisis the treatment team needs to assess the client's immediate life-threatening conditions. These could include lack of blood to any of the major organs, including the brain. After life-threatening issues are resolved, the team can look at levels of pain caused by the ischemia and decide the appropriate medications for handling the pain. Consideration must be given to the risks of substance-use disorders in each client. The goal during a crisis is to prevent as much damage as possible. ICF codes to document the findings are listed in the Systems Affected section.

When the client is not in crisis, the blood can be monitored for prevalence of sickled red blood cells and red blood cell counts. Major organs should also be monitored to be sure they are functioning as well as possible. Preventing organ failure is a major concern. Additional checks will be made to monitor the ongoing use of pain medications. The goal when the client is not in crisis is to maintain the best possible health and prevent another crisis. ICF codes to document the findings are also listed in the Systems Affected section.

It is important to get a self-assessment from the client to help with future treatment (Anie et al., 2012). A self-assessment will help meet the patient where they are and give insight into what they might be feeling. It will also tell the team if education about self-care is required (d250 Managing One's Own Behavior, d570 Looking After One's Health).

Areas of Concern for RT Assessment

The client can be affected in all of the domains (physical, emotional, cognitive, and leisure) and in every one of the Activities and Participation codes. There is a great chance that individuals will have problems with ambulation, coordination, gross motor movement, fatigue (b455 Exercise Tolerance Functions, d4 Mobility) (Ameringer & Smith, 2011), and/or pain (Ballas, 2011). A lower frustration tolerance due to increased pain can be a factor as well (d2 General Tasks and Demands). They are smaller, develop later, and have frequent complications that remove them from school settings, gym class, or being active at recess (d7 Interpersonal Interactions and Relationships, d8 Major Life Areas, d9 Com-

munity, Social, and Civic Life) (Palermo, Riley, & Mitchell, 2008). Individuals with SCD might also have cognitive issues from strokes and SCIs, depending on the severity of the disease (d1 Learning and Applying Knowledge, d3 Communication). The client might have high absenteeism in school (King et al., 2008; Schatz et al., 2009).

ICF Core Set

No ICF Core Set has been developed for Sickle Cell Disease.

Treatment Direction

Whole Team Approach

The whole team works first on solving the acute problems of a crisis. That aspect of treatment can be documented by referring to the ICF code for pain b280 Sensation of Pain and the ICF codes, as listed earlier, that describe the focal point(s) of the current crisis.

When the client is stabilized, the team studies how well the client understands the disease and what needs to be done to avoid future crises. If the client needs more information and is capable of processing it, as documented by ICF codes d250 Managing One's Own Behavior, d570 Looking After One's Health, the team provides education on how to avoid future events, adaptations for deficits, and general health information related to the disease (Pack-Mabien & Haynes, 2009).

The management of SCD in the past was predominantly palliative using symptomatic and preventative approaches. The standard of care for individuals with SCD during vaso-occlusive crisis was to reduce the pain with drugs, typically with opioids. While this approach was effective for some clients, many were under-medicated due to fear of addiction, tolerance, or side effects caused by frequent and long-term use of opioids (Ballas, 2011).

Current standards of care try to prevent vaso-occlusive crisis. Hydroxyurea to make the red blood cells more flexible and blood exchange programs provide blood that is less likely to go into crisis. Hydroxyurea, a cytotoxic agent, reduces the incidence of vaso-occlusive crises by stimulating increased fetal hemoglobin and nitric oxide production; however, its use is limited by side effects, primarily bone marrow suppression, gastrointestinal disturbances, and possible teratogenicity. Frequent blood draws to closely monitor blood conditions are required for this treatment (Charache et al., 1995). It is suggested that early follow-up should be scheduled to prevent readmission within 30 days, which occurs about 20% of the time (Leschke et al., 2012; Sobota et al., 2012). These procedures can be coded as treatment for ICF code b430 Hematological System Functions.

A review of summarized trials of psychosocial interventions as adjuncts to treating SCD was completed by Anie et al. (2012). This article looked at eleven studies, of which six met the required criteria. One study showed that cognitive behavior therapy significantly reduced the affective component of pain (b280 Sensation of Pain). Other interventions included hypnosis and social support procedures where self-empowerment and education were strong facets of the supportive care approach. The effects of these techniques on pain control, quality of life, and healthcare utilization were inconsistent, partly because of inadequate study design. A comprehensive team approach is important to provide continuity of care (Lee et al., 2012).

Recreational Therapy Approach

The general approach to treating SCD in recreational therapy is pain management, adaptation and modification of recreation or community activity, client and family education, and community integration training. Utilizing relaxation and stress management techniques to help the client get though vaso-occlusive crisis along with pharmacologic analgesia can decrease the use of medications and provide a sense of control to the client. A recreational therapist is able to help the client implement techniques that decrease the level of pain to help improve quality of life.

During a crisis, the recreational therapist provides support to the rest of the treatment team in carrying out programs to meet the client's needs. One example is when the client has a fever. The recreational therapist should work with the rest of the medical team to develop guidelines to increase the amount of fluids a client receives via by mouth or IV if symptoms persist. The recreational therapist can monitor fluid intake, while providing opportunities for increased intake during activities. Cellular hydration is important to decrease the severity of the crisis (Okomo & Meremikwu, 2012).

Recreational Therapy Interventions

Clients with SCD are likely to be seen through numerous admissions to acute care hospitals, as well as within community recreation programs. The areas that recreational therapists frequently address with clients with SCD include:

- Normalization of the developmental process that is negatively impacted by inpatient stays (b560 Growth Maintenance Functions)
- Development of skills to cope with pain (b280 Sensation of Pain) and stress (d240 Handling Stress and Other Psychological Demands)
- Development of leisure activities that do not make the sickle cell disease worse (d570 Looking After One's Health)
- Sleep hygiene (b134 Sleep Functions)
- Self-esteem bolstering (b126 Temperament and Personality Functions)
- Internal locus of control, especially with teenagers (b126 Temperament and Personality Functions)

Providing education to help decrease vaso-occlusive crisis related to recreational activities is a major portion of the recreational therapist's responsibility (d250 Managing One's Own Behavior, d570 Looking After One's Health). Previously covered topics and adaptations to solve problems are commonly reviewed (Graff et al., 2012).

Education can also cover coping skills that will help during pain crisis and make everyday stressors easier to handle (d240 Handling Stress and Other Psychological Demands) (Gil et al., 2000). This may include relaxation focusing on diaphragmatic breathing exercises to decrease hypoxia, refocusing, and leisure education (Myrvik, Campbell, & Butcher, 2012; Thomas et al., 1984).

Self-esteem (b126 Temperament and Personality Functions) is important for a client with SCD because there are many limitations caused by the disease. The recreational therapist needs to make sure the client understands that there are things s/he can do to control the disease and activities that s/he can still participate in (d250 Managing One's Own Behavior, d570 Looking After One's Health) (Powers et al., 2002).

When leading community integration, it is important to remember that individuals with SCD have an increased rate of renal dieresis (b620 Urination Functions, d530 Toileting), so be sure restrooms are easily available. The client should be encouraged to wash his/her hands frequently to help prevent infections (d570 Looking After One's Health) and the therapist needs to make sure that direct, unprotected exposure to sunlight is limited if the client is on antibiotics. Community integration trips can be used to have clients demonstrate their learning objectives.

Helping clients understand the importance of getting regular, moderate exercise on a daily basis (d570 Looking After One's Health) is an important role for the recreational therapist. Thirty minutes a day of moderate exercise that avoids exposing the client to increased body temperatures or cold temperatures is important (Waltz et al., 2012; Wendel-Vos et al., 2004). In bad weather a moderate workout at the local gym or walking the mall is appropriate. The recreational therapist should work with the client to find appropriate kinds of exercise.

Other education topics related to appropriate exercise may be given to the client or the client's guardians. These will all help the client to make good decisions about activities and maintain health (d250 Managing One's Own Behavior, d570 Looking After One's Health). The topics include:

Exposure to cold: Clients need to avoid getting cold. That includes dressing appropriately for the weather, including ensuring appropriate protection from rain (d540 Dressing). When there is extreme cold, blood vessels in the extremities constrict, which makes it more likely that sickled red blood cells will be unable to pass through them.

Increased body temperatures: Clients should avoid activities that have the potential to raise their internal body temperatures above 101°F (d570 Looking After One's Health). This includes avoiding hot tubs, saunas, and exercising in hot weather. Environmental heat stress resulting in incomplete heat acclimation could cause dehydration, which increases the risk of a crisis (Okomo & Meremikwu, 2012; Waltz et al., 2012; Yale, Nagib, & Guthrie, 2000).

Competitive sports: Though there is no research that supports an increase in mortality through competitive sports for individuals with SCD, exercise-related deaths do occur at a higher rate,

although they are rare (Tsaras et al., 2009). It is usually not advisable for clients with SCD to engage in a level of exercise that will increase the stress on their bodies. Competitive sports usually require individuals to push themselves physically and often expose them to a variety of severe weather. Youth are also susceptible to peer pressure if they are taken out of a game because of potential risks, hindering their ability to complete the game or workout.

Hypoxia (lack of oxygen reaching the cells): While normal levels of activity are encouraged for clients with sickle cell, excessive levels of activity that lead to lowered levels of oxygen in the blood can precipitate a sickle cell crisis. The types of activities to avoid are strenuous physical exercise, emotional stress, and activities in high altitudes. Scuba diving is also contraindicated (Yale et al., 2000).

Hydration: Consuming adequate amounts of fluids to prevent dehydration is especially important during hot weather. The therapist should provide basic information, such as the location of the drinking fountains in regularly used parks or recreation facilities and the types of foods available at concession stands that count toward hydration, such as soup, Jell-O, puddings, frozen popsicles, and Slurpees. Avoiding environmental causes of dehydration, such as sun exposure and hot temperatures, is another important part of leisure activity planning. When an individual with SCD become dehydrated it causes the cell to lose oxygen and become more rod like (Lew, Etzion, & Bookchin, 2002).

Lower extremity injuries: The recreational therapist who is working with clients in a community setting should look for possible ulcerations of the lower extremity. In inpatient settings, nursing staff will often notice cuts and ulcerations on the lower extremities during their normal physical exam. In either inpatient or outpatient settings the therapist should watch for problems developing on the lower extremities. If the therapist sees cuts, bruises, or blisters on the client's lower extremities during activities, the therapist should report it immediately to the client's primary care provider. With medical care, the duration and frequency of the ulcers decrease (Koshy et al., 1989). Clients should be educated to check their skin frequently for potential problems.

Infection control: The client should be encouraged to wash his/her hands frequently, as this is the main defense against infection. While it is important for clients to avoid hot temperatures or chill from cold or wet weather, being outside usually reduces the exposure to infection (Pack-Mabien & Haynes, 2009).

Photosensitivity: Clients under the age of five years often receive daily prophylactic doses of antibiotics to prevent infections. Often the antibiotics prescribed cause the client to be hypersensitive to sunlight. When working with a client to develop a balanced leisure repertoire, the therapist needs to make sure that direct, unprotected exposure to sunlight is limited. Clients should be instructed to wear a sunscreen of SPF 15 or higher and apply every two hours.

Renal diuresis: Clients usually have an increased rate of renal diuresis causing them to need to use the bathroom more frequently. It also increases the chance of enuresis (Daniel et al., 2010). In planning recreational activities, the therapist should ensure frequent breaks to use the restroom. Also, for camping activities, sensitivity is needed for clients who wet their beds. Extra sleeping bags and quietly waking the child or youth in the middle of the night to use the restroom are appropriate modifications to the activity. It is not appropriate to suggest that the client drink less before going to bed, as the enuresis is not because the client drank too much fluid but because the body processed the fluid less efficiently than normal. When trips are planned, ensure that adequate stops for restroom use and stretching are scheduled (Pack-Mabien & Haynes, 2009). The recreational therapist should instruct the client how advocate for enough stops at restrooms on a trip (b620 Urination Functions, d530 Toileting).

Resources

National Heart, Lung, and Blood Institute
www.nhlbi.nih.gov/health/health-topics/topics/sca/
A comprehensive source of information for the public and professionals regarding sickle cell disease.

Sickle Cell Disease Association of America, Inc.
www.sicklecelldisease.org
Provides resources and information on sickle cell disease.

References

Adams, R. J., Ohene-Frempong K., & Wang W. (2001). Sickle cell and the brain. *Hematology Am Soc Hematol Educ Program 2001*(1), 31-46. doi: 10.1182/asheducation-2001.1.31.

Ameringer, S. & Smith, W. R. (2011). Emerging biobehavioral factors of fatigue in sickle cell disease. *Journal of Nursing Scholarship, 43*(1), 22-29.

Anie, K. A., Grocott, H., White, L., Dzingina, M., Rogers, G., & Cho, G. (2012). Patient self-assessment of hospital pain, mood and health-related quality of life in adults with sickle cell disease. *BMJ Open, 2*(4). doi: 10.1136/bmjopen-2012-001274.

Arya, S. C. & Agarwal, N. (2012). Apropos "complete resolution of sickle cell chronic pain with high-dose vitamin D therapy: A case report and review of the literature". *Journal of Pediatric Hematology and Oncology, 34*(4), e172-173. doi: 10.1097/MPH.0b013e3182441346.

Ballas, S. K. (2011). Update on pain management in sickle cell disease. *Hemoglobin, 35*(5-6), 520-529.

Ballas, S. K., Kesen, M. R., Goldberg, M. F., Lutty, G. A., Dampier, C., Osunkwo, I., & Malik, P. (2012). Beyond the definitions of the phenotypic complications of sickle cell disease: An update on management. *The Scientific World Journal, 2012*, 55. doi: 10.1100/2012/949535.

Berry, P. A., Cross, T. J., Thein, S. L., Portmann, B. C., Wendon, J. A., Karani, J. B., & Bomford, A. (2007). Hepatic dysfunction in sickle cell disease: A new system of classification based on global assessment. *Clinical Gastroenterology and Hepatology, 5*(12), 1469-1476. doi: 10.1016/j.cgh.2007.08.009.

Bolanos-Meade, J. & Brodsky, R. A. (2009). Blood and marrow transplantation for sickle cell disease: Overcoming barriers to success. *Current Opinion in Oncology, 21*(2), 158-161. doi: 10.1097/CCO.0b013e328324ba04.

Centers for Disease Control and Prevention (CDC). (2011). Sickle cell disease (SCD): Symptoms and treatments. Retrieved 06/01/2011, 2011, from http://www.cdc.gov/ncbddd/sicklecell/symptoms.html.

Charache, S., Terrin, M. L., Moore, R. D., Dover, G. J., McMahon, R. P., Barton, F. B., & Eckert, S. V. (1995). Design of the multicenter study of hydroxyurea in sickle cell anemia. Investigators of the multicenter study of hydroxyurea. *Controlled Clinical Trials, 16*(6), 432-446.

Claster, S. & Vichinsky, E. P. (2003). Managing sickle cell disease. *British Medical Journal, 327*(7424), 1151-1155. doi: 10.1136/bmj.327.7424.1151.

Daniel, L. C., Grant, M., Kothare, S. V., Dampier, C., & Barakat, L. P. (2010). Sleep patterns in pediatric sickle cell disease. *Pediatric Blood & Cancer, 55*(3), 501-507. doi: 10.1002/pbc.22564.

DeBaun, M. R., Armstrong, F. D., McKinstry, R. C., Ware, R. E., Vichinsky, E., & Kirkham, F. J. (2012). Silent cerebral infarcts: A review on a prevalent and progressive cause of neurologic injury in sickle cell anemia. *Blood, 119*(20), 4587-4596.

Dekker, L. H., Fijnvandraat, K., Brabin, B. J., & van Hensbroek, M. B. (2012). Micronutrients and sickle cell disease, effects on growth, infection and vaso-occlusive crisis: A systematic review. *Pediatric Blood & Cancer, 59*(2), 211-215.

Ebert, E. C., Nagar, M., & Hagspiel, K. D. (2010). Gastrointestinal and hepatic complications of sickle cell disease. *Clinical Gastroenterology and Hepatology, 8*(6), 483-489. doi: 10.1016/j.cgh.2010.02.016.

Feliu, M. H., Crawford, R. D., Edwards, L., Wellington, C., Wood, M., Whitfield, K. E., & Edwards, C. L. (2011). Neurocognitive testing and functioning in adults sickle cell disease. *Hemoglobin, 35*(5-6), 476-484.

Gil, K. M., Carson, J. W., Sedway, J. A., Porter, L. S., Schaeffer, J. J., & Orringer, E. (2000). Follow-up of coping skills training in adults with sickle cell disease: Analysis of daily pain and coping practice diaries. *Health Psychology, 19*(1), 85-90. doi: 10.1037/0278-6133.19.1.85.

Graff, J. C., Hankins, J., Graves, R. J., Robitaille, K. Y., Roberts, R., Cejda, K., & Porter, J. S. (2012). Exploring family communication about sickle cell disease in adolescence. *Journal of Pediatric Oncology Nursing, 29*(6), 323-336.

Hijmans, C. T., Grootenhuis, M. A., Oosterlaan, J., Heijboer, H., Peters, M., & Fijnvandraat, K. (2011). Neurocognitive deficits in children with sickle cell disease are associated with the severity of anemia. *Pediatric Blood & Cancer, 57*(2), 297-302.

Howard, J., Thomas, V. J., & Rawle, H. M. (2009). Pain management and quality of life in sickle cell disease. *Expert Review of Pharmacoeconomics & Outcomes Research, 9*(4), 347-352. doi: 10.1586/erp.09.32.

Kamani, N. R., Walters, M. C., Carter, S., Aquino, V., Brochstein, J. A., Chaudhury, S., & Shenoy, S. (2012). Unrelated donor cord blood transplantation for children with severe sickle cell disease: Results of one cohort from the phase II study from the Blood and Marrow Transplant Clinical Trials Network (BMT CTN). *Biology of Blood and Marrow Transplantation, 18*(8), 1265-1272.

Kato, G. J., Gladwin, M. T., & Steinberg, M. H. (2007). Deconstructing sickle cell disease: Reappraisal of the role of hemolysis in the development of clinical subphenotypes. *Blood Reviews, 21*(1), 37-47. doi: 10.1016/j.blre.2006.07.001.

King, A. A., DeBaun, M. R., & White, D. A. (2008). Need for cognitive rehabilitation for children with sickle cell disease and strokes. *Expert Review of Neurotherapeutics, 8*(2), 291-296. doi: 10.1586/14737175.8.2.291.

Koshy, M., Entsuah, R., Koranda, A., Kraus, A., Johnson, R., Bellvue, R., & Levy, P. (1989). Leg ulcers in patients with sickle cell disease. *Blood, 74*(4), 1403-1408.

Kryvenko, O. N. & Epstein, J. I. (2012). Pseudocarcinomatous urothelial hyperplasia of the bladder: Clinical findings and follow-up of 70 patients. *Journal of Urology, 7*(12). doi: 10.1016/j.juro.2012.12.005.

Lee, L., Askew, R., Walker, J., Stephen, J., & Robertson-Artwork, A. (2012). Adults with sickle cell disease: An interdisciplinary approach to home care and self-care management with a case study. *Home Healthcare Nurse, 30*(3), 172-183.

Lehmann, G. C., Bell, T. R., Kirkham, F. J., Gavlak, J. C., Ferguson, T. F., Strunk, R. C., & DeBaun, M. R. (2012). Enuresis associated with sleep disordered breathing in children with sickle cell anemia. *Journal of Urology, 188*(4 Suppl), 1572-1576.

Leschke, J., Panepinto, J. A., Nimmer, M., Hoffmann, R. G., Yan, K., & Brousseau, D. C. (2012). Outpatient follow-up and rehospitalizations for sickle cell disease patients. *Pediatric Blood & Cancer, 58*(3), 406-409.

Lew, V. L., Etzion, Z., & Bookchin, R. M. (2002). Dehydration response of sickle cells to sickling-induced Ca++ permeabilization. *Blood, 99*, 2578-2585.

McKerrell, T. D., Cohen, H. W., & Billett, H. H. (2004). The older sickle cell patient. *American Journal of Hematology, 76*(2), 101-106. doi: 10.1002/ajh.20075.

MedlinePlus. (2012, 2/7/12). Sickle cell anemia. Retrieved January 15, 2013, from http://www.nlm.nih.gov/medlineplus/ency/article/000527.htm.

Miller, A. C., & Gladwin, M. T. (2012). Pulmonary complications of sickle cell disease. *American Journal of Respiratory and Critical Care Medicine, 185*(11), 1154-1165. doi: 10.1164/rccm.201111-2082CI.

Myrvik, M. P., Campbell, A. D., & Butcher, J. L. (2012). Single-session biofeedback-assisted relaxation training in children

with sickle cell disease. *Journal of Pediatric Hematology and Oncology, 34*(5), 340-343.

National Heart Lung and Blood Institute (NHLBI). (2011). Sickle cell anemia: Who is at risk? Retrieved June 1, 2011, from http://www.nhlbi.nih.gov/health/dci/Diseases/Sca/SCA_Who IsAtRisk.html.

Okomo, U. & Meremikwu, M. M. (2012). Fluid replacement therapy for acute episodes of pain in people with sickle cell disease. *Cochrane Database of Systematic Reviews 13*(6).

Osei-Yeboah, C. T. & Rodrigues, O. (2011). Renal status of children with sickle cell disease in Accra, Ghana. *Ghana Medical Journal, 45*(4), 155-160.

Osunkwo, I., Ziegler, T. R., Alvarez, J., McCracken, C., Cherry, K., Osunkwo, C. E., & Tangpricha, V. (2012). High dose vitamin D therapy for chronic pain in children and adolescents with sickle cell disease: Results of a randomized double blind pilot study. *British Journal of Haematolgy, 159*(2), 211-215.

Pack-Mabien, A. & Haynes, J., Jr. (2009). A primary care provider's guide to preventive and acute care management of adults and children with sickle cell disease. *Journal of the American Academy of Nurse Practitioners, 21*(5), 250-257. doi: 10.1111/j.1745-7599.2009.00401.x.

Palermo, T. M., Riley, C. A., & Mitchell, B. A. (2008). Daily functioning and quality of life in children with sickle cell disease pain: Relationship with family and neighborhood socioeconomic distress. *Journal of Pain, 9*(9), 833-840. doi: 10.1016/j.jpain.2008.04.002.

Parent, F., Bachir, D., Inamo, J., Lionnet, F., Driss, F., Loko, G., & Simonneau, G. (2011). A hemodynamic study of pulmonary hypertension in sickle cell disease. *New England Journal of Medicine, 365*(1), 44-53. doi: 10.1056/NEJMoa1005565.

Pham, P. T., Pham, P. C., Wilkinson, A. H., & Lew, S. Q. (2000). Renal abnormalities in sickle cell disease. *Kidney International, 57*(1), 1-8. doi: 10.1046/j.1523-1755.2000.00806.x.

Platt, O. S., Brambilla, D. J., Rosse, W. F., Milner, P. F., Castro, O., Steinberg, M. H., & Klug, P. P. (1994). Mortality in sickle cell disease. Life expectancy and risk factors for early death. *New England Journal of Medicine, 330*(23), 1639-1644.

Portocarrero, M. L., Sobral, M. M., Lyra, I., Lordelo, P., & Barroso, U., Jr. (2012). Prevalence of enuresis and daytime urinary incontinence in children and adolescents with sickle cell disease. *Journal of Urology, 187*(3), 1037-1040.

Powers, S., Mitchell, M. J., Graumlich, S. E., Byars, K. C., & Kalinyak, K. A. (2002). Longitudinal assessment of pain, coping, and daily functioning in children with sickle cell disease receiving pain management skills training. *Journal of Clinical Psychology in Medical Settings, 9*(2), 109-119. doi: 10.1023/a:1014940009788.

Ristow, B. & Schiller, N. B. (2011). Pulmonary hypertension in sickle cell disease. *New England Journal of Medicine, 365*, 1645-1646.

Schatz, J., Puffer, E. S., Sanchez, C., Stancil, M., & Roberts, C. W. (2009). Language processing deficits in sickle cell disease in young school-age children. *Developmental Neuropsychology, 34*(1), 122-136. doi: 10.1080/87565640802499191.

Shenoy, S. (2011). Hematopoietic stem cell transplantation for sickle cell disease: Current practice and emerging trends. *Hematology / the Education Program of the American Society of Hematology. American Society of Hematology. Education Program*, 273.

Smith, J. T. (1999). Sickle cell disease. In S. Goldstein & C. R. Reynolds (Eds.), *Handbook of neurodevelopmental and genetic disorders in children* (pp. 368-384). New York: Guilford.

Smith, W. R., Bovbjerg, V. E., Penberthy, L. T., McClish, D. K., Levenson, J. L., Roberts, J. D., & Aisiku, I. P. (2005). Understanding pain and improving management of sickle cell disease: the PiSCES study. *Journal of the National Medical Association, 97*(2), 183-193.

Sobota, A., Graham, D. A., Neufeld, E. J., & Heeney, M. M. (2012). Thirty-day readmission rates following hospitalization for pediatric sickle cell crisis at freestanding children's hospitals: Risk factors and hospital variation. *Pediatric Blood & Cancer, 58*(1), 61-65.

Thomas, J. E., Koshy, M., Patterson, L., Dorn, L., & Thomas, K. (1984). Management of pain in sickle cell disease using biofeedback therapy: A preliminary study. *Biofeedback and Self-Regulation, 9*(4), 413-420.

Tsaras, G., Owusu-Ansah, A., Boateng, F. O., & Amoateng-Adjepong, Y. (2009). Complications associated with sickle cell trait: A brief narrative review. *The American Journal of Medicine, 122*(6), 507-512. doi: 10.1016/j.amjmed.2008.12.020.

Voskaridou, E., Christoulas, D., & Terpos, E. (2012). Sickle-cell disease and the heart: Review of the current literature. *British Journal of Haematolgy, 157*(6), 664-673.

Waltz, X., Hedreville, M., Sinnapah, S., Lamarre, Y., Soter, V., Lemonne, N., & Connes, P. (2012). Delayed beneficial effect of acute exercise on red blood cell aggregate strength in patients with sickle cell anemia. *Clinical Hemorheology and Microcirculation, 52*(1), 15-26. doi: 10.3233/ch-2012-1540.

Wendel-Vos, G. C. W., Schuit, A. J., Feskens, E. J. M., Boshuizen, H. C., Verschuren, W. M. M., Saris, W. H. M., & Kromhout, D. (2004). Physical activity and stroke. A meta-analysis of observational data. *International Journal of Epidemiology, 33*, 787-798.

Wright, J. & Ahmedzai, S. H. (2010). The management of painful crisis in sickle cell disease. *Current Opinion in Supportive and Palliative Care, 4*(2), 97-106. doi: 10.1097/SPC.0b013e328339429a.

Yale, S. H., Nagib, N., & Guthrie, T. (2000). Approach to the vaso-occlusive crisis in adults with sickle cell disease. *American Family Physician, 61*(5), 1349-1356, 1363-1344.

Zemel, B. S., Kawchak, D. A., Ohene-Frempong, K., Schall, J. I., & Stallings, V. A. (2007). Effects of delayed pubertal development, nutritional status, and disease severity on longitudinal patterns of growth failure in children with sickle cell disease. *Pediatric Research, 61*(5 Pt 1), 607-613. doi: 10.1203/pdr.0b013e318045bdca.

34. Spina Bifida

Jo Ann Coco-Ripp

Spina bifida is a birth defect that affects the neural tube. The neural tube is the embryonic structure that eventually develops into the baby's brain, spinal cord, and the tissues that enclose them. Normally, the neural tube forms early and closes by the 28th day after conception. In babies with spina bifida, a portion of the neural tube fails to develop or close properly, causing defects in the spinal cord and in the bones of the spine. There are three types of spina bifida, ranging from mild to severe (Mayo Clinic, 2012):

Spina bifida occulta: An opening in one or more of the vertebrae of the spinal column without apparent damage to the spinal cord. There may be a birthmark or other outward sign in the area. However, most of the time no neurological symptoms occur and there are no other indications of the condition. Occasionally, the opening may be discovered when imaging tests are done for unrelated purposes.

Meningocele: The meninges, or protective covering around the spinal cord, have pushed out through the opening in the vertebrae in a sac called a meningocele. The spinal cord remains intact. This form can be repaired with little or no damage to the nerve pathways. Lasting impact is rare but individuals should be checked regularly for any problems that may be a result of the condition.

Myelomeningocele: This is the most severe form of spina bifida, in which a portion of the spinal cord itself protrudes through the back. In some cases, sacs are covered with skin; in others, tissue and nerves are exposed. Generally, people use the terms spina bifida and myelomeningocele interchangeably. The effects may include muscle weakness, loss of sensation or paralysis below the exposed area of the spine, and loss of bowel and bladder control. In addition, fluid may build up to cause an accumulation in the brain, a condition known as hydrocephalus. This is controlled by a surgical procedure that implants a shunt to relieve the fluid buildup. If a shunt is not implanted, the pressure buildup can cause brain damage, seizures, or blindness. Hydrocephalus may occur without spina bifida, but the two conditions often occur together. Treatment for the fluid buildup and other complications from the more severe forms may require several surgeries throughout childhood (NICHCY National Dissemination Center for Children with Disabilities, 2012).

Incidence/Prevalence in U.S.

It is believed that about 40% of all Americans may have a very minor form of spina bifida, but since they rarely show any symptoms, very few of them ever know that they have it. Together meningocele and myelomeningocele are known as spina bifida manifesta, which translates as spina bifida that can be observed. These occur in approximately one out of every thousand births. Of these infants born with spina bifida manifesta about 96% have myelomeningocele form (NICHCY National Dissemination Center for Children with Disabilities, 2012).

Predominant Age

Spina bifida is a birth defect that affects people for life (Spina Bifida Association of America, 2012). Various impacts may show up as a child develops or during adulthood. The age at which effects of spina bifida manifest themselves is quite unpredictable and very individualized both in terms of age of occurrence and form of manifestation. Results often show up as a person ages due to cumulative effects of activity involving the spine and multiple surgeries.

Causes

The causes of spina bifida are unknown. It appears to result from a combination of genetic and environmental risk factors, such as a family history of neural tube defects and folic acid deficiency (Mayo Clinic, 2012). Recent research has not yet made a definite link to folic acid but exploration is ongoing (Folic acid, 2012).

Systems Affected

The primary body system impacted by spina bifida is the nervous system, including the brain, spinal cord, and supporting tissues. ICF code s1 Structures of the Nervous System can be used to describe the structural defects. The functional consequences to the nervous system will generally be documented with codes in b1 Mental Functions. Secondary impacts may include the muscular system and urinary system as well as other systems, depending on the type and severity of the damage. Possible ICF codes include b6 Genitourinary and Reproductive Functions and b7 Neuromusculoskeletal and Movement-Related Functions.

Three areas of specific impact are explained in more detail. These areas can be described with the same broad set of ICF codes as spina bifida itself.

Hydrocephalus: About 70-90% of children with myelomeningocele develop hydrocephalus, a build-up of fluid in and around the brain (NICHCY National Dissemination Center for Children with Disabilities, 2012). Cerebrospinal fluid cushions and protects the brain and spinal cord. When the fluid is unable to circulate normally, it collects in and around the brain, causing the head to be enlarged. Without treatment, hydrocephalus can cause brain damage and mental retardation (Spina Bifida Association of America, 2012). Doctors usually treat hydrocephalus by surgically inserting a tube called a shunt that drains the excess fluid. The shunt runs under the skin into the chest or abdomen, and the fluid passes harmlessly into the child's body. A newer surgical procedure called endoscopic third ventriculostomy creates a new pathway for draining cerebrospinal fluid. This procedure may be recommended for some children older than six months, including some who experience shunt malfunctions (Gold & Salsberg, 2011).

Chiari II malformation: Nearly all children with myelomeningocele have an abnormal change in the position of the brain (Gold & Salsberg, 2011). The lower part of the brain is located farther down than normal and is partly displaced into the upper part of the spinal canal. This can block the flow of cerebrospinal fluid and contribute to hydrocephalus. In most cases, affected children have no other symptoms, but a small number develop serious problems, such as breathing and swallowing difficulties and upper body weakness (Gold & Salsberg, 2011). In these cases, doctors may recommend surgery to relieve pressure on the brain.

Tethered spinal cord: Most children with myelomeningocele, and a small number with meningocele or spina bifida occulta, have a tethered spinal cord (Mayo Clinic, 2012). This means that the spinal cord does not slide up and down as it should with movement of the spine because it is held in place by surrounding tissue. Some children have no symptoms, but others develop leg weakness, worsening leg function, scoliosis, pain in the back or legs, and changes in bladder function (Gold & Salsberg, 2011). Doctors usually recommend surgery to release the spinal cord from surrounding tissue. After surgery, a child usually returns to his developmental level of functioning (March of Dimes Foundation, 2012).

Secondary Problems

Spina bifida may occasionally cause no symptoms or only minor physical disabilities. More frequently, it leads to varied physical and mental complications. Factors that affect the severity of complications include size and location of the neural tube defect, whether skin covers the affected area, and which spinal nerves come out of the affected area of the spinal cord (Mayo Clinic, 2012).

Examples of complications or secondary conditions associated with spina bifida are latex allergy, obesity, skin problems, gastrointestinal disorders, attaining and retaining mobility, social, educational, and psychological issues (Spina Bifida Association of America, 2012). The first reports of latex allergies in people with spina bifida were in the late 1980s. Today, experts think latex could be a problem for up to 73% of children and youth with spina bifida. No one knows why people are allergic to latex. However, the Spina Bifida Association (2012) has information on latex allergies and a list of products containing latex. Allergies to products can be described with ICF code e115 Products and Technology for Personal Use in Daily Living.

Another health concern with high incidence for persons with spina bifida is obesity and the ramifications resulting from it. Children with hydrocephalus are at a very high risk for developing obesity. Beyond age six at least 50% of children who have spina bifida are overweight, and in adolescence and adulthood over 50% are obese (Spina Bifida Association of America, 2012). Part of the risk of obesity is connected to lack of activity, as it is harder for individuals who have spina bifida to have a physically active lifestyle due to mobility issues. In one cross-sectional study of 203 persons with spina bifida, Dosa et al. (2009) found the obesity rates for adults, particularly women, were much higher than the general population. More frequent hospitalization or other medical problems may also be a limiting factor to staying active. Obesity in turn may contribute to skin breakdown. It often is related to use of assistive devices for mobility, such as braces rubbing on leg areas (Spina Bifida Association of America, 2012). See the chapter on Obesity for information on documenting these issues.

Gastrointestinal disorders, as well as bowel and bladder incontinence issues, may be further complications for children and adults with spina bifida (Gold & Salsberg, 2011; March of Dimes Foundation, 2012). Individual assessment and evaluation is needed to pinpoint levels of need and impact. Issues can be described with ICF codes b515 Digestive Functions, b525 Defecation Functions, and b620 Urination Functions.

People with spina bifida get around in different ways. Depending on the part of the spine impacted, they may walk without any aids or assistance; walk with braces, crutches, or walkers; or use wheelchairs (Centers for Disease Control and Prevention, 2012). A promising treatment (NIH News, 2011) that repairs the spinal cord before birth has been shown to reduce the severity of secondary outcomes related to getting around. Although the likelihood of being able to walk depends on the location of the spinal malformation, children in the prenatal surgery group were more likely to be able to walk without orthotics or crutches (41.9%) than were children in the postnatal surgery group (20.9%). Mobility issues are described with ICF code d4 Mobility.

Spina bifida can affect social, educational, and psychological development. These can be documented with parts of ICF codes b125 Dispositions and Intra-Personal Functions, b126 Temperament and Personality Functions, d1 Learning and Applying Knowledge and d7 Interpersonal Interactions and Relationships.

Social development: In many cases, infants and children with spina bifida require early and frequent hospitalization. This can interrupt normal social development. The challenge is to balance medical needs with the need to let a child develop into a confident, self-sufficient, and independent adult.

Educational issues: The intelligence of individuals with spina bifida varies, just as it does with people in general; however, IQ scores of those with spina bifida cluster in the 70-90 range as opposed to the 100 range for those without it. Affected individuals often have poor short-term memory and poor organizational skills (MOMS, 2011). In some cases, children with spina bifida who also have a history of hydrocephalus experience learning problems. Early intervention with children who experience learning problems can help considerably to prepare them for school (Christopher and Dana Reeve Foundation, n.d.). Additional problems can occur as children with spina bifida get older. Children with myelomeningocele may develop learning disabilities, which can include difficulty paying attention, problems with language and reading comprehension, and trouble learning math (Mayo Clinic, 2012).

Psychological development: Children with special needs of any type often rebel against their disability when they realize it cannot be wished away. They may become depressed, defiant, or withdrawn. Early attention to these issues through peer support groups and/or counseling is often critical to healthy psychological development (MOMS, 2011).

Prognosis

With proper treatment, children with spina bifida can lead full lives. Most do well in school, and many play in sports (Foose & Ardovino, 2008). Because of advances in medicine, about 90% of babies born with spina bifida now live to adulthood, about 80% have normal intelligence, and about 75% play sports and do other fun activities (Spina Bifida Association of America, 2012). Recent studies have showed promising results from repairing the myelomeningocele in utero (Brooks, 2011; Spina Bifida Association, 2012). The procedure may prevent problems after birth and minimize need for shunting.

Assessment

Typical Scope of Team Assessment

Results from three tests during pregnancy may indicate spina bifida. The first test is a blood test during the 16th to 18th weeks of pregnancy, called the alpha-fetoprotein (AFP) screening test. Abnormally high levels of AFP suggest that the fetus has a neural tube defect (Mayo Clinic, 2012). This test is higher in about 75-80% of women who have a fetus with spina bifida (Spina Bifida Association of America, 2012). Confirmation of the AFP screening or further information is gathered from the second test, a fetal ultrasound often called a sonogram, which can show signs of spina bifida such as the open spine. A third test, maternal amniocentesis, takes a small amount of the fluid from the womb through a thin needle to look at protein levels (Mayo Clinic, 2012).

In some cases, spina bifida might not be diagnosed until after the baby is born due to the nature of neural tube defects. The symptoms or results of the defect may not be apparent. After birth, sometimes a hairy patch of skin or dimple on the baby's back indicates spina bifida. This can be confirmed through an image scan, such as an X-ray, MRI, or CT, to get a clearer view of the baby's spine and the bones in the back. Spina bifida occulta might not be diagnosed until late childhood or adulthood, or might never be diagnosed (Centers for Disease Control and Prevention, 2012). Prenatal screening is a personal choice and tests to check for spina bifida and other birth defects yield outcomes that have some unpredictability (Mayo Clinic, 2012).

Myelomeningocele can be seen after the child is born (National Institute of Neurological Disorders and Stroke, 2012). A diagnosis of spina bifida after birth still cannot be certain of the level of severity and impact on the individual. Assessments will be based on individual needs and symptoms. With infants and children, periodic re-assessments are suggested to target impacts of symptoms during development of the child. The choice of assessments depends on the form of spina bifida (March of Dimes Foundation, 2012). Areas for assessment may include:

Quality of life: According to Waters et al. (2009) the shift from a medical or absence of disease understanding of health to an approach that embraces subjective wellness and quality of life includes the need for other ways to assess individuals. The authors reviewed instruments that measure quality of life for individuals with neuro-disabilities and highlighted that different conditions have different quality of life issues and needs. Specific to spina bifida, the authors reviewed a study on children and adolescents by Parkin et al. (1997). Parkin et al. generated over 600 quality of life items through semi-structured interviews with children and adolescents with spina bifida and their parents. They identified items in 10 domains (social, emotional, intellectual, financial, medical, independence, environmental, physical functioning, recreation, and vocation — a mixture of well-being and functional domains). The items were used in the creation of *Spina Bifida Health Related Quality of Life Questionnaire*. Key concerns identified by parents of children with spina bifida revolved around social skills, self-care skills, emotional needs of the children and families, opportunities for independence, and the general public's perception of them. Consequently, Waters et al. (2009) suggested that disability-specific quality of life instruments, specifically the Spina Bifida Health Related Quality of Life Questionnaire, should be considered. Quality of life covers topics similar to the ICF codes. Document with ICF codes when it is appropriate for the treatment setting.

Transitions: Wellness and quality of life approaches embrace the idea that successful transitions from adolescence to adulthood may need to be planned. Specific needs may be targeted to support and smooth the way for more effectively living as an adult with spina bifida. According to information from the Proceedings of the First World Congress on Spina Bifida Research and Care (2009), much of the research related to transitioning from childhood through adolescence included validated measures and the majority used the constructs of activity and participation from the ICF. One measure under development, the *Adolescent Self-Management Independence Survey — version II* (AMIS-II), was used in several of the transition research studies. The development of this instrument has been presented at previous conferences and the current abstract evaluated the measure's psychometric properties using a sample of 135 parent-child dyads from four spina bifida clinics. The age range of the participants was 12 to 25 years. The 17-question AMIS-II demonstrates construct validity and reliability. The instrument has two factors: (1) Self-management: Independent Living, and (2) Self-management: Condition. The tool is administered by interview and measures the amount of independence across multiple domains, including personal care skills such as toileting and taking medications, and independent community living skills such as making and keeping appointments and refilling prescriptions. The AMIS-II was offered as a reliable tool to assess clinically relevant self-management skills in adolescents and young adults with spina bifida (Proceedings from the First World Congress on Spina Bifida Research and Care, 2009). An important ICF code group associated with transitions is d8 Major Life Areas. It is also important to be sure that the patient is aware of his/her rights and knows how to advocate for them. Any issues with advocating for rights can be documented with d940 Human Rights. Document with other ICF codes when it is appropriate for the treatment setting.

Personal care and self-management skills: Personal care and self-management skills are among the general functional skills that may need to be assessed for persons with spina bifida. The impact of spina bifida on functional abilities is very individualized and must be considered uniquely for each person. Due to the wide range and variety of times the symptoms present during a person's life, assessment of functional abilities may be a need during childhood or not until an individual is an adult. Gold and Salsberg (2011) suggest that results from the *Functional Independence Measure for Children* (Wee FIM) can yield helpful information related to self-care. ICF codes d230 Carrying Out Daily Routine, d250 Managing One's Own Behavior, and d5 Self-Care can be used for documenting the required skills.

Screening for use of assistive devices: The abilities vary greatly between individuals. This screening is especially for walking assistance. ICF codes in d4 Mobility may be used, especially d450 Walking.

Hand function: Hand function should be assessed in terms of preference; tactile discrimination; kinesthetic awareness; and ability and speed for performing activities such as page turning, grasp, and manipulation of small objects (Gold, & Salsberg, 2011). ICF codes b260 Proprioceptive Function, b265 Touch Function, b760 Control of Voluntary Movement Functions, d440 Fine Hand Use, and d445 Hand and Arm Use cover these issues.

Social skills: Children and adolescents, particularly individuals who have had several surgeries and hospitalizations or recurring complications, may exhibit social skill deficits from frequent absences or limited opportunities for participation in sports and recreation, thus an analysis of social-emotional functioning may be required (Gold, & Salsberg, 2011). ICF codes d710 Basic Interpersonal Interactions and d720 Complex Interpersonal Interactions cover the skills. Any deficits noted with particular people should be noted with other ICF codes in d7 Interpersonal Interactions and Relationships.

Activity level: For many children and adults with spina bifida, staying active and maintaining a healthy lifestyle remain a challenge. Therefore, the therapist should consider assessing the individual's leisure and recreation interests with a goal of increasing motivation to remain active. Functional abilities to be active can be documented with b130 Energy and Drive Functions. Other ICF codes such as d230 Carrying Out Daily Routine, d910 Community Life, and d920 Recreation and Leisure can document areas where activity deficits may be seen.

Cognition: The more the spinal cord is damaged, the greater the chance that a child will have learning problems. Children with severe hydrocephalus tend to have lower than average IQ scores. Complications from placement of shunts may hinder development of cognitive skills (Foose & Ardovino, 2008; Spina Bifida Association of America, 2008). Abilities in these areas will usually be documented with codes in b140-b189 Specific Mental Functions. Deficits in acquiring learning are documented with d1 Learning and Applying Knowledge.

Assessment baselines are gathered through various methods including direct request, observation within functional task, activity, or community settings, and standardized tools, as well as:

Chart reviews: Thorough reviews from other healthcare evaluations related to mobility, cognitive development, educational needs, and psychosocial issues (Foose, & Ardovino, 2008; Gold, & Salsberg, 2011). A description of joint contractures, joint deformity, neurological level of impairment, self-care skills, extent of pressure sores, cardiovascular fitness, and muscular strength may be some areas found from this review (Gold, & Salsberg, 2011).

Individualized Education Plan (IEP): For the school age child, obtaining results from testing and an IEP will be helpful in overall assessment. A child who is doing well might also benefit from neuropsychological tests that include results from learning about sequencing, organization, and problem solving, as these skills have been found to be a predictor of academic success, especially if discerned prior to fourth grade (Spina Bifida Association of America, 2012).

As a final consideration, the therapist should take into account the classification of spina bifida within the treatment setting. It is often classified as an orthopedic or neurological disability. However, due to the early onset and possible cognitive impairment, some classify it as a developmental disability (Foose, & Ardovino, 2008). These two areas of classification can lead to further assessment support. For example, with spinal cord injuries, assessment for transfer training may be needed; or with intellectual impairment, assessment for receptive and expressive language skills. Even though assessment may be very individualized, being able to target particular areas will be the most effective way to find the specific treatment needed. A full set of deficits that are recorded with ICF codes will allow for complete treatment planning.

Areas of Concern for RT Assessment

Results from RT assessments will vary depending on many factors related to the individual and the setting. Results for children and adolescents will also need to be considered in the context of family involvement. An individual with spina bifida may be seen by a recreational therapist in a school setting, a hospital, a rehabilitation setting, or a community setting. In addition to these settings, sometimes an individual may be seen in a behavioral health setting. Common strengths that may be found are support from family, friends, other professionals such as a teacher, or other persons with spina bifida. These supports should be documented with ICF codes in e3 Support and Relationships. Typical problem areas involve management of secondary issues such as bladder control, latex sensitivity, or learning disabilities and their impact on social skills or self-confidence. Sedentary lifestyles are observed more often than with the typical person, so lack of physical activity is another common area found. Another area of need, primarily for adolescents and young adults, is independent living skills. As the individual with

spina bifida matures, the needs may change to skills and resources for friendship development and healthy leisure time activities. ICF codes to document all of these areas have been discussed.

ICF Core Set

No ICF Core Set has been defined for Spina Bifida.

Treatment Direction

Within 48 hours after birth the exposed nerves and spinal cord are put back into the spinal canal. A shunt may need to be inserted if hydrocephalus occurs. Release of the spinal cord from surrounding tissue may need to be done for some impacts from a tethered spinal cord (March of Dimes Foundation, 2012; Mayo Clinic, 2012).

Ongoing care from the team may involve treatment for bowel and bladder problems, as well as training to use assistive devices (Spina Bifida Association of America, 2012).

Avoiding obesity and maintaining a healthy weight is a challenge that may require ongoing treatment (NICHCY National Dissemination Center for Children with Disabilities, 2012).

Minimizing effects from secondary problems such as latex sensitivity, learning difficulties, and depression are also required throughout the client's life (Spina Bifida Association of America, 2012).

Whole Team Approach

Working with the individual and close family members is the best approach when the person is a child or infant, as advocating for appropriate services in both healthcare and education settings requires a supportive network from family and others. Any lack of support documented with e3 Support and Relationships should be addressed as early in the treatment process as possible (Joseph, 2007; March of Dimes Foundation, 2012; NICHCY National Dissemination Center for Children with Disabilities, 2012). For adolescents and adults, the family involvement may not be as critical because self-advocacy skills can be an effective means to achieve positive outcomes (Gold, & Salsberg, 2011).

Because spina bifida affects so many body systems, it is important that professionals from many areas be consulted to provide up-to-date and comprehensive medical, psychological, and social evaluation, support, and treatment. There are many spina bifida clinics throughout the country that bring the appropriate specialists together to provide the necessary care (Mayo Clinic, 2012; MOMS, 2011).

Recreational Therapy Approach

The focus of recreational therapy generally follows the whole team approach, with a particular focus on maintaining healthy body weight and involvement in physical activity (d570 Looking After One's Health, d920 Recreation and Leisure); development of lifetime sport, recreation, or leisure skills through leisure education and specialized skill development (d920 Recreation and Leisure); and prevention of secondary consequences such as depression (b126 Temperament and Personality Functions). Leger (2005) found that youth with spina bifida who reported high levels of life satisfaction participated in recreation, sport activities, and other aspects of young adult living, yet had concerns for the secondary problems that were part of spina bifida. Thus, the focus for a person with spina bifida would be living well with the disability and preventing the impact of secondary problems (Dickens & McMillen, 2003). Foose and Ardovino (2008) suggest increased sense of self and empowerment through leisure activities (b125 Dispositions and Intra-Personal Functions, b126 Temperament and Personality Functions) can offset frequent complications from surgeries, increased susceptibility to infections, and bladder/bowel dysfunctions. Further, loss of strength (b730 Muscle Power Functions) and inactive lifestyles (d570 Looking After One's Health) from secondary problems can be balanced with an emphasis on physical activity during leisure and recreation (Swann-Guerrero & Mackey, 2008). Motivation to participate in recreation or other socially centered activities may need interventions such as social skills training (b122 Global Psychosocial Functions, b125 Dispositions and Intra-Personal Functions, b126 Temperament and Personality Functions, d7 Interpersonal Interactions and Relationships) or coping skills (d240 Handling Stress and Other Psychological Demands) given the unique stressors of pediatric illness and disability (Gold & Salsberg, 2011).

Recent trends in the research and care of persons with spina bifida can be seen from presentations and sessions at the First and Second World Congresses for Spina Bifida (Abstracts, 2009; Abstracts, 2012; Keynote, 2012; Proceedings, 2009). Several areas of focus discussed at these events included key areas that are commonly addressed by recreational therapists, including:

Transitions: Programs and interventions that support adolescents in making the transition from living with family to independent living are important (e.g., d210 Undertaking a Single Task, d220 Undertaking Multiple Tasks, d230 Carrying Out Daily Routine, d5 Self-Care, d910 Community Life). These may be individual skill development areas or groups that foster interdependent learning.

Physical activity, participation, and health promotion: Individuals who use a wheelchair or other assistive device for ambulation have a greater need to learn skills and techniques to remain physically active as they age. ICF codes that need to be addressed include those in d4 Mobility. Sports, special events, clubs, and recreation skill development (d910 Community Life, d920 Recreation and Leisure) are important. Cognitive behavioral therapy may also be an approach for some individuals who have difficulty with healthy lifestyle development.

Psychosocial and quality of life outcomes: Persons with spina bifida sometimes have a perspective on life that is unique due to spending so much time during childhood in surgery recovery or other issues related to management of physical needs. Coping skills or quality of life issues may be a target area of treatment. Developing assertiveness skills (b125 Dispositions and Intra-Personal Functions), advocacy abilities (d940 Human Rights, d950 Political Life and Citizenship) or moving in a positive direction for psychosocially healthy behaviors (d570 Looking After One's Health) are often needed but sometimes overlooked in the specific treatment plan.

Leisure education programs, specialized camps, health or wellness programs for teens, as well as targeted family sessions, are suggested ways to incorporate information from these international gatherings of leaders in prevention and healthcare focused on spina bifida for recreational therapy (Conference Program, 2012).

From a national research agenda developed specifically for persons with spina bifida, two main areas have elements that relate to recreational therapy practice (Spina Bifida Foundation, n. d.):

Behavioral health: Research on social issues including a variety of challenges, barriers, and ways to improve socialization skills (e.g., d7 Interpersonal Interactions and Relationships), as well as improving family functioning (d760 Family Relationships) is encouraged.

Independence: Targeted elements in this area are increasing capacity for independence, and decreasing barriers, as well as multiple focal points for teaching and learning self-care (d5 Self-Care).

Recreational Therapy Interventions

Interventions frequently used by recreational therapy include leisure education programs, specific skill development, such as wheelchair basketball or other adaptive sports, learning to use adaptive equipment or adapt activities, therapeutic horseback riding, and programs with goals of increasing coping skills (b126 Temperament and Personality Functions, d240 Handling Stress and Other Psychological Demands), social interaction skills (d7 Interpersonal Interactions and Relationships), or self-identity (b122 Global Psychosocial Functions) (Foose & Ardovino, 2008; Gold & Salsberg, 2011; Zabriskie, Lundberg, & Groff, 2005). Increasing motivation (b130 Energy and Drive Functions) to maintain adequate physical activity levels for health is important at every level of a person's development. Verhoef et al. (2007) additionally suggest the inclusion of coping skills (b152 Emotional Functions, d240 Handling Stress and Other Psychological Demands) to offset perceived poor health among young adults with spina bifida. Maintaining muscular function (b730-b749 Muscle Functions) sufficient for daily living skills through activity is often a focus of interventions (Swann-Guerrero & Mackey, 2008). Brinton (2006) recommends swimming and horseback riding as particularly beneficial activities, not only for the advantages from the physical activity but also for the psychosocial benefits from involvement. Zabriskie, Lundberg, and Groff (2005) demonstrated a wide variety of positive outcomes from participation in either alpine skiing or horseback riding programs for a group of individuals with disabilities, which included those with spina bifida. They found the benefits extended beyond learning the specific sport skill and improving physical aspects such as muscular strength (b730 Muscle Power Functions) or balance (b755 Involuntary Movement Reaction

Functions, d415 Maintaining a Body Position). Sports also provided an important context for social interaction and feedback from others (d7 Interpersonal Interactions and Relationships). A programmatic finding from this study also was interesting. Most subjects (96%) chose to participate in the three- or five-week programs instead of a single lesson or experience. Such a finding suggests that participants in this community-based therapeutic recreation and adaptive sport program were willing to commit to, and preferred, longer and more consistent program participation rather than briefer experiences. The implication for recreational therapy intervention planning is that more resources should be committed to programs that promote consistent participation for longer periods of time. Participants are seeking referrals to programs that provide time to develop skills and benefits that a shorter or one-time experience cannot provide.

According to a recent questionnaire study of 179 persons with spina bifida, restrictions in several areas inhibit participation in leisure and other areas (Barf et al., 2009). Perceived specific hindrances included individual physical problems (e.g., b455 Exercise Tolerance Functions), building accessibility (e.g., e150 Design, Construction, and Building Products and Technology of Buildings for Public Use), transportation (d470 Using Transportation), and emotional barriers (b125 Dispositions and Intra-Personal Functions). Barf et al. (2009) recommended more focus be directed to reduction of participation restrictions, especially with respect to leisure activities. Boudos (2009) described a program for increasing participation for teens and young adults in community activities. The program had a transition coordinator who facilitated the changes for 101 persons. After a year, there was a 17% increase in participation across all involved. In this study the internal barrier of motivation (b130 Energy and Drive Functions) appeared to be an inhibiting factor for participants. Information from both of these studies might be used as the foundation to develop a community integration intervention for young adults to gain independence as they transition from living with parents.

Functional Skills

In a study of youth (N=60) with spina bifida, Leger (2005) reported on functional status outcomes using the *Functional Independence Measure* (FIM). The FIM scores indicated the youth were fairly independent even though many had lower item scores, particularly in bladder (b620 Urination Functions) and sphincter control (b525 Defecation Functions) and ability to traverse 14 stairs independently (d460 Moving Around in Different Locations). High scoring areas were self-care (d5 Self-Care) and transfers (d420 Transferring Oneself). Similarly, Dickens and McMillen (2003) stressed that management of varied secondary conditions, which may change at different developmental stages, is crucial to maintaining a high quality of life with spina bifida. They reported some of the common physical challenges reported were pain (b280 Sensation of Pain), skin break-down and pressure sores (d5200 Caring for Skin), mobility limitations (d4 Mobility), latex allergy (e115 Products and Technology for Personal Use in Daily Living), difficulties with endurance (b455 Exercise Tolerance Functions, b740 Muscle Endurance Functions), and difficulties with balance (b755 Involuntary Movement Reaction Functions, d415 Maintaining a Body Position). Due to the nature of spina bifida and the complications that may accompany this condition, the groups also reported physical challenges that differ across the ages. Some individuals between the ages of six and 18 years reported having scoliosis (s760 Structure of Trunk) and breathing difficulties (b440 Respiration Functions) during a time of rapid growth. As youth reach the teen years through young adulthood, many also reported difficulties with weight gain (b530 Weight Maintenance Functions) and concern about sexuality (b640 Sexual Functions, d770 Intimate Relationships).

Primary areas of focus in developing functional skills include:

Muscular ability to walk or use assistive device: Similar to other orthopedic disabilities, people with spina bifida use assistive devices such as walkers, braces, wheelchairs, splints, or crutches (Foose & Ardovino, 2008). Learning how to use the assistive devices correctly and becoming proficient in moving with them (d4 Mobility, especially d465 Moving Around Using Equipment) will improve functional status. Regular physical activity is important for all people, but especially for those with conditions that affect movement, such as spina bifida. The CDC

(2012) recommends 60 minutes of physical activity a day.

Motor function to complete activities of daily living: Encouraging independence at all stages of development is aided by having the necessary physical strength (b730 Muscle Power Functions), coordination (b760 Control of Voluntary Movement Functions), and other motor abilities (d4 Mobility) to complete self-care (d5 Self-Care) and daily tasks (d230 Carrying Out Daily Routine) (Gold & Salsberg, 2011). There may be some self-care skills that are specific to spina bifida, such as bowel and bladder programs (e115 Products and Technology for Personal Use in Daily Living, b620 Urination Functions, b525 Defecation Functions), taking medications (d570 Looking After One's Health), skin care (d5200 Caring for Skin), and transfers (d420 Transferring Oneself). All of these self-care skills will enable individuals with spina bifida to take charge of their health and increase their independence (Dickens & McMillen, 2003).

Problem solving to negotiate community living: For adolescents involved in the public school exceptional child program, when the person with spina bifida reaches 14 years old, both the family and the teen should be involved in the development of a transition plan to ensure that priorities are successfully addressed regarding the youth's transition into post-secondary school, work, and/or independent living (d8 Major Life Areas). This is a specific requirement for the Individualized Education Plan (IEP) and recreational therapy is a related service that can be involved with community living skills. Problem solving skills (d175 Solving Problems) are important for successful transition and part of learning to manage in adulthood (Gold & Salsberg, 2011).

Skills to access transportation, such as adapted vehicle or public systems: In addition to the ability to navigate with personal assistive devices, acquiring skills to use an adapted vehicle or access public transportation systems is necessary for transition to independent living. All of these are aspects of ICF code d4 Mobility. Individuals with spina bifida will become more confident as they gain the skills to access their community. As adults, social isolation (d710 Basic Interpersonal Interactions, d750 Informal Social Relationships) can be a problem (Gold & Salsberg, 2011), thus the more independent a person becomes, the more s/he will find social interaction opportunities presented through work, higher education, or recreation. Self-advocacy (d940 Human Rights) in relation to transportation is a skill that an individual with spina bifida can begin to practice as early as middle school (CDC, 2012).

Coping strategies for impacts from daily stressors and other secondary sources: Foose and Ardovino (2008) state that repeated operations and possible complications from secondary conditions may bring additional and unique stress into the lives of persons with spina bifida. In addition, prolonged absence from school or social isolation as a young adult (Gold & Salsberg, 2011) can add hassles that create the need for enhancing coping techniques. Physical activity and sport involvement can provide one source of coping or stress reduction (d240 Handling Stress and Other Psychological Demands) for persons with spina bifida in addition to the physical (e.g., b455 Exercise Tolerance Functions) and social benefits (d750 Informal Social Relationships) (Brinton, 2006; CDC, 2012; NICHCY, 2012; Swann-Guerrero & Mackey, 2008). Gold and Salsberg (2011) stress that psychosocial needs should be carefully assessed and addressed on an individualized basis at various stages of development with particular attention to transition points such as reintegration from a hospital stay.

Education, Training, and Counseling

According to Fogarty, Hodges, and Wilhite (2007), a key timeframe for increased quality of life is during adolescence. They recommend many strategies that therapists can use to influence youth with spina bifida to increase physical activity (b455 Exercise Tolerance Functions, d570 Looking After One's Health) in their lives such as involvement in adapted sports, support groups, or interest clubs. Other areas of education, training, and counseling might also increase involvement in improved social life (d7 Interpersonal Interactions and Relationships, d910 Community Life). These include exploration of leisure interests, community resources, and adaptive equipment for play or sports (Dickens & McMillen, 2003; Spina Bifida Association of America, 2012). Leisure education sessions are suggested to decrease episodes of depression in persons who have indications of serious problems with mood disorders (b125 Dispositions and Intra-

Personal Functions, b126 Temperament and Personality Functions) (Foose & Ardovino, 2008).

Community Integration

Upon diagnosis of spina bifida, families often become involved in local or national organizations for support, advocacy, and activities (March of Dimes Foundation, 2012; Mayo Clinic, 2012; MOMS, 2011). Many community organizations provide a range of services for children and adults with spina bifida (d910 Community Life, d940 Human Rights). BlazeSports America (BlazeSports, 2011) is an example of one provider that promotes advocacy and positive impacts from involvement at all levels. They have training sessions for individuals, assist with sports competition, and provide consulting services with a recreational therapist in a family format. The National Ability Center (Zabriskie, Lundberg, & Groff, 2005) is another community organization that provides quality, year-round therapeutic recreation programs. Often the referral for a community service provider is made by the therapist in the hospital or through the school district. Community reintegration offered through recreational therapy services at the Rehabilitation Institute of Chicago (2011) is an example of a program that provides treatment and recreation in a community setting.

Health Promotion

Fletcher and Brei (2010) provide a new framework for research, treatment approaches, and health outcomes in the introduction to a special issue of *Developmental Disabilities Research Reviews* that is focused entirely on a multidisciplinary perspective for spina bifida. The authors state that current movement is toward a quality-of-life view rather than a strictly medical model. They also state that individuals with spina bifida are more routinely living into adulthood and longer as adults. This phenomenon means that successful transition from childhood to adulthood is becoming increasingly important. Furthermore, they encourage further research on activities and societal participation for effective healthy lives for persons with spina bifida. Another aspect of health promotion is discussed by Sawin et al. (2009). They focused specifically on self-management issues for adolescent females with spina bifida. They found that assessment and intervention for self-management for this population is critical for transitioning to adulthood and independent living. Liptak, Dosa, and Kennedy (2009) discuss a new way to evaluate transition for youth with spina bifida. They provide helpful information on how they applied the ICF Model with a nationally representative sample of 129 youth over a three-year span. They suggest that data from this approach can lead to interventions that improve transition for youth with spina bifida. Transitions generally involve ICF codes in d5 Self-Care, d7 Interpersonal Interactions and Relationships, and d8 Major Life Areas.

A comprehensive systematic literature review was conducted for the years 2001 to 2009 that focused on any aspect of the ICF in health-related journals (Cerniauskaite et al., 2011). From the criteria of the review, 670 articles remained for the analysis. One interesting result from this review showed that 47 articles used the ICF in context of a specific health condition. The top three conditions among these 47 articles are stroke, multiple sclerosis, and rheumatoid arthritis. Spina bifida was not specifically mentioned in any of the articles. The findings from this systematic review on the ICF suggest future scholarly work, research, and publications on spina bifida include use of ICF as a framework for various aspects of health promotion.

Most of the health promotion emphasis for a person with spina bifida is focused on increased quality of life, such as involvement in sports, recreation, and leisure activities. Management of secondary problems such as obesity due to inactivity or depression is channeled through advocacy of increased physical activity and involvement in a variety of community functions. Essner and Holmbeck (2010) examined the impact of family, peer, and school contexts on depressive symptoms (b126 Temperament and Personality Functions) in youth with spina bifida (N=60 families), as compared with adolescents without spina bifida (N=65 families). Results indicated that adolescents with spina bifida had fewer total positive contexts and less positive experience in peer and school contexts, as compared to typically developing adolescents. Greater total numbers of positive contexts and higher levels of positive experiences in family and school contexts were associated with fewer depressive symptoms for both groups. Positive peer experiences were related to lower depressive symptoms for typically develop-

ing adolescents only. The findings suggest that having fewer positive contexts may place adolescents with spina bifida at risk for higher levels of depressive symptoms (Essner & Holmbeck, 2010). Thus, it is critical to provide motivation for children and adolescents to develop positive social engagements with family and peers (d750 Informal Social Relationships, d760 Family Relationships), if deficits have been found. It is also critical to acquire a variety of physical activity interests, to maintain lifelong health-related quality of life (d570 Looking After One's Health) while living with spina bifida and managing secondary conditions (Leger, 2005; Swann-Guerrero & Mackey, 2008).

Resources

BlazeSports America

www.blazesports.org

BlazeSports America is a 501(c)(3) nonprofit organization resulting from organization efforts for the 1996 Paralympic Games held in Atlanta, GA. Today the organization is a multifaceted, comprehensive service provider that advocates for sports participation opportunities for persons with physical disabilities. It is internationally recognized and serves as an affiliate with many local and regional providers. BlazeSports serves in several capacities with Paralympic committees for specific disability groups. Their website and staff provide cutting edge information and support research for best practices for persons with disabilities and sports participation.

Disabled Sports USA

www.dsusa.org

An organization that promotes sports participation and competition for persons with a variety of disabilities, primarily those with neuromuscular and orthopedic conditions. DSUSA has chapters in all areas of the country and serves as the sanctioning body for Paralympics sports competition. Sports and competition as a foundation for rehabilitation is part of the philosophical foundation of the organization.

Spina Bifida and Hydrocephalus Association of Southern Alberta

www.sbhac.ca

A Canadian association that provides easy-to-find information in layperson's language. There are links to organizations across Canada and a section on sports and recreation resources.

Intermountain Spina Bifida Support Group

utahspinabifida.org/

The Intermountain Spina Bifida Support Group brings together persons with spina bifida, their families, and others who support the efforts in order to connect them to resources through blogs, social gatherings, educational events, and other advocacy support. This group is an example of a state and regional support system for persons with spina bifida.

Christopher and Dana Reeve Foundation

www.christopherreeve.org/site/c.ddJFKRNoFiG/b.40 48063/k.C5D5/Christopher_Reeve_Spinal_Cord_Injury_and_Paralysis_Foundation.htm

Prompted by Christopher Reeve's accident, this foundation began in 1982 with the mission to cure spinal cord injury. Since its beginnings it has evolved into a highly respected foundation that promotes the health and well-being of persons with spinal cord injuries, paralysis, and other mobility impairments through advocacy, research, information, and resources.

Victory Junction Gang Camp

www.victoryjunction.org/

Victory Junction has provided camping and outdoor experiences for a variety of children with chronic medical or disabling conditions since 2004. There is a NASCAR-themed week for children with spina bifida. The camp has American Camp Association and Association of Hole in the Wall Camps accreditations with active involvement by many medical, human service, local persons, and celebrities. The Petty racing family founded the camp, which is located in North Carolina with plans to expand to Kansas soon.

National Center for Physical Activity and Disability (NCPAD)

www.ncpad.org/

An information center concerned with physical activity and disability. The site offers links to valuable topic areas such as disability or condition, research, presentations, videos, references, or programs such as the video *Teens on the Move: An Exercise Video for Teens with Spina Bifida.* www.ncpad.org/videos/fact_sheet.php?sheet=469

Spina Bifida Association

www.spinabifidaassociation.org

A member organization for anyone who lives with the challenges of SB. Since 1973, it has been the only national voluntary health agency solely dedicated to enhancing the lives of those with SB. Its tools are education, advocacy, research, and service. There is information about published research, ongoing studies, and updated findings. The SBA was a co-sponsor of the First and Second World Congresses on Spina Bifida Research and Care. Information from these congresses can be accessed through the SBA website.

Mayo Clinic

www.mayoclinic.com/health/spina-bifida/DS00417

Provides useful, up-to-date information and tools to empower people to manage their own health.

National Institute of Neurological Disorders and Stroke

www.ninds.nih.gov/disorders/spina_bifida/spina_bifida.htm

Offers information aimed at finding ways to treat, prevent, and ultimately cure disorders such as spina bifida.

National Library of Medicine

www.nlm.nih.gov/medlineplus/spinabifida.html

MedlinePlus is the National Institutes of Health web produced by the National Library of Medicine to provide information about diseases, conditions, and wellness issues in easy-to-understand language.

NICHCY National Dissemination Center for Children with Disabilities

www.nichcy.org/Disabilities/Specific/Pages/SpinaBifida.aspx

NICHCY is a central location for information focused on disabilities in children and youth; programs and services for infants, children, and youth with disabilities; IDEA, the nation's special education law; No Child Left Behind, the nation's general education law; and research-based information on effective practices for children with disabilities.

Centers for Disease Control and Prevention

www.cdc.gov/ncbddd/spinabifida/

CDC.gov is CDC's primary online communication channel that provides users with credible, reliable health information.

March of Dimes Foundation

www.marchofdimes.com/default.html

Organization that has a primary focus of prevention and support for parents

References

Abstracts from the First World Congress on Spina Bifida Research and Care. (2009). http://medicalconference.spinabifidaassociation.org/site/c.gn KOKTOtHqE/b.3512717/k.BE78/Home.htm.

Abstracts from the Second World Congress on Spina Bifida Research and Care. (2012). http://www.worldcongressonsb.org/Abstracts/abstracts.

Barf, H. A., Post, M. W. M., Verhoef, M., Jennekens-Schinkel, A., Gooskens, R. H. J. M., & Prevo, A. J. H. (2009). Restrictions in social participation of young adults with spina bifida. *Disability and Rehabilitation, 31*(11), 921-927.

Boudos, R. (2009). Barriers to community participation. In Abstracts from the First World Congress on Spina Bifida Research and Care. http://medicalconference.spinabifidaassociation.org/site/c.gn KOKTOtHqE/b.3512717/k.BE78/Home.htm.

Brinton, L. (2006). Spina bifida and Jean Driscoll. Retrieved from http://www.pelinks4u.org/articles/spinabifida.htm.

BlazeSports. (2011). BlazeSports America programs. Retrieved from http://www.blazesports.org/get-involved/programs/.

Brooks, M. (2011). Prenatal myelomeningocele repair improves outcomes: The MOMS trial. *Medscape Today Medical New.* Retrieved from http://www.medscape.com/viewarticle/737139.

Centers for Disease Control and Prevention (CDC). (2012). Spina bifida. Retrieved from http://www.cdc.gov/ncbddd/spinabifida/index.html.

Cerniauskaite, M., Quintas, R., Boldt, C., Raggi, A., Cieza, A., Bickenbach, J. E., & Leonardi, M. (2011). Systematic literature review on ICF from 2001 to 2009: Its use, implementation and operationalisation. *Disability and Rehabilitation, 33*(4), 281-309.

Christopher and Dana Reeve Foundation. (n.d.). Spina bifida. Retrieved from http://www.christopherreeve.org/atf/cf/%7B3d83418f-b967-4c18-8ada-adc2e5355071%7D/Spina%20Bifida%206-09.PDF.

Conference Program from the Second World Congress on Spina Bifida Research and Care. (2012). http://www.worldcongressonsb.org/.

Dickens, P. & McMillen, J. S. (2003). Growing up with spina bifida: What we have learned: Quality of life and secondary conditions in individuals with spina bifida. The North Carolina Office on Disability and Health. Retrieved from http://www.fpg.unc.edu/~ncodh/pdfs/SpinaBifida.pdf.

Dosa, N. P., Foley, J. T., Eckrich, M., Woodall-Rupp, D., & Liptak, G. S. (2009). Obesity across the lifespan among persons with spina bifida. *Disability and Rehabilitation, 31*(11), 914-920.

Essner, B. S. & Holmbeck, G. N. (2010). The impact of family, peer, and school contexts on depressive symptoms in adolescents with spina bifida. *Rehabilitation Psychology, 55*(4), 340-350. Retrieved 7/14/2011, from REHABDATA database.

Fletcher, J. M. & Brei, T. J. (2010). Introduction: Spina bifida: A multidisciplinary perspective. *Developmental Disabilities Research Review, 16*(1), 1-5. doi: 10.1002/ddrr.101.

Fogarty, E., Hodges, J. S., & Wilhite, B. (2007). Activity patterns of youth with spina bifida. *American Journal of Recreation Therapy, 6*(4), 19-26.

Folic acid. (2012). Retrieved from http://www.spinabifidaassociation.org/site/c.evKRI7OXIoJ8 H/b.8273719/k.2152/Folic_Acid.htm.

Foose, A. & Ardovino, P. (2008). Therapeutic recreation and developmental disabilities. In T. Robertson & T. Long (Eds.), *Foundations of therapeutic recreation* (pp. 127-144). Champaign, IL: Human Kinetics.

Gold, J. T. & Salsberg, D. (2011). Pediatric disorders: Cerebral palsy and spina bifida. In S. R. Flanagan, H. Zaretsky, & A. Moroz (Eds.). *Medical aspects of disability: A handbook for the rehabilitation professional* (4th ed.) (pp 307-347). New York: Springer.

Joseph, D. B. (2007). Current challenges in spina bifida care. *The Scientific World Journal: TSW Urology 7*, 1930-1931. doi: 10.1100/tsw.2007.263.

Keynote Presentations from the Second World Congress on Spina Bifida Research and Care. (2012). Retrieved from http://www.worldcongressonsb.org/Sessions/keynote-presentations.

Leger, R. R. (2005). Severity of illness, functional status, and HRQoL in youth with spina bifida. *Rehabilitation Nursing, 30*(5), 180-188.

Liptak, G., Dosa, N., & Kennedy, J. (2009). Youth with spina bifida and transitions: Using the WHO ICF model in a nationally representative sample. In Abstracts from the First World Congress on Spina Bifida Research and Care (2009). http://medicalconference.spinabifidaassociation.org/site/c.gn KOKTOtHqE/b.3512717/k.BE78/Home.htm.

March of Dimes Foundation. (2012). Birth defects: Spina bifida. Retrieved from http://www.marchofdimes.com/baby/birthdefects_spinabifida .html.

Mayo Clinic. (2012). Causes. Retrieved from http://www.mayoclinic.com/health/spina-bifida/DS00417/DSECTION=causes.

MOMS: Management of Myelomeningocele Study. (2011). Retrieved from http://www.spinabifidamoms.com/english/index.html.

National Institute of Neurological Disorders and Stroke. (2012). NINDS Spina Bifida Information Page. Retrieved from http://www.ninds.nih.gov/disorders/spina_bifida/spina_bifida .htm.

NICHCY National Dissemination Center for Children with Disabilities. (2012). Spina bifida. Retrieved from http://nichcy.org/disability/specific/spinabifida.

NIH News. (2011). Surgery on fetus reduces complications of spina bifida. Retrieved from http://www.nih.gov/news/health/feb2011/nichd-09.htm.

Parkin, P. C., Rosenbaum, P. L., Fehlings, D. L., Van Nie, A., Willan, A. R., & King, D. (1997). Development of a health-related quality of life instrument for use in children with spina bifida. *Quality of Life Research, 6*(2), 123-132.

Proceedings from the First World Congress on Spina Bifida Research and Care. (2009). Retrieved from http://www.cdc.gov/ncbddd/orders/pdfs/207256-A_SpinaBifida_11_13FinalProof.pdf.

Rehabilitation Institute of Chicago (RIC). (2011). Therapeutic recreation programming and services. Retrieved from http://www.ric.org/conditions/therapeutic-rec/programs-services/index.aspx.

Sawin, K. J., Bellin, M. H., Roux, G., Buran, C. F., & Brei, T. J. (2009). The experience of self-management in adolescent women with spina bifida. *Rehabilitation Nursing, 34*, 26-38.

Spina Bifida Association. (2012). The Management of Myelomeningocele Study (MOMS). Retrieved from http://www.spinabifidaassociation.org/site/c.evKRI7OXIoJ8 H/b.8031517/apps/s/content.asp?ct=12059071.

Spina Bifida Association of America. (2012). Health information sheets. Retrieved from http://www.spinabifidaassociation.org/site/c.evKRI7OXIoJ8 H/b.8029553/k.7027/Health_Information_Sheets.htm.

Spina Bifida Association of America. (2012). Latex list. Retrieved from http://www.spinabifidaassociation.org/atf/cf/%7B85f88192-26e1-421e-9e30-4c0ea744a7f0%7D/SBA-LATEXLIST-2012-ENGLISH.PDF.

Spina Bifida Foundation. (n.d.). A National Spina Bifida Research Agenda. Retrieved from http://www.kintera.org/atf/cf/%7BEED435C8-F1A0-4A16-B4D8-A713BBCD9CE4%7D/Research_Agenda1.pdf.

Swann-Guerrero, S. & Mackey, C. (2008). Wellness through physical activity. In T. Robertson & T. Long (Eds.), *Foundations of therapeutic recreation* (pp. 199-216). Champaign, IL: Human Kinetics.

Verhoef, M., Post, M. W. M., Barf, H. A., van Asbeck, F. W. A., Gooskens, R. H. J. M., & Prevo, A. J. H. (2007). Perceived health in young adults with spina bifida. *Developmental Medicine and Child Neurology, 49*, 192-197.

Waters, E., Davis, E., Ronen, G. M., Rosenbaum, P., Livingston, M., & Saigal, S. (2009). Quality of life instruments for children and adolescents with neurodisabilities: How to choose the appropriate instrument. *Developmental Medicine and Child Neurology, 51*, 660-669.

Zabriskie, R. B., Lundberg, N. R., & Groff, D. G. (2005). Quality of life and identity: The benefits of a community-based therapeutic recreation and adaptive sports program. *Therapeutic Recreation Journal, 39*(3), 176-191.

35. Spinal Cord Injury

Nannette M. Vliet and Andrew P. Bogenschutz

The spinal cord is a network of millions of nerve fibers that are responsible for transmitting information from the brain to all parts of the human body and back to the brain. Along with the brain, the spinal cord is part of the central nervous system (CNS), and connects to nerve roots in the peripheral nervous system (PNS). The PNS is outside of the spinal cord and is responsible for communicating information between the body and the CNS.

The spinal cord is divided into ascending and descending tracts. The ascending nerve bundles are responsible for carrying information, such as temperature, joint position, pain, and touch sensations, from the body to the brain. The descending tracts are responsible for communicating information from the brain to the body to initiate movement and control bodily functions. A spinal cord injury (SCI) occurs when the spinal cord is damaged as a result of trauma, disease, or disorder. When the spinal cord is damaged, communication is interrupted and can result in temporary or permanent loss of movement and/or sensation.

Classification of Injury

SCI is classified by level of injury and type of injury. The types of paralysis and related function depend on the level of injury. Where applicable, a syndrome is added to the classification. Each is reviewed below.

Level of Injury

The vertebral column is divided into five segments in descending order starting from the base of the skull: cervical (seven vertebrae with eight cervical nerve roots, C1-C8), thoracic (twelve vertebrae, T1-T12), lumbar (five vertebrae, L1-L5), sacral (five vertebrae, S1-S5) and coccygeal (five fused bones, referred to as the coccygeal). The spinal cord runs through the vertebral column and two nerve roots exit at each vertebra. Damage to the spinal cord or nerves is what is meant by SCI, not damage to the vertebrae. However, in order to classify the area of the spinal cord or nerve impairment, the corresponding vertebra level is identified. For example, in a traumatic event the spinal nerve may have been damaged where it exited the fourth cervical vertebra (C4) even though that vertebra may not have sustained any injury. During the same traumatic event the client may have sustained a vertebral fracture at the C2 level but no nerve damage. The client's correct diagnosis would be a C4 spinal cord injury (s12000 Cervical Spinal Cord) with a C2 fracture (s7102 Bones of Neck Region).

To determine the level of injury (LOI), several tests are performed to assess the vertebral column and spinal cord including x-rays, computerized tomography (CT) scan, and magnetic resonance imaging (MRI) (Mayo Clinic, 2011). This is followed by a neurological exam to determine the level of injury and type of impairment. The neurologic exam consists of a light touch and pinprick test to determine sensory function, and an active range of motion and strength test to determine motor function (Mayo Clinic, 2011). During the neurologic exam, results are recorded on the *International Standards for Neurological Classification of Spinal Cord Injury* (ISNCSCI) form, available from American Spinal Injury Association (2013a). In the light touch test, the evaluator touches the client lightly with his/her finger or touches the client with the rounded end of a closed sterilized safety pin in each of the sensory points indicated on the form to determine intact, altered/diminished, or absent/extinguished sensation. Scoring categories are provided on the form. This is also referred to as assessing dermatomes, which are the areas of skin supplied with nerve fibers by a single spinal nerve root. Diminished or absent sensation in a particular dermatome will identify the nerve damaged and subsequent neurological LOI. This same test is repeated using the sharp safety pin end in the pinprick test to determine if a stronger stimulus can be sensed. The form for these tests is available from American Spinal Injury Association (2013b).

To determine motor function, the individual is instructed to actively move each limb or joint in all possible ranges to determine motor function deficits. While assessing active range of motion, the evaluator simultaneously assesses the strength of the muscles using a modified *Manual Muscle Exam* (MME) through observation of free movement and provision of support and/or resistance, as described below. Although the form requires the evaluator to indicate the MME number (0-5), therapists may be more familiar with the corresponding letters (e.g., 5 = N for Normal). To better assist therapists in understanding the MME, the original MME letter scoring is provided for comparison. Detailed test information is available from American Spinal Injury Association (2013c).

The Manual Muscle Exam uses the following scoring criteria:

Normal: 100% functionality. Score 5 or N: Complete range of motion against gravity with full resistance from examiner.

Good: 75% functionality. Score 4 or G. Complete range of motion against gravity with some resistance.

Fair: 50% functionality. Score 3 or F. Complete range of motion against gravity.

Poor: 25% functionality. Score 2 or P. Complete range of motion with gravity eliminated by examiner support.

Trace: 10% functionality. Score 1 or T. Evidence of contractility.

Zero: 0% functionality. Score 0. No evidence of contractility.

If spasm or contracture exists, place S or C after the grade of a movement that is incomplete for this reason.

Type of Injury

In addition to determining the level of injury, the neurologic exam previously described is the primary method to determine the extent of spinal cord impairment (complete or incomplete). If a client exhibits no motor or sensory function below the level of injury, it is referred to as a complete SCI. If the client exhibits some motor and/or sensory function below the level of injury, it is referred to as an incomplete SCI. An incomplete SCI can be the result of a contusion (bruise) to the spinal cord, a displaced bone, or edema. If the source of the pressure on the spinal cord can be identified early, surgery and/or traction can be utilized to decompress the injured area and may result in increased motor and/or sensory functioning. While early return of function is a good sign, recovery is unpredictable and varies widely. With advances that have been made in acute medical treatment for SCI, incomplete spinal cord injuries are becoming more common, with incomplete SCI increasing from 50.5% of all injuries examined from 1985 to 1990 up to 62.2% of all injuries examined from 2005 to 2011 (National Spinal Cord Injury Statistical Center [NSCISC], 2012).

To provide further classification of type of injury, the American Spinal Injury Association (ASIA) developed the *ASIA Impairment Scale*, which provides five impairment grades (A, B, C, D, and E). In general, a client who has a complete SCI is an ASIA A with no motor or sensory function below the injury level. A client who has an incomplete injury is an ASIA B, C, or D depending upon functional presentation (B = has sensory but no motor function below injury level, C = has motor function below injury level and more than half of key muscles have a muscle grade of 0-2, D = has motor function below injury level and at least half or more of key muscles have a muscle grade of 3 or more). A client who had previous motor and/or sensory deficits but now exhibits no deficits (tests normal in all segments), is an ASIA E.

Types of Paralysis and Related Function

SCI is primarily divided into two types: tetraplegia (formally called quadriplegia), which results from injury C1-C8, and paraplegia, which results from injury to T1-S5. These can be further broken down into complete tetraplegia, incomplete tetraplegia, complete paraplegia, and incomplete paraplegia. Functional abilities of individuals with incomplete injuries will vary depending upon the ASIA grade and extent of damage to the spinal cord. Since 2005, the most frequent neurological category of SCI has been incomplete tetraplegia (40.8%), followed by complete paraplegia (21.6%), incomplete paraplegia (21.4%), and complete tetraplegia (15.8%) (NSCISC, 2012). Trends over time indicate a decreasing occurrence of complete SCI and an increasing prevalence of incomplete injuries, which may be attributed to the provision of earlier interventions to decompress the spine at the LOI, including the increased availability of chemical interventions to reduce edema.

Functional expectations by level, based on a standard complete injury are shown below. Each level of injury will maintain the key muscle actions from the levels preceding it, in addition to the key muscle actions listed for each level. (Adapted from Bryce, 2009; Umphred et al., 2012; and Winnick, 2010). Examples of recreation activities are for illustration purposes only and do not encompass the entire range of activities possible.

C1-C3:

Key muscle actions: limited neck flexion, extension, and rotation.

Functional activity: ventilator or phrenic pacer dependent for breathing with possibility of breathing on own with a C3 SCI; dependent for activities of daily living (ADLs), bowel and bladder care, and transfers, but can verbalize and direct care; modified independent with pressure relief and wheelchair mobility with tilt-in-space power wheelchair utilizing sip-and-puff mechanism or head controls; environmental control units helpful for controlling the home environment; sip-and-puff, mouth-stick, and additional switch adaptations can assist with participation in passive recreation activities including turning pages of a book with a book holder and utilizing a tablet computer with a table-top or wheelchair clamp; possible participation with voice-activated technology with sufficient breath support.

C4:

Key muscle actions: increased control of neck flexion, extension, and rotation; scapula elevation (shoulder shrug); inspiration.

Functional activity: may be ventilator or phrenic pacer dependent for breathing, but most are weaned from mechanical respiration to breathe on their own; dependent for, but can verbally direct, bowel and bladder care, transfers, and most ADLs; however, may be able to contribute to feeding, basic grooming, and basic bathing with use of mobile arm support;

modified independent with pressure relief and wheelchair mobility with tilt-in-space power wheelchair utilizing sip-and-puff mechanism or head controls; environmental control units helpful for controlling the home environment; sip-and-puff activities can include power soccer and riflery; mouth-stick activities can include painting, drawing, and utilizing a tablet computer; may be able to participate in voice-activated technology using a computer.

C5:

Key muscle actions: elbow flexion and supination (can bend arms at elbow and turn palms face up); increased shoulder control, including shoulder flexion, abduction, and extension; and scapular abduction and adduction (can raise arms).

Functional activity: able to breathe on own; dependent but can verbally direct care for bathing, dressing, uneven transfers, and bowel and bladder management; set up to minimal assistance for basic grooming and feeding with use of adaptive equipment, such as mobile arm support, universal cuff with wrist support, plate guard, and Dycem; modified independent with pressure relief and wheelchair mobility with tilt-in-space power wheelchair with arm drive controls; may be able to propel manual chair with modified handrims for short distances on smooth, even surfaces, but with extreme fatigue; may consider power assist wheels for manual wheelchair mobility; maximum assistance for level transfer utilizing transfer board; may be able to drive wheelchair accessible van with lift and hand controls; activity participation can involve simple upper extremity gross motor activities, such as painting, drawing, or utilizing a computer and tablet with adaptive equipment; may be able to participate in increasingly physical activities with assistance and adaptive equipment, such as swimming, outdoor activities, and bowling with a ramp.

C6:

Key muscle actions: increased strength and control of upper extremities, including scapular protraction and elevation, forearm supination, radial wrist extension; tenodesis resulting in thumb and index finger natural opposition with flexion.

Functional activity: increased independence with ADLs and bowel and bladder care with adaptive equipment; males may be able to self-catheterize, while most women require increased assistance;

modified independent with weight shifts, feeding, upper body dressing and washing, and brushing teeth with adaptive equipment; varying levels of assistance required for bowel management and lower body bathing and dressing; power wheelchair mobility recommended, but may utilize manual wheelchair for short distances on smooth surfaces; power assist wheels may be recommended; may require minimal assistance for level sliding board transfers; may be able to drive wheelchair-accessible van with hand controls; increased participation in upper extremity gross motor activities using adaptive equipment, such as cuffs for billiards and golf; may participate in wheelchair sports, such as quad rugby and skiing.

C7-C8:

Key muscle actions: radial and ulnar wrist extension, elbow extension, partial finger extension and thumb abduction, partial finger flexors with C8 SCI.

Functional activity: modified independent with most ADLs with adaptive equipment, including feeding, grooming, bathing, and upper body dressing; possible minimal assistance for lower body dressing; most men and women can be modified independent with bowel and bladder management; modified independent for manual wheelchair mobility and weight shifts; modified independent for transfers and may begin to eliminate transfer board for some level transfers; able to drive a vehicle with hand controls; increased participation in a variety of active recreation activities including wheelchair sports, such as quad rugby, track, and handcycling.

T1-T7:

Key muscle actions: upper extremity muscle function intact; some trunk control and stability.

Functional activity: independent to modified independent with all ADLs, bowel and bladder management, transfers with or without transfer board; manual wheelchair mobility; greater participation in all recreation activities, with and without adaptive equipment including wheelchair basketball, wheelchair tennis, outdoor activities, physical fitness, and weight training.

T8-L1:

Key muscle actions: improved trunk flexion, extension, and rotation.

Functional activity: independent to modified independent with all ADLs, bowel and bladder management, transfers, and manual wheelchair mobility; increased trunk control allows for increased

efficiency and power in propelling wheelchair and greater involvement in unsupported activities; with adaptation, there are few activities that will be off limits; increased participation and independence in higher skill activities, such as kayaking and canoeing.

L2-S5:

Key muscle actions: partial to full control of lower extremities as hip flexors, knee extenders, ankle dorsiflexors, and plantar flexors return with each level of SCI.

Functional activity: increased potential for standing and ambulation with each level of recovery, with long leg and ankle bracing, including knee-ankle-foot orthosis (KAFO), ankle-foot orthosis (AFO), crutches, and/or a cane; increased participation in higher level standing recreation activities such as golf.

Clinical Syndromes

When an individual is diagnosed with an incomplete clinical syndrome, the deficits that the individual will have depend on which part of the spinal cord has been damaged, as well as the level that has been affected. Each clinical syndrome is described below (ASIA, 2002; Field-Fote, 2009).

Anterior cord syndrome: Occurs when there is damage to the anterior portion of the spinal cord, or a reduction in the vascular supply to the anterior portion of the spinal cord, commonly resulting from compression, dislocation of a vertebra, or a cervical disk protrusion. Damage to the anterior spinal cord frequently results in loss of pain sensation, temperature sensation, and motor strength; however, proprioception (the awareness of where a limb is positioned in space), vibration, and the sense of touch are often preserved.

Central cord syndrome: Occurs when there is damage in the central area of the spinal cord, often a result of hyperflexion injuries in the cervical spine, congenital injuries, or degenerative narrowing of the spinal canal. Central cord syndrome is characterized by greater neurological impairments in the upper extremities than the lower extremities. Many individuals will be able to redevelop the ability to walk and may also have normal sexual, bowel, and bladder functions. However, distal weakness and dysfunction in the upper extremities may persist. As a result, individuals are often able to walk but require a power wheelchair for mobility due to safety risks associated with ambulating without complete upper extremity functioning.

Posterior cord syndrome: Occurs when there is damage to the posterior portion of the spinal cord and/or its vascular supply, commonly resulting from posterior impact injuries where the cord is compressed as a result of forces from hyperextension. Posterior cord syndrome frequently results in loss of proprioception, as well as the sense of vibration and deep touch. While motor strength and sensation of pain and temperature are often preserved, the loss of proprioception may prohibit functional ambulation due to a wide-based gait pattern.

Brown-Sequard syndrome: Occurs when there is damage to one lateral side of the spinal cord, frequently caused by a stab or gunshot wound, which results in the loss of voluntary motor control, sensation, and decreased reflexes at the same dermatome level on the side of the damage to the cord. A Brown-Sequard presentation may display a lack of superficial reflexes, clonus (involuntary muscle contractions), and a positive Babinski sign (a reflex when pressure is applied to the foot). On the contra-lateral side of the spinal cord, the individual may display a loss of pain and temperature sensation for several dermatome segments below the LOI.

Incidence/Prevalence in U.S.

There were approximately 270,000 people in the U.S. who were living with SCI in 2012, with approximately 40 cases of new SCI per million population in the U.S. or approximately 12,000 new cases each year (NSCISC, 2012).

Predominant Age

SCI primarily affects younger adults although it can affect a person of any age. For the period between 2005 and 2011, data collected by the National Spinal Cord Injury Association indicates the average age for spinal cord injury is 41 years (NSCISC, 2012).

Causes

Trauma: The main cause of spinal cord injury is trauma. The primary methods of injury are motor vehicle accidents (39.2% of all injuries), falls (28.3% of injuries), violence (14.6% of injuries), and sports related injuries (8.2% of injuries) (NSCISC, 2012). Additional analysis of the National Spinal Cord

Injury Database shows that the percentage of injuries due to falls is increasing over time, while the percentage of injuries caused by sports has decreased (NSCISC, 2012).

Tumor: When a tumor grows on or close to the spinal cord, the pressure that is placed on the cord, as well as the subsequent edema, may cause damage to the spinal cord. Early detection of tumors leading to early surgical intervention can help reduce the pressure, resulting in better prognosis for maintaining or regaining full sensation and motor control (National Institute for Neurological Disorders and Stroke [NINDS], 2011).

Transverse myelitis (TM): TM is an acute inflammatory process that typically results from an infectious agent that causes damage to neural tissues. TM is a rare disease that affects approximately one to four individuals per million population and does not have a hereditary influence or gender specificity. Approximately one third of all individuals with TM will make close to a full recovery, while another third will have moderate impairment, and the final third will have severe impairment as a result of the inflammation (NINDS, 2011).

Guillain-Barré syndrome (GBS): GBS results from an acute inflammatory process, which demyelinates nerves in the PNS. GBS is a rare disorder that affects one in 100,000 people (NINDS, 2011). GBS typically presents as an ascending myelopathy, where damage spreads to higher levels of the spinal cord unless contained through use of drugs to reduce inflammation (Field-Fote, 2009).

Systems Affected

SCI affects the nervous system, including motor and/or sensory functions. The physical damage to the spinal cord can be recorded using ICF codes in s120 Spinal Cord and Related Structures. Pain is recorded with ICF code b280 Sensation of Pain. Functional losses can be recorded with the diagnostic systems described earlier or with ICF codes in the Body Functions section starting with b260 Proprioceptive Function and potentially including many of the rest of the codes.

Secondary Problems

Concurrent impairment of nerve innervations to other body structures and functions results in increased risk of additional medical complications for individuals with SCI. Some of the more common secondary complications include:

Autonomic dysreflexia or hyperreflexia (AD): AD is a life threatening rise in blood pressure (b420 Blood Pressure Functions), that can occur in individuals with a LOI at or above T6 when there is a negative stimulus within or outside of the body below the level of injury (Consortium for Spinal Cord Medicine [CSCM], 1997; Juknis, Cooper, & Oksana, 2012). During an episode of AD, the presence of a negative stimulus triggers a sympathetic response surge that cannot be moderated by the parasympathetic system secondary to the damage caused by the SCI. When symptoms of AD arise, including a pounding headache due to high blood pressure, stuffy nose, profuse sweating above the LOI, the presence of goose bumps, change in vision, such as blurred vision or seeing spots, and/or feeling flushed and apprehensive (CSCM, 1997; Juknis, Cooper, & Oksana, 2012), the source of irritation must be located and alleviated or the individual could suffer a stroke or even death. The most common cause of AD is a bladder issue, be it an overfull bladder, a kinked catheter, or a bladder/kidney infection. Other common causes include impacted bowel; irritation to the skin from causes as diverse as clothing or shoes that are too tight, sunburn, a pressure sore, an ingrown toenail, and pressure from sharp object; or additional outside stimuli from medical testing, procedures, bone injury, etc. (CSCM, 1997; Juknis et al., 2012; Rabchevsky & Kitzman, 2011). Resolving AD generally begins with sitting the individual as upright as possible and looking for the source of the problem. Lying down is avoided because it will contribute to an increase in blood pressure. The search for the irritation evolves into a process of loosening and/or removing any tight clothing or other items, including shirts, pants, shoes, catheter tubes, abdominal binders, etc., tracking the individual's blood pressure, catheterizing the individual to remove any excess urine, checking for bowel impaction or constipation, and searching for any other signs of irritation, such as sitting on an object, development of a skin sore, etc. If this series of steps does not resolve the dysreflexic episode, then medication may be necessary (CSCM, 1997; Juknis et al., 2012). Individuals with SCIs must be educated on the signs and symptoms of AD and be able to direct medical or other individuals on how to provide treatment.

Because AD only occurs in individuals with SCI, it is not familiar to many hospital personnel and paramedics. For this reason, those who are susceptible to AD should carry a card that describes causes and treatment procedures in the event of an emergency (CSCM, 1997).

Pressure ulcers (decubitus ulcers, skin sores): The human skin relies on the flow of oxygen through the body's blood supply to remain healthy. When too much pressure builds up on the skin in a particular area, the flow of blood to that area is halted and the skin begins to die, resulting in pressure ulcers (Kawasaki & Warms, 2007). Because most individuals with SCI have impaired sensation below the LOI, the brain cannot tell the body to move and relieve pressure from body parts, thereby restoring blow flow and oxygenation of the skin. For example, when sitting for a long period of time, the flow of oxygen to the buttocks is cut off, resulting in a feeling of numbness and/or "pins and needles." This triggers an individual with full sensation to change positions, relieving the symptoms and restoring the flow of oxygen. An individual with SCI does not get this message and subsequently does not know to remove the pressure, which is first seen as a red spot on the skin area affected. If pressure is not consistently alleviated through shifting body positions and timed weight shifts, the seemingly innocuous red spot can lead to skin breakdown, eventually moving its way through muscle and into the bone, potentially resulting in a life threatening bone infection. There are four stages of pressure sore development which involve progressive deterioration of the skin and its underlying tissue, muscles, and bones if treatment is not sought. These stages are characterized as follows: Stage 1: a red spot or discoloration at the site of the sore, without a break in the skin; Stage 2: an open sore created by the breaking of the top layer of the skin, Stage 3: the wound continually deepens, breaking through an individual's second level of skin to the underlying fat tissue, and finally, Stage 4: the breakdown reaches through fat tissue to the underlying muscle and possibly affects the bone as well (Kawasaki & Warms, 2007). See the chapter on Pressure Ulcers for more information and ICF codes to use for scoring the effects of pressure ulcers. While pressure ulcers are highly preventable with education and the implementation of movement and pressure relief strategies, it is estimated that 34% of individuals in acute care and rehabilitation (Verschueren et al., 2011), and 25-30% of individuals within five years post injury (Juknis et al., 2012) will be affected by pressure ulcers. Pressure ulcers are also the second most common reason for rehospitalization in individuals living with SCI, with a prevalence rate of 15-30% (Gelis et al., 2009). The most commonly affected areas of skin are the bony prominences of the body (buttocks, ankles, elbows, hips, knees, shoulder blades), with the most noted occurrences seen in the sacrum, ischium, and the heel (Verschueren et al., 2011). Aside from pressure build up, other risk factors that contribute to the development of pressure ulcers include shearing and or scraping of the skin (e.g., skin movement over bone across rough surfaces, minor abrasions), excessive moisture, primarily from bladder or bowel accidents, and history of additional pressure ulcers (Verschueren et al., 2011; Juknis et al., 2012). Maintaining a healthy lifestyle with regular exercise, proper nutrition, and cessation of smoking is referenced in the literature as a preventative measure for avoiding pressure ulcers (Gelis et al., 2009). Even so, the most important contributing factor to the prevention of pressure ulcers remains proper education of the individual by healthcare providers. The individuals or their care team need to be sure to implement weight-shifting every 20-30 minutes (leaning forward in wheelchair, leaning to alternating sides of the wheelchair, maintaining a wheelie position, or lifting buttocks off of wheelchair seat by pushing up with arms on wheelchair armrests), turning clients every two hours during sleep, and proper positioning while sitting and lying to remove pressure from the risk areas (Gelis et al., 2009; Juknis et al., 2012).

Respiratory complications: Injuries to the upper thoracic and cervical spinal cord impact the respiratory muscles (diaphragm, intercostal muscles, and abdominal muscles) that aid in taking deep breaths and in coughing, leading to a wide occurrence of respiratory complications in individuals with SCI (b440 Respiration Functions, b445 Respiratory Muscle Functions, b450 Additional Respiratory Functions). While pneumonia has been documented to be the leading cause of death among individuals with SCI (NSCISC, 2012), atelectasis (s430 Structure of Respiratory System), or the collapse of part or all of a lung, is the most common respiratory complication among individuals in the acute phase of

a cervical spinal cord injury, affecting approximately 37% of those individuals (Ditunno et al., 2012). Additionally, the importance of attending to respiratory issues from initiation of trauma life support, and continuing through acute care and rehabilitation management cannot be underestimated. It is imperative that healthcare professionals are diligent about recognizing respiratory difficulties as well as encouraging the individual to engage in regular respiratory care. Being proactive in an individual's efforts to reduce fluid build-up in the lungs through techniques such as wearing an abdominal binder, using cough assist techniques, and suctioning and obtaining annual flu vaccinations recommended by the CDC are key prevention tactics to prevent these severe respiratory complications (Ditunno et al., 2012; Juknis et al., 2012).

Spasticity or spastic hypertonia: The interruption of messages to the reflex center of the brain may result in the overcompensation of the spinal cord reflex system, leading to spasticity (b750 Motor Reflex Functions, b765 Involuntary Movement Functions, b780 Sensations Related to Muscles and Movement Functions). Spasticity affects approximately 65-78% of individuals living with chronic SCI, and is characterized by uncontrollable, jerky movements, abnormal increased tone in a muscle group, overactive reflexes, and/or involuntary bending or straightening of muscles (Reyes & Chiodo, 2011). Treatment of spasticity depends on how many muscle groups are affected in addition to the level of interference the spasms may cause in activities and participation. The occurrence of spasms could potentially be pain free, with the nature of the spasm providing assistance in performing daily life tasks. In these circumstances, an individual's spasticity can be managed with a daily range of motion, stretching routine. However, spasms can also be extremely painful (b280 Sensation of Pain), limiting functional abilities and potentially causing safety issues if body positioning and stability are compromised. When spasticity becomes an impediment to functional mobility, independence, or quality of life, treatment can include oral drug therapy, electrical stimulation, and other pharmacological and surgical intervention strategies (Elbasiouny et al., 2010).

Temperature regulation: In general, individuals with a complete SCI will be impacted by thermoregulation issues (b550 Thermoregulatory Functions). Individuals with SCIs above T6 will be most impacted (Cesario & Darouiche, 2003). Due to both the disruption in the sympathetic nervous system and the body's damaged sensory functioning, an individual is at risk for decreased body core temperature as well as the inability to regulate body temperature. This dysfunction leads to the body's inability to effectively sweat to cool the body in situations of high heat, and the body's inability to send normal temperature sensations to the brain, resulting in feeling cold in normal temperatures (Young, 2006). During hot weather conditions, where hyperthermia may be a risk, individuals should take precautions, such as drinking plenty of fluids, being aware of heat tolerance, using spray bottles to cool down, and staying in shaded areas when outside (Louis Calder Memorial Library, 2009). To address issues of hypothermia, an individual must monitor core body temperature and avoid situations of sudden, significant changes in environment (Young, 2006). Both hypothermia and hyperthermia can be fatal conditions.

Heterotopic ossification (HO): HO, the growth of new bone in soft tissue areas, affects 10-53% of individuals with SCI. It begins primarily in the first two to three weeks post injury, with the most notable occurrences happening at the two-month mark following acquisition of an SCI (Teasell et al., 2010). For individuals with SCI, HO is most likely to occur in the hips, knees, and shoulders. Symptoms may include redness and warmth in the affected area, joint and muscle pain, reduced range of motion in the affected joint, edema, and a low-grade fever. If left untreated, HO can cause decreased range of motion and contractures (b710 Mobility of Joint Functions, b780 Sensations Related to Muscles and Movement Functions), leading to significant functional limitations. While limited conclusions have been drawn on absolute primary prevention methods, muscle stretching and joint mobilization, along with careful monitoring by the individual's physician has been recommended (Teasell et al., 2010).

Deep vein thrombosis (DVT): A DVT occurs when a blood clot forms in a vein, most commonly in the lower extremities (b415 Blood Vessel Functions). If a DVT is not recognized and precautions taken, the DVT may break away from the lower extremities and travel to the lungs, causing a life threatening pulmonary embolism (Medline Plus, n.d.). As a result of SCI and the related immobility, the rate of blood flow to the lower extremities is decreased, increasing the likelihood of a DVT. Individuals in the acute and early rehabilitation phases of spinal cord injury care are at the highest risk of developing a DVT, with the risk potential peaking at seven to ten days (Popa et al., 2010). It is critical that individuals and care professionals are diligent in watching for the signs of DVT, which may include increased skin temperature, lower extremity swelling, pain, tenderness, and possible skin discoloration (Popa et al., 2010). Practice guidelines indicate that anticoagulation medication be administered to patients within 72 hours after SCI and continue approximately eight to twelve weeks (Juknis et al., 2012). Additional prevention strategies include mobilization through range of motion exercises, physical therapy, and the use of compression stockings (Popa et al., 2010).

Orthostatic (postural) hypotension: Orthostatic hypotension is a decrease in systolic blood pressure of more than 20 mm Hg and/or a decrease in diastolic blood pressure of more than 10 mm HG when changing from the supine to an upright position (b420 Blood Pressure Functions) (Shatzer, 2009). It can result in dizziness, lightheadedness, possible fainting or brief loss of consciousness, fatigue, headache, nausea, pallor, perioral and facial numbness, and blurred vision (Popa et al., 2010; Krassioukov et al., 2009; Shatzer, 2009). The most significant results are usually coded with ICF code b110 Consciousness Functions. With the damage sustained by the autonomic nervous system after a SCI, blood will tend to pool in the lower extremities or lower abdomen; therefore, a quick change of position, such as getting into a seated position after lying down for an extended period of time, can cause orthostatic hypotension (Krassioukov et al., 2009). There is a higher prevalence rate of orthostatic hypertension in individuals with tetraplegia (82%) than paraplegia (50%) (Krassioukov et al., 2009). Orthostatic hypotension generally resolves over time without the need for long-term medical treatment (Shatzer, 2009). Treatment interventions include an elastic abdominal binder and/or lower limb compression stockings (watch for formation of pressure ulcers), decreased seat-back angle in a recliner wheelchair from near supine gradually to full upright as tolerated, gradually raising the head of bed before getting out of bed, salt tablets, and medications (Shatzer, 2009).

Prognosis

Currently there is no cure for SCI, although there have been advances made in pharmacology and research studies utilizing human embryonic stem cells. Pharmacology trials have shown that administering methylprednisolone (a high dose steroid) within eight hours of injury improves recovery by approximately 20% due to the ability of methylprednisolone to decrease the edema in the spinal cord, thus reducing pressure and preserving function (Bracken, 2012). Edema is one of the primary causes of secondary damage to the spinal cord and takes weeks or even months to dissipate completely even with early administration of steroids (Borgens & Liu-Snyder, 2012). Individuals who have signals that are consistent with spinal cord edema or hemorrhage on MRI imaging have been shown to have worse functional outcomes (Wilson et al., 2012).

An average individual can expect to have function return for approximately 18 months, or sometimes longer, following initial injury (Fawcett et al., 2007). Only a small portion of individuals will make a full recovery from injury, with most people having permanent loss of some motor and/or sensory function (Fawcett et al., 2007).

The life expectancy for an individual with a SCI is slightly below the average for individuals without a SCI, with higher mortality rates being seen during the first year following the initial SCI, specifically for those who have high tetraplegia and are ventilator dependent (Charlifue, Jah, & Lammertse, 2010). The primary reasons for the shorter life expectancies within the first year following SCI are pneumonia and septicemia (NSCISC, 2012). There is also an increased risk to be hospitalized as a result of secondary conditions, including urinary tract infections, autonomic dysreflexia, skin breakdown, pneumonia, depression, and substance abuse (Charlifue, Jah, & Lammertse, 2010).

Assessment

Typical Scope of Team Assessment

Assessment of a SCI is an ongoing process that begins with admission to an acute care program and progresses through rehabilitation and outpatient treatment. Each team member participates in the assessment process with the goal of maximizing independence and quality of life.

After medical stability is achieved, the assessment process begins by identifying the level of injury and ASIA classification, as described earlier, along with identifying any secondary physical, cognitive, or sensory injuries that may have been sustained.

The treatment team must also consider the emotional well-being of the individual, watching for signs of depression, anxiety, and other related issues. These may be documented with ICF codes b125 Dispositions and Intra-Personal Functions, b126 Temperament and Personality Functions, b130 Energy and Drive Functions, and b152 Emotional Functions.

Areas of Concern for RT Assessment

With the overall goal of recreational therapy interventions being restoration of the maximum possible levels of physical, emotional, and social skills through participation in a physically and socially active leisure lifestyle, the assessment process must go beyond evaluating an individual's physical functioning in collaboration with the physical therapist and occupational therapist. The recreational therapist must also get a basic sense of the individual's premorbid leisure lifestyle.

Rehabilitation professionals must also consider the meaning of participation for the individual, including what living in their own environments with a changed self looks and feels like (Ripat & Woodgate, 2012). With this understanding, the RT must also place assessment emphasis on a variety of psychosocial factors. Since most SCIs result from a traumatic injury, individuals generally have little knowledge of disability, including its social, physical, emotional, and financial impacts. The RT gets a sense of the individual's knowledge level regarding issues such as accessibility, transportation, disability rights, community services, and resources. It is also important to address the psychosocial and emotional needs and resources of the individual. The RT will evaluate the importance the individual places on an active leisure lifestyle (both physical and social) and begin to search for potential recreation options post discharge (Ackerman, Kedersha, & Vliet, 2002). ICF codes that can be used to document deficits in the individual include d240 Handling Stress and Other Psychological Demands, d4 Mobility, d620

Acquisition of Goods and Services, d730 Relating with Strangers, d870 Economic Self-Sufficiency, d910 Community Life, d920 Recreation and Leisure, and d940 Human Rights. Deficits in the community can be documented with ICF codes in e3 Support and Relationships, e4 Attitudes, and e5 Services, Systems, and Policies.

ICF Core Set

A brief and comprehensive ICF Core Set for Spinal Cord Injury is available.

Treatment Direction

Whole Team Approach

Shared communication between all members of the treatment team, which may include a physician/physiatrist, case manager, social worker, recreational therapist, physical therapist, occupational therapist, psychologist, client, family, and caregivers, is critical and must be ongoing to most effectively and efficiently achieve client goals. The roles of team members vary as the individual progresses through the continuum of care.

Acute care phase: During this phase, the team focus is on medical management to stabilize the individual and reduce subsequent injury to the spinal cord (s120 Spinal Cord and Related Structures). Discharge placement post medical stability, whether to the home or to a rehabilitation facility, is explored and initiated. Conversations with the individual and caregivers begin about potential home modifications, if the goal is to return home, and future caregiving needs (e3 Support and Relationships, e5 Services, Systems, and Policies). Prevention of secondary problems also becomes a priority during the early stages of treatment. Treatment of secondary problems should be documented with the associated ICF codes. Treatment team members also begin educating the individual and family about the injury itself as well as realistic goals and expectations (Ackerman et al., 2002).

Rehabilitation phase: This phase is marked by the individual becoming a more active participant in the recovery process. The focus moves away from medical stability to maximizing functional independence. Many SCI treatment teams follow a critical pathway of functional expectations for specific levels of SCI that guide the treatment plan. The ultimate goal for SCI rehabilitation is discharge to the least restrictive environment with maximum independence, quality of life, and safety. Recent literature suggests that to provide competent and comprehensive care during rehabilitation, an interdisciplinary, holistic approach that extends beyond medical stability and physiological consequences, to include consideration of social, psychological, and functional independence is critical (Emerich, Parsons, & Stein, 2012). Recommendations may be made for additional services post in-patient rehabilitation, such as a day program and/or additional outpatient services. Any combination of the treatment team may be involved in these services with the goal being to refine the more advanced skills as the individual transitions away from the safety of the rehabilitation center back to the realities of the home and community environment (Ackerman et al., 2002). The ICF codes in the RT areas of concern during the assessment process can be used to document the treatment provided.

Day program/outpatient therapies: As the length of stay for inpatient rehabilitation continues to decrease, the need for outpatient therapy to hone skills and return to successful community living becomes greater. Results from a five-year research project funded by the National Institute on Disability and Rehabilitation Research (the SCIRehab Project), and involving six SCI-specific rehabilitation programs, found that approximately 44% of the total hours of rehabilitation received by individuals after sustaining a SCI occurred post discharge from an inpatient rehabilitation center (Backus et al., 2013).

Recreational Therapy Approach

The recreational therapist supports the overall team approach with a focus on the development of a well-rounded, healthy leisure lifestyle for post discharge that promotes health, continued recovery, quality of life, and well-being. While past research has drawn relationships between the role of recreational therapy concepts (including leisure time physical activity, sports and outdoor participation, social skills, social support, perceived barriers, and leisure in general) to adjustment to disability, quality of life, and life satisfaction post injury, efforts to describe not only recreational therapy interventions, but also the measurable outcomes of these interventions have just recently been undertaken. Using a practice-based evidence approach, the SCIRehab

Project is paving the way to evidence-based practice guidelines for all SCI rehabilitation professionals, including recreational therapy (Whiteneck et al., 2009).

Recreational Therapy Interventions

The greatest direct evidence of recreational therapy interventions and their corresponding outcomes has come from the SCIRehab Project (Cahow et al., 2009). In the SCIRehab Project, recreational therapy SCI rehabilitation professionals from six U.S. rehabilitation centers developed a uniform documentation system to describe the details of SCI recreational therapy sessions. The use of a consistent approach across the rehabilitation centers allowed the recreational therapists to track and describe the most utilized approaches to, and content of, recreational therapy SCI treatment. Information was gathered on 1,500 clients and was used to develop a recreational therapy taxonomy. Intervention categories in the taxonomy include leisure education and counseling, leisure skill and knowledge development, outings (including leisure skill and general community outings), and social activity. Within these overall categories, specific priority topic areas were identified. Specific content of the recreational therapy taxonomy can be found in the SCIRehab literature (Cahow et al., 2009; Gassaway et al., 2011). It should be carefully reviewed and utilized by recreational therapists working in SCI rehabilitation. Some of the important focus areas include:

Functional skills: Functional skills training may include wheelchair mobility skills (e.g., d460 Moving Around in Different Locations, d465 Moving Around Using Equipment), with specific emphasis on community mobility and problem solving (d175 Solving Problems), as well as leisure skill development. The skills should include, at a minimum, identification of strategies for cardiovascular and physical endurance and strength (e.g., d570 Looking After One's Health), and adapted recreation (d920 Recreation and Leisure, e115 Products and Technology for Personal Use in Daily Living, e140 Products and Technology for Culture, Recreation, and Sport). Individuals should be educated about recreation options, methods of activity adaptation, and, if appropriate equipment is available, specific skill interventions and practice of the skills taught. Finally, the provision of resources cannot be overlooked, including visual reminders of how to perform the skill, safety issues, community resources, vendors, and potential funding for equipment.

Education, training, and counseling: Recreational therapy programs should have a formal leisure education program to educate individuals about stigma (e4 Attitudes), stress management (d240 Handling Stress and Other Psychological Demands), advocacy (e.g., d950 Political Life and Citizenship), disability rights (e.g., d940 Human Rights), accessibility (e.g., e150 Design, Construction, and Building Products and Technology of Buildings for Public Use), problem solving (d175 Solving Problems), time management (d230 Carrying Out Daily Routine), and consequences of inactivity (e.g., d570 Looking After One's Health). Any deficits in ICF code b164 Higher-Level Cognitive Functions should be addressed before training in specific skills begins. The RT also works with the individual to counteract the effects of anxiety and depression following injury. ICF codes that may be cited include (b125 Dispositions and Intra-Personal Functions, b126 Temperament and Personality Functions, b130 Energy and Drive Functions, and b152 Emotional Functions. It is only when all of these topics are addressed and other treatment team approaches are applied that adjustment to disability can begin.

Community integration: Individual and/or group outings, as well as family training outings, will help to ensure that the individual can transfer the education, problem solving, and skills they have been taught in the hospital or rehabilitation setting to the real-world environment. Outings offer the RT the opportunity to evaluate the individual's level of functional independence, specific leisure and community skills, assertiveness, safety awareness, and overall adaptation to disability, social stigma, and accessibility issues. Any deficits that were noted in ICF codes d240 Handling Stress and Other Psychological Demands, d4 Mobility, d620 Acquisition of Goods and Services, d730 Relating with Strangers, d870 Economic Self-Sufficiency, d910 Community Life, d920 Recreation and Leisure, d940 Human Rights, e3 Support and Relationships, e4 Attitudes, and e5 Services, Systems, and Policies can be addressed on these outings.

Health promotion: While health promotion is not specifically mentioned in the recreational therapy taxonomy, the education received through a formal leisure education and counseling program and on community outings infuses concepts of health-promoting behaviors for successfully living with SCI. These apply not only to overall life quality and satisfaction, but also to the prevention of secondary medical complications. The importance of health promotion (e.g., d570 Looking After One's Health) is often overlooked during rehabilitation. The information individuals and families need to comprehend immediately after injury, during rehabilitation, and upon discharge can be overwhelming. There never seems to be time to talk about health promotion. However, as highlighted in Healthy People 2020, health promotion strategies and eliminating health disparities among individuals with disabilities should be addressed (Healthy People 2020, n.d.). Leisure education programs in rehabilitation can be an ideal mechanism to provide knowledge, skills, and abilities in using leisure for health promotion and health behavior change. Using the Healthy Living though Leisure model as a framework, the recreational therapist can build or expand leisure education programs that focus on lifestyle changes that promote health through recreation and are also grounded in health behavior change and leisure theory (Coyle, Shank, & Vliet, 2010). This individualized model allows the recreational therapist to move the individual through four stages of behavior change: (1) becoming informed about the concepts of health and wellness, leisure as promoting health, and assessing his/her own wellness; (2) evaluating motivation and readiness to change; (3) putting plans into action, whereby individuals start making healthy decisions about physically and socially active leisure, and begin to become competent in skill development, resource utilization, and the negotiation of barriers; and (4) providing support systems and strategies to ensure the behavioral change.

Using the practice-based evidence approach, the SCIRehab Project highlights how the types of intervention used by the different rehabilitation disciplines, along with the time spent receiving each discipline's service, impacted overall rehabilitation outcomes at discharge and at one year post injury. Areas of focus included functional independence, discharge placement, the occurrence of medical complications and subsequent re-hospitalizations, and a return to positive participation in life (Whiteneck et al., 2008). After the documentation of recreational therapy intervention types and analysis of content according to the recreational therapy taxonomy, initial outcomes of recreational therapy services are positive. Recreational therapy was proven not only to be an active service in SCI rehabilitation, but also a discipline whose interventions positively contributed to patient outcomes at discharge and one year post injury.

Recreational therapy services were provided to 94% of the individuals in SCI rehabilitation, with an average of 18 hours of recreational therapy treatment time per patient. In the recreational therapy taxonomy areas, approximately 76% of the patients participated in a community outing, 22% participated in specific leisure skill outings, and 80% engaged in leisure skill development in the rehabilitation center (Gassaway et al., 2011). The level and content of recreational therapy involvement was impacted by the level of SCI and the completeness of the injury. Individuals with preservation of motor function below the level of SCI (ASIA D incomplete) spent the least amount of time receiving recreational therapy treatment, and individuals with tetraplegia spent more time than individuals with paraplegia on community outing interventions. Finally, the content of sessions took a slightly different focus for individuals with high tetraplegia (C1-C4) than for those with low tetraplegia and paraplegia. Recreational therapy outings and in-center interventions with individuals with high cervical injuries focused more on the individuals being assertive (b126 Temperament and Personality Functions) and directing their care (d570 Looking After One's Health), including verbalizing their needs to family and caregivers and participating in family training sessions (d760 Family Relationships). Leisure skills sessions with individuals in these groupings also focused less on independent participation in the preferred activity and more on exposure to adaptive equipment (e115 Products and Technology for Personal Use in Daily Living, e120 Products and Technology for Personal Indoor and Outdoor Mobility and Transportation) and education about options and resources for participation (d920 Recreation and Leisure) (Gassaway et al., 2011).

Overall, it has been documented that more time spent participating in recreational therapy interventions during inpatient rehabilitation is positively associated with outcomes in the areas of functional independence, participation, decreased secondary complications, and discharge to home (Gassaway et al., 2011). More specifically, the findings of the SCIRehab project indicate the value of time spent in specific interventions and achievement of these outcome indicators. Cahow et al. (2012) found the following correlations between RT interventions and outcomes: Increased time spent on leisure skill outings and in CTRS-led classes and increased time that the CTRS spent on patient assessment both were positively associated with higher FIM motor scores at discharge from rehabilitation. Increased time spent in leisure education and counseling was positively correlated with an increased likelihood of discharge to and residing at home one year post injury and higher physical independence scores at discharge. Increased time spent in community outings led by the CTRS was positively correlated with higher social integration and mobility scores from the *Craig Handicap Assessment and Reporting Technique* (CHART). Increased time spent on leisure skill outings was positively correlated with less re-hospitalization at the one-year mark post injury. Increased time spent on community outings was positively correlated with decreased pressure ulcers and was a strong predictor of sports involvement and outdoor activities one year post discharge. Time spent in activity-related sessions, including sports, aquatics, outdoor activities, creative expression, and gardening was a strong predictor of active participation in each respective activity one year post discharge.

Backus et al. (2013) found that receiving RT services post discharge were positively correlated with higher scores on the *Satisfaction with Life Scale* and increased social integration, as measured by the CHART. Increased time in RT, along with post discharge peer support, was positively correlated with increased likelihood of return to school or work one year post injury.

Recreational therapy services are, and will continue to be, a solid force in successful community reintegration following SCI. The potential for recreational therapy involvement and outcomes post inpatient rehabilitation discharge is great. Additional research is needed on the outcomes of recreational therapy services in outpatient settings (Backus et al., 2013), as well as the contributions of recreational therapy on active participation in life beyond the one-year-post-injury time frame. Cahow and colleagues (2012) argue that the magnitude of recreational therapy's interventions may not be truly felt until well after the one-year-post-injury mark, when individuals living with SCI have completed formal therapy and have established everyday routines.

Resources

National Spinal Cord Injury Association (NSCIA)
www.spinalcord.org
The NSCIA is a membership organization in the United Spinal Association whose mission is to improve the quality of life for individuals living with spinal cord injury and disorders. This website provides valuable resources on research and publications, advocacy efforts, support resources for families and individuals with SCI, including information for local chapters of NSCIA, and a wealth of information on the technical and practical aspects of living with SCI.

American Spinal Injury Association (ASIA)
www.asia-spinalinjury.org
ASIA is a membership organization for professionals in the field of spinal cord injury medicine whose overall mission is to promote standards of healthcare excellence for individuals with spinal cord injury, while providing education to members, individuals with SCI and their families, and other healthcare professionals. The organization is also highly involved in research activities aimed at preventing SCI, reducing disability associated with SCI, and improving quality of care.

Paralyzed Veterans of America (PVA)
www.pva.org
PVA is a veteran's service organization whose aim is to ensure that veterans living with spinal cord injuries have the resources and support to live full, productive lives. While their mission of providing advocacy for quality healthcare, research, and disability rights is focused on U.S. veterans, their publications and online resources are open to all. The PVA also administers and funds the Consortium for Spinal Cord Medicine, whose goal is to provide evidence-based practice guidelines for the management of spinal cord injury. The Consortium for Spinal Cord Medicine provides free, downloadable, practical consumer guides on several important issues surrounding living with a spinal cord injury.

References

Ackerman, P., Kedersha, K., & Vliet, N. (2002). Every step of the way. Care management of the patient with a spinal cord injury. *Care Management, 8*, 23-27.

American Spinal Injury Association. (2002). International standards for neurological classification of spinal cord injury. *J Spinal Cord Medicine, 26*(Supp 1), S50-S56.

American Spinal Injury Association. (2010). 2009 Review and revisions of the international standards for neurological classification of spinal cord injury. *J Spinal Cord Medicine, 33*(4), 346-52.

American Spinal Injury Association. (2013a). International Standards for Neurological Classification of SCI (ISNCSCI). Retrieved from http://www.asia-spinalinjury.org/elearning/ASIA_ISCOS_high.pdf.

American Spinal Injury Association. (2013b). International Standards for Classification of SCI: Key sensory points. Retrieved from http://www.asia-spinalinjury.org/elearning/Key_Sensory_Points.pdf.

American Spinal Injury Association. (2013c). International Standards for Classification of SCI: Motor exam guide. Retrieved from http://www.asia-spinalinjury.org/elearning/Motor_Exam_Guide.pdf.

Backus, D., Gassaway, J., Smout, R. J., Hsieh, C. H., Heinemann, A. W., DeJong, G., & Horn, S. (2013). Relation between inpatient and postdischarge services and outcomes 1 year postinjury in people with traumatic spinal cord injury. *Archives of Physical Medicine and Rehabilitation, 94*(4), S165-S174.

Borgens, R. & Liu-Snyder, P. (2012). Understanding secondary injury. *The Quarterly Review of Biology, 87*(2), 89-127.

Bracken, M. (2012). Steroids for acute spinal cord injury. *Cochrane Database of Systematic Reviews (Online),* 1CD001046. doi: 10.1002/14651858.CD001046.pub2.

Bryce, T. N. (2009). *Spinal cord injury: Rehabilitation medicine quick reference.* Demos Medical.

Cahow, C., Skolnick, S., Joyce, J., Jug, J., Dragon, C., & Gassaway, J. (2009). SCIRehab Project Series: The therapeutic recreation taxonomy. *The Journal of Spinal Cord Medicine, 32*(3), 298-306.

Cahow, C., Gassaway, J., Rider, C., Joyce, J., Bogenshutz, A., Edens, K., Kreider, S. E. D., & Whiteneck, G. (2012). Relationship of therapeutic recreation inpatient rehabilitation interventions and patient characteristics to outcomes following spinal cord injury: The SCIRehab Project. *The Journal of Spinal Cord Medicine, 35*(6), 547-564.

Cesario, M. D. & Darouiche, R. O. (2003). Temperature regulation in spinal cord disease. Retrieved from www.ncbi.nlm.nih.gov/books/NBK9412/.

Charlifue S., Jah, A., & Lammertse, D. (2010). Aging with spinal cord injury. *Phys Med Rehabil Clin N Am, 21*(2), 383-402.

Consortium for Spinal Cord Medicine. (1997). *Autonomic dysreflexia: What you should know, a guide for people with spinal cord injury.* Washington, DC: Paralyzed Veterans of America.

Coyle, C. P., Shank, J. W., & Vliet, N. M. (2010). Leisure and rehabilitation. In L. Payne, B. Ainsworth, & G. Godbey (Eds.), *Leisure, health, and wellness: Making the connections* (pp. 264-277). State College, PA: Venture Publishing, Inc.

Ditunno, J. F., Cardenas, D. D., Formal, C., & Dalal, K. (2009). Advances in the rehabilitation management of acute spinal cord injury. In Verhaagen & J. W. McDonald III (Eds.), *Handbook of clinical neurology, vol 109 (3rd series) spinal cord injury* (pp. 181-195). San Diego, CA: Elsevier Science and Technology Books retrieved from http://www.sciencedirect.com.libproxy.temple.edu/science/handbooks/00729752/109.

Elbasiouny, S. M., Moroz, D., Bakr, M. M., & Mushahwar, V. (2010). Management of spasticity after spinal cord injury:

Current techniques and future directions. *Neurorehabilitation and Neural Repair, 24*(1), 23-33.

Emerich, L., Parsons, K. C., & Stein, A. (2012) Competent care for persons with spinal cord injury and dysfunction in acute inpatient rehabilitation. *Top Spinal Cord Inj Rehabil, 18*(2), 149-166.

Fawcett, J., Curt, A., Steeves, J., Coleman, W., Tuszynski, M., Lammertse, D., & ... Short, D. (2007). Guidelines for the conduct of clinical trials for spinal cord injury as developed by the ICCP panel: Spontaneous recovery after spinal cord injury and statistical power needed for therapeutic clinical trials. *Spinal Cord, 45*(3), 190-205.

Field-Fote, E. C. (Ed.). (2009). *Spinal Cord Injury Rehabilitation.* Philadelphia: F. A. Davis.

Gassaway, J., Dijkers, M., Rider, C., Edens, K., Cahow, C., & Joyce, J. (2011). Therapeutic recreation treatment time during inpatient rehabilitation. *The Journal of Spinal Cord Medicine, 34*(2), 176-185.

Gelis, A., Dupeyron, A., Legros, P., Benaim, C., Pelissier, J., & Fattal, C. (2009). Pressure ulcer risk factors in persons with spinal cord injury: Part 2: The chronic stage. *Spinal Cord, 47*, 651-661.

Healthy People 2020. (n.d.). Disability and Health. Retrieved from http://www.healthypeople.gov/2020/topicsobjectives2020/overview.aspx?topicid=9.

Juknis, N., Cooper, J. M., & Oksana, O. (2012). The changing landscape of spinal cord injury. *Handbook of Clinical Neurology, 109*, 149-66.

Juknis, N., Cooper, J. M., & Volshteyn, O. (2009). The changing landscape of spinal cord injury. In J. Verhaagen & J. W. McDonald III (Eds.), *Handbook of clinical neurology, vol 109 (3rd series) spinal cord injury* (pp. 149-166). San Diego, CA: Elsevier Science and Technology Books retrieved from http://www.sciencedirect.com.libproxy.temple.edu/science/handbooks/00729752/109.

Kawasaki, G. & Warms, C. (2007). Staying healthy after spinal cord injury: Taking care of pressure sores [Brochure]. Northwest Regional Spinal Cord Injury System.

Krassioukov, A., End, J. J., Warburton, D. E., & Teasell, R. (2009). A systematic review of the management of orthostatic hypotension after spinal cord injury. *Archives of Physical Medicine and Rehabilitation, 90*(5), 876-885.

Louis Calder Memorial Library of the University of Miami/Jackson Memorial Medical Center. (2009). Other complications of spinal cord injury: Hyperthermia. Retrieved from http://calder.med.miami.edu/pointis/hype.html.

Mayo Clinic. (2011). Spinal cord injury: Tests and diagnosis. Retrieved from http://www.mayoclinic.com/health/spinal-cord-injury/DS00460/DSECTION=tests-and-diagnosis.

Medline Plus. (n.d.). Deep vein thrombosis. Retrieved from http://www.nlm.nih.gov/medlineplus/deepveinthrombosis.html.

National Institute for Neurological Disorders and Stroke. (2011, Aug. 3). NINDS Brain and Spinal Tumors Information Page. Retrieved from http://www.ninds.nih.gov/disorders/brainandspinaltumors/brainandspinaltumors.htm.

National Institute for Neurological Disorders and Stroke. (2011, July 1). NINDS transverse myelitis information page. Retrieved from http://www.ninds.nih.gov/disorders/transversemyelitis/transversemyelitis.htm.

National Institute for Neurological Disorders and Stroke. (2011, Aug. 16). Guillain-Barré syndrome fact sheet. Retrieved from http://www.ninds.nih.gov/disorders/gbs/detail_gbs.htm.

National Spinal Cord Injury Statistical Center. (2012). Facts and figures at a glance. Retrieved from https://www.nscisc.uab.edu/.

Popa, C., Popa, F., Grigorean, V. T., Onose, G., Sandu, A. M., Popescu, M., Burnei, G., Strambu, V., & Sinescu, C. (2010).

Vascular dysfunctions following spinal cord injury. *Journal of Medicine and Life, 3*(3), 275-285. Retrieved from www.ncbi.nlm.nih.gov/pmc/articles/PMC3019008/.

Rabchevsky, A. & Kitzman, P. H. (2011). Latest approaches for the treatment of spasticity and autonomic dysreflexia in chronic spinal cord injury. *Neurotherapeutics: The Journal of the American Society for Experimental Neurotherapeutics, 8*, 274-282.

Reyes, M. R. & Chiodo, A. (2011). Spasticity and spinal cord injury. Retrieved from http://www.msktc.org/sci/factsheets/Spasticity.

Ripat, J. D. & Woodgate, R. L. (2012). Self-perceived participation among adults with spinal cord injury: A grounded theory study. *Spinal Cord, 50*, 908-914.

Shatzer, M. M. (2009). Autonomic nervous system issues: Orthostatic hypotension. In Bryce, T. N., *Spinal cord injury: Rehabilitation medicine quick reference*. Demos Medical.

Teasell, R. W., Mehta, S., Aubut, J. L., Ashe, M. C., Sequeira, K., Macaluso, S., & Tu, L. (2010). A systematic review of the therapeutic interventions for heterotopic ossification after spinal cord injury. *Spinal Cord, 48*, 512-521.

Umphred, D. A., Roller, M. L., Burton, G. U., & Lazaro, R. T. (2012). *Umphred's neurological rehabilitation*. Elsevier Health Sciences.

Verschueren, J. H. M., Post, M. W. M., de Groot, S., van der Woude, L. H. V., van Asbeck, F. W. A., & Roi, M. (2011). Occurrence and predictors of pressure ulcers during primary in-patient spinal cord injury rehabilitation. *Spinal Cord, 49*, 106-112.

Whiteneck, G., Gassaway, J., Dijkers, M., & Jha, A. (2008). New approach to study the contents and outcomes of spinal cord injury rehabilitation: The SCIRehab Project. *The Journal of Spinal Cord Medicine, 32*(3), 251-259.

Wilson, J., Grossman, R., Frankowski, R., Kiss, A., Davis, A., Kulkarni, A., & … Fehlings, M. (2012). A clinical prediction model for long-term functional outcome after traumatic spinal cord injury based on acute clinical and imaging factors. *Journal of Neurotrauma, 29*(13), 2263-2271. doi: 10.1089/neu.2012.2417.

Winnick, J. P. (2010). *Adapted physical education and sport*. Human Kinetics.

Yarkony, G. M. & Heinemann, A. W. (1995). Pressure ulcers. In S. L. Stover, J. A. DeLisa, & G. G. Whiteneck (Eds.), *Spinal cord injury: Clinical outcomes from the model systems* (pp. 100-19). Gaithersburg, MD: Aspen Publishers.

Young, W. (2006). Hypothermia and poikilothermia in spinal cord injury. Retrieved from http://sci.rutgers.edu/forum/showthread.php?t=62059.

36. Substance-Related Disorders

Stephanie Wood, J. Randal Wyble, and Jodie Charters

Substance-related disorders involve the use of substances in ways that can be harmful to the person taking the substance, other people in the person's life, and the person's community. For the person, negative physical, psychological, mental, interpersonal, and work- or school-related effects can be experienced (Centers for Disease Control and Prevention, 2010). Substance use can also take a toll on those who are in a relationship with the person who is using substances, as they may sacrifice their own goals to support and protect the person (MDSC, 2009; Wood & Tirone, 2013). The community can experience the harmful effects of substance use through increased criminal behavior, including actions taken to have access to the drug of choice, increased mental health care needs, family dysfunction, workplace absenteeism, etc.

The prevention and treatment of substance-related disorders can occur in a variety of healthcare settings from detoxification units to community based offices, using a variety of approaches from abstinence to harm reduction, in partnership with supports, such as family, mental health agencies, Alcoholics Anonymous, Narcotics Anonymous, and community leisure or recreation facilities, with the intention of facilitating a change process that supports the person who is harmfully involved, the affected others, and the community to reach their optimal health.

The *Diagnostic and Statistical Manual of Mental Disorders* (5th ed.) describes substance-related disorders. The *DSM-5* covers 10 separate classes of drugs: alcohol; caffeine; cannabis; hallucinogens (divided into arylcyclohexylamines and all others); inhalants; opioids; sedatives, hypnotics, and anxiolytics; amphetamines, cocaine, and other stimulants; tobacco; and other or unknown substances. Although the actions of the classes of drugs on the brain are different, all of the drugs have the common property

of directly activating the brain's reward system. Excessive use of substances can cause two kinds of problems, as outlined in the *DSM-5*, substance use disorder and substance-induced disorder. The substance-induced disorders are further divided into intoxication and withdrawal (APA, 2013). Each of the classes of drugs has its own list of criteria for diagnosing the disorders related to the class. Because alcohol is one of the most widely used substances, we will use it as the example for describing the diagnostic procedure.

Substance use disorder looks at the problems associated with ongoing use of the substance. (In the *DSM-IV-TR* these were called substance dependence and substance abuse, but they were combined because the distinction did not seem to be useful.) There are 11 criteria for each of the classes of drugs covered in the *DSM-5*.

The first four cover impaired control and ask (1) Was more of the drug taken than intended? (2) Are there persistent desires or unsuccessful efforts to reduce use? (3) Is a great deal of time spent being sure the substance is available? (4) Is there a strong craving for the substance?

The next three criteria cover social impairment. (5) Does use result in a failure to fulfill major role obligations? (6) Does the person continue to use the substance even though it creates recurrent social problems? (7) Are important activities given up because of use?

The risk of use is explored in the next two criteria. (8) Is the substance used in ways that are physically dangerous? (9) Does the person continue to use even though use is making some problem worse?

The last two criteria are pharmacological. (10) Is the person developing a tolerance? (11) Is there evidence of withdrawal?

It is considered a clinically significant impairment if two or more of the eleven criteria are met (APA, 2013).

Substance-induced disorders are divided into intoxication and withdrawal. Intoxication requires meeting four criteria: recent ingestion or exposure to the substance, clinically significant behavioral or psychological changes, one or more of a set of symptoms specific to the substance, and the signs must not be attributable to another condition or disorder. For alcohol the symptoms include slurred speech, unsteady gait, stupor, and others. Withdrawal is diagnosed when these four criteria are met: cessation or reduction in use or exposure, substance-specific symptoms, the symptoms are causing significant distress or impairment, and the symptoms can't be attributed to another condition or disorder. The symptoms for alcohol include hand tremor, nausea, transient hallucinations, and others (APA, 2013).

Sometimes substance use will cause conditions that appear to be psychiatric disorders. These are diagnosed as the psychiatric condition, for example, substance/medication-induced psychotic disorder. The term "addiction" is no longer used, according to the *DSM-5* (APA, 2013).

Incidence/Prevalence

In North America, the incidence and prevalence of substance use varies, particularly regarding the types of substances used. Geographical and cultural factors influence access, availability, and trends in use. Data collected in the U.S. and Canada look at the use of the following substances: alcohol, cannabis/marijuana, cocaine (including crack), heroin, hallucinogens, inhalants, pain relievers/pain killers (e.g., Percodan®, Demerol®, OxyContin®), tranquilizers, stimulants (e.g., speed, ecstasy, methamphetamine, crystal meth, Ritalin®, Adderall®, Dexedrine®), and sedatives (e.g., Valium®, Ativan®, Xanax®) (Health Canada, 2012; Substance Abuse and Mental Health Services Administration [SAMHSA], 2012). U.S. data from the 2011 National Survey on Drug Use and Health show eight percent of those surveyed identified substance dependence or abuse (SAMHSA, 2012).

Alcohol continues to be the substance of choice in North America. The culture of alcohol use in the U.S. and Canada continues to support overconsump-

tion (Giesbrecht et al., 2011). Of those who identified as having either substance dependence or abuse in the past year, 70% were diagnosed with alcohol dependence or abuse, 11% were diagnosed with dependence or abuse related to a combination of alcohol and illicit drugs, and 19% were diagnosed with dependence or abuse related to one or more of the classes of illicit drugs. Cannabis/marijuana, including hashish, is the most common illicit drug of choice (SAMHSA, 2012).

Those who are unemployed were more likely to engage in substance use (SAMHSA, 2012). Men are more likely than women to report use of alcohol and drugs (Health Canada, 2012; SAMHSA, 2012). The only exception to this was with the use of pain relievers and sedatives, which was shown to be more likely in women (Health Canada, 2012). Those with less than high school education had a higher incidence of drug-related dependency or abuse, but not alcohol-related dependency or abuse when compared to those with a high school degree or greater (SAMHSA, 2012).

Different substances have different rates of treatment. The *DSM-5* (American Psychiatric Association, 2013) identifies criteria for those needing treatment for alcohol use disorders. In the U.S., of those who met the criteria, 8.5% received treatment per the 2010 survey data. Of those identified as needing treatment for illicit drugs, with criteria similar to the alcohol criteria, 18.8% received treatment. The major limiting factor for those who were identified as needing but not receiving treatment for all substances was that more than 90% of the people with the substance use disorder did not feel there was a need for treatment (SAMHSA, 2012).

Predominant Age

Substance use (including alcohol and drugs) can occur at any age. Problematic substance use can occur any time across the lifespan, and those seeking support or treatment will represent a wide age range. That said, North Americans begin engaging in substance use at a young age. In Canada, the average age of initiation of use for cannabis is 15.6 years of age and for alcohol, 16.0 years of age (Health Canada, 2012). U.S. data suggests a diagnosis of substance abuse and dependency is more likely to occur between the ages of 18-25 (18.6%) as opposed to those aged 12-17 (6.9%) or those 26 years old or older (6.3%). For both alcohol and illicit drug dependency and abuse, those aged 26 years old or older who were identified as needing treatment were more likely to receive treatment than those in the younger age groups (SAMHSA, 2012).

Causes

Five general areas have been identified as causes of substance related disorders:

Familial, social, or cultural factors: Problems with substance use is more likely when a person's primary family, social, and/or cultural network tolerates, approves, and/or models substance abuse and related behaviors. This primary network generally shifts from family environment to friends during adolescence and early adulthood (Bahr, Marcos, & Maughan, 1995; Conger & Rueter, 1996).

Personality factors: Substance use problems are more likely in those experiencing depression, high levels of stress, challenges in self-regulating behavior, and/or having poor coping skills. Considerable research links personality disorder problems with substance use (Leventhal & Schmitz, 2006; Sher, Bartholow, & Wood, 2000).

Cognitive factors: Substance use produces a positive effect that reinforces the continued or increased use of substances, particularly if the individual also has positive expectancies related to the effects of the substance. Individuals may have a specific expectation that substance use will reduce negative emotional states (Leventhal & Schmitz, 2006).

Genetic factors: A person who has a parent with a substance use problem is at a greater risk for developing a substance use problem even when social factors are controlled for (Kaprio et al., 1987; van den Bree et al., 1998). This may be because genetically vulnerable individuals inherit a greater sensitivity to the positive psychopharmacological effects of substances (Uhl et al., 1993).

Biological factors: Particular neurotransmitters, including dopamine and serotonin, affect the reward pathways of the brain. Research shows that substance use can artificially influence the function of the neurotransmitters to the extent that it becomes difficult for the reward system of the brain to be stimulated naturally (Genetic Science Learning Center, 2011).

Systems Affected

Substance use exists on a continuum (Health Canada, 2000). Hazards and consequences of use are not universal and harmful involvement with one substance does not necessarily lead to harmful involvement with another. Most North Americans use some form of mood-altering substance without experiencing harm (Health Canada, 2000). The type, quantity, frequency, and route of administration of a substance influence the impact it has on those using it. Their medical, emotional, and physical health and level of tolerance also have an impact.

Exploring the potential impact of a substance on the whole person is important. For example, smoking marijuana or tobacco causes lung damage (b440 Respiration Functions, s430 Structure of Respiratory System) and alcohol use can impact liver function (s560 Structure of Liver). Other substances have different effects, which the RT will need to understand when working with a client with a particular substance use disorder. Beyond the physical aspects, it is equally important to understand how the substance use impacts relationships (d710 Basic Interpersonal Interactions), employment (d840-d859 Work and Employment), and personal health practices (d570 Looking After One's Health).

For those who experience harm, the impact can be felt both directly and indirectly across the spectrum of health.

Physical health concerns include illness, injuries, hyperactivity of the autonomic nervous system, and physical damage to the body (Centers for Disease Control and Prevention, 2010). Possible ICF codes include b110 Consciousness Functions, b235 Vestibular Functions, b4 Functions of the Cardiovascular, Hematological, Immunological, and Respiratory Systems, b750-b789 Movement Functions, s110 Structure of Brain, and s4 Structures of the Cardiovascular, Immunological, and Respiratory Systems.

Mental health concerns include anxiety, depression, loss of motivation, anger, agitation, and irritability (American Psychiatric Association, 2013). ICF codes include b122 Global Psychosocial Functions, b125 Dispositions and Intra-Personal Functions, b126 Temperament and Personality Functions, and b130 Energy and Drive Functions.

Social health concerns include strained or unhappy relationships with the possibility of a breakdown (d7 Interpersonal Interactions and Relationships), as well as problems at work or school (d8 Major Life Areas) (Gruber & Taylor, 2006).

Cognitive health concerns may include short-term confusion, learning problems, and memory loss (Carpenter, 2001). ICF codes include b117 Intellectual Functions, b140 Attention Functions, b144 Memory Functions, b160 Thought Functions, b163 Basic Cognitive Functions, and b164 Higher-Level Cognitive Functions, leading to deficits in d1 Learning and Applying Knowledge. In rare cases, hallucinations (b156 Perceptual Functions) and delusions (b160 Thought Functions) are possible (American Psychiatric Association, 2013).

Additional problems may include poor impulse control, poor judgment, and poor sleep quality with frequent disruptions in the sleep/wake cycle and insomnia. Related ICF codes include b130 Energy and Drive Functions, b134 Sleep Functions, and b164 Higher-Level Cognitive Functions.

Lifestyle issues may include financial instability, unemployment, homelessness, traffic accidents, conflict with the law, food insecurity, poor nutritional intake, and poor dental hygiene. ICF codes include d2 General Tasks and Demands, d5 Self-Care, d6 Domestic Life, and d8 Major Life Areas. Furthermore, violence and crime are sometimes associated with substance use. Substance use does not cause violence, but it may influence it (Deitch, Koutsenok, & Ruiz, 2000). Victims and perpetrators of violence may be using substances when a crime is committed, and crimes may occur to generate revenue to support substance use.

Secondary Problems

Others affected: A person's substance use may impact those around them, including family, friends, co-workers, and classmates. Research shows one third of Canadians report personal, physical, or emotional harm because of another's involvement with alcohol (Adlaf, Begin, & Sawka, 2005; MDSC, 2009). The impact of substance use upon others affected is important (Gruber & Taylor, 2006; Suman & Nagalakshmi, 1996). They may experience isolation (Forsbrey, Frabutt, & Smith, 2005; Gaudia, 1987; Lorenz & Yaffee, 1989; Velleman et al., 1993), social life restrictions (Velleman et al., 1993), dissatisfying relationships (Kahler, McCrady, & Epstein, 2003; Velleman et al., 1993), public

embarrassment (Velleman et al., 1993), a disruption of routines or family celebrations (Velleman et al., 1993), feelings of shame (Gaudia, 1987), anger and resentment (Lorenz & Yaffee, 1989; Velleman et al., 1993), the burden of multiple roles or changing roles (Suman & Nagalakshmi, 1996; Velleman et al., 1993), depression (Lorenz & Yaffee, 1989), guilt or responsibility (Lorenz & Yaffee, 1989), changes in physical health (Lorenz & Yaffee, 1989; Velleman et al., 1993), financial instability (Gaudia, 1987; Kirby et al., 2005) and violence (Adlaf et al., 2005; Velleman et al., 1993). Affected others often demonstrate great strength and adaptability. Generally, their actions that allow their loved ones to survive through provision of shelter, money, food, emotional support, and protection are done to protect both the person harmfully involved with substance use and themselves. These strategies make sense in the short term, but long term often drastically impact the others' lives. They will often give up important aspects of their lives, one of which is leisure. It is essential to work with and support concerned significant others to find long-term solutions and explore their own leisure, personal empowerment, and ability to take time for themselves. When the person with the diagnosis is the only concern, the relevant ICF codes can be found in d7 Interpersonal Interactions and Relationships and scored for the person. When treatment involves the whole support structure, ICF codes in d7 Interpersonal Interactions and Relationships are scored for all the people involved. In addition, deficits in the behaviors of the support group should be documented. Codependency, seen as a deficit in ICF code d710 Basic Interpersonal Interactions, is the primary problem to look for.

Concurrent disorders or dual diagnosis: It is not uncommon for people with substance use problems to also experience mental health concerns. Research shows more than 50% of those seeking help for their substance use also have a mental illness (37% for people with alcohol use problems and 53% for people with drug use problems) (CCSA, 2009). Furthermore, 15-20% of those seeking mental health services report problematic substance use (CCSA, 2009; MDSC, 2009). This trend does not improve over time: of seniors with a substance abuse problem 25-50% also have a mental illness (MDSC, 2009). Treatment for people experiencing concurrent disorders can be complicated and complex; frequent relapse and reoccurring crises tend to be the norm (CCSA, 2009). In addition to the increased challenges of coping with their circumstances and the stigma of both problematic substance use and mental illness, clients with concurrent disorders more often experience higher rates of unemployment, relationship difficulties, social anxiety, poverty, homelessness, social marginalization, and, in some cases, conflict with the law (CCSA, 2009). See chapters on the particular concurrent disorder for information on assessment and treatment.

Other disorders associated with substance use: Other disorders are listed below. See chapters on the particular disorder for information on assessment and treatment.

People with anxiety disorders have a two to five times greater risk of having substance use problems. At least 75% of people with both an anxiety disorder and substance use problem will develop the anxiety disorder first (CCSA, 2009).

The risk for developing a substance use problem is increased for those with attention-deficit/hyperactivity disorder, particularly when there has been no early intervention (CCSA, 2009).

Characterized by unusual changes in mood, the largest group of mental health conditions is referred to as mood disorders (with the most common being major depressive disorder, bipolar disorder, dysthymia, and cyclothymia). Substance use and mood disorders have a strong correlation; those with substance use problems are more likely to experience a mood disorder and those with mood disorders, particularly bipolar disorder, are more likely to use substances (CCSA, 2009).

Psychosis is often characterized by delusions and/or hallucinations. Schizophrenia is the most commonly diagnosed form of psychosis. The impact of these conditions presents challenges for functioning in society. Rates of substance use are much higher among people experiencing psychosis compared to the general population. Those diagnosed with schizophrenia are five times more likely to experience substance use problems (six times more for illicit drugs and three more times for alcohol) (CCSA, 2009) and 80% of people diagnosed with schizophrenia report experiencing a substance use problem at some point during their lifetime (MDSC, 2009). Substance use makes the diagnosis of

psychosis challenging. Substance use can increase the onset of psychosis and worsen the symptoms and course of the illness (CCSA, 2009). Tobacco, followed by cannabis, is the most-used substance by people diagnosed with psychosis. People with schizophrenia are two to three times more likely to smoke cigarettes than the general population — 58-88% are smokers (CCSA, 2009). Furthermore, heavy cannabis users are six times more likely to be diagnosed with schizophrenia than those who do not use cannabis.

Those with a diagnosis of substance use and antisocial personality disorder have been shown to have less life satisfaction and be more impulsive, more isolated, and more depressed than people with antisocial personality disorder alone.

Prognosis

The prognosis of harmful substance use is unclear. When clients access a program, it typically falls into one of two categories — inpatient and outpatient. Inpatient services may include withdrawal management or detoxification and structured treatment programs. Outpatient services may include day withdrawal management services, one-on-one counseling, psycho-education and group therapy, treatment for concerned significant others, workplace or school counseling, etc. Residential treatment facilities or sober/clean living environments may also be included in this category although some may operate in a closed-group format.

Many treatments suggest complete abstinence as the goal for substance use treatment, but this may not be the goal of a client. A harm reduction route, such as controlled drinking, may be an option. Client goals and outcomes can be influenced by gender, readiness to change, extent and impact of use, reasons for use, coping skills, the quality and comprehensive nature of programs offered, other health conditions, polysubstance use, environmental factors, and social support networks, including significant others, peers, and professionals.

Change exists on a continuum (Prochaska & Velicer, 1997). The transtheoretical model, more commonly referred to as a stages of change model, demonstrates the thought process behind making change (DiClemente & Prochaska, 1998). The stages of change are pre-contemplation (not yet acknowledging a behavior to change), contemplation (acknowledging there is a problem but not yet ready or sure if they want to change), preparation (getting ready to change), action (changing the behavior), and maintenance (maintaining the behavior change). Relapse can occur at any place across the continuum of change and is a natural part of the process. In the event of a relapse, with the individual returning to a previous stage of change, such as moving from action to pre-contemplation, it is important to remember that the individual is not back at step one. Instead that person has gained information and experiences that s/he may draw upon, should s/he choose to move forward with the changes that were initially made. Social support networks are important to help cope with relapses and prevent them from occurring. Success should be defined by the client's self-identified treatment goals. Abstinence should not be the only marker of success. A harm-reduction approach may be helpful for identifying and celebrating success in treatment.

Assessment

The assessment process for substance intoxication and substance withdrawal is very different from the process for assessing substance use disorders.

For intoxication and withdrawal the concerns are largely medical. The patient needs to be assessed for life-threatening medical conditions related to the substance. The question is, what do we need to do to keep this person alive and get the substance out of his/her system?

For substance use disorders, the questions are different. The team first asks whether there really is a problem by using the DSM-5 criteria. If so, readiness, willingness, and confidence to change are crucial for motivating initial and then sustained behavior change. Consequently, in partnership with the client, the team will assess a client's motivation to make a change related to substance use by using the stages of change model or a similar measure. Determining and reinforcing extrinsic and, more importantly, intrinsic motivation to change may involve exploring the harmful impact of substance use on the person's life. Aspects to ask the client about include loved ones, finances, leisure, school or employment, conflict with the law, physical health, and mental health. Many clients may not engage with treatment before they experience what is referred to in 12-Step circles as "hitting bottom" which involves a significant

negative impact on many areas of a person's life. Following the assessment of motivation the team looks for the most effective way to support the client's change based upon the client's readiness and motivation level, including working to motivate individuals with substance use disorders who are ambivalent to change. Because a recreational therapist is not involved in the medical issues of intoxication and withdrawal, the following discussion will look at the details of what the team and recreational therapist do to assess substance-related disorders.

Typical Scope of Team Assessment

The connection between trauma and substance use is evident in research and practice. It is not uncommon for people with substance use problems to have a history of physical or sexual abuse (CCSA, 2009; Health Canada, 2000). Substance use is often an attempt to cope with or escape the impact of traumatic events. Those who use substances to avoid normal anxiety and sadness may establish a pattern of behavior that can be hard to change. They may believe they cannot function without their substance(s) of choice (Health Canada, 2000). Often this is a strategy that works in the short term. In fact it makes sense that someone would look to find ways to minimize the impact of the traumatic event. But in the long term it becomes increasingly problematic. Increases in alcohol and drug use may lead to new traumatic experiences that then fuel the cycle of coping with substance use (CCSA, 2009). The team assessment focuses on identifying possible causes of substance abuse including social or familial issues, personality factors, cognitive beliefs, and biological or genetic factors. It includes exploration of the client's medical history, history of abuse, relationships with family, friends, and coworkers, social supports, environmental factors, and mental health. ICF codes to record findings related to intrapersonal and interpersonal systems were discussed earlier.

Quality social support resources can be extremely important in coping with traumatic, stressful, or anxiety-provoking events or situations (CCSA, 2009). The team needs to understand the kinds of support the person will have when undergoing treatment. Deficits in support should be documented with ICF codes under e3 Support and Relationships. Issues related to the community where the client lives may also be documented with e5 Services, Systems, and Policies.

Areas of Concern for RT Assessment

The recreational therapist needs to understand the underlying cause of the substance use, any co-occurring health diagnoses, the client's insight into the current role of leisure, and the client's hopes for the future role of leisure. Some of this will come from the team, but recreational therapists possess the skills and training to explore leisure in depth. Assessment findings related to the client's leisure awareness and leisure skills will additionally help to identify recreational therapy interventions to help build a foundation for positive leisure in life. Areas of concern include the ability to identify interests and values, the ability to plan for free time, and skills at problem solving to overcome barriers to leisure. The findings will vary depending upon the assessment questions and the rapport between the client and therapist. Findings can be recorded using the ICF codes discussed previously.

ICF Core Set

No ICF Core Set has been defined for Substance-Related Disorders.

Treatment Direction

When the diagnosis is substance intoxication or substance withdrawal, the treatment is to provide a safe environment for the client to detoxify and to facilitate conversations that could motivate the client to engage in further treatments as it relates to an additional diagnosis of substance use disorder.

A diagnosis of a substance use disorder is identified and treatment usually begins when the ongoing use of substances has resulted in a person failing to fulfill major roles related to work, school, or home (American Psychiatric Association, 2013). From a client's perspective, treatment is generally sought when they are having problems in one or more of the areas known commonly as the four Ls — love (relationships), living (health), livelihood (employment or, in the case of students, education), and legal (problems which may be directly or indirectly related to the use of substances).

Treatment can occur in different settings including inpatient, outpatient, and residential settings. The type of treatment could include a variety of ap-proaches including but not limited to medications, cognitive behavioral therapy, family therapy, motivational interviewing, and therapeutic communities (National Institute on Drug Abuse, 2009). Ideally, the setting and type of services utilized are determined by the needs of the individual client at a given point in their treatment. Treatment programs should offer ongoing multidisciplinary assessments and approaches to meet the individual needs of the client (Sadock & Sadock, 2003). Realistically, however, the client's resources and ability to access services also impacts the setting and type of treatment they receive. For example, a client may benefit from a structured inpatient program but be unable to access it due to financial constraints or responsibilities such as employment or caregiving.

Treatment approaches vary according to each organization's mandate but typically fall into one of two approaches: abstinence or harm reduction.

In general, an abstinence-based approach is informed by a disease-based framework where abstinence is viewed as an immediate intervention. In this approach, problematic substance use is seen as a progressive, chronic disease that cannot be cured, although it is possible to enter recovery (National Institute on Alcohol Abuse and Alcoholism, 2007). Those with substance use disorders are seen as unable to control their use and therefore are encouraged to abstain from their substance of choice indefinitely. One problem with some abstinence-based approaches is the assumption that all of the documented problems will go away if the person stops using the substance. Given the wide range of problems that are often found, this is not a reasonable assumption. Treatment needs to consider addressing all the significant deficits found during the assessment process.

Harm-reduction-based treatment takes a different approach. According to Tatarsky (1998) harm reduction

> accepts active substance use as a fact and assumes that substance users must be engaged where they are, not where the provider thinks they should be. It recognizes that substance use and its consequences vary along a continuum of harmful effects for the user and the community and that behaviour generally changes by small incremental steps (p.10).

When implemented within policy and programs, clients in a harm-reduction program are not required to immediately halt their use (CAMH, 2009). Although abstinence may be included as part of a harm-reduction approach, the underlying premise is that clients choose the option that makes the most sense for them given the context of their lives. Harm reduction may include a reduction in use, but it is more focused on a reduction in harms related or associated with the use.

Treatment can also vary depending on the organization's integration, alignment, or partnership with mental health services. Concurrent disorders (also known as co-occurring or dual diagnosis) have been described as a major problem in North America (CCSA, 2009). These were discussed in the section on secondary problems.

Whole Team Approach

Treatment for substance use disorders occurs across a continuum. From talking to a family physician to entering a structured residential program, the decision to enter treatment is often difficult. The whole team approach involves healthcare professionals, the client, and any significant others the client chooses to have involved. The makeup of the team and the emphasis of treatment may vary in response to the client's need at any point in the treatment process. In general, following the person's entry into treatment for a substance use disorder, the care will consist of interventions focused on detoxification, recovery, and maintenance (SAMHSA, 2011).

Entering treatment: For some, entering treatment follows some type of an event and/or client insight into the harms caused by use. These can be internal or external motivations. Most clients will enter treatment for external reasons; finding internal motivators is important to maintaining and sustaining recovery goals. Examples of a motivator could be the loss of something important, usually a relationship or employment, or an employer making treatment a condition of continued employment. Other clients enter treatment because of a medical crisis brought on by intoxication or withdrawal. Whether the client makes a decision to stop using a substance or is forced to stop using it because of a crisis, the next step in treatment is detoxification.

Detoxification: Sudden discontinuation of substance use after a physiological dependence has developed can lead to severe health issues. The process for detoxification will vary depending on the specific substance and only occurs if a physiological dependency has developed. In general, detoxification is a medical process designed to help the client be safe as they cope with the physiological dependency and associated withdrawal symptoms that occur in response to discontinuing the use of the substance. The end result is to have the client's body free and clean of the substance. This phase of treatment addresses ICF codes that were used to document the immediate harm caused by the latest episode of use.

Recovery: At this point clients may or may not have a healthy support system in place. The depth and length of a rehabilitation program will vary depending on the needs of the client. The desired outcome of rehabilitation is to teach clients needed skills in order to meet their goal related to substance use. Ultimately, this goal is focused on reducing the risk of harm that would result from continued use at the current level. Frequently, but not always, this goal focuses on abstaining from any substance use. If this is the case, an important aspect of rehabilitation often suggested is ongoing involvement in a 12-Step program such as Alcoholics or Narcotics Anonymous. However, the goal of reducing the risk of harm from continued substance use may stop short of abstinence and instead be focused on developing non-harmful patterns of substance use (Barry, 1999). The decision to pursue abstinence or a harm-reduction-based approach is made with consideration of the client's motivation level, substance use patterns, and the philosophy of the treatment program. ICF codes related to this phase include consideration of codes related to the physical harm the substance use is causing (for example b110 Consciousness Functions, b235 Vestibular Functions, b4 Functions of the Cardiovascular, Hematological, Immunological, and Respiratory Systems, b750-b789 Movement Functions, s110 Structure of Brain, and s4 Structures of the Cardiovascular, Immunological, and Respiratory Systems), functional deficits in mental and emotional processing (b122 Global Psychosocial Functions, b125 Dispositions and Intra-Personal Functions, b126 Temperament and Personality Functions, b130 Energy and Drive Functions, b134 Sleep Functions, and b164 Higher-Level Cognitive

Functions, d240 Handling Stress and Other Psychological Demands), areas where the use is causing harm in relationships (d6 Domestic Life, d7 Interpersonal Interactions and Relationships, and d8 Major Life Areas), and any deficits noted in the client's support structure (e3 Support and Relationships).

Recreational Therapy Approach

Recreational therapists work in many of the settings identified above and provide interventions throughout the recovery process. Recreational therapists usually work as part of a multidisciplinary treatment team. Other disciplines on the team will vary according to the setting, but may include psychiatrists, nurses, psychologists, social workers, counselors, music therapists, art therapists, drama therapists, occupational therapists, technicians, pharmacists, vocational counselors, and spiritual advisors. Interventions may be individually based, but are more likely to be group based. They may also be facilitated unidisciplinary or multidisciplinary.

Recreational Therapy Interventions

The focus of the interventions provided are determined as a result of an initial recreational therapy assessment, which identifies the strengths, challenges, needs, and goals of the client as related to the recovery process.

Role of Leisure

A major focus is placed on the role that leisure can play in enhancing the likelihood of success in recovery, including coping and stress management (d240 Handling Stress and Other Psychological Demands), developing healthy lifestyles (d570 Looking After One's Health), and building positive relationships (d7 Interpersonal Interactions and Relationships) (Faulkner, 1991; Carruthers & Hood, 1992; Carruthers, 1999; Carruthers & Hood, 2002; Arai et al., 2008). Leisure involvement allows clients to learn about themselves, develop self-awareness, find acceptance with where they are, and learn to celebrate their successes (Hood, 2003). Specific recreational therapy interventions for clients making changes to their substance use commonly explore coping (d240 Handling Stress and Other Psychological Demands), goal setting (d163 Thinking), leisure planning (d920 Recreation and Leisure),

safety planning (d571 Looking After One's Safety), managing emotions (e.g., d720 Complex Interpersonal Interactions, d250 Managing One's Own Behavior), connecting with social supports (d7 Interpersonal Interactions and Relationships), and practicing social skills (d710 Basic Interpersonal Interactions). Each is further described below.

Coping: Research has drawn connections between leisure and coping (Bedini & Guinan, 1996; Coleman & Iso-Ahola, 1993; Iwasaki, 2006; Iwasaki, MacKay, & Mactavish, 2005; Iwasaki et al., 2006; Kleiber, Hutchinson, & Williams, 2002). Participation in either active or social leisure encourages coping with stress (d240 Handling Stress and Other Psychological Demands) through leisure's ability to connect participants to positive social supports (e3 Support and Relationships) and opportunities to experience self-determination (Coleman & Iso-Ahola, 1993; Iwasaki et al., 2006; Wijndaele, 2007).

Goal setting: Setting leisure goals can provide a structure for future leisure plans. Whether applying for a library card, meeting a friend, or training for a marathon, helping clients to understand how to identify and set clear, measurable, and achievable leisure goals can make the difference between achievable and unachievable leisure outcomes. Before clients set a goal, they need to have support to explore their leisure needs. For many clients, the concept of leisure is perceived as something that is not for them, especially if it has been positioned as a reward. If leisure is viewed as a reward, then clients in recovery might think they can only have those experiences when all of their "wrongdoings" have been fixed. The role of a recreational therapist is to reposition leisure as a tool for coping within the recovery process, and a tool for connecting with themselves, their supports, and their community in a positive way. Leisure can help clients who are making changes in their substance use to see themselves differently and help them find meaning in their life (Hood, 2003). For some clients, leisure will have been rarely experienced without their substance of choice. Recreational therapy supports a process of developing leisure awareness through the exploration of interests, benefits, values, attitudes, barriers, resources, and goal setting. Clients are encouraged to find interests and activities they find meaningful, enjoyable, and rejuvenating (Hood, 2003; McCracken, 1991). ICF codes that can be addressed with this technique include b126 Temperament and Personality Functions, b130 Energy and Drive Functions, d163 Thinking, d7 Interpersonal Interactions and Relationships, and d920 Recreation and Leisure.

Leisure planning: Planning leisure that takes into consideration goals, current resources, and safety requirements is potentially a new way for persons harmfully involved to think about leisure. It is often reassuring when clients learn that leisure takes thought and skill and that it is normal for it to be challenging when starting out. The challenge begins when clients "break up" with their substance, which acted as a constant leisure activity, a dependable leisure partner, and came with a culture of use whose rules were understood. For many clients it is hard to imagine how they could ever have fun again without their substance. Learning to experience leisure without the use of substances can be extremely challenging (Hood, 2003). Recreational therapists design programs that will not only appeal to clients, but also incorporate the element of choice, which can provide opportunities to practice self-determination (d2 General Tasks and Demands). Choice can mean having a variety of activity options available or having flexibility in an activity for clients to determine the extent of their participation based on their goals. Programs that are facilitated in a treatment agency are ideal for leisure exploration in a structured environment. Programs that are facilitated in the community are ideal for experiencing realistic successes and challenges that can be supported and debriefed in a safe manner. It also helps with transitions to independent living if a client can replicate a leisure experience without the formal support of an agency.

Safety planning: For clients in recovery an important element of experiencing positive leisure is safety planning. Clients may need to develop strategies to negotiate the social, physical, mental, and environmental factors that can influence the achievement of their leisure goals. What the safety concerns are, and what the safety plan will look like, will be unique to each client. There are various types of safety, including (1) social safety (focuses on reducing risk associated with relationships), (2) physical safety (focuses on reducing risk associated with activity demands), (3) emotional safety (focuses on reducing risk associated with overwhelming feelings and emotions), and (4) environmental safety (focuses on reducing the risk associated with places). Any of these factors can trigger a craving and/or an unsafe experience. It is valuable to provide clients with the opportunity to plan how to keep themselves safe. For example, a client may set a goal to develop personal boundaries that aid in avoiding or minimizing exposure to situations where they feel unsafe, developing self-confidence and assertiveness skills, and/or understanding personal needs related to having positive leisure experiences and then developing skills to obtain such needs. Some of the ICF codes that can be cited for safety planning include b126 Temperament and Personality Functions, b130 Energy and Drive Functions, d240 Handling Stress and Other Psychological Demands, d250 Managing One's Own Behavior, d570 Looking After One's Health, d710 Basic Interpersonal Interactions, and d720 Complex Interpersonal Interactions.

Managing emotions: Learning how to manage feelings and emotions related to leisure participation can be important for clients. It involves learning how to deal with feelings that come when anticipating an activity, being in the activity, and ending the activity (b125 Dispositions and Intra-Personal Functions, b126 Temperament and Personality Functions, b130 Energy and Drive Functions). Emotions experienced can include excitement, fear, exhilaration, disappointment, connectedness, and loneliness. Getting support to understand those emotions provides the opportunity to develop skills to manage them, which enables the leisure experience to continue to be an area of positive growth.

Connecting with social supports: Connecting with social supports through community leisure opportunities, including the exploration of personally relevant, age-appropriate, and accessible leisure, is important (Klitzing, 2004; Hebblethwaite & Pedlar, 2005). A sense of belonging is crucial to health and has strong benefits for recovery. The leisure of some clients may be so intertwined with their substance use that when they stop, they are unsure of what activities are available and how to have fun at this life stage. Social supports, including recovery groups related to support for substance use, can be extremely important and may be explored (Hale, Hannum, & Espelage, 2005). The self-management principles developed in self-help groups and the value of learning from those who may have had shared experiences should not be overlooked (Lorig & Holman, 2003). ICF codes that can be the target of this kind of treatment include many of the codes in d7 Interpersonal Interactions and Relationships, especially d710 Basic Interpersonal Interactions.

Practicing social skills: Clients need the chance to practice social skills (d710 Basic Interpersonal Interactions). For many clients their socialization has occurred in settings that have been strongly connected to their harmful involvement with substances. Having the opportunity to practice socializing while not using substances is important.

The idea that clients have a right to healthy leisure may meet with resistance. With its many benefits, leisure can act as a tool for managing stress, experiencing joy, developing healthier coping skills, fostering positive connections with self and others, and more. Clients often feel like they don't deserve to have fun. Leisure is more than an easy filler for time gaps in schedules and a reward for good behavior. It is a meaningful and safe context within which clients can explore new ways of connecting with themselves and others.

Functional Skills

Everyone's experience with harmful involvement is unique. Specific functional skills to be explored will depend on the needs of the client. Examples may include controlling impulses, managing emotions, building relationships, and setting and respecting boundaries. Influencing factors may include the type of substance used, length of time used, route of administration, previous and current coping mechanisms, cultural factors, the way someone was raised, co-occurring conditions or injuries, and history of trauma. ICF codes that are cited during the assessment process form the basis for treatment. Functional skills that need to be improved may include b125 Dispositions and Intra-Personal Functions, b126 Temperament and Personality Functions, b130 Energy and Drive Functions, d710 Basic Interpersonal Interactions, d760 Family Relationships, and e3 Support and Relationships.

Education, Training, and Counseling

To make sustained behavior change, clients will need support with motivation, behavior modification, and emotion management, including confidence and handling stress. It is important not to confuse a client's readiness for change with their confidence in their ability to do so. Although the approach taken to change behavior may be influenced by the goals of the agency, it is important for recreational therapists to be familiar with evidence-based practices that support behavior change including motivational interviewing (MI), cognitive behavior therapy (CBT) and the transtheoretical model (stages of change) (Baker et al., 2012; Dutra et al., 2008). ICF codes that may be a target of motivational work include b125 Dispositions and Intra-Personal Functions, b126 Temperament and Personality Functions, b130 Energy and Drive Functions, d240 Handling Stress and Other Psychological Demands, and d250 Managing One's Own Behavior.

Community Integration

Clients accessing treatment for substance use will require varying degrees of support for community integration. Although client contact may occur in an inpatient hospital setting for withdrawal management or multi-day structured treatment most clients will come from, return to, or remain in a community setting while seeking treatment. In addition to the personal changes clients may be looking to make, clients may also be working towards making changes to their external environment including people they interact with, places they go, and things they do (d7 Interpersonal Interactions and Relationships, e3 Support and Relationships).

When a client decides to make changes, this does not mean their external environment is ready to support this change. It is important to help clients connect to personally meaningful opportunities in their community that support the health and lifestyle changes they are making, particularly those that continue to enhance the client's quality of life. This is why integrating the development and delivery of leisure education and recreation programs in community settings (d910 Community Life) is crucial to maintaining recovery goals. RTs bring people out of the clinical setting and into the community setting to learn and practice their skills. They present a variety of leisure opportunities to match the diverse interests of the people accessing services. Although cost may not always be a constraint for clients, finding affordable, low cost, or free community options for participation is important. Prior to participating in a public event or activity, the

RT needs to discuss with the group how to respect and maintain everyone's anonymity and confidentiality. Finally, RTs present options that give everyone the opportunity to explore in a safe, supportive environment.

Health Promotion

Health promotion related to harmful involvement with substance use is complex. Its goal is to empower individuals and communities to take responsibility for the improvement and maintenance of their health. Recreational therapists promote health utilizing both downstream and upstream approaches. Downstream interventions focus on the client's individual needs. Upstream interventions focus on population-wide influences on health such as policy work, collaborating with communities, or targeted social marketing campaigns to increase awareness and education, all while focused on the connection between leisure and health. Some possible upstream interventions for recreational therapists concerned with substance use include eliminating sponsorship of municipal recreation facilitates by companies that produce alcohol and providing community recreation alternatives to substance abuse. Such efforts may be justified from the assessment and treatment of a particular client if ICF codes e3 Support and Relationships and e5 Services, Systems, and Policies were identified as concerns.

Currently, the most visible work of recreational therapy is provided downstream in the treatment and intervention phases. With that said, however, work in the treatment and intervention phases can incorporate upstream health promotion approaches by focusing on determinants of health when planning programs; focusing on client's emotional, physical, and social safety in programming; advocating for access and availability to affordable housing; connecting with meaningful free and low-cost recreation opportunities; etc. Strong communities mobilizing change are an essential component to reducing alcohol- and drug-related harms. Availability of and engagement in meaningful leisure is integral to the health of individuals, families, communities, and society as a whole.

Resources

Canadian Centre on Substance Abuse (CCSA)
www.ccsa.ca

CCSA provides national leadership and evidence-informed analysis and advice to mobilize collaborative efforts to reduce alcohol and other drug-related harms. Their website provides links to information on a variety of relevant topics including substances and addictions, treatment, drug strategies, enforcement, harm reduction, populations, settings, and prevention.

Centre for Addictions and Mental Health (CAMH)
www.camh.net

As Canada's largest mental health and addictions teaching hospital, the CAMH website offers practical, evidence-based publications and resources related to substance use and addictions, mental health, concurrent disorders, trauma, policy research, clinical tools, and health promotion.

National Institute on Drug Abuse (NIDA)
www.drugabuse.gov

NIDA offers resources for medical and health professionals, researchers, parents, teachers, students, and young adults. They provide strategic support and conduct research across a broad range of disciplines and ensure rapid and effective dissemination and use of the results of that research to significantly improve prevention and treatment and to inform policy as it relates to drug abuse and addiction.

Substance Abuse and Mental Health Services Administration (SAMHSA)
www.samhsa.gov

SAMHSA aims to reduce the impact of substance abuse and mental illness on America's communities. Their website offers information on research, publications, grant opportunities, and more. They believe recovery is possible, treatment works, and advocate the importance of behavioral health and prevention.

References

Adlaf, E. M., Begin, P., & Sawka, E. (Eds.). (2005). *Canadian Addiction Survey (CAS): A national survey of Canadians' use of alcohol and other drugs: Prevalence of use and related harms: Detailed report*. Ottawa: Canadian Centre on Substance Abuse.

Arai, S., Griffin, J., Miatello, A., & Greig, C. L. (2008). Leisure and recreation involvement in the context of healing from trauma. *Therapeutic Recreation Journal, 42*(1), 37-55.

American Psychiatric Association. (2013). *Diagnostic and statistical manual of mental disorders* (5th ed.). Washington, DC: American Psychiatric Publishing.

Bahr, S. J., Marcos, A. C., & Maughan, S. L. (1995). Family, educational and peer influences on the alcohol use of female and male adolescents. *Journal of Studies on Alcohol, 56*, 457-469.

Baker, A. L., Thornton, L. K., Hiles, S., Hides, L., & Lubman, D. I. (2012). Psychological interventions for alcohol misuse among people with co-occurring depression or anxiety disorders: A systematic review. *Journal of Affective Disorders, 139*(3), 217-229.

Barry, K. L. (1999). *Brief interventions and brief therapies for substance abuse*. Rockville, MD: U.S. Department of Health and Human Services.

Bedini, L. A. & Guinan, D. M. (1996). "If I could just be selfish…": Caregivers' perceptions of their entitlement to leisure. *Leisure Sciences, 18*, 227-239.

Canadian Centre on Substance Abuse (CCSA). (2009). *Substance abuse in Canada: Concurrent disorders*. Ottawa, ON: Canadian Centre on Substance Abuse.

Carpenter, S. (2001). Cognition is central to drug addiction. *Monitor on Psychology, 32*(6). Retrieved from www.apa.org/monitor/jun01/cogcentral.aspx.

Carruthers, C. (1999). Pathological gambling: Implications for therapeutic recreation practice. *Therapeutic Recreation Journal, 33*(4), 287-303.

Carruthers, C. P. & Hood, C. D. (1992). Alcoholics and children of alcoholics: The role of leisure in recovery. *Journal of Physical Education, Recreation & Dance, 63*(4), 48-51.

Carruthers, C. P. & Hood, C. D. (2002). Coping skills program for individuals with alcoholism. *Therapeutic Recreation Journal, 36*(2), 154-171.

Centers for Disease Control and Prevention. (2010). Fact sheets: Alcohol use and health. Retrieved from www.cdc.gov/alcohol/fact-sheets/alcohol-use.htm.

Centre for Mental Health and Addiction (CAMH). (2009). Harm reduction: Its meaning and application for substance use issues position statement. Retrieved December 2010 from www.camh.net/Public_policy/Public_policy_papers/harmred uctionposition.html.

Coleman, D. & Iso-Ahola, S. E. (1993). Leisure and health: The role of social support and self-determination. *Journal of Leisure Research, 25*(2), 111-128.

Conger, R. D. & Rueter, M. A. (1996). Siblings, parents and peers: A longitudinal study of social influences in adolescent risk for alcohol use and abuse. *Advances in Applied Developmental Psychology, 10*, 1-30.

Deitch, D., Koutsenok, I., & Ruiz, A. (2000). The relationship between crime and drugs: What we have learned in recent decades. *Journal of Psychoactive Drugs, 32*(4), 391-397.

DiClemente, C. C. & Prochaska, J. O. (1998). Toward a comprehensive transtheoretical model of change: Stages of change and addictive behaviors. In W.R. Miller & N. Heather (Eds.). *Treating addictive behaviors* (2nd ed.). New York: Plenum Press.

Dutra, L., Stathopoulou, G., Basen, S. L., Leyro, T. M., Powers, M. B., & Otto, M. W. (2008). A meta-analytic review of psychosocial interventions for substance use disorders. *The American Journal of Psychiatry, 165*(2), 179-87.

Faulkner, R. W. (1991). *Therapeutic recreation protocol for treatment of substance addictions*. State College, PA: Venture Publishing, Inc.

Forsbrey, A., Frabutt, J., & Smith, H. (2005). Social isolation among caregivers of court-involved youths: A qualitative investigation. *Journal of Addictions and Offender Counseling, 25*(2), 97-113.

Gaudia, R. (1987). Effects of compulsive gambling on the family. *Social Work*, May/June, 254-256.

Genetic Science Learning Center. (2011) Beyond the reward pathway. Learn Genetics. Retrieved from http://learn.genetics.utah.edu/content/addiction/reward/pathw ays.html.

Giesbrecht, N., Stockwell, T., Kendall, P., Strang, R., & Thomas, G. (2011). Alcohol in Canada: Reducing the toll through

focused interventions and public health policies. *Canadian Medical Association Journal, 183*(4), 450-455.

Gruber, K. J. & Taylor, M. (2006). A family perspective for substance abuse: Implications from the literature. *Journal of Social Work Practice in the Addictions, 6*(1), 1-29.

Hale, C. J., Hannum, J. W., & Espelage, D. L. (2005). Social support and physical health: The importance of belonging. *Journal of American College Health, 53*(6), 276-284.

Health Canada. (2012). Canadian alcohol and drug use monitoring survey. Retrieved from www.hc-sc.gc.ca/hc-ps/drugs-drogues/stat/_2010/summary-sommaire-eng.php.

Health Canada. (2000). *Straight facts about drugs and drug abuse*. Ottawa, ON: Queen's Press.

Hebblethwaite, S. & Pedlar, A. (2005). Community integration for older adults with mental health issues: Implications for therapeutic recreation. *Therapeutic Recreation Journal, 39*(4), 264-276.

Hood, C. (2003). Women in recovery from alcoholism: The place of leisure. *Leisure Sciences, 25*(1), 51-79.

Iwasaki, Y. (2006). Counteracting stress through leisure coping: A prospective health study. *Psychology, Health & Medicine, 11*(2), 209-220.

Iwasaki, Y., MacKay, K., & Mactavish, J. (2005). Gender-based analysis of coping with stress among professional managers: Leisure coping and non-leisure coping. *Journal of Leisure Research, 37*(1), 1-28.

Iwasaki, Y., MacKay, K., Mactavish, J., Ristock, J., & Bartlett, J. (2006). Voices from the margins: Stress, active living, and leisure as a contributor to coping with stress. *Leisure Sciences, 28*, 163-180.

Kahler, C. W., McCrady, B. S., & Epstein, E. E. (2003). Sources of distress among women in treatment with their alcoholic partners. *Journal of Substance Abuse Treatment, 24*(3), 257-265.

Kaprio, J., Koskenvuo, M., Langinvainio, H., Romanov, K., Sarna, S., & Rose, R. J. (1987). Genetic influences on use and abuse of alcohol: A study of 5638 adult Finnish twin brothers. *Alcohol Clinical Experimental Research, 11*, 349-356.

Kirby, K. C., Dugosh, K. L., Benishek, L. A., & Harrington, V. M. (2005). The significant other checklist: Measuring the problems experienced by family members of drug users. *Addictive Behaviors, 30*(1), 29-47.

Kleiber, D. A., Hutchinson, S. L., & Williams, R. (2002). Leisure as a resource in transcending negative life events: Self-protection, self-restoration, and personal transformation. *Leisure Sciences, 24*, 219-235.

Klitzing, S. W. (2004). Women who are homeless: Leisure and affiliation. *Therapeutic Recreation Journal, 38*(4), 348-365.

Leventhal, A. M. & Schmitz, J. M. (2006). The role of drug use outcome expectancies in substance abuse risk: An interactional-transformational model. *Addictive Behaviors, 31*(11), 2038-2062.

Lorig, K. R. & Holman, H. R. (2003). Self-management education: History, definition, outcomes, and mechanisms. *Annals of Behavioral Medicine, 26*(1), 1-7.

Lorenz, V. C. & Yaffee, R. A. (1989). Pathological gambling: Psychosomatic, emotional marital difficulties as reported by the spouse. *The Journal of Gambling Behavior, 4*(1), 13-26.

McCracken, J. L. (1991). Creativity and leisure for recovering alcoholics. *Alcoholism Treatment Quarterly, 8*(3), 83-89.

Mood Disorders Society of Canada (MDSC). (2009). Quick facts: Mental health and addiction in Canada, third edition. Guelph, ON: Mood Disorders Society of Canada.

National Institute on Drug Abuse. (2009). *Principles of drug addiction treatment: A research- based guide* (2nd ed.) (NIH Publication No. 09 — 4180). Rockville, MD: Author.

National Institute on Alcohol Abuse and Alcoholism. (2007). FAQ for the general public: Is alcoholism a disease? Retrieved January 14, 2011 from http://www.niaaa.nih.gov/FAQs/General-English/Pages/default.aspx.

Prochaska, J. O & Velicer, W. F. (1997). The transtheoretical model of health behavior change. *American Journal of Health Promotion, 12*(1), 38-48.

Sadock, B. & Sadock, V. (2003). *Kaplan & Sadock's synopsis of psychiatry* (9th ed.). New York, New York: Lippincott Williams & Wilkins.

Sher, K. J., Bartholow, B. D., & Wood, M. D. (2000). Personality and substance use disorders: A prospective study. *Journal of Consulting and Clinical Psychology, 68*(5), 818-829.

Substance Abuse and Mental Health Services Administration (SAMHSA). (2012). *Results from the 2011 national survey on drug use and health: Volume I. Summary of national findings* (NSDUH Series H-44, HHS Publication No. SMA 12-4713). Rockville, MD: author.

Suman, L. N. & Nagalakshmi, S. V. (1996). Family dysfunction in alcoholic families. *Indian Journal of Clinical Psychology, 23*(2), 117-121.

Tatarsky, A. (1998). An integrative approach to harm reduction psychotherapy: A case of problem drinking secondary to depression. *Psychotherapy in Practice, 4*(1), 9-24.

Uhl, G., Blum, K., Noble, E., & Smith, S. (1993). Substance abuse vulnerability and D2 receptor genes. *Trends in Neurosciences, 16*(3), 83-88.

van den Bree, M. B. M., Johnson, E. O., Neale, M. C., & Pickens, R. W. (1998). Genetic and environmental influences on drug use and abuse/dependence in male and female twins. *Drug and Alcohol Dependence, 52*(3), 231-241.

Velleman, R., Bennett, G., Miller, T., Orford, J., Rigby, K., & Tod, A. (1993). The families of problem drug users: A study of 50 close relatives. *Addiction, 88*, 1281-1289.

Wood, S. & Tirone, S. (2013). The leisure of women caring for people harmfully involved with alcohol, drugs, and gambling. *Journal of Leisure Research, 45*(5), 583-601.

Wijndaele, K. (2007). Association between leisure time physical activity and stress, social support and coping: A cluster-analytical approach. *Psychology of Sport and Exercise, 8*(4), 425-440.

37. Total Joint Replacement

Heather R. Porter

Total joint replacement (TJR) is the removal of a diseased or damaged joint and the implantation of an artificial joint called a prosthesis. This procedure can be done for any joint of the body including knees, hips, ankles, toes, fingers, wrists, elbows, and shoulders. This chapter covers total hip replacement (THR) and total knee replacement (TKR) since these are the most common procedures. These are also referred to as total hip arthroplasty (THA) and total knee arthroplasty (TKA).

The typical client has a history of osteoarthritis, rheumatoid arthritis, or traumatic joint injury and presents with severe joint pain during activity and rest (Singh, 2011). The client's ability to perform daily life tasks and to sleep is substantially impaired due to the pain. Other symptoms may include disabling stiffness, swelling, locking, and giving way. All conservative treatment measures, such as medication, assistive devices, therapy, bracing, and weight loss are exhausted before considering TJR (Palmer, 2014).

Clients who have a THR or TKR will need to follow specific precautions, which are listed in the Treatment Direction section. Other common joint surgeries that a therapist will see in a rehabilitation setting may also follow these precautions.

To clarify the differences in these surgeries, a description of four primary hip and knee surgeries are provided (Crepeau, Cohn, & Schell, 2003).

Hip fracture with closed reduction: This is a break in any portion of the femur that can be manipulated into its natural position without major surgery. The client must follow weight-bearing (WB) precautions established by the surgeon and total hip precautions (THP).

Total hip replacement (THR) or *total hip arthroplasty* (THA): This is the surgical removal of a diseased or injured hip joint, which is replaced with a prosthetic appliance. If the articular surfaces of both the acetabulum and the femur are replaced, the prosthesis is considered a total hip arthroplasty. If the femoral head is replaced and the acetabulum is not altered, the prosthesis is considered a hip hemiarthroplasty or partial hip replacement. The client must follow WB precautions and THP.

Hip fracture with open reduction and internal fixation (ORIF): This is a surgical procedure that uses wires, screws, or pins applied directly to the fractured bone segments to keep them in place. This therapist must clarify if THP, modified THP, or WB restrictions were ordered by the surgeon.

Total knee replacement (TKR) or *total knee arthroplasty* (TKA): This is the implantation of a device to substitute for damaged joint surfaces. Related terms come from the type of prosthesis. Unicompartment or hemiarthroplasty is partial replacement of the joint. Hemiarthroplasty replaces the diseased component. Typically, active movement of the knee is encouraged during all activities after the surgery. Twisting motions that put undue stress on the joint should be avoided. WB restrictions may also be prescribed.

Components of the Replacement

Components of the THR include the acetabulum component that is held in place by screws, spikes, a special cement, or cementless design (as described later in this chapter). It is typically made out of plastic and may have a metal backing. The second component of the prosthesis is the femoral stem that is also held in place with cement or has a cementless design. It is typically made out of metal or ceramic.

During a TKR, the end of the femur (upper leg bone) is removed and replaced with a metal shell called the femoral component. The end of the tibia (lower leg bone) is also removed and replaced with a channeled plastic piece with a metal stem called the tibial component. Depending on the condition of the kneecap portion of the knee joint, a plastic "button" may also be added under the kneecap surface. This is called the patellar component. The components are typically made out of plastic and metal. They are held in place with cement or have a cementless design.

Cemented vs. Uncemented Prosthesis

Rasul (2012) describes the differences as follows: Cemented joint replacement is a procedure in which bone cement (polymethylmethacrylate — PMMA) is used to fix the prosthesis in place. It is most frequently used for older adults who are less active. It is also used for those who have osteoporosis. Pain relief and enhanced joint mobility are noticeable immediately after surgery. The cement can loosen over time and sometimes bits of cement break off and cause further pain or joint damage.

Ingrowth or cementless joint replacement is done by pressing the prosthesis into place so it holds with friction. The prosthesis is covered with a textured metal or special bone-like substance, which allows bone to grow into the prosthesis, thus negating the need for cement to hold it in place. This procedure is based on a fracture-healing model. It may last longer than a cemented prosthesis because there is no cement that can loosen. It is used frequently in younger, more active clients. There is extended recovery time, however, when compared to the cemented prosthesis, because of the length of time for the natural bone to grow and attach to the prosthesis.

Primary vs. Revision Surgery

Primary joint replacement or arthroplasty refers to the first replacement surgery. Revision refers to a second or succeeding surgery performed usually for an unstable, loose, or painful joint replacement.

Contraindications for Undergoing a THR or TKR

There are several contraindications for joint replacement. These include active local or systemic infection or other medical conditions that preclude safe anesthesia and the demands of surgery and rehabilitation, severe neuropathic joint disease, severe vascular disease, any process that is rapidly destroying bone, rapidly progressive neurological diseases, or the absence or relative insufficiency of the abductor musculature for THR (Iannotti & Parker, 2013, Marya & Bawari, 2010). Overweight or obesity is also considered a relative contraindication (Marya & Bawari, 2010).

Joint replacements should be delayed as long as possible for manual laborers, athletes, or overweight or obese persons because increased stress on the prosthesis leads to a higher mechanical failure rate and subsequent revision (Marya & Bawari, 2010).

Incidence/Prevalence in U.S.

Approximately 600,000 total knee replacements (American Association of Orthopaedic Surgeons [AAOS], 2011a) and 285,000 total hip replacements (AAOS, 2011b) are performed each year in the U.S.

Predominant Age

About two-thirds of all THR procedures are performed in individuals who are older than 65, with 62% of all THR procedures in the U.S. being performed on women (Kauffman, Barr, & Moran, 2007). The most common age group for TKR is 65-84 (Kaplan, 2005).

Causes

Rheumatoid arthritis, osteoarthritis, or a traumatic joint injury can cause severe joint damage resulting in pain and limited function. When non-surgical interventions fail to manage these issues, a total joint replacement may become a viable option.

Systems Affected

The primary system affected is the musculoskeletal system (s750 Structure of Lower Extremity). Functional issues are usually coded with b280 Sensation of Pain, b710 Mobility of Joint Functions, b770 Gait Pattern Functions, and aspects of d4 Mobility. However other bodily systems can be affected positively as a secondary effect of surgery. These include increased activity due to decreased joint pain and the resulting increase in muscle function (b7 Neuromusculoskeletal and Movement-Related Functions) and cardiopulmonary endurance (b4 Functions of the Cardiovascular, Hematological, Immunological, and Respiratory Systems).

Secondary Problems

There is less than a one percent mortality rate for knee and hip replacement surgery. Some of the possible complications from surgery include deep vein thrombosis and pulmonary emboli, wound healing problems, wound and deep tissue infection often associated with diabetes mellitus and obesity, pneumonia, myocardial infarction, joint instability or malalignment, hip dislocation if THP are not maintained, urinary tract infection, nausea and vomiting usually related to pain medication, nerve damage, blood vessel injury, and loss of appetite. Associated risks of anesthesia include heart, lung, kidney, and liver damage. Long-range complications of joint replacement surgery include prosthetic loosening and wear.

Secondary Problems from Surgery

Palmer (2014), AAOS (2011a), and Werner and Brown (2012) describe the following secondary problems:

Pain: Reduced by long-acting narcotic analgesics. Attention to side effects is imperative.

Bowel and bladder functions: Constipation caused by decreased mobility, post-anesthesia effects, or a side effect of narcotic analgesics is a frequent complaint.

Nutrition and hydration: Elderly clients are at risk for malnutrition and dehydration due to physical limitations and/or cognitive deficits. Dehydration can lead to acute metabolic or renal problems.

Blood clots: Blood thinners are commonly prescribed to decrease risks of developing a blood clot. Warning signs of blood clots include increased calf pain, tenderness or redness above or below the knee, and increased swelling of calf, ankle, and foot. Warning signs of a pulmonary embolism, a blood clot that breaks loose and travels to the lungs, include sudden shortness of breath, sudden onset of chest pain, and localized chest pain with coughing.

Infection: Commonly caused by bacteria that enter the blood stream via dental procedures, urinary tract infections, and skin infections. The bacteria may lodge around the hip or knee and causes infection that is very difficult to treat. Consequently, after having a TKR or THP, preventive antibiotics are prescribed before undergoing dental or surgical procedures that could allow bacteria to enter the bloodstream.

Falls: Following the surgery, clients are at a higher risk for falls until balance, flexibility, and strength are improved. Falls precautions should be followed.

Hip stability (in THR only): The total hip prosthesis can become dislocated in one percent to 10% of THRs and up to 28% in total hip revisions. The majority of dislocations occur within the first three months after surgery. Risk factors for dislocation include being female, due to muscle mass, strength, and differences in soft tissues caused by genetics and hormones; having previous hip surgery; and surgical factors. The dislocation may be corrected through non-surgical or surgical procedures.

Leg-length inequality (in THR only): The surgeon may need to slightly lengthen or shorten the leg to maximize stability and biomechanics of the hip, consequently some clients may need to wear a shoe with a lift to attain leg-length equality.

Prognosis

THR

On average, recovery from a THR can take three to six months (National Institute of Arthritis and Musculoskeletal and Skin Diseases [NIAMSD], 2014). The total hip prosthesis lasts approximately 15 years in 95% of people who undergo a THR. Total hip revisions are commonly performed 15-20 years after the original procedure, once the prosthesis becomes worn (NIAMSD, 2014). Revisions are not as successful as the initial THR; consequently all available options are typically explored prior to undergoing a hip revision (NIAMSD, 2014).

TKR

A rapid and substantial improvement in pain, functional status, and overall health-related quality of life is seen in about 90% of clients who undergo a TKR (AAOS, 2011a). The best predictor of range of motion following total knee replacement is the preoperative range of motion (AAOS, 2011a). Kneeling is usually uncomfortable, but it is not harmful (AAOS, 2011a). The client may feel a soft clicking of the metal and plastic with knee flexion or walking. These usually diminish over time (AAOS, 2011a). Clients might also experience some numbness in the skin around the incision (AAOS, 2011a). Long-term studies of TKR show a 90% plus prosthesis survival rate at 15-year follow-ups (AAOS, 2011a).

The proportion of patients with good-to-excellent outcomes declines with each successive revision.

Factors that increase a client's risk of needing revision surgery include being 55 years of age or younger, male gender, diagnosis of OA, obesity, and presence of comorbid conditions (NIH, 2003). Obesity puts the replaced knee at an increased risk of loosening or dislocation and younger clients, who are more physically active than older adults, have increased risk of trauma and stress to the replaced knee.

Both THR and TKR

The client must be cleared by the surgeon to resume driving. The surgeon bases this decision on muscle control to provide adequate reaction time for braking and accelerating, joint flexion and extension to comfortably sit in the car and operate the brake and gas pedal, and stability of the joint surgery. Many surgeons do not want the client to be in a vehicle for several weeks (typically six weeks) after surgery, other than the car ride home from the healthcare facility.

Clients need to avoid excessive physical activity as defined by their surgeon. Excessive activity or weight may accelerate this normal wear and cause the replacement to loosen and become painful (AAOS, 2011a).

Expected activity after surgery: recreational walking, swimming, golf, driving, light hiking, recreational biking, ballroom dancing, normal stair climbing.

Activity exceeding usual recommendations after surgery: vigorous walking or hiking, skiing, tennis, repetitive lifting exceeding 50 pounds, repetitive aerobic stair climbing.

Dangerous activity after surgery: jogging or running, contact sports, jumping sports, high impact aerobics.

Metal components of the joint replacement may activate metal detectors at airports and other buildings that require such security. The client should request a card from his/her surgeon that verifies joint replacement surgery and alert security personnel prior to going through a metal detector.

Clients with joint replacements should alert their doctors and dentists that they have an artificial joint. These joints are at risk for infection by bacteria introduced by any invasive procedures such as surgery, dental or gum work, urological and endo-scopic procedures, as well as from infections elsewhere in the body (AAOS, 2011a, 2011b).

Sexual activity may be contraindicated until the two-month follow-up appointment with the surgeon (AAOS, 2011a, 2011b).

Assessment

Prior to approval and acceptance of joint replacement surgery, the orthopedic surgeon conducts an assessment (Rasul, 2012; AAOS, 2011a, 2011b). The surgeon will take medical history to gather information about general health and the extent of hip or knee pain (b280 Sensation of Pain) and how it affects the ability to perform daily activities (b455 Exercise Tolerance Functions, b710 Mobility of Joint Functions, b715 Stability of Joint Functions, b730 Muscle Power Functions, d4 Mobility). A thorough physical examination that includes the assessment of the hip's or knee's mobility, strength, and alignment will be given. X-rays or MRIs will be used to determine the extent of damage or deformity in the hip or knee (s750 Structure of Lower Extremity). Blood tests or other tests will be given to determine the condition of the bone and soft tissues of joint (b415 Blood Vessel Functions, b430 Hematological System Functions).

Typical Scope of Team Assessment

Clients who receive inpatient rehabilitation services are evaluated primarily in the following areas: replaced joint range of motion without breaking precautions, functional abilities to perform life tasks, knowledge and application of joint and weight-bearing precautions, and adjustment to situation (d230 Carrying Out Daily Routine, d4 Mobility).

Discharge is recommended only when wound healing is satisfactory, knee flexion of 90° has been achieved, the patient is considered to be safe and supported in the home environment, and no complications are present. Anticlotting medication is often continued at home for a period of time.

Not all clients who undergo a THR or TKR will receive inpatient rehabilitation services. Some clients skip inpatient rehab and receive in-home and outpatient therapy services only. These clients typically are younger clients who do not have a significant past medical history that requires close monitoring, do not present with any mental or cognitive deficits that would impact their ability to adhere to precautions and exercise regime, and possess the motivation and initiative to follow through with the surgeon's directions (e120 Products and Technology for Personal Indoor and Outdoor Mobility and Transportation, e340 Personal Care Providers and Personal Assistants).

Areas of Concern for RT Assessment

A history of progressive inactivity is most common as clients adapt their lifestyle to meet the challenges of living with joint pain and limited joint function. Some of the complications of this type of adaptation include pulmonary, cardiac, and muscular deconditioning, increased weight, poor nutrition, depression, loss of a healthy leisure lifestyle, and social isolation. Relevant ICF codes might include b130 Energy and Drive Functions, b152 Emotional Functions, b280 Sensation of Pain, b710 Mobility of Joint Functions, b715 Stability of Joint Functions, b730 Muscle Power Functions, b735 Muscle Tone Functions, b740 Muscle Endurance Functions, b770 Gait Pattern Functions, d230 Carrying Out Daily Routine, d4 Mobility, and d570 Looking After One's Health. Often pain and limited joint function has caused the patient to stop healthy recreation and leisure pursuits. When this is the case, the RT should cite code d920 Recreation and Leisure and plan as part of treatment to provide information on leisure activities that will promote joint health and general fitness. Other deficits the recreational therapist should note include the sets of skills described in ICF codes d2 General Tasks and Demands and d5 Self-Care.

ICF Core Set

An ICF Core Set for the general diagnosis of TJR (or the specific diagnoses of THP or TKR) has not yet been published. ICF Core Sets that might be helpful in identifying relevant ICF codes include Arthritis, Musculoskeletal Conditions, and Osteoarthritis.

Treatment Direction

Clients who have a THR or TKR will need to follow specific precautions and parameters. Weight-bearing precautions apply to both THR and TKR. Total hip precautions apply to THR.

Weight-Bearing Precautions

Weight-bearing precautions are set by the surgeon or physician for a variety of conditions, such as total hip or knee replacements, fractures, or sprains. Specific weight-bearing precautions are written in the client's medical record and must be followed to prevent injury and promote healing. Changes will be made to less restrictive weight-bearing precautions as healing occurs. There are five levels of weight bearing (Cooper, 2006):

Non-weight bearing (NWB): May not put any weight on the identified extremities. If the restriction involves both lower extremities, activity is limited to those completed while sitting or in bed. May complete transfers using a transfer board.

Touchdown weight bearing (TDWB) or *toe-touch weight bearing* (TTWB): The majority of the client's weight bearing must be through the client's arms on the walking device and the unaffected extremity. Weight bearing on the involved extremity is limited to using the toes to make contact with floor, primarily to maintain balance. TTWB is not as much weight as the client can carry on his/her toes. The affected extremity can bear approximately 10% of normal weight. Physical therapists recommend strategies for safe walking and prescribe a mobility device to help clients adhere to weight-bearing precautions. Close collaboration between the physical therapist and other allied health professionals is essential so that the client is able to engage in functional activity safely and effectively while using the device.

Partial weight bearing (PWB): This typically refers to bearing 50% of the client's body weight on the involved extremity. It is frequently estimated by the client and therapist and requires sustained effort and attention. Note that when walking, a normal gait puts 100% of the client's weight on the extremity when it is the only limb on the ground. This would not be allowed with partial weight bearing.

Weight bearing as tolerated (WBAT): The amount of weight put on the extremity is left to the discretion of the client based on his/her level of comfort.

Full weight bearing (FWB): No restrictions on amount of weight put on the extremity. Client can put all of his/her weight on the extremity.

Total Hip Precautions

After a total hip replacement or hip fracture with a closed reduction, total hip precautions (THP) must be followed until the soft tissue has healed adequately and the surgeon removes the precautions, typically about 12 weeks post surgery (Zachazewski & Quillen, 2008). THP are designed to protect the hip joint and avoid injury, such as dislocation. The usual precautions include (Cooper, 2006; Kennon, 2008):

- Do not flex the involved hip beyond 90°. This means the client will have to sit on elevated chairs or toilet seats to maintain precautions and cannot bend over from the hips to reach objects or tie shoes. A reacher is required.
- Do not turn the leg inwards so the hips are rotated internally.
- Do not rotate the trunk in a way that may result in an internal hip rotation.
- Do not turn the feet excessively inward or outward. The patient cannot pivot on the operated leg.
- Do not cross the legs at the ankles or knees.
- Do not lie or roll onto the uninvolved side.
- Place a pillow between the legs when lying on the involved side.
- An abduction wedge pillow is commonly used during waking hours to prevent internal rotation of the hip. The "V" shaped abduction pillow is placed between the legs and Velcroed around the thighs to hold it in place. Sometimes clients are instructed to wear it when sleeping to prevent breaking hip precautions.

For some clients, individualized precautions may be prescribed by the surgeon. Inpatient rehabilitation therapists must be diligent about checking the client-specific THP set by the surgeon.

Other Recovery Issues

All care must take into account surgical precautions related to keeping the surgery site protected. These include no immersion in water, bandages to prevent irritation from clothing, support stockings to decrease the risk of deep vein thrombosis, and observation of the site to detect early signs of infection. Ice is used to reduce swelling, heat to increase range of motion. Appropriate diet promotes proper tissue healing. Exercise programs are established by physical therapists to restore muscle strength and reduce scarring (b415 Blood Vessel Functions, b430 Hematological System Functions, b710 Mobility of Joint Functions, b715 Stability of Joint Functions, b730 Muscle Power Functions, b735 Muscle Tone Functions, b740 Muscle Endurance Functions, b770 Gait Pattern Functions).

The goal is to prevent further complications from the surgery, as described in the Secondary Problems section and restore function to the treated leg.

TKR

The surgeon prescribes specific weight-bearing precautions, a knee immobilizer, and a schedule to wear a continuous passive motion (CPM) machine. The knee immobilizer is a soft Velcro brace from the ankle to the middle thigh. The patient wears it after a TKR until quadriceps strength is regained. In certain situations, careful resistive or gradual range of motion exercises are initiated (Rasul, 2012). The CPM machine is placed on the affected leg when the client is in bed to gently bend and straighten the knee without the assistance of the client. It can assist with managing edema, enhancing range of motion, and improving venous circulation thus decreasing risks of deep vein thrombosis.

THR

The surgeon prescribes specific weight-bearing precautions, total hip precautions, and an abduction wedge pillow.

Whole Team Approach

Due to the short length of the inpatient rehabilitation stay, the team's primary focus is on increasing range of motion within precautions for the replaced joint, restoring functional skills to complete life tasks (d230 Carrying Out Daily Routine), walking (d450 Walking), educating the client on how to maintain precautions after discharge through adaptation and modification of activities, increasing the client's awareness of the benefits of exercise in achieving optimal outcomes, developing a home exercise program (b730 Muscle Power Functions, b735 Muscle Tone Functions, b740 Muscle Endurance Functions), and identifying resources to solve problems with life tasks (e115 Products and Technology for Personal Use in Daily Living).

Recreational Therapy Approach

Recreational therapists address the issues noted in the whole team approach as it pertains to engagement in recreation, leisure, play, and community activities. Participation in active, enjoyable activities within limitations can help improve strength and range of motion, as well as aid in better sleep, reduction of pain, maintenance of a positive attitude, and healthy weight loss. Therapists additionally address systemic issues, such as environmental and personal factors, that affect the client's ability to continue such involvement post discharge.

Recreational Therapy Interventions

The following interventions are commonly used for clients with joint replacements.

Benefits of leisure: Clients are educated about the importance of active leisure for recovery and health promotion with particular attention to enhancing range of motion and muscle strength (b710 Mobility of Joint Functions, b730 Muscle Power Functions, b735 Muscle Tone Functions, b740 Muscle Endurance Functions, d570 Looking After One's Health).

Physical leisure activity: Exercise options are reviewed and explored for recovery and long-term health promotion, especially when a deficit in appropriate leisure activities is noted during the assessment (d920 Recreation and Leisure, d570 Looking After One's Health).

Functional mobility skills: Recreational therapists address the development of functional mobility skills within specific recreational and community activities that will be part of the client's lifestyle after discharge. These skills may be needed to address deficits noted in d2 General Tasks and Demands, d4 Mobility, and d5 Self-Care.

Community problem solving and resource awareness: Resource awareness education goes hand-in-hand with community problem solving since knowledge of resources and how to access them are essential skills to problem solve for barriers. These may include community accessibility training, energy conservation training, and personal and community leisure resource awareness. ICF codes related to the problems that may need to be solved include d4 Mobility, d940 Human Rights, and e140 Products and Technology for Culture, Recreation, and Sport.

Resources

American Association of Orthopaedic Surgeons

www.aaos.org

Therapists might find the TKR and THR exercise guides helpful.

THR Exercise Guide:

orthoinfo.aaos.org/topic.cfm?topic=A00303

TKR Exercise Guide:

orthoinfo.aaos.org/topic.cfm?topic=A00301

Arthritis Foundation

www.arthritis.org

The largest national nonprofit organization that supports the more than 100 types of arthritis and related conditions.

References

American Association of Orthopaedic Surgeons. (2011a). Total knee replacement. Retrieved from http://orthoinfo.aaos.org/topic.cfm?topic=A00389.

American Association of Orthopaedic Surgeons. (2011b). Total hip replacement. Retrieved from http://orthoinfo.aaos.org/topic.cfm?topic=A00377.

Cooper, G. (2006). *Essential physical medicine and rehabilitation*. New York, NY: Springer Publishing Company.

Crepeau, E., Cohn, E., & Schell, B. (2003). *Willard and Spackman's occupational therapy* (10th ed.). Philadelphia, PA: Lippincott Williams & Wilkins.

Iannotti, J. P. & Parker, R. (2013). *The netter collection of medical illustrations: Musculoskeletal system, volume 6, part II, spine and lower limb 2*. Philadelphia, PA: Elsevier Health Sciences.

Kaplan, R. (2005). *Physical medicine and rehabilitation review: Pearls of wisdom, 2nd edition*. New York: McGraw-Hill Education.

Kennon, R. (2008). *Hip and knee surgery: A patient's guide to hip replacement, hip resurfacing, knee replacement, and knee arthroscopy*. Raleigh, NC: Lulu Press, Inc.

Kauffman, T. L., Barr, J. O., & Moran, M. L. (2007). *Geriatric rehabilitation manual*. Philadelphia, PA: Elsevier Health Sciences.

Marya, S. K. S. & Bawari, R. K. (2010). *Total hip replacement surgery: Principles and techniques*. London: JP Medical Ltd.

National Institute of Arthritis and Musculoskeletal and Skin Diseases. (2014). Questions and answers about hip replacements. Retrieved from http://www.niams.nih.gov/Health_Info/Hip_Replacement/.

National Institutes of Health. (2003). NIH consensus development conference on total knee replacement. Retrieved from http://consensus.nih.gov/2003/2003totalkneereplacement117html.htm.

Palmer, S. (2014). Total knee arthroplasty. Retrieved from http://emedicine.medscape.com/article/1250275-overview.

Rasul, A. (2012). Total joint replacement rehabilitation. Retrieved from http://emedicine.medscape.com/article/320061-overview.

Singh, J. (2011). Epidemiology of knee and hip arthroplasty: A systemic review. *The Open Orthopaedics Journal, 5*, 80-85.

Werner, B. C. & Brown, T. E. (2012). Instability after total hip arthroplasty. *World Journal of Orthopedics. 3*(8), 122-130.

Zachazewski, J. E. & Quillen, W. S. (2008). *Pathology and intervention in musculoskeletal rehabilitation*. Philadelphia, PA: Elsevier Health Sciences.

38. Traumatic Brain Injury

Donna L. Long, Donna L. Gregory, and Heather R. Porter

A traumatic brain injury (TBI) is a form of acquired brain injury that occurs from a direct trauma to the brain. It can be caused by a blow or jolt to the head or a penetrating injury, such as a gunshot wound, that causes damage to the brain. Not all jolts or blows to the head result in a TBI.

TBIs are classified as mild, moderate, or severe depending on the extent of damage to the brain. Mild TBI is also called concussion or minor brain injury. It occurs when an impact or forceful motion of the head results in a brief alteration of mental status, such as confusion or disorientation, loss of memory for events immediately before or after the injury, or brief loss of consciousness. Individuals are classified as having a mild TBI if they have a Glasgow Coma Scale (GCS) score of 13-15 and have symptoms of headache, fatigue, sleep disturbance, irritability, sensitivity to noise or light, balance problems, decreased concentration or attention, decreased speed of thinking, memory problems, nausea, blurry vision, dizziness, depression, anxiety, emotional mood swings, and/or seizures (CDC, 2010a; Brain Injury Association of America, 2011). See the Assessment section below for more information about GCS. Frequently people who sustain a mild TBI fail to recognize the potential severity of their injury and do not receive medical care at the time of injury. They may present to their primary care physician days, weeks, or even months after the injury with complaints of persistent symptoms.

Individuals are classified as having a moderate TBI when there is a loss of consciousness, along with persistent confusion and functional impairments in one or more of the cognitive, physical, emotional, or behavioral domains, along with a GCS score of 8-12 (Brain Injury Association of America, 2011).

Individuals are classified has having a severe TBI when there is a prolonged unconscious state or coma with a GCS score less than 8 (Brain Injury Association of America, 2011).

The most common types of TBI are discussed below.

Blast injuries: Traumatic brain injuries caused by explosions (bTBI) have significantly increased over the past few years, largely attributed to improvised explosive devices used by terrorists and insurgents in Iraq and Afghanistan. The use of body armor is allowing soldiers to survive blasts that would otherwise be fatal. Blast induced TBIs have been called the signature wound of the Afghanistan and Iraq wars. Studies are underway to better understand the effects of blast injuries, but we still have a lot to learn. Early evidence suggests that closed TBI and blast TBI (bTBI) may produce very similar symptoms, including cognitive impairment. One discrete feature that may result from bTBI is an increased risk for hearing loss and tinnitus (a continuous noise or ringing in the ear). Individuals who sustain a bTBI may also have post-traumatic stress disorder (PTSD) symptoms (Hicks et al., 2010).

Acceleration-deceleration injury or shearing injury: This type of injury is caused when the body is traveling at a high speed and then comes to an abrupt stop, as in a motor vehicle accident or a fall, producing diffuse axonal injury (DAI). It results in a widespread brain injury to many axons in numerous parts of the brain (NINDS, 2011a). This leads to a breakdown of communication within the brain and affects processing for the connections that remain. There are three reaction movements that occur during acceleration-deceleration events: (1) The direct impact of the brain and skull, as when the head hits the dashboard, causes a contusion on the frontal lobes of the brain resulting in a focal brain injury. (2) The impact bounces the brain around in the skull causing more contusions. (3) After the brain tissue crashes against the inside of the skull at impact, a bounce back motion occurs that throws the head and brain in the opposite direction, causing a second bruise on the opposite side of the brain resulting in extensive diffuse and focal bruising from the tearing and stretching throughout the brain. The first injury is referred to as a "coup." The return injury is a "contrecoup."

Penetrating injuries: This type of injury, also referred to as an open head injury, is an injury to the brain that results from a foreign object penetrating the skull and entering the brain (CDC, 2012). Penetrating injuries can be caused by bone fragments from a skull fracture, firearms, or sharp objects such as a knife.

Shaken baby syndrome: This is a serious brain injury that occurs when an infant or toddler is forcefully shaken. It causes coup-contrecoup damage, destroys a child's brain cells, and prevents his or her brain from getting enough oxygen (NINDS, 2011a).

Incidence/Prevalence

It is estimated 1.7 million TBIs occur each year in the United States (CDC, 2011a) of which one million are children and youth from motor vehicle accidents, sports, falls, brain tumors, and abuse (Laatsch et al., 2007). Approximately 75% of TBIs that occur each year are classified as mild and the remaining 25% are classified as moderate to severe (CDC, 2011a). The CDC data does not include soldiers injured in Iraq or Afghanistan who were treated in military or VA hospitals. However, a Congressional Research Service Report for Congress (Fischer, 2009) indicated that from 2003 to 2007 over 43,000 soldiers were diagnosed with TBI.

Predominant Age

The CDC (2011b) states that children from birth to four years, older adolescents 15-19, and older adults aged 65 years and older are most likely to sustain a TBI. Males are twice as likely as females to experience a TBI. The highest rate of TBI-related hospitalizations occur among adults 75 years and older.

Causes

TBI is largely preventable. According to the CDC (2010b), a keen awareness of safety and more state laws requiring people to wear seatbelts in the car and helmets while riding bikes or motorcycles has

decreased the number of TBIs in the U.S. Primary causes of TBI are shown below (CDC, 2010b, NINDS, 2011a):

- Falls are the leading cause of TBI (35.2%). It is suggested that an increase in fall-related TBIs is related to people living longer. These people have decreased agility and their balance is affected by some prescription medications.
- Motor vehicle accidents account for 17.3% of reported TBIs and result in the largest number of TBI-related deaths at 31.8%.
- Being struck by or colliding with a moving or stationary object accounts for 16.5% of reported TBIs and is the second leading cause of TBI among children ages 0-14 accounting for 25% of reported injuries in children.
- Assault accounts for 10% of reported TBIs. Based on data collected by the TBI Model System program (Salisbury, Novack, & Brunner 2004) injuries caused by gunshot wounds occur more frequently in males between the ages of 20 and 24 who are unmarried, unemployed, and living alone at the time of injury.
- Half of TBI incidents involve alcohol use.

Systems Affected

The primary system affected is the structure of the brain (s110 Structure of Brain). Any part of the brain may be affected. Since the brain controls and regulates voluntary and involuntary body functions, there can be a wide spectrum of dysfunction. Below is a list of the most common impairments (NINDS, 2011a).

Physical changes: These may include impairments such as weakness (b730 Muscle Power Functions, b740 Muscle Endurance Functions, b455 Exercise Tolerance Functions), muscle tone and coordination problems (b735 Muscle Tone Functions, b760 Control of Voluntary Movement Functions), full or partial paralysis (b730 Muscle Power Functions), balance difficulties (b755 Involuntary Movement Reaction Functions, d4 Mobility), and/or fatigue (b455 Exercise Tolerance Functions).

Cognitive changes: These may include impairments in arousal and attention (b110 Consciousness Functions, b114 Orientation Functions, b140 Attention Functions), initiation (b130 Energy and Drive Functions), and memory (b144 Memory

Functions). Problem solving (d175 Solving Problems) and the whole set of functions in b164 Higher-Level Cognitive Functions may be affected including, judgment, organization and planning, time management, abstract reasoning, and insight. Other cognitive changes may be noticed in reading (d166 Reading), writing (d170 Writing), language and communication (b167 Mental Functions of Language), new learning (d130-d159 Basic Learning), and/or confabulation (b160 Thought Functions).

Emotional and behavioral changes: These may include difficulty with social skills, such as an inability to empathize with others or poor pragmatics (d710 Basic Interpersonal Interactions), inappropriate or self-centered behavior (d710 Basic Interpersonal Interactions), disinhibited behavior, and other emotional-behavioral issues such as irritability, agitation, frustration, flat affect, depression, and/or anxiety (b152 Emotional Functions).

Secondary Problems

Secondary problems of a traumatic brain injury include several that cause further damage to the structure of the brain (s110 Structure of Brain). Functional changes for these additional traumas are similar to what was described in the Systems Affected section.

Anoxic injury: An injury to that results from an absence of oxygen to the brain (Idyll Arbor, 2001).

Hypoxic injury: An injury that results from a decrease of oxygen to the brain (NINDS, 2010).

Cranial nerve dysfunction: Twelve pairs of cranial nerves emerge from the brain. Injury to one or more of the cranial nerves may occur after a TBI resulting in impairments in taste, smell, or visual, auditory, or vestibular function (Whyte et al., 2004).

Edema: Swelling and excess fluid in the brain (Idyll Arbor, 2001).

Hematomas: A collection or pooling of blood that can increase intracranial pressure (ICP). Three types of hematomas can cause injury to the brain (Mayo Foundation for Medical Education and Research, 2011): (1) subdural hematoma where blood vessels rupture between the brain and the dura (membranes that cover the brain), (2) epidural or extradural hematoma where blood vessels rupture between the dura and the skull, and (3) intracerebral or intraparenchymal hematoma, which is bleeding within the brain itself. ICP is controlled by surgery.

Hydrocephalus: Hydrocephalus or ventricular enlargement occurs when cerebral spinal fluid (CSF) accumulates in the brain resulting in dilation of the cerebral ventricles (spaces in the brain) and an increase in intercranial pressure (NINDS, 2011b). Symptoms of hydrocephalus, such as incontinence, gait disorder, and dementia, are often difficult to detect in severely impaired patients. Failure to improve or deterioration of cognitive or behavioral function may be indicative of hydrocephalus (Whyte et al., 2010).

Other secondary problems, which lead to additional diagnosis categories include:

Heterotopic ossification (HO): HO is the formation of bone where bone does not usually form in soft tissues (Simonsen et al., 2007). Its etiology is unknown and occurs in approximately 10-20% of individuals with severe TBI in predominantly proximal joints of the upper and lower extremities (Simonsen et al., 2007). Symptoms of HO may include pain, warmth, swelling, and contracture formation. Medical management and treatment options including nonsteroidal anti-inflammatory medications, radiation, and/or surgery to remove the HO (Whyte et al., 2004; Whyte et al., 2010). Use ICF code b710 Mobility of Joint Functions.

Seizures: Post-traumatic seizures, recurrent seizures, and epilepsy are known complications of TBI (Whyte et al., 2010). Seizures may develop immediately, within 24 hours, or more than one week after the injury. According to the National Institute of Neurological Disorders and Stroke (2011a), about 25% of patients with brain contusions or hematomas and about 50% of patients with penetrating head injuries will develop seizures that occur within the first 24 hours of the injury. The risk of new seizure development is greatest during the first two years following a TBI (Whyte et al., 2010). See the chapter on Epilepsy for more information about documenting seizure activity.

Prognosis

A systematic review of the literature on mild TBI showed that the prognosis is favorable. In the majority of cases, children and adults were found to have none to little short-term or long-term deficits one to three months post injury (Carroll et al., 2004). In regards to severe TBI, a study of 846 cases of severe TBI (GCS ≤ 8) was analyzed over the course of one year (Jiang et al., 2004). Findings indicated that after one year, 31.56% had good recovery, 14.07% had moderate recovery, 24.35% had severe disability, 0.59% were in vegetative state, and 29.43% had died. This somewhat "U" shaped prognosis for severe TBI was also reported by Maas, Stocchetti, and Bullock (2008) for both moderate and severe TBI.

The most powerful independent prognostic variables include age, GCS motor score, pupillary response, and CT characteristics (Maas, Stocchetti, & Bullock, 2008). Length and severity of a coma, length of post-traumatic amnesia, and age are also predictors of long-term outcomes (NINDS, 2011a). As a general rule, the longer one remains in a coma or state of post-traumatic amnesia, the more severe the brain injury (NINDS, 2011a). In regards to age, individuals over 60 or under the age of two have the worst prognosis, even if they sustain the same injury as someone not in those age groups (Lenrow, n.d.). Other factors that influence prognosis are extent of injury and location of injury (NINDS, 2011a).

In addition to the above prognostic variables, the brain's ability to adapt to injury must be considered. The brain may find different pathways to send and receive information or create new pathways (Lenrow, n.d.). The brain will try to recover, but in order for that to happen, it must be stimulated. Although about 85% of recovery occurs in the first six months (Maas et al., 2008), further recovery can be seen months and even years after initial injury (NINDS, 2011a). Additional research and advances in technology will help to improve the quality of diagnosis and prognosis.

Assessment

Typical Scope of Team Assessment

There are several scales used for assessment of brain injury: the *Glasgow Coma Scale* (GCS), the *Rancho Los Amigos Levels of Cognitive Functioning Scale* (called Rancho Scale for short), the Disability Rating Scale (DRS), and the Functional Independence Measure (FIM) supplemented by the Functional Assessment Measure (FAM). The results from each of these scales can be translated to ICF codes, if required.

The *Glasgow Coma Scale* is a brief assessment of the level of consciousness and the severity of injury. The highest possible score is a 15 and the lowest possible score is a three. A score of 13-15 is considered a mild brain injury, 9-12 a moderate brain injury, and eight or less a severe brain injury (burlingame & Blaschko, 2010). A score of three to eight indicates that the person is in a severe coma and a score of three indicates that the person is in a vegetative state. There are three subcategories in the GCS: (1) Eyes Open (E), (2) Best Verbal Response (V), and (3) Best Motor Response (M). The score is written so that each function is described (e.g. E4 + V4 + M6 = 14) (burlingame & Blaschko, 2010).

The *Rancho Los Amigos Levels of Cognitive Functioning Scale* (Rancho Scale for short) is an eight-level scale that helps identify the cognitive level of functioning after a traumatic brain injury (burlingame & Blaschko, 2010). It was designed to measure and track a person's recovery through behavioral observation. Level 1 is the lowest possible cognitive score (no response to stimuli, coma) and Level 8 is the highest possible score (purposeful and appropriate) (burlingame & Blaschko, 2010). Rancho Los Amigos Hospital has developed a 10-level scale, however, they recommend that the revised scale not be used until further validity and reliability of the tool are established (Burton, 2003).

The *Disability Rating Scale* (DRS) was developed specifically for use with TBI to assess functional changes throughout the recovery process. The DRS consists of eight items divided into four categories: (1) arousal and awareness, (2) cognitive ability to handle self-care functions, (3) physical dependence upon others, and (4) psychosocial adaptability for work, housework, or school. Scoring the scale produces a quantitative measure of the level of disability: 0 (none), 1 (mild), 2-3 (partial), 4-6 (moderate), 7-11 (moderately severe), 12-16 (severe), 17-21 (extremely severe), 22-24 (vegetative state), 25-29 (extreme vegetative state) (Rapport et al., 1982).

The *Functional Independence Measure* (FIM) was designed as a tool to collect data for comparison of rehabilitation outcomes across the continuum of healthcare. The FIM consists of 18-items designed to assess the person's degree of disability and burden of care. Items are rated on a seven-point scale, with 1 = total assist (<25% independence), 2 = maximal assist (25-50% independence), 3 = moderate assist (50-75% independence), 4 = minimal assist (>75% independence), 5 = supervision or setup (setup of needed items, standby, cueing or coaxing without physical contact), 6 = modified independence (assistive device and/or more than a reasonable time), and 7 = complete independence (100% independence) (Chumney et al., 2010).

The *Functional Assessment Measure* (FAM) was developed to supplement the FIM. The purpose of the FAM is to address the major functional areas that are not emphasized directly in the FIM, including cognitive, behavioral, communication, and community functioning measures (Wright, 2000). The FAM consists of an additional 12 items and uses a seven-point scale modeled after the FIM. It is important to note that the FAM items do not stand alone, but are intended to be added to the 18 items of the FIM. The total 30-item scale combination is referred to as the FIM (18) + FAM (12) (Wright, 2000).

Areas of Concern for RT Assessment

Common findings include physical, cognitive, social, visual-perceptual, and emotional impairments that affect the person's ability to function optimally in work (d840-d859 Work and Employment), school (d810-d839 Education), home (d630-d649 Household Tasks), and community environments (d6 Domestic Life, d7 Interpersonal Interactions and Relationships, and d9 Community, Social, and Civic Life) (Whyte et al., 2004). All ICF Activity & Participation codes have two qualifiers dedicated to scoring the person's ability to function in his/her real-life community environment. Other findings include a history of alcohol use, which is the most common risk factor for TBI (d570 Looking After One's Health); deficits in cognition (b1 Mental Functions, d1 Learning and Applying Knowledge); changes in behavior, mood, and personality (b125 Dispositions and Intra-Personal Functions, b126 Temperament and Personality Functions, b130 Energy and Drive Functions); impairments in ADLs, such as self-care, toileting, mobility, feeding/swallowing, and basic communication (d2 General Tasks and Demands, d3 Communication, d4 Mobility, and d5 Self-Care); and limitations with complex skills related to time management (b164 Higher-Level Cognitive Functions, d230 Carrying Out Daily Routine), community mobility (d460 Moving Around in Different Locations, d465 Moving Around Using Equipment), and school (d810-d839 Education) or vocational tasks

(d840-d859 Work and Employment). Some over-learned skills, however, may present outside of anticipated abilities (Porter & burlingame, 2006). Over-learned skills may "shine through" even though the person has deficits in this area. Because it is over-learned, it is more automatic. For example, a person who has been involved in the hobby of woodworking for many years may have problems with sequencing, but when presented with a simple wood project, he is able to sequence the steps involved without difficulty.

Substantial decreases in leisure and community participation post TBI are a major issue (d920 Recreation and Leisure, d910 Community Life). For example, Wise et al. (2010) conducted a one-year longitudinal study on adults with moderate to severe TBI (n=160) and found that at one year 81% of the participants did not return to pre-injury levels of leisure engagement. Sixty percent were moderately to severely bothered by this change. They reported a reduction of almost 50% in the number of leisure activities post injury, along with an increase in engagement in more isolative home-based, non-social activities, and engagement in fewer sports and outdoor activities. Interestingly, none of the participants reported using any adaptive or special equipment for recreation (e140 Products and Technology for Culture, Recreation, and Sport; e115 Products and Technology for Personal Use in Daily Living). Primary reasons reported for the change in leisure activities included balance (b755 Involuntary Movement Reaction Functions, d415 Maintaining a Body Position), coordination (b760 Control of Voluntary Movement Functions), physical impairment (b7 Neuromusculoskeletal and Movement-Related Functions), fatigue (b455 Exercise Tolerance Functions, vision issues (b210 Seeing Functions), and cautiousness (b125 Dispositions and Intra-Personal Functions, b126 Temperament and Personality Functions). Those that returned to pre-injury levels of leisure engagement did so within four months post injury. The authors propose that perhaps we should rethink the way we approach the trajectory of rehabilitation for those with TBI. There is much emphasis on return to work as a marker for successful rehabilitation, yet the numbers of those with moderate to severe TBI who return to stable employment remain low. Using participation in purposeful, goal-oriented leisure activities as a bridge to the greater demands of the workplace may be more effective.

A literature review by Temkin et al. (2009) supports the above study, finding that individuals with moderate to severe TBI have disrupted leisure and recreation (d920 Recreation and Leisure) engagement for many years after injury, along with significant decreases in quality of life, social relationships (d730-d779 Particular Interpersonal Relationships), and independent living (choose specific ICF Activities & Participation codes that relate to the task). They additionally found that by one year post injury, psychosocial problems appear to be greater than problems in basic activities of daily living, highlighting the importance of psychosocial rehabilitation (b125 Dispositions and Intra-Personal Functions, b126 Temperament and Personality Functions, b130 Energy and Drive Functions, d240 Handling Stress and Other Psychological Demands, d250 Managing One's Own Behavior, d350-d369 Conversation and Use of Communication Devices and Techniques, d7 Interpersonal Interactions and Relationships, d910 Community Life, d920 Recreation and Leisure, d930 Religion and Spirituality).

Along with documenting the condition of the patient, the recreational therapist should document the level of support that is available to the patient from friends and family (e3 Support and Relationships). Support for the patient during the recovery process is a necessary part of recovery for a moderate to severe TBI.

ICF Core Set

A brief and comprehensive ICF Core Set for Traumatic Brain Injury is available.

Treatment Direction

Whole Team Approach

The initial treatment direction is to prevent further damage to the structure of the brain and provide an environment where the brain can heal (s110 Structure of Brain). During the initial weeks of inpatient rehabilitation, the team primarily focuses on restoration of skills through graduated tasks and repetition based on the theories of brain plasticity. The last weeks of the person's rehabilitation focuses on transitioning the individual into his/her discharge environment. This includes teaching the person and

caregiver, as appropriate, compensatory strategies and techniques to facilitate the recovery process post discharge.

Recreational Therapy Approach

Recreational therapy supports the team approach with the interventions described below.

Recreational Therapy Interventions

Recreational therapy treatment interventions are designed to address impairments in the cognitive, physical, social/emotional, visual/perceptual, and psychological domains. Several interventions related to cognitive, physical, and social/emotional functioning are discussed below. Modalities used to address dysfunction, whenever possible, should be activities that are going to be part of the person's activity pattern after discharge. This functional approach should be taken because individuals with TBI often have difficulty generalizing learned skills to a different context.

Cognitive Interventions

An outline of the *Rancho Los Amigos Levels of Cognitive Functioning Scale* grouped into four different stages, along with the general treatment guidelines that accompany each stage is shown below. Cognitive retraining strategies are used to promote restoration of the cognitive skills.

Rancho 1 (coma stage): The person at this level does not respond to sounds, sight, touch, or movement. Although it is unclear if it helps to improve cognitive function at this stage, therapists often use sensory stimulation as an intervention to monitor progression to the next stage (b110 Consciousness Functions, b156 Perceptual Functions). "Incidental reports on functional MRI studies show [however] that external stimuli can be processed in the human cortex of some vegetative patients, and that even spoken commands might elicit appropriate cortical responses that are indistinguishable from normal human responses" (Maas, Stocchetti, & Bullock, 2008, p 735). Consequently, the person "might hear, see, and realize a lot more than is commonly thought, and the concept that a vegetative state might be a worse outcome than death has become uncertain" (Maas, Stocchetti, & Bullock, 2008, p 735).

Rancho II, III (low arousal stage): Individuals begin to respond to sensory stimulation (b110

Consciousness Functions, b156 Perceptual Functions). Therapists try to elicit purposeful responses and one-step direction following (d210 Undertaking a Single Task) by providing stimuli to invoke spontaneous responses, such as handing the person a deck of cards to encourage a "shuffling" response or tossing the person a ball to encourage a catch/throw response. Therapy is done in a quiet environment with minimal distractions to encourage focus on the task at hand (b140 Attention Functions). Therapists might also begin to address orientation (b114 Orientation Functions).

Rancho IV, V, VI (post-traumatic amnesia stage): Individuals are disoriented and may be agitated and restless (b147 Psychomotor Functions). Therapy is provided in a quiet environment with minimal distractions. The goal is to gradually improve the person's basic cognitive processes in the areas of attention (b140 Attention Functions), memory (b144 Memory Functions), and orientation (b114 Orientation Functions). Therapy sessions start out short (e.g., two 15-minute sessions) and become longer (e.g., one 30-minute session) as tolerance allows. The therapist gently redirects the person back to the task at hand should s/he become distracted. Modalities chosen reflect the person's interests to maximize attention, motivation, and willingness to participate in the task (d210 Undertaking a Single Task). The therapist should be flexible within the specific modality and change modalities as required to keep the person's attention. Other strategies to improve the ability to direct and maintain focused attention include manipulation of environmental stimuli and activity structure. The therapist should start with simple tasks and then increase the complexity of the tasks in a controlled, hierarchal manner (Ashley et al., 2010). Breaking down tasks and activities into smaller, more manageable components through task analysis will help to improve learning (Persel & Persel, 2010). For individuals with severe memory impairments, Errorless Learning (EL) can be an effective learning strategy. The principle of EL is that individuals should be prevented from making mistakes during learning (Pitel et al., 2006). Individuals with severe memory impairments often do not benefit from trial and error learning because they are unable to recall their errors and the correct responses. The EL technique ensures that the individual avoids repeating the errors, thus learns

only the correct response. This technique has been used effectively to teach individuals with severe memory impairments new information, specific skills, or procedures (Cohen et al., 2010; Clare & Jones, 2008).

Rancho VII, VIII (post-confusional stage): Individuals are oriented x4 (person, place, time, circumstance) and do not exhibit agitation or restless behavior. Individuals typically have problems with higher-level cognitive skills (b164 Higher-Level Cognitive Functions, d160-d179 Applying Knowledge), such as problem solving, reasoning, organizing and planning, and decision-making, along with memory impairments (b144 Memory Functions). They also become overloaded and decompensate in stressful situations (d240 Handling Stress and Other Psychological Demands). The therapist addresses restoration of skills through graduated tasks and repetition, using EL techniques if appropriate. The therapist also teaches the individual and family compensatory strategies (e3 Support and Relationships) to manage impairments. Individuals with memory impairments might respond well to the of use external aids such as memory books, appointment diaries, notebooks, and to-do lists as compensatory strategies for functional day-to-day memory problems. These aids can use technology, such as mobile phones and electronic devices, as appropriate (Rees et al., 2007). Integration training, family training, and social skills training (e.g., d710-d729 General Interpersonal Interactions, d155 Acquiring Skills, d230 Carrying Out Daily Routine) are emphasized.

Physical Interventions

The Neuro-Developmental Treatment (NDT/Bobath) is a common approach to physical skill restoration that focuses on the development of balanced and symmetrical movements rather than on compensatory movements or learned nonuse of limbs (Bryan, Harrington, & Elliott, 2010). Recreational therapists can become certified in NDT through courses offered by the NDT Association. Places of employment often host NDT certification courses and cover the cost of the course as a way to advance the skill set of its therapists.

As previously reviewed, individuals with a TBI are at a significant risk for engagement in only sedentary activities (d570 Looking After One's Health, d920 Recreation and Leisure). Engagement in regular, moderate physical activity affords many benefits (b455 Exercise Tolerance Functions), yet it is challenging for this population. In a study of 384 adults with TBI, Driver (2008) found that affect was a significant mediator to engagement in physical activity. The authors recommended that:

> [r]ehabilitation specialists must create activity programs and environments that facilitate the development and fostering of positive affect... facilitating mastery experiences, increasing social support, and enhancing positive affective experiences. While these suggestions are not a "revolutionary" concept, rehabilitation typically occurs in a therapeutic environment rather than an environment where individuals participate in groups, make choices, or have fun. (p. 303)

Recreational therapy can play a major role in physical activity promotion in this population as the above recommendations to include improvement in affect (b125 Dispositions and Intra-Personal Functions, b126 Temperament and Personality Functions, b152 Emotional Functions) are underlying principles of the profession.

Social/Behavioral Interventions

Social and behavioral changes post TBI are common. Behaviors described in this section should be added to the patient's assessment and designated for treatment as appropriate. Most of the behaviors will be seen as deficits in ICF codes b122 Global Psychosocial Functions, b125 Dispositions and Intra-Personal Functions, b126 Temperament and Personality Functions, b152 Emotional Functions, b160 Thought Functions, and b164 Higher-Level Cognitive Functions. Observations might include confabulation, delusions, lability, and reduced anger control.

These deficits can also lead to particular behaviors, such as those associated with ICF codes d710 Basic Interpersonal Interactions and d720 Complex Interpersonal Interactions. Behaviors may include physical and verbal aggression, destructive behaviors, disinhibition, poor social judgment, sexual disinhibition, and unacceptable social conduct.

Other issues that may need to be documented include elopement (d571 Looking After One's Safety), impulsiveness (b130 Energy and Drive Functions), perseveration (b147 Psychomotor Functions), and agitation (b147 Psychomotor Functions) (Yody et al., 2000; Ylvisaker, Harvey, & Feeney, 2003).

Individuals might also present with a pseudode-pressed personality "associated with dorsolateral or dorsomedial prefrontal lesions... characterized by some combination of reduced initiation, apathy, lack of drive, loss of interest, lethargy, slowness, inattentiveness, reduced spontaneity, unconcern, lack of emotional reactivity, dullness, poor grooming, and perseveration" (Ylvisaker et al., 2003, p. 8) (b130 Energy and Drive Functions, b125 Dispositions and Intra-Personal Functions, b126 Temperament and Personality Functions). Cognitive impairments, such as memory, problem solving, and self-awareness, can also directly affect social-behavioral skills contributing to difficulty in forming and maintaining relationships (d720 Complex Interpersonal Interactions) and also leading to feelings of failure and frustration by the individual (Ylvisaker et al., 2003). And finally, environmental factors, premorbid patterns, and other psychological causes, such as depression, can also impact social behaviors (Yody et al., 2000).

Unwanted behaviors can have a negative impact on family dynamics and functioning, rehabilitation and discharge outcomes, quality of life, and community integration in all segments of life (Yody et al., 2000). Changing unwanted behaviors is not a simple task because individuals with TBI often lack insight into their own behaviors and the consequences of such behaviors (Yody et al., 2000). Consequently, social and behavioral skills, which have been documented during initial assessment or ongoing treatment as having deficits, need to be re-learned, reinforced, and supported.

A technique called applied behavior analysis (ABA) aids in decreasing the frequency, intensity, and duration of unwanted behaviors. It is based in behavioral theory and is team oriented. ABA is a contingency management approach that is based on the principle that behaviors increase or decrease in frequency as a result of positive and negative consequences. In other words, ABA involves the management and modification of behavior by manipulating the consequences (Ylvisaker et al., 2007). ABA plans are often initiated and implemented in a rehabilitation setting and then carried over into the person's real-life settings (Yody et al.,

2000). Creating a positive learning environment to increase success and decrease the risk of a behavioral episode is promoted. Strategies recommended by Persel & Persel (2010) include: allow rest time; keep the environment simple; minimize distractions and interruptions; keep instructions simple; give feedback; set clear and realistic goals; be calm and redirect to task; provide choices, but limit choice as needed not to overwhelm the person; decrease chance of failure (keep success rate above 80% to ensure challenge but avoid frustration); vary activities to maintain interest, attention, and motivation; overplan; and analyze and break down tasks into smaller steps to increase opportunities for participation and completion of various steps. Recreational therapists are integral members of the ABA plan, contributing to the identification of realistic consequences in leisure and community settings that could serve to reinforce desired behaviors.

Another technique is Positive Behavior Support (PBS). PBS has been used in a variety of settings, such as schools and residential facilities, with various populations including developmental disabilities, emotional disorders, and behavioral disorders (Gardner et al., 2003). According to Ylvisaker et al. (2003), PBS

> … focuses on enhancing individuals' quality of life by teaching useful and effective behaviors and by redesigning environments so that the person can achieve meaningful goals in a way that is efficient and also consistent with the needs of others… [A] guiding assumption behind PBS is that when individuals' needs are effectively met and quality of life correspondingly enhanced, problem behaviors substantially decrease in the absence of targeted response-deceleration interventions. (p. 11)

With an increased focus on holistic supports, PBS reflects a shift from the medical paradigm to a more holistic, support-oriented paradigm promoted by the ICF (Ylvisaker et al., 2003). It utilizes antecedent-focused, support-oriented interventions that revolve around environmental design and behavioral skill instruction (Gardner et al., 2003, Ylvisaker et al., 2003). For example, the environment is modified to reduce the risk of the unwanted behavior through the utilization of structured routines; positive communication, choice, and control; engagement in meaningful activities and roles; positive rewards and reinforcement of desirable behaviors; engagement in satisfying social relationships; engagement in meaningful recreation and leisure; participation in meaningful community activities; and the development of a positive sense of self (Gardner et al., 2003; Ylvisaker et al., 2003).

Resources

Brain Injury Association of America
www.biausa.org/
Dedicated to increasing access to quality healthcare and raising awareness and understanding of brain injury through advocacy, education, and research. Provides help, hope, and healing for individuals who live with brain injury, their families, and the professionals who serve them.

References

Ashley, M. J., Leal, R., Mehta, Z., Ashley, J. G., & Ashley, M. J. (2010). Cognitive disorders: Diagnosis and treatment in traumatic brain injury. In M. J. Ashley (Ed.). *Traumatic brain injury rehabilitation, treatment, and case management,* (pp. 583-615). Boca Raton, FL: CRC Press.

Brain Injury Association of America. (2011). About brain injury. Accessed via website http://www.biausa.org/about-brain-injury.htm#types.

Bryan, V. L., Harrington, D. W., & Elliott, M. G. (2010). Management of residual physical deficits. In M. J. Ashley (Ed.). *Traumatic brain injury rehabilitation, treatment, and case management,* (pp. 583-615). Boca Raton, FL: CRC Press.

burlingame, j. & Blaschko, T. M. (2010). *Assessment tools for recreational therapy and related fields, 4th edition.* Enumclaw, WA: Idyll Arbor, Inc.

Burton W. (2003). *Comments on the revision of the Rancho Los Amigos Levels of Cognitive Functioning Scale.* Downey, CA: Rancho Los Amigo National Rehabilitation Hospital.

Carroll, L., Cassidy, D., Peloso, P., Borg, J., von Holst, H., Holm, L., Paniak, C., & Pepin, M. (2004). Prognosis for mild traumatic brain injury: Results from the WHO collaborating centre task force on mild traumatic brain injury. *J Rehabil Med, Suppl. 43,* 84-105.

Centers for Disease Control and Prevention. (2012). Injury prevention and control: Traumatic brain injury: Traumatic Brain Injury. Accessed via website http://www.cdc.gov/TraumaticBrainInjury/severe.html.

Centers for Disease Control and Prevention. (2011a). Injury Prevention and Control: Traumatic Brain Injury: Traumatic Brain Injury. Accessed via website http://www.cdc.gov/TraumaticBrainInjury/index.html.

Centers for Disease Control and Prevention. (2011b). Injury Prevention and Control: Traumatic Brain Injury: How many people have TBI? Accessed via website http://www.cdc.gov/traumaticbraininjury/statistics.html#A.

Centers for Disease Control and Prevention. (2010a). Injury Prevention and Control: Traumatic Brain Injury: Concussion. Accessed via website http://www.cdc.gov/concussion/signs_symptoms.html.

Centers for Disease Control and Prevention. (2010b). Injury prevention and control: Traumatic brain injury: Causes. Accessed via website http://www.cdc.gov/TraumaticBrainInjury/causes.html.

Chumney, D., Nollinger, K., Shesko, K., Skop, K., Spencer, M., & Newton, R. A. (2010). Ability of functional independence measure to accurately predict functional outcome of stroke-specific population: Systematic review. *Journal of Rehabilitation Research & Development, 47*(1), 17-30.

Clare, L. & Jones, S. P. (2008). Errorless Learning in the rehabilitation of memory impairment: A critical review. *Neuropsychological Review 18,* 1-23.

Cohen, M., Ylvisaker, C., Hamilton, J., Kemp, L., & Claiman, B. (2010). Errorless learning of functional life skills in an individual with three aetiologies of severe memory and executive function impairment. *Neuropsychological Rehabilitation, 20*(3), 355-376.

Driver, S. (2008). Development of a conceptual model to predict physical activity participation in adults with brain injuries. *Adaptive Physical Activity Quarterly, 25,* 289-307.

Fischer, H. (2009). *United States military casualty statistics: Operation Iraqi Freedom and Operation Enduring Freedom.* Congressional Research Service, access via website http://www.dtic.mil/cgi-bin/GetTRDoc?AD=ADA498363 & Location=U2 & doc=GetTRDoc.pdf.

Gardner, R., Bird, F., Maguire, H., Carreiro, R., & Abenaim, N. (2003). Intensive positive behavior supports for adolescents with acquired brain injury: Long term outcomes in community settings. *Journal of Head Trauma Rehabilitation, 18*(1), 52-74.

Haskings, E. C., Cicerone, K., Dams-O'Connor, K, Eberle, R., Langenbahn, D, & Shapiro-Rosenbaum, A. (2012). *Cognitive rehabilitation manual: Translating evidence-based recommendations into practice.* Reston, VA: ACRM Publishing.

Hicks, R. R., Fertig, S. J., Derocher, R. E., Koroshetz, W. J., & Pancrazio, J. J. (2010). Neurological effects of blast injury. *Journal of TRAUMA Injury, Infection and Critical Care, 68*(5), 1257-1262.

Idyll Arbor. (2001). *Idyll Arbor's therapy dictionary, 2nd edition.* Enumclaw, WA: Idyll Arbor, Inc.

Jiang, J., Gao, G., Li, W., Yu, M., & Zhu, C. (2004). Early indicators of prognosis in 846 cases of severe traumatic brain injury. *Journal of Neurotrauma, 19*(7), 869-874.

Laatsch, L., Harrington, D., Holz, G., Marcantuono, J., Mozzoni, M., Walsh, V., & Hersey, K. (2007). An evidence-based review of cognitive and behavioral rehabilitation treatment studies in children with acquired brain injury. *Journal of Head Trauma Rehabilitation, 22*(4), 248-256.

Lenrow, D. (n.d.). Treatment for traumatic brain injury: Recovery. Accessed via website http://www.traumaticbraininjury.com/content/treatmentsfor/recovery.html.

Maas, A., Stocchetti, N., & Bullock, R. (2008). Moderate and severe traumatic brain injury in adults. *Lancet Neurol, 7,* 728-741.

Mayo Foundation for Medical Education and Research. (2011). Intracranial hematoma. Accessed via website http://www.mayoclinic.com/health/intracranial-hematoma/DS00330/DSECTION=causes.

National Institute of Neurological Disorders and Stroke, National Institute of Health. (2010). Neurological effects of blast injury. *Journal of TRAUMA Injury, Infection and Critical Care, 68*(5), 1257-1263.

National Institute of Neurological Disorders and Stroke, National Institute of Health. (2011a). What immediate post-injury complications can occur from a TBI? Traumatic brain injury:

Hope through research. Accessed via website http://www.ninds.nih.gov/disorders/tbi/detail_tbi.htm#170003218.

National Institute of Neurological Disorders and Stroke. (2011b). Hydrocephalus fact sheet. Accessed via website http://www.ninds.nih.gov/disorders/hydrocephalus/detail_hydrocephalus.htm.

Persel, C. S. & Persel, C. H. (2010). The use of applied behavior analysis in traumatic brain injury rehabilitation. In M. J. Ashley (Ed.). *Traumatic brain injury rehabilitation, treatment, and case management.* (pp. 583-615). Boca Raton, FL: CRC Press.

Pitel, A., Beaunieux, H., LeBaron, N., Joyeux, F., Desgranges, B., & Eustache, F. (2006). Two case studies in the application of errorless learning techniques in memory impaired patients with additional executive deficits. *Brain Injury, 20*(10), 1099-1110.

Porter, H. & burlingame, j. (2006). *Recreational therapy handbook of practice: ICF-based diagnosis and treatment.* Enumclaw, WA: Idyll Arbor, Inc.

Rapport, M., Hall, K., Hopkins, K., Belleza, T. & Cope, D. N. (1982). Disability rating scale for severe head trauma: Coma to community. *Archives of Physical Medicine and Rehabilitation, 63,* 118-123.

Rees, L., Marshall, S., Hartridge, C., Mackie, D., & Weiser, M. (2007). Cognitive interventions post acquired brain injury. *Brain Injury, 21*(2), 161-200.

Salisbury, D., Novack, T., & Brunner, R. (2004). TBI inform — Traumatic brain injury caused by violence. Traumatic Brain Injury Model System Information Network. Accessed via website http://main.uab.edu/tbi/show.asp?durki=85704.

Simonsen, L., Sonne-Holm, S., Krasheninnikoff, M., & Engberg, A. (2007). Symptomatic heterotopic ossification after very severe traumatic brain injury in 114 patients: Incidence and risk factors. *Injury, 38*(10), 1146-1150.

Temkin, N., Corrigan, J., Dikmen, S., Machamer, J. (2009). Social functioning after traumatic brain injury. *J Head Trauma Rehabil, 24*(6), 460-467.

Whyte, J., Ponsford, J., Watanabe, T., & Hart, T. (2010). Traumatic brain injury. In DeLisa et al. (Eds.). *Rehabilitation medicine: Principles and practices,* 5th ed., pp. 575-623. Philadelphia: Lippincott Williams & Wilkins.

Whyte, J., Hart, T., Laborde, A., & Rosenthal, M. (2004). Rehabilitation issues in traumatic brain injury. In DeLisa et al. (Eds.). *Rehabilitation medicine: Principles and practices,* 4th ed., pp. 1677-1713. Philadelphia: Lippincott.

Wise, E., Mathews-Dalton, C., Dikmen, S., Temkin, N. Machamer, J., Bell, K., & Powell, J. (2010). Impact of traumatic brain injury on participation in leisure activities. *Arch Phys Med Rehabili, 91,* 1357-1362.

Wright, J. (2000). The functional assessment measure. The Center for Outcome Measurement in Brain Injury, accessed via website http://www.tbims.org/combi/FAM/index.html.

Ylvisaker, M., Jacobs, H., & Feeney, T. (2003). Positive supports for people who experience behavioral and cognitive disability after brain injury: A review. *Journal of Head Trauma Rehabilitation, 18*(1), 7-32.

Ylvisaker, M., Turkstra, L., Coehlo, C., Yorkston, K., Kennedy, M., Sohlberg, M., & Avery, J. (2007). Behavioural interventions for children and adults with behavior disorders after TBI: A systematic review of the evidence. *Brain Injury, 21*(8), 769-805.

Yody, B., Schaub, C, Conway, J., Peters, S., Strauss, D., Helsinger, S. (2000). Applied behavior management and acquired brain injury: Approaches and assessment. *Journal of Head Trauma, 15*(4), 1041-1060.

39. Visual Impairments and Blindness

Tara L. Perry

Challenges to understanding visual impairment and blindness include the inconsistency of definitions used to classify levels of vision loss, the diversity of causes, and the individual differences in how people experience and are impacted by visual impairment and blindness. The ICF classifies vision in terms of b210 Seeing Functions, b215 Functions of Structures Adjoining the Eye, s220 Structure of Eyeball, and s230 Structures Around the Eye. Given the broad range of potential changes in vision functions and structures, content in this section is primarily limited to a description of what is most commonly meant when individuals are identified as visually impaired or blind and addresses the two criteria used in defining visual impairment and blindness, visual acuity (b2100 Visual Acuity Functions) and visual field (b2101 Visual Field Functions).

Normal eyesight is recognized as a visual acuity of 20/20, which means that an individual with normal vision can see small details at 20 feet away. If a person has a visual acuity of 20/50, for example, that person would see the same detail at 20 feet away that person with normal eyesight would see from 50 feet away. Visual field, or degrees of peripheral vision, indicates how well a person sees side to side and up and down. Normal peripheral vision is approximately 90 degrees lateral and 60 degrees medial, superior, and inferior. In the United States, visual impairment is defined as a visual acuity of 20/40 or less with the best correction. This level of visual impairment can cause difficulties for a person, such as being limited to a restricted driver's license in most states (Centers for Disease Control and Prevention [CDC], 2011; Friedman et al., 2008). Low vision, a term less frequently seen in vision loss definitions, is significant visual impairment with visual acuity between 20/70 and 20/200 that is not correctable (Smith et al., 2005). The definition of legal blindness, which is used to determine rehabilitation and other vision

services, is a visual acuity of 20/200 or less in the better eye with best correction or a visual field extent of 20 degrees or less in diameter (CDC, 2009a, 2011; Friedman et al., 2008).

Alternatively, the *International Statistical Classification of Diseases and Related Health Problems* (ICD) defines low vision as less than 20/60 but better than or equal to 20/200 or 20 degrees or less in the best eye with the best correction. The ICD defines blindness as 20/400 or less than 10 degrees in the best eye with the best correction (World Health Organization [WHO], 2009).

Visual impairment and blindness are also often described by their etiology with primary causes including diabetic retinopathy and age-related diseases such as macular degeneration, glaucoma, and cataract (CDC, 2009b, 2011; Prevent Blindness America, 2012). With the variety of criteria used to define visual impairment and blindness, as well as a diverse etiology, it is important for practitioners to understand these contexts, and how individuals' functioning and quality of life may be impacted.

Incidence/Prevalence in U.S.

Visual impairment and blindness are among the 10 most common causes of disability in the U.S. (Bailey et al., 2006; CDC, 2009a). An estimated 21 million Americans are visually impaired (CDC, 2009a; U.S. Dept. of Health and Human Services [USDHHS], 2008). Approximately 14 million Americans 12 years and older have visual impairment, defined as distance visual acuity of 20/50 or worse, and 11 million could improve their vision to 20/40 or better through refractive correction (Vitale, Cotch, & Sperduto, 2006). In 2007, the rate of blindness and visual impairment among children and adolescents under 18 years old was 25 per 1,000 population (USDHHS, 2008). Over one half of the children who are visually impaired in the U.S. also

417

have multiple disabilities (Di Stefano et al., 2006). Approximately 3.4 million Americans over 40 are affected by visual impairment, with one million of those classified as blind (CDC, 2009a, 2011; Friedman et al., 2008; Saaddine et al., 2004).

Based on 2000 Census data, for persons over 40 macular degeneration was the leading cause of blindness among white persons (54.4% of the cases); glaucoma and cataract accounted for 60% of blindness for black persons; and cataract was the leading cause of bi-lateral vision loss (visual acuity of 20/40 or less) for white, black, and Hispanic persons (Congdon et al., 2004). Half of the estimated 61 million adults in the U.S. who were classified as being at high risk for serious vision loss visited an eye doctor in the past 12 months (CDC, 2009c). Prevalence of persons who have low vision or are blind is expected to increase by 70% by 2020 (Congdon et al., 2004) and double by 2030 (Prevent Blindness America, 2012).

Predominant Age

While visual impairment and blindness can affect a person at any age, there is a dramatic relationship between age and vision impairment (Di Stefano et al., 2006), as shown in these selected statistics. Blindness or low vision affects approximately one in 28 Americans older than 40 years (Congdon et al., 2004). More than two thirds of adults who are visually impaired are 65 and older (Di Stefano et al., 2006). Prevalence of visual impairment and blindness increases rapidly with age, particularly after age 75 (Friedman et al., 2008).

Causes

There are a variety of ocular and cortical causes of visual impairment and blindness. While ocular visual impairments are caused by diseases or conditions affecting the eye, cortical (also referred to as cerebral or neurological) visual impairments (CVI) are caused by injury or structural differences in the brain (Roman-Lantzy, 2010). CVI is diagnosed when there is (1) an eye exam that is either normal or cannot explain the degree of diminished functional vision, (2) a history of a significant congenital or acquired brain injury or neurologic disorder, and (3) the presence of the unique visual behaviors associated with CVI, such as attraction to specific colors, difficulties with visual fields, difficulties with

visually complex arrays, the inability to visually attend to novel targets, and difficulties viewing targets at a distance (Roman-Lantzy, 2010).

According to the CDC (2009b), common eye diseases that cause visual impairment and blindness include the following:

Refractive errors: The most frequent refractive error eye problems in the U.S. include myopia (nearsightedness), hyperopia (farsightedness), astigmatism (distorted vision at all distances), and presbyopia (loss of close vision).

Age-related macular degeneration (AMD): AMD is a retinal eye disease associated with aging that results in damaged sharp and central vision. AMD is the leading cause of permanent impairment in reading and close-up vision. When the macula is affected, central vision needed for reading and driving is impacted. AMD is referred to as either wet or dry. Wet AMD occurs when abnormal blood vessels begin to grow under the macula, causing blood and fluid leakage, leading to rapidly decreased central vision. Dry AMD, which accounts for approximately 70-90% of AMD cases, occurs when the macula thins over time, resulting in a gradual blurring of central vision (CDC, 2009b).

Cataract: Cataract is the clouding of the eye's lens that can occur at any age due to a variety of causes. It is the leading cause of blindness worldwide and vision loss in the U.S. Treatment for the removal of cataract is widely available; however, reasons cited by the CDC for a lack of treatment include insurance coverage, treatment costs, patient choice, and lack of awareness.

Diabetic retinopathy (DR): DR is the leading cause of blindness in the U.S. and a complication of diabetes mellitus. DR causes progressive damage to the blood vessels of the retina, the light-sensitive tissue at the back of the eye. There are four progressive stages to DR including mild nonproliferative retinopathy (microaneurysms), moderate nonproliferative retinopathy (blockage in some retinal vessels), severe nonproliferative retinopathy (more blocked vessels that deprive the retina of blood supply which leads to growing new blood vessels), and proliferative retinopathy (most advanced stage) (CDC, 2009b).

Glaucoma: Glaucoma occurs with either normal eye pressure or a rise in the normal fluid pressure, resulting in damage to the optic nerve. The group of diseases that cause glaucoma can lead to vision loss or blindness. Early treatment is the best prevention of vision loss. Two types of glaucoma can occur. Open angle glaucoma progresses gradually and results in severe vision loss, often before the patient is aware of the amount of loss. Closed angle glaucoma occurs suddenly and is painful, often causing patients to seek medical help prior to permanent damage (CDC, 2009b).

Amblyopia: Commonly referred to as "lazy eye," amblyopia occurs when the brain and an eye do not work together, causing reduced vision in that eye. Conditions causing amblyopia include strabismus; more nearsightedness, farsightedness, or astigmatism in one eye or the other; and cataract. Untreated, it is the most common cause of one-eye vision impairment in children and young and middle-aged adults, impacting two to three percent of the population (CDC, 2009b).

Strabismus: This imbalance in the positioning of the two eyes causes a lack of coordination between the eyes. The eyes may cross in (esotropia) or turn out (exotropia). Strabismus occurs mostly in children, and the cause is typically unknown (CDC, 2009b).

Diplopia (double vision): There are two types of diplopia: monocular and binocular. Monocular diplopia is caused by an optical aberration, such as a cataract, and the second image persists even when one eye is covered. Binocular diplopia results from misalignment of the eyes caused by a lesion in the central nervous system, ocular motor nerve, neuromuscular junction, or extraocular muscle. With binocular diplopia, the second image does not persist when one eye is covered. Placing a patch over one eye to remove the second image can be helpful. Alternating between the right and left eye each day keeps the eyes balanced. Depth perception impairment will be evident when only one eye is used for vision (American Academy of Ophthalmology, 2013).

Visual field impairments: Visual field impairments can include visual neglect (lack of awareness of one side of the environment) or field loss (loss of vision in a specific area of the visual field) (Porter & burlingame, 2006).

Quality of vision impairments: Impairments that affect quality of vision include: (1) night blindness or hyposensitivity to light making it difficult to see when it is dark; (2) photophobia or hypersensitivity to daylight making it difficult to see during the day; (3) color blindness, a partial inability to distinguish certain colors, usually red from green, or a total inability to see color; (4) floaters; (5) stray lights; and (6) seeing stars or flashes (Porter & burlingame, 2006).

Systems Affected

The body structures affected are listed in ICF codes s220 Structure of Eyeball and s230 Structures Around the Eye. The therapist can use the following correlations for coding: s2203 Retina could be used to address diabetic retinopathy and macular degeneration; s2204 Lens of Eyeball would address cataract; and s2202 Iris or s2205 Vitreous Body would address glaucoma (Hendershot, Placek, & Goodman, 2006). Seeing functions are addressed in b210 Seeing Functions and b215 Functions of Structures Adjoining the Eye. Deficits in seeing function can be noted in detail using the subcodes.

Secondary Problems

The research on visual impairment and blindness does not make clear distinctions between secondary and comorbid conditions, and comorbidity is reported more often. For example, depression (b126 Temperament and Personality Functions) is reported as a secondary and comorbid condition to visual impairment and blindness. Other comorbid conditions that occur with visual impairment and blindness include diabetes, hearing impairment, stroke, falls, and cognitive decline (CDC, 2009a).

There are also particular comorbid conditions associated with visual impairment and age. According to Crews and Campbell (2001), persons with visual impairments aged 70 and older reported stroke, osteoporosis, depression, and cognitive disorientation twice as often as persons without visual impairment. If these problems are noted, the recreational therapist will need to look at other diagnoses for additional information about assessment and treatment.

As well, persons with visual impairments have higher rates of diabetes, arthritis, hypertension, heart disease, hearing impairment, and falls. Data analyzed from the National Health Interview Survey (NHIS) also indicated that older persons with visual impairment or blindness experience more limitations in activities including difficulty walking, getting into or out of a chair or bed, getting outside, getting to outside places, preparing meals, shopping for groceries, doing light housework, managing money, and managing medications (Crews & Campbell, 2001).

The study also found that participation was limited in older persons with visual impairment or blindness. They were less likely to get together with neighbors or friends, talk on the phone, go to church, eat out, or attend movies or sports events. These same older persons reported that they were less likely to exercise, less active than a year ago, and experienced poorer health (Crews & Campbell, 2001). Holbrook et al. (2009) reported low physical activity levels for adults with visual impairment or blindness. Young and middle-aged adults did not meet recommended daily quantity or intensity levels of physical activity to provide health-producing benefits. This sedentary lifestyle is a health problem for persons with visual impairment or blindness, providing the potential for the onset of secondary conditions associated with physical inactivity and obesity.

Prognosis

Visual impairment and blindness may or may not be correctable. In the cases that are not correctable, the prognosis is based on the person's ability to achieve healthy psychosocial adjustment and adapt to his/her situation. Several factors, including the amount and type of vision loss, age, comorbid or secondary conditions, resources, support, psychosocial adjustment, and environmental facilitators or barriers, are likely to influence how well individuals adjust to and live with visual impairment or blindness. One view is that visual impairment leads to a compromised quality of life due to inability to drive, read, keep track of bills, and travel in unfamiliar places (CDC, 2009a). In contrast, according to the National Federation of the Blind (NFB) (2012), if an individual "has proper training and opportunity, blindness can be reduced to a physical nuisance," and people who are blind can lead fully functional and independent lives.

Many of the factors that impact the prognosis for persons with visual impairment or blindness can be mitigated. For example, mobility, a person's ability to move around, can be facilitated through the combination of good orientation skills and use of a long cane or guide dog. Adaptive technology can aid an individual in accomplishing work, domestic,

recreational, and/or personal tasks. For example, individuals with visual impairment or blindness can read, conduct work, shop, pay bills, play games and cards, and engage in social networking activities with the aid of diverse adaptive technologies including computers, low vision aids, and/or modified products. When an individual achieves psychosocial adjustment, s/he is able to identify needs and gain the resources and support needed to meet those needs.

Factors such as attitudes of others and physical environments may also facilitate or inhibit an individual with visual impairment or blindness. The relationship of age and comorbidity is more complex; persons who are visually impaired or blind and 70 and older report having comorbid conditions, lower functioning in activities, decreased participation, decreased exercise, lower health status, and increased depression (Crews & Campbell, 2001; Crews, Jones, & Kim, 2006). It may be concluded that the prognosis for individuals with visual impairment or blindness may be very positive, provided the individual can gain adaptive skills, adjust well, and have access to needed support and resources. However, to the degree these factors are not provided or available, the prognosis will be less positive.

Assessment

Typical Scope of Team Assessment

Assessment may be one of the first steps in preventing visual impairment and blindness. If a therapy team is providing services to individuals at risk for potentially blinding diseases, including diabetic retinopathy or age-related diseases, screening for these causes of vision loss is important. The current impetus of several agencies that work toward decreasing the incidence of avoidable visual impairment and blindness (e.g., CDC, NEI, Prevent Blindness America, USDHHS, and WHO) is to increase screening, early detection, and treatment for persons affected by potentially blinding conditions. According to WHO (2012), "Globally, up to 80 percent of visual impairment and blindness in adults is preventable or treatable." However, the CDC (2009a) reports that only two thirds of persons with diabetes receive screening for diabetic retinopathy, though the screening measures are effective and affordable; cataract surgery can restore vision, yet unoperated senile cataracts are a major cause of blindness among U.S. African Americans; and approximately half of individuals with glaucoma are undiagnosed even though early detection and treatment can prevent vision loss.

Once an individual does have a visual impairment or blindness, assessment may be conducted to determine rehabilitation services that may assist the person in adjustment. A variety of vision rehabilitation services are available to help people cope with vision loss. These services include clinical assessments, vision rehabilitation therapy, orientation and mobility training, counseling, and other support services. However, access to these services has been limited due to inadequate referral rates from optometrists and ophthalmologists, a lack of awareness by persons with visual impairment about the availability of services, and financial and physical barriers (Di Stefano et al., 2006). ICF codes for describing the condition are b210 Seeing Functions, b215 Functions of Structures Adjoining the Eye, s220 Structure of Eyeball, and s230 Structures Around the Eye. Deficits in access to services may be documented with ICF codes that include d460 Moving Around in Different Locations, d470 Using Transportation, d570 Looking After One's Health, d740 Formal Relationships, e355 Health Professionals, e450 Individual Attitudes of Health Professionals, and e580 Health Services, Systems, and Policies.

Areas of Concern for RT Assessment

Recreational therapists do not directly assess the structural impairments of the eye but rather assess the client's level of visual functioning. The level of visual functioning is documented in order to assist therapists in identifying strengths or limitations of the client and to guide any needed accommodations or modifications for treatment interventions. For example, the *Functional Assessment of Characteristics for Therapeutic Recreation, Revised* (FACTR-R) and the *Idyll Arbor Activity Assessment* (IAAA) both require that the therapist note the level of visual function, whether vision is correctable, and if the patient actually uses the correction (burlingame & Blaschko, 2010). Therapists may also note changes in vision and provide this assessment information to an appropriate team member.

Skills and resources that may help a client adjust to visual impairment or blindness should also be assessed. A recreational therapist should assess the client's ability to function in clinical, home, and community settings. Some areas to assess include psychosocial adjustment (b126 Temperament and Personality Functions); physical activity (b455 Exercise Tolerance Functions); ability to comprehend written instructions (d166 Reading); basic problem solving ability (d175 Solving Problems); ability to perform activities of daily living (d230 Carrying Out Daily Routine); ability to handle problems (d240 Handling Stress and Other Psychological Demands); communication issues (d315 Communicating with — Receiving — Nonverbal Messages); balance, mobility, and other issues related to moving around during activities and in the community to get to activities (d4 Mobility); issues with self-care (d5 Self-Care, d630-d649 Household Tasks); access to goods and services (d620 Acquisition of Goods and Services); interactions with others (d7 Interpersonal Interactions and Relationships, d910 Community Life); skills required for leisure activities (d920 Recreation and Leisure); cases where needed technology is not available (e1 Products and Technology); how much assistance others will be able to provide (e3 Support and Relationships); and attitudes of others (e4 Attitudes).

ICF Core Set

No ICF Core Set has been developed for Visual Impairments or Blindness.

Treatment Direction

Whole Team Approach

It is essential to provide comprehensive eye examinations for those 65 years and older at high risk for visual impairment and blindness and for those with diabetes (Saaddine et al., 2004). Appropriate medical or surgical treatments can then be provided. In regard to the approach to rehabilitation services for those patients already experiencing visual impairment or blindness, Crews and Campbell (2001) indicate that rehabilitation services need to be more complex, beyond the traditional provision of mobility and low vision aids, and recognize the importance of exercise and general physical and mental health.

RT Approach

Recreational therapists do not correct visual impairments or blindness. Rather, individualized treatment is provided to assist in adjusting to vision loss in ways that promote increased function, independence, health, and quality of life. For example, recreational therapists may address adjustment, effective coping, exposure to and education about adaptive equipment and technology, compensatory strategies, community integration, social interaction skills, assertiveness training, and involvement in physical activity. RTs should also identify contextual factors that could potentially facilitate or inhibit participation, such as attitudes of others, physical features in the natural or human environment, and personal values, and find ways to overcome identified barriers.

Recreational Therapy Interventions

The following interventions are representative of common practices in working with persons with visual impairment or blindness. At this time, there is very little research on the efficacy of varied interventions specific to this population, and further research needs to be conducted to support and improve professional practice.

Functional Skills

Individuals with visual impairment or blindness will vary in their functional skills. One skill that will be required as a basis for all the others is problem solving (d175 Solving Problems). RTs should be sure to teach basic problem solving skills before looking at teaching ways to solve specific problems. Some specific skills which may be addressed after basic problem solving include:

Orientation and mobility: Persons who are visually impaired or blind need effective orientation and mobility skills to safely, purposefully, and independently travel in and through diverse environments. "Orientation skills enable people with visual impairments to use sensory information to know their location in different settings, and mobility skills enable them to travel in different areas" (Minnesota State Academy for the Blind, 2013). Recreational therapists can assist individuals who are visually impaired or blind by providing effective descriptive information about various environments, such as describing a room, path of travel, or outdoor area, with sufficient and relevant detail to allow the individual to understand his/her surroundings. The recreational therapist may also use the sighted guide

technique to assist the individual in exploring the environment. It is important to ask the individual what assistance, if any, is needed for orientation and mobility in a given environment. Individuals with visual impairment or blindness who are skilled in orientation and mobility will often indicate what information is needed and how they wish to proceed. Recreational therapists may work collaboratively with trained orientation and mobility specialists to better assess and provide assistance to individuals with visual impairments or blindness. Individuals who need to improve their orientation and mobility skills should be referred to an orientation and mobility specialist. ICF codes that are addressed by this kind of intervention include d4 Mobility, d710 Basic Interpersonal Interactions I asking for help, and e1 Products and Technology.

Self-care: Functional self-care skills may present challenges for individuals experiencing the onset of visual impairment or blindness. They must adapt to performing daily tasks of self-care without visual input. For example, it is difficult to orient to where food is on a plate and coordinate the use of utensils. Pouring liquids into containers, particularly hot liquids, may also be challenging. Recreational therapists can assist individuals in developing adaptive skills and behaviors to accomplish these types of self-care tasks in an effective manner. For example orienting individuals to locations of foods on their plates, using the clock method, is an adaptive technique which may make eating easier. Recreational therapists can consult with other vision specialists to provide assistance with self-care skills. ICF codes addressed are found in d5 Self-Care and d6 Domestic Life.

Communication: Communication skills are an integral component of social skills. Individuals with effective social skills are able to engage with others and recognize and utilize socially normative behaviors such as shaking hands, making eye contact, and interpreting gestures. For example, a person who is visually impaired or blind, due to a lack of visual input, may not know that someone has extended a hand for a handshake. Therefore, the person who is blind may not respond. Often, persons who are visually impaired or blind are taught to put their hands out first to offer to shake, so they do not miss the extended hand of the other person. Eye contact is also an important normative behavior, particularly in some cultures. Even though a person who is blind cannot see the other person, s/he can attempt to make eye contact by following the person's voice when speaking. This may not result in targeted eye contact, but the attempt may be appreciated by the person who can see. ICF codes addressed include d315 Communicating with — Receiving — Nonverbal Messages, d335 Producing Nonverbal Messages, and d7104 Social Cues in Relationships).

Reading: Reading is an important means of accessing information. Individuals with visual impairment or blindness may require alternative formats including large print, Braille, audio, and/or digital formats. These adaptations are in response to documented deficits in b210 Seeing Functions and d166 Reading. A variety of assistive technologies (e130 Products and Technology for Education), such as software programs that convert text to speech, scanners, reading devices, magnifiers, Braillers, etc., may be used to facilitate reading.

Leisure skills: Leisure skill development and participation (d910 Community Life; d920 Recreation and Leisure), community resource development, and healthy leisure development are all important functional skills. They are discussed later as part of Health Promotion.

Facilitators and barriers: RTs concentrate on identification of environmental facilitators or barriers such as products and technology (e1 Products and Technology); physical environment (e2 Natural Environment and Human-Made Changes to Environment, especially e2201 Animals, e240 Light, and e250 Sound); support and relationships (e3 Support and Relationships); attitudes (e4 Attitudes); and services, systems, or policies (e5 Services, Systems, and Policies). Focus should be placed on minimizing or resolving barriers and maximizing or strengthening facilitators to improve participation and quality of life.

Education, Training, and Counseling

Americans with Disabilities Act (ADA): RTs can provide education about the Americans with Disabilities Act (ADA) to facilitate awareness of civil and legal rights regarding access to facilities and programs. Some relevant sections of the ADA for persons with visual impairment or blindness may include employment, access to public transportation and goods and services provided by state and local governments, access to goods and services available to the general public, and communications. The ADA addresses the use of service animals, accessibility standards (e.g., texturing of surfaces, Braille and raised lettering for identifying locations), access to programs and services, and provision of materials in alternative formats. ICF codes that document the need for this information are included in e2 Natural Environment and Human-Made Changes to Environment.

Leisure counseling: Leisure counseling is provided as needed to facilitate psychosocial adjustment (b126 Temperament and Personality Functions, d240 Handling Stress and Other Psychological Demands) and optimal participation that promotes health and quality of life (d570 Looking After One's Health). Individuals with visual impairment or blindness will encounter different issues in adapting to their vision loss. Some common psychosocial adjustment issues can include decreased self-efficacy; increased potential for depression as a comorbid or secondary condition (b126 Temperament and Personality Functions); changes in vision and functional capacities, particularly for individuals with degenerative eye conditions (b210 Seeing Functions); potential for increased social isolation due to reduced access to information, opportunities, transportation, etc. (d460 Moving Around in Different Locations, d470 Using Transportation, d710 Basic Interpersonal Interactions); and societal and individual attitudes that may be limiting (e4 Attitudes). Any of these issues could impact an individual's leisure choices, engagement level, satisfaction, and overall view of quality of life.

Lifestyle: Lifestyle alteration education with particular attention to physical inactivity patterns and obesity is important. Specifically for those with diabetic retinopathy, education can assist with altering patterns to promote better diet and exercise for diabetes management (d570 Looking After One's Health).

Adaptive technology: Adaptive technology training can teach effective use of assistive technology products to facilitate participation and independence in home, work, and community settings (e1 Products and Technology). Examples of helpful adaptive technology may include computers with adapted software to convert text to Braille or speech; smart phones with a variety of relevant applications; talking products such as watches, clocks, GPS units, scales, thermostats, and calculators; Braille and other labeling systems for food, clothes, and other items; Braille, large print, and audio books; and Braille or large print scrabble, cards, etc.

Compensatory strategies: Compensatory strategies include training for visual impairments, such as using an anchor for left neglect, turning head to compensate for visual field loss, alternate patching for diplopia, and labeling the color of clothing for color vision impairment (e.g., e115 Products and Technology for Personal Use in Daily Living).

Assertiveness training: Assertiveness training (b126 Temperament and Personality Functions) facilitates asking for assistance, seeking directions, and responding effectively to diverse people and situations (d730 Relating with Strangers). It is essential that individuals with visual impairment or blindness are able to ask relevant questions of others to gain information about environments, changing circumstances, etc. For example, a person with visual impairment or blindness may encounter construction on a known path of travel and, therefore, need to ask a stranger about the circumstances to gain information and determine a safe alternate route. A person who is visually impaired or blind may need assistance identifying items while shopping and may ask another shopper or seek help from someone in customer service.

Community Integration

Community integration sessions for clients with visual impairment or blindness assist the client in using functional skills effectively and working within the real home, work, community, or recreation environment. Helpful integration outings may include sessions that address:

Community functioning: RTs can improve the level of functioning in the community by teaching clients how to move around (d450 Walking, d460 Moving Around in Different Locations); ask for directions (d730 Relating with Strangers); access goods and services (d620 Acquisition of Goods and Services, d470 Using Transportation, d920 Recreation and Leisure, d930 Religion and Spirituality); problem solving (d175 Solving Problems); and using assistive technology (e1 Products and Technology).

Transportation: RTs can address the client's skill and comfort level with accessing and using private

and public transportation and to use it effectively to get to and from activities (d470 Using Transportation).

Safety: RTs can teach clients how to deal with emergencies and safety issues (d240 Handling Stress and Other Psychological Demands). They can address mobility concerns or safety hazards that may occur in moving around (d4 Mobility) and teach the clients what to do if they get lost or disoriented about directions or the route (d470 Using Transportation).

Equipment: RTs can provide information and training for equipment to facilitate independence in the community such as a long cane or laser cane, GPS unit, or cell phone (e1 Products and Technology).

Health Promotion

Physical activity programs increase client awareness of the benefits of physical activity for health, address the consequences to inactivity such as obesity and resulting secondary conditions, and raise quantity and quality levels of physical activity. Exercise basics address ICF codes b455 Exercise Tolerance Functions and d570 Looking After One's Health to prevent secondary conditions and promote health. Coping with stress addresses ICF code d240 Handling Stress and Other Psychological Demands, emphasizes positive mental health, and potentially addresses depression (b126 Temperament and Personality Functions).

Resources

American Foundation for the Blind

www.afb.org

This national non-profit specifically prioritizes broadening access to technology, elevating the quality of information and tools for professionals who serve persons with vision loss, and promoting independent and healthy living for people with vision loss by providing them and their families with relevant and timely resources. AFB offers resources for individuals, families, seniors, and professionals. AFB publishes the *Journal of Visual Impairment and Blindness*, a primary source for research and practice-based articles.

National Center for Physical Activity and Disability

www.ncpad.org

The NCPAD website provides information and resources to enable people with disabilities to be as physically active as they choose to be. Links to newsletters, adapted sports, research, videos, and accessibility assist individuals and professionals in promoting and facilitating physical activity.

Academy for Certification of Vision Rehabilitation & Education Professions

www.acvrep.org

Recreational therapists who are interested in additional certifications related to vision impairments can explore certifications available through this organization. Certifications include Certified Low Vision Therapist, Certified Orientation and Mobility Specialist, and Certified Vision Rehabilitation Therapist.

Note

The views expressed in this chapter are those of the author and do not represent the views of the Federal Energy Regulatory Commission.

References

American Academy of Ophthalmology. (2013). Diplopia. Accessed via website http://www.aao.org/theeyeshaveit/disturbances/diplopia.cfm.

Bailey, R. N., Indian, R. W., Zhang, X., Geiss, L. S., Duenas, M. R., & Saaddine, J. B. (2006). Visual impairment and eye care among older adults — 5 states. *Morbidity and Mortality Weekly Report, 55*(49), 1321-1325. Retrieved from http://www.cdc.gov/mmwr/preview/mmwrhtml/mm5549a1.htm#top.

burlingame, j. & Blaschko, T. M. (2010). *Assessment tools for recreational therapy and related fields* (4th ed.). Ravensdale, WA: Idyll Arbor.

Centers for Disease Control and Prevention. (2011). Blindness and vision impairment: What's the problem? Retrieved October 28, 2012 from http://www.cdc.gov/healthcommunication/ToolsTemplates/EntertainmentEd/Tips/Blindness.html

Centers for Disease Control and Prevention. (2009a). Vision Health Initiative (VHI) — Vision loss: A public health problem. Retrieved October 28, 2012 from http://www.cdc.gov/ vision health/ basic_information/vision_loss.htm.

Centers for Disease Control and Prevention. (2009b). Vision Health Initiative (VHI) — Basic information: Common eye disorders. Retrieved October 28, 2012 from http://www.cdc.gov/visionhealth/basic_information/eye_disorders.htm.

Centers for Disease Control and Prevention. (2009c). Vision Health Initiative (VHI) — Vision loss: National data. Retrieved October 28, 2012 from http://www.cdc.gov/visionhealth/data/national.htm.

Congdon, N., O'Colmain, B., Klaver, C., Klein, R., Mun-Oz, B., Friedman, D, & Hyman, L. (2004). Causes and prevalence of visual impairment among adults in the United States. *Archives of Ophthalmology, 122*, 477-485. Retrieved from www.archophthalmol.com.

Crews, J. E. & Campbell, V. A. (2001). Health conditions, activity limitations, and participation restrictions among older people with visual impairments. *Journal of Visual Impairment and Blindness, 95*(8), 453-467. Retrieved from http://web.ebscohostcom/ehost/pdfviewer/pdfviewer?vid=3 & hid=107 & sid=bbcab04e-8a8b-43d8-b6af-06452e132fad%40sessionmgr112.

Crews, J. E., Jones, G. C., & Kim, J. H. (2006). Double jeopardy: The effects of comorbid conditions among older people with vision loss. *Journal of Visual Impairment and Blindness, 100*, 824-848. Retrieved from http://web.ebscohost.com/ehost/pdfviewer/pdfviewer?vid=3 & hid=107 & sid=bbcab04e-8a8b-43d8-b6af-06452e132fad%40sessionmgr112.

Di Stefano, A. F., Huebner, K., Garber, M., & Smith, A. J. (2006). Community services, needs, and resources in visual impairment: A 21st century public health perspective. *Journal of Visual Impairment and Blindness, 100*, 793-805. Retrieved from http://web.ebscohost.com/ehost/pdfviewer/pdfviewer?vid=3 & hid=107 & sid=bbcab04e-8a8b-43d8-b6af-06452e132fad%40sessionmgr112.

Friedman, D., Congdon, N., Kempen, J., & Tielsch, J. (2008). Vision problems in the U.S.: Prevalence of adult vision impairment and age-related eye disease in America, 2008 update to the 4th edition. Retrieved from http://www.preventblindness.org/vpus/.

Hendershot, G. E., Placek, P. J., & Goodman, N. (2006). Taming the beast: Measuring vision-related disability using the International Classification of Functioning. *Journal of Visual Impairment and Blindness, 100*, 806-823. Retrieved from http://web.ebscohost.com/ehost/pdfviewer/pdfviewer?vid=3 & hid=107 & sid=bbcab04e-8a8b-43d8-b6af-06452e132fad%40sessionmgr112.

Holbrook, E. A., Caputo, J. L., Perry, T. L., Fuller, D. K., & Morgan, D. (2009). Physical activity, body composition, and perceived quality of life of adults with visual impairment. *Journal of Visual Impairment and Blindness, 103*(1), 17-29. Retrieved from http://web.ebscohost.com/ehost/pdfviewer/pdfviewer?vid=3 & hid=107 & sid=bbcab04e-8a8b-43d8-b6af-06452e132fad%40sessionmgr112.

Minnesota State Academy for the Blind. (2013). Orientation and mobility: Definition. Retrieved January 25, 2013 from http://www.msab.state.mn.us/Programs/orientationmobility/index.asp.

National Eye Institute. (2012). A national plan 1999-2003: Report of the visual impairment and ITS rehabilitation panel. Retrieved January 18, 2013 from http://www.nei.nih.gov/resources/strategicplans/neiplan/frm_impairment.asp.

National Federation of the Blind. (2012). NFB — Voice of the nation's blind. Retrieved October 29, 2012 from https://nfb.org/.

Prevent Blindness America. (2012). Vision problems in the U.S. Retrieved October 28, 2012 from http://www.visionproblemsus.org/introduction.html.

Porter, H. & burlingame, j. (2006). *Recreational therapy handbook of practice: ICF-based diagnosis and treatment.* Enumclaw, WA: Idyll Arbor, Inc.

Roman-Lantzy, C. (2010). Teaching orientation and mobility to students with cortical visual impairment. In W. R. Wiener, R. L. Welsh, & B. B. Blasch (eds.). *Foundations of orientation and mobility* (3rd ed.), (pp. 667-714). New York, NY: American Foundation for the Blind.

Saaddine, J., Benjamin, S., Pan, L., Venkat Narayan, K. M., Tierney, E., Kanjilal, S., & Geiss, L. (2004). Prevalence of visual impairment and selected eye diseases among persons aged ≥50 years with and without diabetes — United States, 2002. *Morbidity and Mortality Weekly Report, 53*(45), 1069-

1071. Retrieved from http://www.cdc.gov/mmwr/preview/mmwrhtml/mm5345a3.htm#top.

Smith, R. W., Austin, D. R., Kennedy, D. W., Youngkhill, L., & Hutchinson, P. (2005). Disabling conditions. In *Inclusive and special recreation: Opportunities for persons with disabilities* (5th ed.) (pp. 54-84). Boston: McGraw-Hill.

U.S. Department of Health and Human Services. (2008). *Healthy People 2010 progress review: Vision and hearing.* Retrieved October 3, 2010 from http://www.healthypeople.gov/data/2010prog/focus28/default.htm.

Vitale, S., Cotch, M. F., & Sperduto, R. D. (2006). Prevalence of visual impairment in the United States. *Journal of the American Medical Association, 295*(18), 2158-2163. Retrieved from http://jama.ama-assn.org/cgi/reprint/295/18/2158.

World Health Organization. (2012). 10 facts about blindness. Retrieved October 29, 2012 from http://www.who.int/features/factfiles/blindness/blindness_facts/en/index9.html.

World Health Organization. (2009). 10 facts about blindness. Retrieved October 3, 2010 from h.who.int/features/factfiles/blindness/ en/index.html.

Appendix: ICF Core Sets

In an effort to make the ICF easier to use, common ICF codes that are used for specific conditions and populations have been grouped together into core sets. The development of each core set went through a rigorous process that included many healthcare centers conducting empirical studies to identify common problems related to the health condition, a systematic literature review on problems associated with the health condition, surveys to identify problems considered to be relevant by experts who treat individuals with the health condition, a qualitative study to identify problems from the point of view of individuals who have the particular health condition, and a structured decision making and consensus process at an international conference to develop the first version of the core set (Bickenbach, Cieza, Rauch, & Stucki, 2012).

The following core sets have been reprinted with permission from the ICF Research Branch. For more information about the ICF Research Branch or to ask specific questions about the ICF Core Sets, visit the website www.icf-research-branch.org. There is an ICF Core Set manual and a corresponding ICF-based documentation form online at www.icf-core-sets.org (Bickenbach, Cieza, Rauch, & Stucki, 2012).

The evaluation of the core sets is an ongoing process and more core sets are currently being developed. Clinicians should use the ICF Core Sets to steer the evaluation process. Every client is an individual and will present with varied problems. Consequently, it is imperative that clinicians do not limit their evaluation process to only those categories listed in each core set.

Generic Core Set
Grill et al. (2011)

Minimal Generic Set

Body Functions

b130	Energy and Drive Functions
b152	Emotional Functions
b280	Sensation of Pain

d230	Carrying Out Daily Routine
d450	Walking
d455	Moving Around
d850	Remunerative Employment

Clinical Generic Set

Body Functions

b130	Energy and Drive Functions
b134	Sleep Functions
b152	Emotional Functions
d230	Carrying Out Daily Routine
b280	Sensation of Pain
b455	Exercise Tolerance Functions
b640	Sexual Functions
b710	Mobility of Joint Functions
b730	Muscle Power Functions

Activities and Participation

d240	Handling Stress and Other Psychological Demands
d450	Walking
d455	Moving Around
d470	Using Transportation
d510	Washing Oneself
d540	Dressing
d570	Looking After One's Health
d640	Doing Housework
d660	Assisting Others
d710	Basic Interpersonal Interactions
d770	Intimate Relationships
d850	Remunerative Employment
d920	Recreation and Leisure

Arthritis
Grill et al. (2007)

Brief ICF Core Set for Acute Arthritis

Body Functions

b126	Temperament and Personality Functions
b130	Energy and Drive Functions
b134	Sleep Functions
b152	Emotional Functions
b280	Sensation of Pain
b415	Blood Vessel Functions
b430	Hematological System Functions
b440	Respiration Functions
b455	Exercise Tolerance Functions
b710	Mobility of Joint Functions
b715	Stability of Joint Functions
b730	Muscle Power Functions
b780	Sensations Related to Muscles and Movement Functions

Body Structures

s220	Structure of Eyeball
s710	Structure of Head and Neck Region
s720	Structure of Shoulder Region
s730	Structure of Upper Extremity
s740	Structure of Pelvic Region
s750	Structure of Lower Extremity
s760	Structure of Trunk
s770	Additional Musculoskeletal Structures Related to Movement
s810	Structure of Areas of Skin

Activities & Participation

d230	Carrying Out Daily Routine
d410	Changing Basic Body Position
d440	Fine Hand Use
d445	Hand and Arm Use
d450	Walking
d510	Washing Oneself
d530	Toileting
d540	Dressing
d550	Eating
d845	Acquiring, Keeping, and Terminating a Job

Environmental Factors

e110	Products or Substances for Personal Consumption
e115	Products and Technology for Personal Use in Daily Living
e120	Products and Technology for Personal Indoor and Outdoor Mobility and Transportation
e340	Personal Care Providers and Personal Assistants
e355	Health Professionals
e410	Individual Attitudes of Immediate Family Members
e580	Health Services, Systems, and Policies

Comprehensive ICF Core Set for Acute Arthritis

Body Functions

b126	Temperament and Personality Functions
b130	Energy and Drive Functions
b134	Sleep Functions
b152	Emotional Functions
b280	Sensation of Pain
b415	Blood Vessel Functions
b430	Hematological System Functions
b435	Immunological System Functions
b440	Respiration Functions
b455	Exercise Tolerance Functions
b710	Mobility of Joint Functions
b715	Stability of Joint Functions
b720	Mobility of Bone Functions
b730	Muscle Power Functions
b735	Muscle Tone Functions
b740	Muscle Endurance Functions
b770	Gait Pattern Functions
b780	Sensations Related to Muscles and Movement Functions

Body Structures

s220	Structure of Eyeball
s230	Structures Around the Eye
s420	Structure of Immune System
s430	Structure of Respiratory System
s710	Structure of Head and Neck Region
s720	Structure of Shoulder Region
s730	Structure of Upper Extremity
s740	Structure of Pelvic Region
s750	Structure of Lower Extremity
s760	Structure of Trunk
s770	Additional Musculoskeletal Structures Related to Movement
s810	Structure of Areas of Skin
s830	Structure of Nails

Activities and Participation

d230	Carrying Out Daily Routine
d240	Handling Stress and Other Psychological Demands
d410	Changing Basic Body Position
d415	Maintaining a Body Position
d420	Transferring Oneself
d430	Lifting and Carrying Objects
d435	Moving Objects with Lower Extremities
d440	Fine Hand Use
d445	Hand and Arm Use
d450	Walking
d460	Moving Around in Different Locations
d465	Moving Around Using Equipment
d470	Using Transportation
d510	Washing Oneself
d520	Caring for Body Parts
d530	Toileting
d540	Dressing
d550	Eating
d560	Drinking
d620	Acquisition of Goods and Services
d630	Preparing Meals
d640	Doing Housework
d650	Caring for Household Objects
d660	Assisting Others
d770	Intimate Relationships
d840	Apprenticeship (Work Preparation)
d845	Acquiring, Keeping, and Terminating a Job
d850	Remunerative Employment

Environmental Factors

e110	Products or Substances for Personal Consumption
e115	Products and Technology for Personal Use in Daily Living
e120	Products and Technology for Personal Indoor and Outdoor Mobility and Transportation
e125	Products and Technology for Communication
e135	Products and Technology for Employment
e150	Design, Construction, and Building Products and Technology of Buildings for Public Use
e155	Design, Construction, and Building Products and Technology of Buildings for Private Use
e225	Climate
e245	Time-Related Changes
e310	Immediate Family
e320	Friends
e340	Personal Care Providers and Personal Assistants
e355	Health Professionals
e410	Individual Attitudes of Immediate Family Members
e420	Individual Attitudes of Friends
e440	Individual Attitudes of Personal Care Providers and Personal Assistants
e450	Individual Attitudes of Health Professionals
e570	Social Security Services, Systems, and Policies
e575	General Social Support Services, Systems, and Policies
e580	Health Services, Systems, and Policies

Ankylosing Spondylitis

Boonen et al (2007)

Brief ICF Core Set for Ankylosing Spondylitis

Body Functions

b130	Energy and Drive Functions
b134	Sleep Functions
b152	Emotional Functions
b455	Exercise Tolerance Functions
b710	Mobility of Joint Functions
b780	Sensations Related to Muscles and Movement Functions

Body Structures

s740	Structure of Pelvic Region
s750	Structure of Lower Extremity
s760	Structure of Trunk
s770	Additional Musculoskeletal Structures Related to Movement

Activities & Participation

d230	Carrying Out Daily Routine
d410	Changing Basic Body Position
d450	Walking
d475	Driving
d760	Family Relationships
d845	Acquiring, Keeping, and Terminating a Job
d850	Remunerative Employment
d920	Recreation and Leisure

Environmental Factors

e110	Products or Substances for Personal Consumption
e3	Support and Relationships

Comprehensive ICF Core Set for Ankylosing Spondylitis

Body Functions

b130	Energy and Drive Functions
b1300	Energy Level
b1301	Motivation
b134	Sleep Functions
b152	Emotional Functions
b210	Seeing Functions
b280	Sensation of Pain
b28010	Pain in Head and Neck
b28011	Pain in Chest
b28013	Pain in Neck
b28014	Pain in Upper Limb
b28015	Pain in Lower limb
b28016	Pain in Joints
b28018	Pain in Body Part, Other Specified
b440	Respiration Functions
b4402	Depth of Respiration
b455	Exercise Tolerance Functions
b640	Sexual Functions
b710	Mobility of Joint Functions
b740	Muscle Endurance Functions
b770	Gait Pattern Functions
b780	Sensations Related to Muscles and Movement Functions
b7800	Sensation of Muscle Stiffness

Body Structures

s220	Structure of Eyeball
s2202	Structure of Iris
s430	Structure of Respiratory System
s4302	Structure of Thoracic Region
s720	Structure of Shoulder Region
s740	Structure of Pelvic Region
s750	Structure of Lower Extremity
s75001	Hip Joint
s75011	Knee Joint
s75021	Ankle Joint and Joints of Foot and Toes
s760	Structure of Trunk
s7600	Structure of Vertebral Column
s76000	Cervical Vertebral Column
s76001	Thoracic Vertebral Column
s76002	Lumbar Vertebral Column
s770	Additional Musculoskeletal Structures Related to Movement
s7700	Bones
s7702	Muscles
s7703	Extra-Articular Ligaments, Fasciae

Activities & Participation

d230	Carrying Out Daily Routine
d240	Handling Stress and Other Psychological Demands
d410	Changing Basic Body Position
d415	Maintaining a Body Position
d430	Lifting and Carrying Objects
d450	Walking
d455	Moving Around
d470	Using Transportation
d475	Driving
d510	Washing Oneself
d520	Caring for Body Parts
d530	Toileting
d540	Dressing
d570	Looking After One's Health
d620	Acquisition of Goods and Services
d640	Doing Housework
d660	Assisting Others
d760	Family Relationships
d770	Intimate Relationships
d845	Acquiring, Keeping, and Terminating a Job
d870	Economic Self-Sufficiency
d910	Community Life
d920	Recreation and Leisure

Environmental Factors

e110	Products or Substances for Personal Consumption
e1101	Drugs
e115	Products and Technology for Personal Use in Daily Living
e120	Products and Technology for Personal Indoor and Outdoor Mobility and Transportation
e135	Products and Technology for Employment
e150	Design, Construction, and Building Products and Technology of Buildings for Public Use
e225	Climate
e3	Support and Relationships
e4	Attitudes
e540	Transportation Services, Systems, and Policies
e570	Social Security Services, Systems, and Policies
e575	General Social Support Services, Systems, and Policies
e580	Health Services, Systems, and Policies
e590	Labor and Employment Services, Systems, and Policies

Bipolar Disorder

Vieta et al. (2007)

Brief ICF Core Set for Bipolar Disorder

Body Functions

b126	Temperament and Personality Functions
b130	Energy and Drive Functions
b134	Sleep Functions
b140	Attention Functions
b144	Memory Functions
b152	Emotional Functions
b160	Thought Functions

Activities & Participation

d175	Solving Problems
d230	Carrying Out Daily Routine
d240	Handling Stress and Other Psychological Demands
d570	Looking After One's Health
d760	Family Relationships
d770	Intimate Relationships
d845	Acquiring, Keeping, and Terminating a Job

Environmental Factors

e1101	Drugs
e320	Friends
e355	Health Professionals
e410	Individual Attitudes of Immediate Family Members
e460	Societal Attitudes

Comprehensive ICF Core Set for Bipolar Disorder

Body Functions

b126	Temperament and Personality Functions
b130	Energy and Drive Functions
b134	Sleep Functions
b140	Attention Functions
b144	Memory Functions
b147	Psychomotor Functions
b152	Emotional Functions
b156	Perceptual Functions
b160	Thought Functions
b164	Higher-Level Cognitive Functions
b280	Sensation of Pain
b330	Fluency and Rhythm of Speech Functions
b530	Weight Maintenance Functions
b640	Sexual Functions

Activities & Participation

d175	Solving Problems
d177	Making Decisions
d210	Undertaking a Single Task
d220	Undertaking Multiple Tasks
d230	Carrying Out Daily Routine
d240	Handling Stress and Other Psychological Demands
d570	Looking After One's Health
d710	Basic Interpersonal Interactions
d720	Complex Interpersonal Interactions
d760	Family Relationships
d770	Intimate Relationships
d845	Acquiring, Keeping, and Terminating a Job
d870	Economic Self-Sufficiency
d920	Recreation and Leisure

Environmental Factors

e1101	Drugs
e310	Immediate Family
e320	Friends
e355	Health Professionals
e410	Individual Attitudes of Immediate Family Members
e420	Individual Attitudes of Friends
e450	Individual Attitudes of Health Professionals
e460	Societal Attitudes
e570	Social Security Services, Systems, and Policies
e580	Health Services, Systems, and Policies

Breast Cancer

Brach et al. 2004

Brief ICF Core Set for Breast Cancer

Body Functions

b130	Energy and Drive Functions
b134	Sleep Functions
b152	Emotional Functions
b180	Experience of Self and Time Functions
b280	Sensation of Pain
b435	Immunological System Functions
b640	Sexual Functions
b710	Mobility of Joint Functions

Body Structures

s420	Structure of Immune System
s630	Structure of Reproductive System
s720	Structure of Shoulder Region

Activities & Participation

d230	Carrying Out Daily Routine
d240	Handling Stress and Other Psychological Demands
d430	Lifting and Carrying Objects
d445	Hand and Arm Use
d640	Doing Housework
d760	Family Relationships
d770	Intimate Relationships
d850	Remunerative Employment

Environmental Factors

e115	Products and Technology for Personal Use in Daily Living
e310	Immediate Family
e320	Friends
e355	Health Professionals
e410	Individual Attitudes of Immediate Family Members
e420	Individual Attitudes of Friends
e450	Individual Attitudes of Health Professionals
e570	Social Security Services, Systems, and Policies
e580	Health Services, Systems, and Policies
e590	Labor and Employment Services, Systems, and Policies

Comprehensive ICF Core Set for Breast Cancer

Body Functions

b126	Temperament and Personality Functions
b130	Energy and Drive Functions
b134	Sleep Functions
b152	Emotional Functions
b180	Experience of Self and Time Functions
b1801	Body Image

b265	Touch Function
b280	Sensation of Pain
b2801	Pain in Body Part
b435	Immunological System Functions
b4352	Functions of Lymphatic Vessels
b4353	Functions of Lymph Nodes
b455	Exercise Tolerance Functions
b530	Weight Maintenance Functions
b640	Sexual Functions
b650	Menstruation Functions
b660	Procreation Functions
b670	Sensations Associated with Genital and Reproductive Functions
b710	Mobility of Joint Functions
b720	Mobility of Bone Functions
b730	Muscle Power Functions
b740	Muscle Endurance Functions
b780	Sensations Related to Muscles and Movement Functions
b810	Protective Functions of the Skin
b820	Repair Functions of the Skin
b840	Sensation Related to the Skin

Body Structures

s420	Structure of Immune System
s4200	Lymphatic Vessels
s4201	Lymphatic Nodes
s630	Structure of Reproductive System
s6302	Breast and Nipple
s720	Structure of Shoulder Region
s730	Structure of Upper Extremity
s760	Structure of Trunk
s810	Structure of Areas of Skin

Activities & Participation

d177	Making Decisions
d230	Carrying Out Daily Routine
d240	Handling Stress and Other Psychological Demands
d430	Lifting and Carrying Objects
d445	Hand and Arm Use
d510	Washing Oneself
d520	Caring for Body Parts
d540	Dressing
d550	Eating
d560	Drinking
d570	Looking After One's Health
d620	Acquisition of Goods and Services
d630	Preparing Meals
d640	Doing Housework
d650	Caring for Household Objects
d660	Assisting Others
d720	Complex Interpersonal Interactions
d750	Informal Social Relationships
d760	Family Relationships
d770	Intimate Relationships
d850	Remunerative Employment
d920	Recreation and Leisure

Environmental Factors

e110	Products or Substances for Personal Consumption
e115	Products and Technology for Personal Use in Daily Living
e165	Assets
e225	Climate
e310	Immediate Family
e315	Extended Family

e320	Friends
e325	Acquaintances, Peers, Colleagues, Neighbors, and Community Members
e340	Personal Care Providers and Personal Assistants
e355	Health Professionals
e410	Individual Attitudes of Immediate Family Members
e415	Individual Attitudes of Extended Family Members
e420	Individual Attitudes of Friends
e425	Individual Attitudes of Acquaintances, Peers, Colleagues, Neighbors, and Community Members
e440	Individual Attitudes of Personal Care Providers and Personal Assistants
e450	Individual Attitudes of Health Professionals
e465	Social Norms, Practices, and Ideologies
e540	Transportation Services, Systems, and Policies
e555	Associations and Organizational Services, Systems, and Policies
e570	Social Security Services, Systems, and Policies
e575	General Social Support Services, Systems, and Policies
e580	Health Services, Systems, and Policies
e590	Labor and Employment Services, Systems, and Policies

Cardiopulmonary Conditions

Boldt et al. (2005) and Wildner et al. (2005)

Brief ICF Core Set for Cardiopulmonary Conditions for Acute Care

Body Functions

b110	Consciousness Functions
b130	Energy and Drive Functions
b280	Sensation of Pain
b415	Blood Vessel Functions
b420	Blood Pressure Functions
b435	Immunological System Functions
b440	Respiration Functions
b445	Respiratory Muscle Functions
b450	Additional Respiratory Functions
b455	Exercise Tolerance Functions
b460	Sensations Associated with Cardiovascular and Respiratory Functions
b510	Ingestion Functions

Body Structures

s760	Structure of Trunk
s810	Structure of Areas of Skin

Activities & Participation

d330	Speaking
d410	Changing Basic Body Position
d415	Maintaining a Body Position
d420	Transferring Oneself
d450	Walking
d510	Washing Oneself
d520	Caring for Body Parts
d530	Toileting
d540	Dressing

Environmental Factors

e110	Products or Substances for Personal Consumption
e115	Products and Technology for Personal Use in Daily Living
e120	Products and Technology for Personal Indoor and Outdoor Mobility and Transportation

e250	Sound
e260	Air Quality
e310	Immediate Family
e570	Social Security Services, Systems, and Policies
e580	Health Services, Systems, and Policies

Brief ICF Core Set for Cardiopulmonary Conditions for Post-Acute Care

Body Functions

b110	Consciousness Functions
b114	Orientation Functions
b130	Energy and Drive Functions
b134	Sleep Functions
b140	Attention Functions
b260	Proprioceptive Function
b410	Heart Functions
b430	Hematological System Functions
b450	Additional Respiratory Functions
b510	Ingestion Functions
b810	Protective Functions of the Skin
b820	Repair Functions of the Skin

Body Structures

s430	Structure of Respiratory System

Activities & Participation

d177	Making Decisions
d240	Handling Stress and Other Psychological Demands
d410	Changing Basic Body Position
d420	Transferring Oneself
d450	Walking
d460	Moving Around in Different Locations
d465	Moving Around Using Equipment
d540	Dressing
d910	Community Life

Environmental Factors

e110	Products or Substances for Personal Consumption
e115	Products and Technology for Personal Use in Daily Living
e125	Products and Technology for Communication
e155	Design, Construction, and Building Products and Technology of Buildings for Private Use
e245	Time-Related Changes
e250	Sound
e415	Individual Attitudes of Extended Family Members
e420	Individual Attitudes of Friends
e455	Individual Attitudes of Health-Related Professionals
e465	Social Norms, Practices, and Ideologies

Comprehensive ICF Core Set for Cardiopulmonary Conditions for Care

Body Functions

b110	Consciousness Functions
b114	Orientation Functions
b130	Energy and Drive Functions
b134	Sleep Functions
b280	Sensation of Pain
b410	Heart Functions
b415	Blood Vessel Functions
b420	Blood Pressure Functions
b430	Hematological System Functions

b435	Immunological System Functions
b440	Respiration Functions
b445	Respiratory Muscle Functions
b450	Additional Respiratory Functions
b455	Exercise Tolerance Functions
b460	Sensations Associated with Cardiovascular and Respiratory Functions
b510	Ingestion Functions
b545	Water, Mineral, and Electrolyte Balance Functions
b610	Urinary Excretory Functions
b710	Mobility of Joint Functions
b730	Muscle Power Functions
b820	Repair Functions of the Skin

Body Structures

s760	Structure of Trunk
s810	Structure of Areas of Skin

Activities & Participation

d240	Handling Stress and Other Psychological Demands
d330	Speaking
d410	Changing Basic Body Position
d415	Maintaining a Body Position
d420	Transferring Oneself
d450	Walking
d510	Washing Oneself
d520	Caring for Body Parts
d530	Toileting
d540	Dressing

Environmental Factors

e110	Products or Substances for Personal Consumption
e115	Products and Technology for Personal Use in Daily Living
e120	Products and Technology for Personal Indoor and Outdoor Mobility and Transportation
e250	Sound
e260	Air Quality
e310	Immediate Family
e320	Friends
e355	Health Professionals
e410	Individual Attitudes of Immediate Family Members
e420	Individual Attitudes of Friends
e450	Individual Attitudes of Health Professionals
e570	Social Security Services, Systems, and Policies
e580	Health Services, Systems, and Policies

Comprehensive ICF Core Set for Cardiopulmonary Conditions for Post-Acute Care

Body Functions

b110	Consciousness Functions
b114	Orientation Functions
b130	Energy and Drive Functions
b134	Sleep Functions
b140	Attention Functions
b144	Memory Functions
b152	Emotional Functions
b260	Proprioceptive Function
b280	Sensation of Pain
b310	Voice Functions
b410	Heart Functions
b415	Blood Vessel Functions
b420	Blood Pressure Functions
b430	Hematological System Functions

b435	Immunological System Functions
b440	Respiration Functions
b445	Respiratory Muscle Functions
b450	Additional Respiratory Functions
b455	Exercise Tolerance Functions
b460	Sensations Associated with Cardiovascular and Respiratory Functions
b510	Ingestion Functions
b525	Defecation Functions
b530	Weight Maintenance Functions
b545	Water, Mineral, and Electrolyte Balance Functions
b610	Urinary Excretory Functions
b620	Urination Functions
b710	Mobility of Joint Functions
b730	Muscle Power Functions
b740	Muscle Endurance Functions
b760	Control of Voluntary Movement Functions
b780	Sensations Related to Muscles and Movement Functions
b810	Protective Functions of the Skin
b820	Repair Functions of the Skin

Body Structures

s410	Structure of Cardiovascular System
s430	Structure of Respiratory System
s760	Structure of Trunk
s810	Structure of Areas of Skin

Activities & Participation

d155	Acquiring Skills
d177	Making Decisions
d230	Carrying Out Daily Routine
d240	Handling Stress and Other Psychological Demands
d410	Changing Basic Body Position
d415	Maintaining a Body Position
d420	Transferring Oneself
d430	Lifting and Carrying Objects
d440	Fine Hand Use
d445	Hand and Arm Use
d450	Walking
d460	Moving Around in Different Locations
d465	Moving Around Using Equipment
d510	Washing Oneself
d520	Caring for Body Parts
d530	Toileting
d540	Dressing
d550	Eating
d560	Drinking
d570	Looking After One's Health
d760	Family Relationships
d870	Economic Self-Sufficiency
d910	Community Life

Environmental Factors

e110	Products or Substances for Personal Consumption
e115	Products and Technology for Personal Use in Daily Living
e120	Products and Technology for Personal Indoor and Outdoor Mobility and Transportation
e125	Products and Technology for Communication
e150	Design, Construction, and Building Products and Technology of Buildings for Public Use
e155	Design, Construction, and Building Products and Technology of Buildings for Private Use
e245	Time-Related Changes
e250	Sound

e260	Air Quality
e310	Immediate Family
e315	Extended Family
e320	Friends
e355	Health Professionals
e360	Other Professionals
e410	Individual Attitudes of Immediate Family Members
e415	Individual Attitudes of Extended Family Members
e420	Individual Attitudes of Friends
e450	Individual Attitudes of Health Professionals
e455	Individual Attitudes of Health-Related Professionals
e465	Social Norms, Practices, and Ideologies
e555	Associations and Organizational Services, Systems, and Policies
e570	Social Security Services, Systems, and Policies
e575	General Social Support Services, Systems, and Policies
e580	Health Services, Systems, and Policies

Cerebrovascular Accident

Geyh et al. (2004)

Brief ICF Core Set for CVA

Body Functions

b110	Consciousness Functions
b114	Orientation Functions
b167	Mental Functions of Language
b730	Muscle Power Functions

Body Structures

s110	Structure of Brain

Activities & Participation

d330	Speaking
d450	Walking
d530	Toileting
d550	Eating

Environmental Factors

e310	Immediate Family

Comprehensive ICF Core Set for CVA

Body Functions

b110	Consciousness Functions
b114	Orientation Functions
b117	Intellectual Functions
b126	Temperament and Personality Functions
b130	Energy and Drive Functions
b134	Sleep Functions
b140	Attention Functions
b144	Memory Functions
b152	Emotional Functions
b156	Perceptual Functions
b164	Higher-Level Cognitive Functions
b167	Mental Functions of Language
b172	Calculation Functions
b176	Mental Functions of Sequencing Complex Movements
b180	Experience of Self and Time Functions
b210	Seeing Functions
b215	Functions of Structure Adjoining the Eye
b260	Proprioceptive Function
b265	Touch Function

b270	Sensory Functions Related to Temperature and Other Stimuli
b280	Sensation of Pain
b310	Voice Functions
b320	Articulation Functions
b330	Fluency and Rhythm of Speech Functions
b410	Heart Functions
b415	Blood Vessel Functions
b420	Blood Pressure Functions
b455	Exercise Tolerance Functions
b510	Ingestion Functions
b525	Defecation Functions
b620	Urination Functions
b640	Sexual Functions
b710	Mobility of Joint Functions
b715	Stability of Joint Functions
b730	Muscle Power Functions
b735	Muscle Tone Functions
b740	Muscle Endurance Functions
b750	Motor Reflex Functions
b755	Involuntary Movement Reaction Functions
b760	Control of Voluntary Movement Functions
b770	Gait Pattern Functions

Body Structures

s110	Structure of Brain
s410	Structure of Cardiovascular System
s720	Structure of Shoulder Region
s730	Structure of Upper Extremity
s750	Structure of Lower Extremity

Activities & Participation

d115	Listening
d155	Acquiring Skills
d160	Focusing Attention
d166	Reading
d170	Writing
d172	Calculating
d175	Solving Problems
d210	Undertaking a Single Task
d220	Undertaking Multiple Tasks
d230	Carrying Out Daily Routine
d240	Handling Stress and Other Psychological Demands
d310	Communicating with — Receiving — Spoken Messages
d315	Communicating with — Receiving — Nonverbal Messages
d325	Communicating with — Receiving — Written Messages
d330	Speaking
d335	Producing Nonverbal Messages
d345	Writing Messages
d350	Conversation
d360	Using Communication Devices and Techniques
d410	Changing Basic Body Position
d415	Maintaining a Body Position
d420	Transferring Oneself
d430	Lifting and Carrying Objects
d440	Fine Hand Use
d445	Hand and Arm Use
d450	Walking
d455	Moving Around
d460	Moving Around in Different Locations
d465	Moving Around Using Equipment
d470	Using Transportation
d475	Driving
d510	Washing Oneself
d520	Caring for Body Parts
d530	Toileting
d540	Dressing
d550	Eating
d570	Looking After One's Health
d620	Acquisition of Goods and Services
d630	Preparing Meals
d640	Doing Housework
d710	Basic Interpersonal Interactions
d750	Informal Social Relationships
d760	Family Relationships
d770	Intimate Relationships
d845	Acquiring, Keeping, and Terminating a Job
d850	Remunerative Employment
d855	Non-Remunerative Employment
d860	Basic Economic Transactions
d870	Economic Self-Sufficiency
d910	Community Life
d920	Recreation and Leisure

Environmental Factors

e110	Products or Substances for Personal Consumption
e115	Products and Technology for Personal Use in Daily Living
e120	Products and Technology for Personal Indoor and Outdoor Mobility and Transportation
e125	Products and Technology for Communication
e135	Products and Technology for Employment
e150	Design, Construction, and Building Products and Technology of Buildings for Public Use
e155	Design, Construction, and Building Products and Technology of Buildings for Private Use
e165	Assets
e210	Physical Geography
e310	Immediate Family
e315	Extended Family
e320	Friends
e325	Acquaintances, Peers, Colleagues, Neighbors, and Community Members
e340	Personal Care Providers and Personal Assistants
e355	Health Professionals
e360	Other Professionals
e410	Individual Attitudes of Immediate Family Members
e420	Individual Attitudes of Friends
e425	Individual Attitudes of Acquaintances, Peers, Colleagues, Neighbors, and Community Members
e440	Individual Attitudes of Personal Care Providers and Personal Assistants
e450	Individual Attitudes of Health Professionals
e455	Individual Attitudes of Health-Related Professionals
e460	Societal Attitudes
e515	Architecture and Construction Services, Systems, and Policies
e525	Housing Services, Systems, and Policies
e535	Communication Services, Systems, and Policies
e540	Transportation Services, Systems, and Policies
e550	Legal Services, Systems, and Policies
e555	Associations and Organizational Services, Systems, and Policies
e570	Social Security Services, Systems, and Policies
e575	General Social Support Services, Systems, and Policies
e580	Health Services, Systems, and Policies
e590	Labor and Employment Services, Systems, and Policies

Chronic Ischemic Heart Disease

Cieza, Stucki, Geyh, et al. (2004)

Brief ICF Core Set for Chronic Ischemic Heart Disease

Body Functions

b130	Energy and Drive Functions
b152	Emotional Functions
b280	Sensation of Pain
b410	Heart Functions
b415	Blood Vessel Functions
b420	Blood Pressure Functions
b455	Exercise Tolerance Functions
b460	Sensations Associated with Cardiovascular and Respiratory Functions
b730	Muscle Power Functions
b740	Muscle Endurance Functions

Body Structures

s410	Structure of Cardiovascular System

Activities & Participation

d230	Carrying Out Daily Routine
d240	Handling Stress and Other Psychological Demands
d450	Walking
d455	Moving Around
d570	Looking After One's Health
d620	Acquisition of Goods and Services
d760	Family Relationships
d770	Intimate Relationships
d850	Remunerative Employment

Environmental Factors

e110	Products or Substances for Personal Consumption
e310	Immediate Family
e320	Friends
e325	Acquaintances, Peers, Colleagues, Neighbors, and Community Members
e355	Health Professionals
e410	Individual Attitudes of Immediate Family Members
e570	Social Security Services, Systems, and Policies

Comprehensive ICF Core Set for Chronic Ischemic Heart Disease

Body Functions

b130	Energy and Drive Functions
b134	Sleep Functions
b152	Emotional Functions
b280	Sensation of Pain
b410	Heart Functions
b415	Blood Vessel Functions
b440	Respiration Functions
b455	Exercise Tolerance Functions
b460	Sensations Associated with Cardiovascular and Respiratory Functions
b530	Weight Maintenance Functions
b640	Sexual Functions
b730	Muscle Power Functions
b740	Muscle Endurance Functions

Body Structures

s410	Structure of Cardiovascular System

Activities & Participation

d230	Carrying Out Daily Routine
d240	Handling Stress and Other Psychological Demands
d430	Lifting and Carrying Objects
d450	Walking
d455	Moving Around
d460	Moving Around in Different Locations
d470	Using Transportation
d475	Driving
d480	Riding Animals for Transportation
d570	Looking After One's Health
d620	Acquisition of Goods and Services
d630	Preparing Meals
d640	Doing Housework
d760	Family Relationships
d770	Intimate Relationships
d850	Remunerative Employment
d920	Recreation and Leisure

Environmental Factors

e110	Products or Substances for Personal Consumption
e115	Products and Technology for Personal Use in Daily Living
e125	Products and Technology for Communication
e135	Products and Technology for Employment
e140	Products and Technology for Culture, Recreation, and Sport
e150	Design, Construction, and Building Products and Technology of Buildings for Public Use
e155	Design, Construction, and Building Products and Technology of Buildings for Private Use
e225	Climate
e260	Air Quality
e310	Immediate Family
e315	Extended Family
e320	Friends
e325	Acquaintances, Peers, Colleagues, Neighbors, and Community Members
e330	People in Positions of Authority
e340	Personal Care Providers and Personal Assistants
e355	Health Professionals
e360	Other Professionals
e410	Individual Attitudes of Immediate Family Members
e415	Individual Attitudes of Extended Family Members
e420	Individual Attitudes of Friends
e425	Individual Attitudes of Acquaintances, Peers, Colleagues, Neighbors, and Community Members
e430	Individual Attitudes of People in Positions of Authority
e440	Individual Attitudes of Personal Care Providers and Personal Assistants
e450	Individual Attitudes of Health Professionals
e455	Individual Attitudes of Health-Related Professionals
e460	Societal Attitudes
e570	Social Security Services, Systems, and Policies
e580	Health Services, Systems, and Policies
e590	Labor and Employment Services, Systems, and Policies

Chronic Pain

Cieza, Stucki, Weigl, Kullmann, et al. (2004)

Brief ICF Core Set for Chronic Pain

Body Functions

b130	Energy and Drive Functions

b134	Sleep Functions
b147	Psychomotor Functions
b152	Emotional Functions
b1602	Content of Thought
b280	Sensation of Pain
b455	Exercise Tolerance Functions
b730	Muscle Power Functions
b760	Control of Voluntary Movement Functions

Activities & Participation

d175	Solving Problems
d230	Carrying Out Daily Routine
d240	Handling Stress and Other Psychological Demands
d430	Lifting and Carrying Objects
d450	Walking
d640	Doing Housework
d760	Family Relationships
d770	Intimate Relationships
d850	Remunerative Employment
d920	Recreation and Leisure

Environmental Factors

e1101	Drugs
e310	Immediate Family
e355	Health Professionals
e410	Individual Attitudes of Immediate Family Members
e570	Social Security Services, Systems, and Policies

Comprehensive ICF Core Set for Chronic Pain

Body Functions

b122	Global Psychosocial Functions
b126	Temperament and Personality Functions
b130	Energy and Drive Functions
b134	Sleep Functions
b140	Attention Functions
b147	Psychomotor Functions
b152	Emotional Functions
b1602	Content of Thought
b164	Higher-Level Cognitive Functions
b180	Experience of Self and Time Functions
b260	Proprioceptive Function
b265	Touch Function
b270	Sensory Functions Related to Temperature and Other Stimuli
b280	Sensation of Pain
b430	Hematological System Functions
b455	Exercise Tolerance Functions
b640	Sexual Functions
b710	Mobility of Joint Functions
b730	Muscle Power Functions
b735	Muscle Tone Functions
b740	Muscle Endurance Functions
b760	Control of Voluntary Movement Functions
b780	Sensations Related to Muscles and Movement Functions

Body Structures

s770	Additional Musculoskeletal Structures Related to Movement

Activities & Participation

d160	Focusing Attention
d175	Solving Problems
d220	Undertaking Multiple Tasks
d230	Carrying Out Daily Routine

d240	Handling Stress and Other Psychological Demands
d410	Changing Basic Body Position
d415	Maintaining a Body Position
d430	Lifting and Carrying Objects
d450	Walking
d455	Moving Around
d470	Using Transportation
d475	Driving
d510	Washing Oneself
d540	Dressing
d570	Looking After One's Health
d620	Acquisition of Goods and Services
d640	Doing Housework
d650	Caring for Household Objects
d660	Assisting Others
d720	Complex Interpersonal Interactions
d760	Family Relationships
d770	Intimate Relationships
d845	Acquiring, Keeping, and Terminating a Job
d850	Remunerative Employment
d855	Non-Remunerative Employment
d910	Community Life
d920	Recreation and Leisure

Environmental Factors

e1101	Drugs
e310	Immediate Family
e325	Acquaintances, Peers, Colleagues, Neighbors, and Community Members
e355	Health Professionals
e410	Individual Attitudes of Immediate Family Members
e420	Individual Attitudes of Friends
e425	Individual Attitudes of Acquaintances, Peers, Colleagues, Neighbors, and Community Members
e430	Individual Attitudes of People in Positions of Authority
e450	Individual Attitudes of Health Professionals
e455	Individual Attitudes of Health-Related Professionals
e460	Societal Attitudes
e465	Social Norms, Practices, and Ideologies
e570	Social Security Services, Systems, and Policies
e575	General Social Support Services, Systems, and Policies
e580	Health Services, Systems, and Policies
e590	Labor and Employment Services, Systems, and Policies

Depression

Cieza, Chatterji, et al. (2004)

Brief ICF Core Set for Depression

Body Functions

b1263	Psychic Stability
b1265	Optimism
b1300	Energy Level
b1301	Motivation
b1302	Appetite
b140	Attention Functions
b147	Psychomotor Functions
b1521	Regulation of Emotion
b1522	Range of Emotion

Activities & Participation

d163	Thinking
d175	Solving Problems
d177	Making Decisions
d2301	Managing Daily Routine

d2303	Managing One's Own Activity Level
d240	Handling Stress and Other Psychological Demands
d350	Conversation
d510	Washing Oneself
d570	Looking After One's Health
d760	Family Relationships
d770	Intimate Relationships
d845	Acquiring, Keeping, and Terminating a Job

Environmental Factors

e1101	Drugs
e310	Immediate Family
e320	Friends
e325	Acquaintances, Peers, Colleagues, Neighbors, and Community Members
e355	Health Professionals
e410	Individual Attitudes of Immediate Family Members
e415	Individual Attitudes of Extended Family Members
e420	Individual Attitudes of Friends
e450	Individual Attitudes of Health Professionals
e580	Health Services, Systems, and Policies

Comprehensive ICF Core Set for Depression

Body Functions

b117	Intellectual Functions
b126	Temperament and Personality Functions
b1260	Extraversion
b1261	Agreeableness
b1262	Conscientiousness
b1263	Psychic Stability
b1265	Optimism
b1266	Confidence
b130	Energy and Drive Functions
b1300	Energy Level
b1301	Motivation
b1302	Appetite
b1304	Impulse Control
b134	Sleep Functions
b1340	Amount of Sleep
b1341	Onset of Sleep
b1342	Maintenance of Sleep
b1343	Quality of Sleep
b1344	Functions Involving the Sleep Cycle
b140	Attention Functions
b144	Memory Functions
b147	Psychomotor Functions
b152	Emotional Functions
b1520	Appropriateness of Emotion
b1521	Regulation of Emotion
b1522	Range of Emotion
b160	Thought Functions
b1600	Pace of Thought
b1601	Form of Thought
b1602	Content of Thought
b1603	Control of Thought
b164	Higher-Level Cognitive Functions
b1641	Organization and Planning
b1642	Time Management
b1644	Insight
b1645	Judgment
b180	Experience of Self and Time Functions
b1800	Experience of Self
b1801	Body Image
b280	Sensation of Pain

b460	Sensations Associated with Cardiovascular and Respiratory Functions
b530	Weight Maintenance Functions
b535	Sensations Associated with the Digestive System
b640	Sexual Functions
b780	Sensations Related to Muscles and Movement Functions

Activities & Participation

d110	Watching
d115	Listening
d163	Thinking
d166	Reading
d175	Solving Problems
d177	Making Decisions
d210	Undertaking a Single Task
d220	Undertaking Multiple Tasks
d230	Carrying Out Daily Routine
d2301	Managing Daily Routine
d2302	Completing the Daily Routine
d2303	Managing One's Own Activity Level
d240	Handling Stress and Other Psychological Demands
d310	Communicating with — Receiving — Spoken Messages
d315	Communicating with — Receiving — Nonverbal Messages
d330	Speaking
d335	Producing Nonverbal Messages
d350	Conversation
d355	Discussion
d470	Using Transportation (car, bus, train, plane, etc.)
d475	Driving (riding bicycle and motorbike, driving car, riding animals, etc.)
d510	Washing Oneself
d520	Caring for Body Parts
d540	Dressing
d550	Eating
d560	Drinking
d570	Looking After One's Health
d620	Acquisition of Goods and Services
d630	Preparing Meals
d640	Doing Housework
d650	Caring for Household Objects
d660	Assisting Others
d710	Basic Interpersonal Interactions
d720	Complex Interpersonal Interactions
d730	Relating with Strangers
d750	Informal Social Relationships
d760	Family Relationships
d770	Intimate Relationships
d830	Higher Education
d845	Acquiring, Keeping, and Terminating a Job
d850	Remunerative Employment
d860	Basic Economic Transactions
d865	Complex Economic Transactions
d870	Economic Self-Sufficiency
d910	Community Life
d920	Recreation and Leisure
d930	Religion and Spirituality
d950	Political Life and Citizenship

Environmental Factors

e1101	Drugs
e165	Assets
e225	Climate
e240	Light
e245	Time-Related Changes

e250	Sound
e310	Immediate Family
e320	Friends
e325	Acquaintances, Peers, Colleagues, Neighbors, and Community Members
e330	People in Positions of Authority
e340	Personal Care Providers and Personal Assistants
e355	Health Professionals
e360	Other Professionals
e410	Individual Attitudes of Immediate Family Members
e415	Individual Attitudes of Extended Family Members
e420	Individual Attitudes of Friends
e425	Individual Attitudes of Acquaintances, Peers, Colleagues, Neighbors, and Community Members
e430	Individual Attitudes of People in Positions of Authority
e440	Individual Attitudes of Personal Care Providers and Personal Assistants
e450	Individual Attitudes of Health Professionals
e455	Individual Attitudes of Health-Related Professionals
e460	Societal Attitudes
e465	Social Norms, Practices, and Ideologies
e525	Housing Services, Systems, and Policies
e570	Social Security Services, Systems, and Policies
e575	General Social Support Services, Systems, and Policies
e580	Health Services, Systems, and Policies
e590	Labor and Employment Services, Systems, and Policies

Diabetes Mellitus

Ruof et al. (2004)

Brief ICF Core Set for Diabetes Mellitus

Body Functions

b130	Energy and Drive Functions
b210	Seeing Functions
b270	Sensory Functions Related to Temperature and Other Stimuli
b410	Heart Functions
b415	Blood Vessel Functions
b420	Blood Pressure Functions
b455	Exercise Tolerance Functions
b530	Weight Maintenance Functions
b540	General Metabolic Functions
b545	Water, Mineral, and Electrolyte Balance Functions
b610	Urinary Excretory Functions

Body Structures

s220	Structure of Eyeball
s410	Structure of Cardiovascular System
s550	Structure of Pancreas
s610	Structure of Urinary System
s750	Structure of Lower Extremity

Activities & Participation

d240	Handling Stress and Other Psychological Demands
d450	Walking
d520	Caring for Body Parts
d570	Looking After One's Health

Environmental Factors

e110	Products or Substances for Personal Consumption
e115	Products and Technology for Personal Use in Daily Living
e310	Immediate Family
e355	Health Professionals

e465	Social Norms, Practices, and Ideologies
e570	Social Security Services, Systems, and Policies
e580	Health Services, Systems, and Policies
e585	Education and Training Services, Systems, and Policies

Comprehensive ICF Core Set for Diabetes Mellitus

Body Functions

b110	Consciousness Functions
b130	Energy and Drive Functions
b1300	Energy Level
b1302	Appetite
b134	Sleep Functions
b140	Attention Functions
b152	Emotional Functions
b210	Seeing Functions
b260	Proprioceptive Function
b265	Touch Function
b270	Sensory Functions Related to Temperature and Other Stimuli
b280	Sensation of Pain
b410	Heart Functions
b415	Blood Vessel Functions
b420	Blood Pressure Functions
b430	Hematological System Functions
b435	Immunological System Functions
b455	Exercise Tolerance Functions
b4550	General Physical Endurance
b4551	Aerobic Capacity
b4552	Fatiguability
b515	Digestive Functions
b530	Weight Maintenance Functions
b540	General Metabolic Functions
b545	Water, Mineral, and Electrolyte Balance Functions
b555	Endocrine Gland Functions
b610	Urinary Excretory Functions
b620	Urination Functions
b630	Sensations Associated with Urinary Functions
b640	Sexual Functions
b660	Procreation Functions
b710	Mobility of Joint Functions
b730	Muscle Power Functions
b810	Protective Functions of the Skin
b820	Repair Functions of the Skin
b840	Sensation Related to the Skin

Body Structures

s140	Structure of Sympathetic Nervous System
s150	Structure of Parasympathetic Nervous System
s220	Structure of Eyeball
s410	Structure of Cardiovascular System
s4100	Heart
s4101	Arteries
s4102	Veins
s4103	Capillaries
s550	Structure of Pancreas
s610	Structure of Urinary System
s6100	Kidneys
s630	Structure of Reproductive System
s750	Structure of Lower Extremity
s7502	Structure of Ankle and Foot
s810	Structure of Areas of Skin
s830	Structure of Nails

Activities & Participation

d240	Handling Stress and Other Psychological Demands
d440	Fine Hand Use
d450	Walking
d455	Moving Around
d475	Driving
d520	Caring for Body Parts
d570	Looking After One's Health
d620	Acquisition of Goods and Services
d630	Preparing Meals
d750	Informal Social Relationships
d760	Family Relationships
d770	Intimate Relationships
d845	Acquiring, Keeping, and Terminating a Job
d850	Remunerative Employment
d920	Recreation and Leisure
d9201	Sports
d9204	Hobbies
d9205	Socializing

Environmental Factors

e110	Products or Substances for Personal Consumption
e115	Products and Technology for Personal Use in Daily Living
e310	Immediate Family
e315	Extended Family
e320	Friends
e325	Acquaintances, Peers, Colleagues, Neighbors, and Community Members
e330	People in Positions of Authority
e340	Personal Care Providers and Personal Assistants
e355	Health Professionals
e360	Other Professionals
e410	Individual Attitudes of Immediate Family Members
e415	Individual Attitudes of Extended Family Members
e420	Individual Attitudes of Friends
e425	Individual Attitudes of Acquaintances, Peers, Colleagues, Neighbors, and Community Members
e430	Individual Attitudes of People in Positions of Authority
e440	Individual Attitudes of Personal Care Providers and Personal Assistants
e450	Individual Attitudes of Health Professionals
e455	Individual Attitudes of Health-Related Professionals
e465	Social Norms, Practices, and Ideologies
e510	Services, Systems, and Policies for the Production of Consumer Goods
e550	Legal Services, Systems, and Policies
e555	Associations and Organizational Services, Systems, and Policies
e560	Media Services, Systems, and Policies
e570	Social Security Services, Systems, and Policies
e575	General Social Support Services, Systems, and Policies
e580	Health Services, Systems, and Policies
e585	Education and Training Services, Systems, and Policies
e590	Labor and Employment Services, Systems, and Policies
e595	Political Services, Systems, and Policies

Geriatric Patients

Grill, Hermes, et al. (2005)

Brief ICF Core Set for Geriatric Patients for Post-Acute Care

Body Functions

b134	Sleep Functions
b435	Immunological System Functions
b455	Exercise Tolerance Functions
b460	Sensations Associated with Cardiovascular and Respiratory Functions
b620	Urination Functions
b630	Sensations Associated with Urinary Functions
b765	Involuntary Movement Functions

Body Structures

s110	Structure of Brain
s320	Structure of Mouth
s430	Structure of Respiratory System
s610	Structure of Urinary System
s720	Structure of Shoulder Region
s750	Structure of Lower Extremity
s770	Additional Musculoskeletal Structures Related to Movement

Activities & Participation

d230	Carrying Out Daily Routine
d360	Using Communication Devices and Techniques
d410	Changing Basic Body Position
d415	Maintaining a Body Position
d420	Transferring Oneself
d450	Walking
d460	Moving Around in Different Locations
d465	Moving Around Using Equipment
d510	Washing Oneself
d520	Caring for Body Parts
d530	Toileting
d550	Eating
d570	Looking After One's Health
d760	Family Relationships
d860	Basic Economic Transactions

Environmental Factors

e110	Products or Substances for Personal Consumption
e245	Time-Related Changes
e330	People in Positions of Authority
e355	Health Professionals
e425	Individual Attitudes of Acquaintances, Peers, Colleagues, Neighbors, and Community Members
e450	Individual Attitudes of Health Professionals
e460	Societal Attitudes
e465	Social Norms, Practices, and Ideologies
e570	Social Security Services, Systems, and Policies

Comprehensive ICF Core Set for Geriatric Patients for Post-Acute Care

Body Functions

b110	Consciousness Functions
b114	Orientation Functions
b117	Intellectual Functions
b130	Energy and Drive Functions
b134	Sleep Functions

b140   Attention Functions
b144   Memory Functions
b147   Psychomotor Functions
b152   Emotional Functions
b156   Perceptual Functions
b167   Mental Functions of Language
b176   Mental Functions of Sequencing Complex Movements
b180   Experience of Self and Time Functions
b210   Seeing Functions
b215   Functions of Structures Adjoining the Eye
b230   Hearing Functions
b240   Sensations Associated with Hearing and Vestibular Functions
b260   Proprioceptive Function
b265   Touch Function
b270   Sensory Functions Related to Temperature and Other Stimuli
b280   Sensation of Pain
b320   Articulation Functions
b410   Heart Functions
b415   Blood Vessel Functions
b420   Blood Pressure Functions
b430   Hematological System Functions
b435   Immunological System Functions
b440   Respiration Functions
b450   Additional Respiratory Functions
b455   Exercise Tolerance Functions
b460   Sensations Associated with Cardiovascular and Respiratory Functions
b510   Ingestion Functions
b525   Defecation Functions
b530   Weight Maintenance Functions
b535   Sensations Associated with the Digestive System
b540   General Metabolic Functions
b545   Water, Mineral, and Electrolyte Balance Functions
b620   Urination Functions
b630   Sensations Associated with Urinary Functions
b710   Mobility of Joint Functions
b715   Stability of Joint Functions
b730   Muscle Power Functions
b735   Muscle Tone Functions
b755   Involuntary Movement Reaction Functions
b760   Control of Voluntary Movement Functions
b765   Involuntary Movement Functions
b770   Gait Pattern Functions
b780   Sensations Related to Muscles and Movement Functions
b810   Protective Functions of the Skin
b820   Repair Functions of the Skin
b840   Sensation Related to the Skin

Body Structures

s110   Structure of Brain
s120   Spinal Cord and Related Structures
s320   Structure of Mouth
s410   Structure of Cardiovascular System
s430   Structure of Respiratory System
s610   Structure of Urinary System
s620   Structure of Pelvic Floor
s710   Structure of Head and Neck Region
s720   Structure of Shoulder Region
s740   Structure of Pelvic Region
s750   Structure of Lower Extremity
s760   Structure of Trunk
s770   Additional Musculoskeletal Structures Related to Movement

s810   Structure of Areas of Skin

Activities & Participation

d130   Copying
d155   Acquiring Skills
d177   Making Decisions
d230   Carrying Out Daily Routine
d240   Handling Stress and Other Psychological Demands
d310   Communicating with — Receiving — Spoken Messages
d315   Communicating with — Receiving — Nonverbal Messages
d330   Speaking
d335   Producing Nonverbal Messages
d360   Using Communication Devices and Techniques
d410   Changing Basic Body Position
d415   Maintaining a Body Position
d420   Transferring Oneself
d440   Fine Hand Use
d445   Hand and Arm Use
d450   Walking
d460   Moving Around in Different Locations
d465   Moving Around Using Equipment
d510   Washing Oneself
d520   Caring for Body Parts
d530   Toileting
d540   Dressing
d550   Eating
d560   Drinking
d570   Looking After One's Health
d760   Family Relationships
d770   Intimate Relationships
d860   Basic Economic Transactions
d930   Religion and Spirituality
d940   Human Rights

Environmental Factors

e110   Products or Substances for Personal Consumption
e115   Products and Technology for Personal Use in Daily Living
e120   Products and Technology for Personal Indoor and Outdoor Mobility and Transportation
e125   Products and Technology for Communication
e140   Products and Technology for Culture, Recreation, and Sport
e145   Products and Technology for the Practice of Religion and Spirituality
e150   Design, Construction, and Building Products and Technology of Buildings for Public Use
e240   Light
e245   Time-Related Changes
e250   Sound
e310   Immediate Family
e315   Extended Family
e320   Friends
e325   Acquaintances, Peers, Colleagues, Neighbors, and Community Members
e330   People in Positions of Authority
e355   Health Professionals
e360   Other Professionals
e410   Individual Attitudes of Immediate Family Members
e415   Individual Attitudes of Extended Family Members
e420   Individual Attitudes of Friends
e425   Individual Attitudes of Acquaintances, Peers, Colleagues, Neighbors, and Community Members
e430   Individual Attitudes of People in Positions of Authority
e450   Individual Attitudes of Health Professionals

e455	Individual Attitudes of Health-Related Professionals
e460	Societal Attitudes
e465	Social Norms, Practices, and Ideologies
e570	Social Security Services, Systems, and Policies
e580	Health Services, Systems, and Policies

Hand Conditions

Rudolf et al. (2012)

Brief ICF Core Set for Hand Conditions

Body Functions

b152	Emotional Functions
b265	Touch Function
b270	Sensory Functions Related to Temperature and Other Stimuli
b280	Sensation of Pain
b710	Mobility of Joint Functions
b715	Stability of Joint Functions
b730	Muscle Power Functions
b760	Control of Voluntary Movement Functions
b810	Protective Functions of the Skin

Body Structures

s120	Spinal Cord and Related Structures
s720	Structure of Shoulder Region
s730	Structure of Upper Extremity

Activities & Participation

d230	Carrying Out Daily Routine
d430	Lifting and Carrying Objects
d440	Fine Hand Use
d445	Hand and Arm Use
d5	Self-Care
d6	Domestic Life
d7	Interpersonal Interactions and Relationships
d840-d859	Work and Employment

Environmental Factors

e1	Products and Technology
e3	Support and Relationships
e5	Services, Systems, and Policies

Comprehensive ICF Core Set for Hand Conditions

Body Functions

b134	Sleep Functions
b152	Emotional Functions
b1801	Body Image
b260	Proprioceptive Function
b265	Touch Function
b2700	Sensitivity to Temperature
b2701	Sensitivity to Vibration
b2702	Sensitivity to Pressure
b2703	Sensitivity to a Noxious Stimulus
b280	Sensation of Pain
b415	Blood Vessel Functions
b7100	Mobility of Single Joint
b7101	Mobility of Several Joints
b715	Stability of Joint Functions
b720	Mobility of Bone Functions
b7300	Power of Isolated Muscles and Muscle Groups
b7301	Power of Muscles of One Limb
b735	Muscle Tone Functions

b740	Muscle Endurance Functions
b760	Control of Voluntary Movement Functions
b765	Involuntary Movement Functions
b780	Sensations Related to Muscles and Movement Functions
b810	Protective Functions of the Skin
b820	Repair Functions of the Skin
b830	Other Functions of the Skin
b840	Sensation Related to the Skin
b860	Functions of Nails

Body Structures

s120	Spinal Cord and Related Structures
s410	Structure of Cardiovascular System
s710	Structure of Head and Neck Region
s720	Structure of Shoulder Region
s7300	Structure of Upper Arm
s7301	Structure of Forearm
s7302	Structure of Hand
s770	Additional Musculoskeletal Structures Related to Movement
s810	Structure of Areas of Skin
s830	Structure of Nails

Activities & Participation

d170	Writing
d230	Carrying Out Daily Routine
d360	Using Communication Devices and Techniques
d410	Changing Basic Body Position
d420	Transferring Oneself
d430	Lifting and Carrying Objects
d4400	Picking Up
d4401	Grasping
d4402	Manipulating
d4403	Releasing
d4408	Fine Hand Use, Other Specified
d4450	Pulling
d4451	Pushing
d4452	Reaching
d4453	Turning or Twisting the Hands or Arms
d4454	Throwing
d4455	Catching
d4458	Hand and Arm Use, Other Specified
d455	Moving Around
d465	Moving Around Using Equipment
d470	Using Transportation
d475	Driving
d510	Washing Oneself
d520	Caring for Body Parts
d530	Toileting
d540	Dressing
d550	Eating
d560	Drinking
d570	Looking After One's Health
d620	Acquisition of Goods and Services
d630	Preparing Meals
d640	Doing Housework
d650	Caring for Household Objects
d660	Assisting Others
d7	Interpersonal Interactions and Relationships
d810-d839	Education
d840-d859	Work and Employment
d920	Recreation and Leisure

Environmental Factors

e110	Products or Substances for Personal Consumption

e115 Products and Technology for Personal Use in Daily Living
e120 Products and Technology for Personal Indoor and Outdoor Mobility and Transportation
e125 Products and Technology for Communication
e130 Products and Technology for Education
e135 Products and Technology for Employment
e140 Products and Technology for Culture, Recreation, and Sport
e150 Design, Construction, and Building Products and Technology of Buildings for Public Use
e155 Design, Construction, and Building Products and Technology of Buildings for Private Use
e165 Assets
e225 Climate
e310 Immediate Family
e315 Extended Family
e320 Friends
e325 Acquaintances, Peers, Colleagues, Neighbors, and Community Members
e330 People in Positions of Authority
e335 People in Subordinate Positions
e340 Personal Care Providers and Personal Assistants
e345 Strangers
e355 Health Professionals
e360 Other Professionals
e410 Individual Attitudes of Immediate Family Members
e420 Individual Attitudes of Friends
e425 Individual Attitudes of Acquaintances, Peers, Colleagues, Neighbors, and Community Members
e430 Individual Attitudes of People in Positions of Authority
e440 Individual Attitudes of Personal Care Providers and Personal Assistants
e445 Individual Attitudes of Strangers
e450 Individual Attitudes of Health Professionals
e455 Individual Attitudes of Health-Related Professionals
e460 Societal Attitudes
e465 Social Norms, Practices, and Ideologies
e525 Housing Services, Systems, and Policies
e530 Utilities Services, Systems and Policies
e535 Communication Services, Systems, and Policies
e540 Transportation Services, Systems, and Policies
e550 Legal Services, Systems, and Policies
e555 Associations and Organizational Services, Systems, and Policies
e570 Social Security Services, Systems, and Policies
e575 General Social Support Services, Systems, and Policies
e580 Health Services, Systems, and Policies
e585 Education and Training Services, Systems, and Policies
e590 Labor and Employment Services, Systems, and Policies

Head and Neck Cancer

Tschiesner et al. (2010)

Brief ICF Core Set for Head and Neck Cancer

Body Functions
b130 Energy and Drive Functions
b152 Emotional Functions
b280 Sensation of Pain
b310 Voice Functions
b440 Respiration Functions
b510 Ingestion Functions

Body Structures
s320 Structure of Mouth
s330 Structure of Pharynx
s340 Structure of Larynx
s710 Structure of Head and Neck Region

Activities and Participation
d230 Carrying Out Daily Routine
d330 Speaking
d550 Eating
d560 Drinking
d760 Family Relationships
d870 Economic Self-Sufficiency

Environmental Factors
e110 Products or Substances for Personal Consumption
e310 Immediate Family
e355 Health Professionals

Comprehensive ICF Core Set for Head and Neck Cancer

Body Functions
b117 Intellectual Functions
b126 Temperament and Personality Functions
b130 Energy and Drive Functions
b134 Sleep Functions
b152 Emotional Functions
b1801 Body Image
b230 Hearing Functions
b240 Sensations Associated with Hearing and Vestibular Functions
b250 Taste Function
b255 Smell Function
b280 Sensation of Pain
b310 Voice Functions
b320 Articulation Functions
b435 Immunological System Functions
b440 Respiration Functions
b455 Exercise Tolerance Functions
b5100 Sucking
b5101 Biting
b5102 Chewing
b5103 Manipulation of Food in the Mouth
b5104 Salivation
b51050 Oral Swallowing
b51051 Pharyngeal Swallowing
b51052 Esophageal Swallowing
b51058 Swallowing, Other Specified
b51059 Swallowing, Unspecified
b530 Weight Maintenance Functions
b535 Sensations Associated with the Digestive System
b555 Endocrine Gland Functions
b640 Sexual Functions
b710 Mobility of Joint Functions
b730 Muscle Power Functions
b810 Protective Functions of the Skin
b820 Repair Functions of the Skin

Body Structures
s1106 Structure of Cranial Nerves
s3200 Teeth
s3201 Gums
s32020 Hard Palate
s32021 Soft Palate

s3203	Tongue
s3204	Structure of Lips
s3208	Structure of Mouth, Other Specified
s3209	Structure of Mouth, Unspecified
s3300	Nasal Pharynx
s3301	Oral Pharynx
s3308	Structure of Pharynx, Other Specified
s3309	Structure of Pharynx, Unspecified
s3400	Vocal Folds
s3408	Structure of Larynx, Other Specified
s3409	Structure of Larynx, Unspecified
s410	Structure of Cardiovascular System
s420	Structure of Immune System
s4300	Trachea
s4301	Lungs
s510	Structure of Salivary Glands
s520	Structure of Esophagus
s7101	Bones of Face
s7103	Joints of Head and Neck Region
s7104	Muscles of Head and neck Region
s7105	Ligaments and Fasciae of Head and Neck Region
s7108	Structure of Head and Neck Region, Other Specified
s7109	Structure of Head and Neck Region, Unspecified
s720	Structure of Shoulder Region
s7301	Structure of Forearm
s750	Structure of Lower Extremity
s760	Structure of Trunk
s810	Structure of Areas of Skin

Activities and Participation

d230	Carrying Out Daily Routine
d240	Handling Stress and Other Psychological Demands
d330	Speaking
d350	Conversation
d360	Using Communication Devices and Techniques
d415	Maintaining a Body Position
d430	Lifting and Carrying Objects
d460	Moving Around in Different Locations
d470	Using Transportation
d475	Driving
d510	Washing Oneself
d520	Caring for Body Parts
d550	Eating
d560	Drinking
d570	Looking After One's Health
d640	Doing Housework
d710	Basic Interpersonal Interactions
d720	Complex Interpersonal Interactions
d750	Informal Social Relationships
d760	Family Relationships
d770	Intimate Relationships
d845	Acquiring, Keeping, and Terminating a Job
d910	Community Life
d920	Recreation and Leisure
d930	Religion and Spirituality

Environmental factors

e1100	Food
e1101	Drugs
e115	Products and Technology for Personal Use in Daily Living
e125	Products and Technology for Communication
e165	Assets
e310	Immediate Family
e320	Friends
e340	Personal Care Providers and Personal Assistants

e355	Health Professionals
e410	Individual Attitudes of Immediate Family Members
e460	Societal Attitudes
e525	Housing Services, Systems, and Policies
e535	Communication Services, Systems, and Policies
e555	Associations and Organizational Services, Systems, and Policies
e570	Social Security Services, Systems, and Policies
e575	General Social Support Services, Systems, and Policies
e580	Health Services, Systems, and Policies
e585	Education and Training Services, Systems, and Policies
e590	Labor and Employment Services, Systems, and Policies

Hearing Loss

paper not yet submitted

Brief ICF Core Set for Hearing Loss

Body functions

b126	Temperament and Personality Functions
b140	Attention Functions
b144	Memory Functions
b152	Emotional Functions
b210	Seeing Functions
b230	Hearing Functions
b240	Sensations Associated with Hearing and Vestibular Functions

Body structures

s110	Structure of Brain
s240	Structure of External Ear
s250	Structure of Middle Ear
s260	Structure of Inner Ear

Activities and participation

d115	Listening
d240	Handling Stress and Other Psychological Demands
d310	Communicating with — Receiving — Spoken Messages
d350	Conversation
d360	Using Communication Devices and Techniques
d760	Family Relationships
d820	School Education
d850	Remunerative Employment
d910	Community Life

Environmental factors

e125	Products and Technology for Communication
e250	Sound
e310	Immediate Family
e355	Health Professionals
e410	Individual Attitudes of Immediate Family Members
e460	Societal Attitudes
e580	Health Services, Systems, and Policies

Comprehensive ICF Core Set for Hearing Loss

Body functions

b117	Intellectual Functions
b126	Temperament and Personality Functions
b1300	Energy Level
b1301	Motivation
b140	Attention Functions
b144	Memory Functions
b152	Emotional Functions

b1560	Auditory Perception
b1561	Visual Perception
b164	Higher-Level Cognitive Functions
b167	Mental Functions of Language
b210	Seeing Functions
b2300	Sound Detection
b2301	Sound Discrimination
b2302	Localization of Sound Source
b2304	Speech Discrimination
b235	Vestibular Functions
b240	Sensations Associated with Hearing and Vestibular Functions
b280	Sensation of Pain
b310	Voice Functions
b320	Articulation Functions
b330	Fluency and Rhythm of Speech Functions

Body structures

s110	Structure of Brain
s240	Structure of External Ear
s250	Structure of Middle Ear
s260	Structure of Inner Ear
s710	Structure of Head and Neck Region

Activities and participation

d110	Watching
d115	Listening
d140	Learning to Read
d155	Acquiring Skills
d160	Focusing Attention
d175	Solving Problems
d220	Undertaking Multiple Tasks
d240	Handling Stress and Other Psychological Demands
d310	Communicating with — Receiving — Spoken Messages
d315	Communicating with — Receiving — Nonverbal Messages
d330	Speaking
d3503	Conversing with One Person
d3504	Conversing with Many People
d355	Discussion
d360	Using Communication Devices and Techniques
d440	Fine Hand Use
d470	Using Transportation
d475	Driving
d620	Acquisition of Goods and Services
d660	Assisting Others
d710	Basic Interpersonal Interactions
d720	Complex Interpersonal Interactions
d730	Relating with Strangers
d740	Formal Relationships
d750	Informal Social Relationships
d760	Family Relationships
d770	Intimate Relationships
d810	Informal Education
d820	School Education
d825	Vocational Training
d830	Higher Education
d840	Apprenticeship (Work Preparation)
d845	Acquiring, Keeping, and Terminating a Job
d850	Remunerative Employment
d855	Non-Remunerative Employment
d860	Basic Economic Transactions
d870	Economic Self-Sufficiency
d910	Community Life
d920	Recreation and Leisure
d930	Religion and Spirituality
d940	Human Rights
d950	Political Life and Citizenship

Environmental factors

e115	Products and Technology for Personal Use in Daily Living
e120	Products and Technology for Personal Indoor and Outdoor Mobility and Transportation
e125	Products and Technology for Communication
e130	Products and Technology for Education
e135	Products and Technology for Employment
e140	Products and Technology for Culture, Recreation, and Sport
e145	Products and Technology for the Practice of Religion and Spirituality
e150	Design, Construction, and Building Products and Technology of Buildings for Public Use
e155	Design, Construction, and Building Products and Technology of Buildings for Private Use
e225	Climate
e240	Light
e2500	Sound Intensity
e2501	Sound Quality
e310	Immediate Family
e315	Extended Family
e320	Friends
e325	Acquaintances, Peers, Colleagues, Neighbors, and Community Members
e330	People in Positions of Authority
e335	People in Subordinate Positions
e340	Personal Care Providers and Personal Assistants
e345	Strangers
e350	Domesticated Animals
e355	Health Professionals
e360	Other Professionals
e410	Individual Attitudes of Immediate Family Members
e415	Individual Attitudes of Extended Family Members
e420	Individual Attitudes of Friends
e425	Individual Attitudes of Acquaintances, Peers, Colleagues, Neighbors, and Community Members
e430	Individual Attitudes of People in Positions of Authority
e440	Individual Attitudes of Personal Care Providers and Personal Assistants
e445	Individual Attitudes of Strangers
e450	Individual Attitudes of Health Professionals
e455	Individual Attitudes of Health-Related Professionals
e460	Societal Attitudes
e465	Social Norms, Practices, and Ideologies
e515	Architecture and Construction Services, Systems, and Policies
e525	Housing Services, Systems, and Policies
e535	Communication Services, Systems, and Policies
e540	Transportation Services, Systems, and Policies
e545	Civil Protection Services, Systems, and Policies
e550	Legal Services, Systems, and Policies
e555	Associations and Organizational Services, Systems, and Policies
e560	Media Services, Systems, and Policies
e570	Social Security Services, Systems, and Policies
e575	General Social Support Services, Systems, and Policies
e580	Health Services, Systems, and Policies
e585	Education and Training Services, Systems, and Policies
e590	Labor and Employment Services, Systems, and Policies

Inflammatory Bowel Disease

Peyrin-Biroulet et al. (2010)

Brief ICF Core Set for Inflammatory Bowel Disease

Body Functions

b130	Energy and Drive Functions
b134	Sleep Functions
b152	Emotional Functions
b1801	Body Image
b28012	Pain in Stomach or Abdomen
b515	Digestive Functions
b525	Defecation Functions

Body Structures

s540	Structure of Intestine
s770	Additional Musculoskeletal Structures Related to Movement

Activities & Participation

d5301	Regulating Defecation
d570	Looking After One's Health
d7	Interpersonal Interactions and Relationships
d810-d839	Education
d840-d859	Work and Employment

Environmental Factors

e110	Products or Substances for Personal Consumption
e310	Immediate Family
e355	Health Professionals
e570	Social Security Services, Systems, and Policies
e580	Health Services, Systems, and Policies

Comprehensive ICF Core Set for Inflammatory Bowel Diseases

Body Functions

b130	Energy and Drive Functions
b134	Sleep Functions
b152	Emotional Functions
b1801	Body Image
b28012	Pain in Stomach or Abdomen
b28016	Pain in Joints
b430	Hematological System Functions
b435	Immunological System Functions
b515	Digestive Functions
b525	Defecation Functions
b530	Weight Maintenance Functions
b535	Sensations Associated with the Digestive System
b545	Water, Mineral, and Electrolyte Balance Functions
b640	Sexual Functions
b660	Procreation Functions
b810	Protective Functions of the Skin

Body Structures

s540	Structure of Intestine
s770	Additional Musculoskeletal Structures Related to Movement

Activities & Participation

d230	Carrying Out Daily Routine
d5301	Regulating Defecation
d570	Looking After One's Health
d7	Interpersonal Interactions and Relationships

d810-d839	Education
d840-d859	Work and Employment
d920	Recreation and Leisure

Environmental Factors

e110	Products or Substances for Personal Consumption
e1501	Design, Construction, and Building Products and Technology for Gaining Access to Facilities inside Buildings for Public Use
e310	Immediate Family
e320	Friends
e355	Health Professionals
e410	Individual Attitudes of Immediate Family Members
e420	Individual Attitudes of Friends
e425	Individual Attitudes of Acquaintances, Peers, Colleagues, Neighbors, and Community Members
e450	Individual Attitudes of Health Professionals
e570	Social Security Services, Systems, and Policies
e580	Health Services, Systems, and Policies

Low Back Pain

Cieza, Stucki, Weigl, Disler, et al. (2004)

Brief ICF Core Set for Low Back Pain

Body Functions

b130	Energy and Drive Functions
b134	Sleep Functions
b152	Emotional Functions
b280	Sensation of Pain
b455	Exercise Tolerance Functions
b710	Mobility of Joint Functions
b715	Stability of Joint Functions
b730	Muscle Power Functions
b735	Muscle Tone Functions
b740	Muscle Endurance Functions

Body Structures

s120	Spinal Cord and Related Structures
s760	Structure of Trunk
s770	Additional Musculoskeletal Structures Related to Movement

Activities & Participation

d240	Handling Stress and Other Psychological Demands
d410	Changing Basic Body Position
d415	Maintaining a Body Position
d430	Lifting and Carrying Objects
d450	Walking
d530	Toileting
d540	Dressing
d640	Doing Housework
d760	Family Relationships
d845	Acquiring, Keeping, and Terminating a Job
d850	Remunerative Employment
d859	Work and Employment, Other Specified and Unspecified

Environmental Factors

e110	Products or Substances for Personal Consumption
e135	Products and Technology for Employment
e155	Design, Construction, and Building Products and Technology of Buildings for Private Use
e310	Immediate Family
e355	Health Professionals

e410	Individual Attitudes of Immediate Family Members
e450	Individual Attitudes of Health Professionals
e550	Legal Services, Systems, and Policies
e570	Social Security Services, Systems, and Policies
e580	Health Services, Systems, and Policies

Comprehensive ICF Core Set for Low Back Pain

Body Functions

b126	Temperament and Personality Functions
b130	Energy and Drive Functions
b134	Sleep Functions
b152	Emotional Functions
b180	Experience of Self and Time Functions
b260	Proprioceptive Function
b280	Sensation of Pain
b455	Exercise Tolerance Functions
b620	Urination Functions
b640	Sexual Functions
b710	Mobility of Joint Functions
b715	Stability of Joint Functions
b720	Mobility of Bone Functions
b730	Muscle Power Functions
b735	Muscle Tone Functions
b740	Muscle Endurance Functions
b750	Motor Reflex Functions
b770	Gait Pattern Functions
b780	Sensations Related to Muscles and Movement Functions

Body Structures

s120	Spinal Cord and Related Structures
s740	Structure of Pelvic Region
s750	Structure of Lower Extremity
s760	Structure of Trunk
s770	Additional Musculoskeletal Structures Related to Movement

Activities & Participation

d240	Handling Stress and Other Psychological Demands
d410	Changing Basic Body Position
d415	Maintaining a Body Position
d420	Transferring Oneself
d430	Lifting and Carrying Objects
d445	Hand and Arm Use
d450	Walking
d455	Moving Around
d460	Moving Around in Different Locations
d465	Moving Around Using Equipment
d470	Using Transportation
d475	Driving
d510	Washing Oneself
d530	Toileting
d540	Dressing
d570	Looking After One's Health
d620	Acquisition of Goods and Services
d630	Preparing Meals
d640	Doing Housework
d650	Caring for Household Objects
d660	Assisting Others
d710	Basic Interpersonal Interactions
d760	Family Relationships
d770	Intimate Relationships
d845	Acquiring, Keeping, and Terminating a Job
d850	Remunerative Employment

d859	Work and Employment, Other Specified and Unspecified
d910	Community Life
d920	Recreation and Leisure

Environmental Factors

e110	Products or Substances for Personal Consumption
e120	Products and Technology for Personal Indoor and Outdoor Mobility and Transportation
e135	Products and Technology for Employment
e150	Design, Construction, and Building Products and Technology of Buildings for Public Use
e155	Design, Construction, and Building Products and Technology of Buildings for Private Use
e225	Climate
e255	Vibration
e310	Immediate Family
e325	Acquaintances, Peers, Colleagues, Neighbors, and Community Members
e330	People in Positions of Authority
e355	Health Professionals
e360	Other Professionals
e410	Individual Attitudes of Immediate Family Members
e425	Individual Attitudes of Acquaintances, Peers, Colleagues, Neighbors, and Community Members
e450	Individual Attitudes of Health Professionals
e455	Individual Attitudes of Health-Related Professionals
e460	Societal Attitudes
e465	Social Norms, Practices, and Ideologies
e540	Transportation Services, Systems, and Policies
e550	Legal Services, Systems, and Policies
e570	Social Security Services, Systems, and Policies
e575	General Social Support Services, Systems, and Policies
e580	Health Services, Systems, and Policies
e585	Education and Training Services, Systems, and Policies
e590	Labor and Employment Services, Systems, and Policies

Multiple Sclerosis

Coenen et al. (2011)

Brief ICF Core Set for Multiple Sclerosis

Body Functions

b130	Energy and Drive Functions
b152	Emotional Functions
b164	Higher-Level Cognitive Functions
b210	Seeing Functions
b280	Sensation of Pain
b620	Urination Functions
b730	Muscle Power Functions
b770	Gait Pattern Functions

Body Structures

s110	Structure of Brain
s120	Spinal Cord and Related Structures

Activities & Participation

d175	Solving Problems
d230	Carrying Out Daily Routine
d450	Walking
d760	Family Relationships
d850	Remunerative Employment

Environmental Factors

e310	Immediate Family

e355	Health Professionals
e410	Individual Attitudes of Immediate Family Members
e580	Health Services, Systems, and Policies

Comprehensive ICF Core Set for Multiple Sclerosis

Body Functions

b114	Orientation Functions
b126	Temperament and Personality Functions
b1300	Energy Level
b1301	Motivation
b1308	Energy and Drive Functions, Other Specified (fatigue)
b134	Sleep Functions
b140	Attention Functions
b144	Memory Functions
b152	Emotional Functions
b156	Perceptual Functions
b164	Higher-Level Cognitive Functions
b210	Seeing Functions
b235	Vestibular Functions
b260	Proprioceptive Function
b265	Touch Function
b270	Sensory Functions Related to Temperature and Other Stimuli
b280	Sensation of Pain
b310	Voice Functions
b320	Articulation Functions
b330	Fluency and Rhythm of Speech Functions
b445	Respiratory Muscle Functions
b455	Exercise Tolerance Functions
b5104	Salivation
b5105	Swallowing
b525	Defecation Functions
b5500	Body Temperature
b5508	Thermoregulatory Functions, Other Specified (sensitivity to heat)
b5508	Thermoregulatory Functions, Other Specified (sensitivity to cold)
b620	Urination Functions
b640	Sexual Functions
b710	Mobility of Joint Functions
b730	Muscle Power Functions
b735	Muscle Tone Functions
b740	Muscle Endurance Functions
b750	Motor Reflex Functions
b760	Control of Voluntary Movement Functions
b7650	Involuntary Contractions of Muscles
b7651	Tremor
b770	Gait Pattern Functions
b780	Sensations Related to Muscles and Movement Functions

Body Structures

s110	Structure of Brain
s120	Spinal Cord and Related Structures
s610	Structure of Urinary System
s730	Structure of Upper Extremity
s750	Structure of Lower Extremity
s760	Structure of Trunk
s810	Structure of Areas of Skin

Activities & Participation

d110	Watching
d155	Acquiring Skills
d160	Focusing Attention
d163	Thinking
d166	Reading
d170	Writing
d175	Solving Problems
d177	Making Decisions
d210	Undertaking a Single Task
d220	Undertaking Multiple Tasks
d230	Carrying Out Daily Routine
d240	Handling Stress and Other Psychological Demands
d330	Speaking
d350	Conversation
d360	Using Communication Devices and Techniques
d410	Changing Basic Body Position
d415	Maintaining a Body Position
d420	Transferring Oneself
d430	Lifting and Carrying Objects
d440	Fine Hand Use
d445	Hand and Arm Use
d450	Walking
d455	Moving Around
d460	Moving Around in Different Locations
d465	Moving Around Using Equipment
d470	Using Transportation
d475	Driving
d510	Washing Oneself
d520	Caring for Body Parts
d530	Toileting
d540	Dressing
d550	Eating
d560	Drinking
d570	Looking After One's Health
d620	Acquisition of Goods and Services
d630	Preparing Meals
d640	Doing Housework
d650	Caring for Household Objects
d660	Assisting Others
d710	Basic Interpersonal Interactions
d720	Complex Interpersonal Interactions
d750	Informal Social Relationships
d760	Family Relationships
d770	Intimate Relationships
d825	Vocational Training
d830	Higher Education
d845	Acquiring, Keeping, and Terminating a Job
d850	Remunerative Employment
d860	Basic Economic Transactions
d870	Economic Self-Sufficiency
d910	Community Life
d920	Recreation and Leisure
d930	Religion and Spirituality

Environmental Factors

e1101	Drugs
e1108	Products or Substances for Personal Consumption, Other Specified (special formulations of food to maintain safety and nutrition)
e115	Products and Technology for Personal Use in Daily Living
e120	Products and Technology for Personal Indoor and Outdoor Mobility and Transportation
e125	Products and Technology for Communication
e135	Products and Technology for Employment
e150	Design, Construction, and Building Products and Technology of Buildings for Public Use
e155	Design, Construction, and Building Products and Technology of Buildings for Private Use

e165	Assets
e2250	Temperature
e2251	Humidity
e2253	Precipitation
e310	Immediate Family
e315	Extended Family
e320	Friends
e325	Acquaintances, Peers, Colleagues, Neighbors, and Community Members
e330	People in Positions of Authority
e340	Personal Care Providers and Personal Assistants
e355	Health Professionals
e360	Other Professionals
e410	Individual Attitudes of Immediate Family Members
e415	Individual Attitudes of Extended Family Members
e420	Individual Attitudes of Friends
e425	Individual Attitudes of Acquaintances, Peers, Colleagues, Neighbors, and Community Members
e430	Individual Attitudes of People in Positions of Authority
e440	Individual Attitudes of Personal Care Providers and Personal Assistants
e450	Individual Attitudes of Health Professionals
e460	Societal Attitudes
e515	Architecture and Construction Services, Systems, and Policies
e525	Housing Services, Systems, and Policies
e540	Transportation Services, Systems, and Policies
e550	Legal Services, Systems, and Policies
e555	Associations and Organizational Services, Systems, and Policies
e570	Social Security Services, Systems, and Policies
e575	General Social Support Services, Systems, and Policies
e580	Health Services, Systems, and Policies
e585	Education and Training Services, Systems, and Policies
e590	Labor and Employment Services, Systems, and Policies

Musculoskeletal Conditions

Scheuringer et al. (2005) and Stoll et al. (2005)

Brief ICF Core Set for Musculoskeletal Conditions for Acute Care

Body Functions

b130	Energy and Drive Functions
b152	Emotional Functions
b415	Blood Vessel Functions
b440	Respiration Functions
b455	Exercise Tolerance Functions
b525	Defecation Functions
b620	Urination Functions
b710	Mobility of Joint Functions
b735	Muscle Tone Functions

Body Structures

s410	Structure of Cardiovascular System
s710	Structure of Head and Neck Region
s730	Structure of Upper Extremity
s740	Structure of Pelvic Region
s760	Structure of Trunk
s810	Structure of Areas of Skin

Activities & Participation

d240	Handling Stress and Other Psychological Demands
d410	Changing Basic Body Position
d415	Maintaining a Body Position
d420	Transferring Oneself
d450	Walking
d510	Washing Oneself
d520	Caring for Body Parts
d530	Toileting
d550	Eating

Environmental Factors

e110	Products or Substances for Personal Consumption
e355	Health Professionals
e420	Individual Attitudes of Friends

Brief ICF Core Set for Musculoskeletal Conditions for Post-Acute Care

Body Functions

b134	Sleep Functions
b260	Proprioceptive Function
b280	Sensation of Pain
b435	Immunological System Functions
b530	Weight Maintenance Functions
b620	Urination Functions
b730	Muscle Power Functions
b740	Muscle Endurance Functions
b755	Involuntary Movement Reaction Functions
b780	Sensations Related to Muscles and Movement Functions

Activities & Participation

d155	Acquiring Skills
d177	Making Decisions
d230	Carrying Out Daily Routine
d240	Handling Stress and Other Psychological Demands
d410	Changing Basic Body Position
d415	Maintaining a Body Position
d430	Lifting and Carrying Objects
d445	Hand and Arm Use
d450	Walking
d465	Moving Around Using Equipment
d510	Washing Oneself
d520	Caring for Body Parts
d530	Toileting
d540	Dressing
d550	Eating

Environmental Factors

e110	Products or Substances for Personal Consumption
e115	Products and Technology for Personal Use in Daily Living
e120	Products and Technology for Personal Indoor and Outdoor Mobility and Transportation
e225	Climate
e355	Health Professionals
e450	Individual Attitudes of Health Professionals

Comprehensive ICF Core Set for Musculoskeletal Conditions for Acute Care

Body Functions

b110	Consciousness Functions
b130	Energy and Drive Functions
b134	Sleep Functions
b152	Emotional Functions

b180	Experience of Self and Time Functions
b260	Proprioceptive Function
b280	Sensation of Pain
b415	Blood Vessel Functions
b440	Respiration Functions
b455	Exercise Tolerance Functions
b525	Defecation Functions
b620	Urination Functions
b710	Mobility of Joint Functions
b715	Stability of Joint Functions
b730	Muscle Power Functions
b735	Muscle Tone Functions
b820	Repair Functions of the Skin

Body Structures

s410	Structure of Cardiovascular System
s430	Structure of Respiratory System
s710	Structure of Head and Neck Region
s720	Structure of Shoulder Region
s730	Structure of Upper Extremity
s740	Structure of Pelvic Region
s750	Structure of Lower Extremity
s760	Structure of Trunk
s810	Structure of Areas of Skin

Activities & Participation

d240	Handling Stress and Other Psychological Demands
d410	Changing Basic Body Position
d415	Maintaining a Body Position
d420	Transferring Oneself
d445	Hand and Arm Use
d450	Walking
d510	Washing Oneself
d520	Caring for Body Parts
d530	Toileting
d550	Eating
d760	Family Relationships

Environmental Factors

e110	Products or Substances for Personal Consumption
e115	Products and Technology for Personal Use in Daily Living
e120	Products and Technology for Personal Indoor and Outdoor Mobility and Transportation
e150	Design, Construction, and Building Products and Technology of Buildings for Public Use
e310	Immediate Family
e320	Friends
e355	Health Professionals
e410	Individual Attitudes of Immediate Family Members
e420	Individual Attitudes of Friends
e450	Individual Attitudes of Health Professionals
e580	Health Services, Systems, and Policies

Comprehensive ICF Core Set Musculoskeletal Conditions for Post-Acute Care

Body Functions

b130	Energy and Drive Functions
b134	Sleep Functions
b152	Emotional Functions
b260	Proprioceptive Function
b270	Sensory Functions Related to Temperature and Other Stimuli
b280	Sensation of Pain

b415	Blood Vessel Functions
b435	Immunological System Functions
b440	Respiration Functions
b455	Exercise Tolerance Functions
b525	Defecation Functions
b530	Weight Maintenance Functions
b620	Urination Functions
b710	Mobility of Joint Functions
b715	Stability of Joint Functions
b730	Muscle Power Functions
b735	Muscle Tone Functions
b740	Muscle Endurance Functions
b755	Involuntary Movement Reaction Functions
b760	Control of Voluntary Movement Functions
b770	Gait Pattern Functions
b780	Sensations Related to Muscles and Movement Functions
b810	Protective Functions of the Skin

Body Structures

s710	Structure of Head and Neck Region
s720	Structure of Shoulder Region
s730	Structure of Upper Extremity
s740	Structure of Pelvic Region
s750	Structure of Lower Extremity
s760	Structure of Trunk
s810	Structure of Areas of Skin

Activities & Participation

d155	Acquiring Skills
d177	Making Decisions
d230	Carrying Out Daily Routine
d240	Handling Stress and Other Psychological Demands
d310	Communicating with — Receiving — Spoken Messages
d410	Changing Basic Body Position
d415	Maintaining a Body Position
d420	Transferring Oneself
d430	Lifting and Carrying Objects
d440	Fine Hand Use
d445	Hand and Arm Use
d450	Walking
d460	Moving Around in Different Locations
d465	Moving Around Using Equipment
d510	Washing Oneself
d520	Caring for Body Parts
d530	Toileting
d540	Dressing
d550	Eating
d560	Drinking
d570	Looking After One's Health
d760	Family Relationships

Environmental Factors

e110	Products or Substances for Personal Consumption
e115	Products and Technology for Personal Use in Daily Living
e120	Products and Technology for Personal Indoor and Outdoor Mobility and Transportation
e125	Products and Technology for Communication
e150	Design, Construction, and Building Products and Technology of Buildings for Public Use
e225	Climate
e310	Immediate Family
e320	Friends
e340	Personal Care Providers and Personal Assistants
e355	Health Professionals

e410   Individual Attitudes of Immediate Family Members
e420   Individual Attitudes of Friends
e430   Individual Attitudes of People in Positions of Authority
e440   Individual Attitudes of Personal Care Providers and Personal Assistants
e450   Individual Attitudes of Health Professionals
e555   Associations and Organizational Services, Systems, and Policies
e575   General Social Support Services, Systems, and Policies
e580   Health Services, Systems, and Policies

Neurological Conditions

Ewert et al. (2005); Grill, Ewert, et al. (2005); and Stier-Jarmer et al. (2005)

Brief ICF Core Set for Neurological Conditions for Acute Care

Body functions
b110   Consciousness Functions
b140   Attention Functions
b167   Mental Functions of Language
b215   Functions of Structures Adjoining the Eye
b235   Vestibular Functions
b240   Sensations Associated with Hearing and Vestibular Functions
b270   Sensory Functions Related to Temperature and Other Stimuli
b415   Blood Vessel Functions
b430   Hematological System Functions
b440   Respiration Functions
b525   Defecation Functions
b535   Sensations Associated with the Digestive System
b710   Mobility of Joint Functions

Body Structures
s110   Structure of Brain
s120   Spinal Cord and Related Structures
s710   Structure of Head and Neck Region

Activities and Participation
d360   Using Communication Devices and Techniques
d410   Changing Basic Body Position
d415   Maintaining a Body Position
d420   Transferring Oneself
d465   Moving Around Using Equipment
d510   Washing Oneself
d520   Caring for Body Parts
d530   Toileting
d540   Dressing
d550   Eating
d560   Drinking
d760   Family Relationships

Environmental Factors
e120   Products and Technology for Personal Indoor and Outdoor Mobility and Transportation
e315   Extended Family
e465   Social Norms, Practices, and Ideologies
e550   Legal Services, Systems, and Policies
e570   Social Security Services, Systems, and Policies

Brief ICF Core Set for Neurological Conditions for Post Acute Care

Body Functions
b126   Temperament and Personality Functions
b130   Energy and Drive Functions
b160   Thought Functions
b164   Higher-Level Cognitive Functions
b167   Mental Functions of Language
b210   Seeing Functions
b420   Blood Pressure Functions
b450   Additional Respiratory Functions
b510   Ingestion Functions
b530   Weight Maintenance Functions
b550   Thermoregulatory Functions
b620   Urination Functions
b740   Muscle Endurance Functions
b770   Gait Pattern Functions

Body Structures
s410   Structure of Cardiovascular System
s730   Structure of Upper Extremity

Activities & Participation
d115   Listening
d155   Acquiring Skills
d170   Writing
d175   Solving Problems
d410   Changing Basic Body Position
d420   Transferring Oneself
d440   Fine Hand Use
d450   Walking
d460   Moving Around in Different Locations
d465   Moving Around Using Equipment
d520   Caring for Body Parts
d530   Toileting
d540   Dressing
d550   Eating
d560   Drinking

Environmental Factors
e110   Products or Substances for Personal Consumption
e115   Products and Technology for Personal Use in Daily Living
e120   Products and Technology for Personal Indoor and Outdoor Mobility and Transportation
e125   Products and Technology for Communication
e355   Health Professionals
e415   Individual Attitudes of Extended Family Members
e550   Legal Services, Systems, and Policies

Comprehensive ICF Core Set for Neurological Conditions for Acute Care

Body Functions
b110   Consciousness Functions
b114   Orientation Functions
b130   Energy and Drive Functions
b134   Sleep Functions
b140   Attention Functions
b147   Psychomotor Functions
b152   Emotional Functions
b156   Perceptual Functions
b167   Mental Functions of Language
b180   Experience of Self and Time Functions

b210	Seeing Functions
b215	Functions of Structures Adjoining the Eye
b230	Hearing Functions
b235	Vestibular Functions
b240	Sensations Associated with Hearing and Vestibular Functions
b260	Proprioceptive Function
b265	Touch Function
b270	Sensory Functions Related to Temperature and Other Stimuli
b280	Sensation of Pain
b310	Voice Functions
b410	Heart Functions
b415	Blood Vessel Functions
b420	Blood Pressure Functions
b430	Hematological System Functions
b435	Immunological System Functions
b440	Respiration Functions
b450	Additional Respiratory Functions
b455	Exercise Tolerance Functions
b510	Ingestion Functions
b525	Defecation Functions
b535	Sensations Associated with the Digestive System
b540	General Metabolic Functions
b545	Water, Mineral, and Electrolyte Balance Functions
b620	Urination Functions
b710	Mobility of Joint Functions
b715	Stability of Joint Functions
b730	Muscle Power Functions
b735	Muscle Tone Functions
b755	Involuntary Movement Reaction Functions
b760	Control of Voluntary Movement Functions
b810	Protective Functions of the Skin

body Structures

s110	Structure of Brain
s120	Spinal Cord and Related Structures
s410	Structure of Cardiovascular System
s430	Structure of Respiratory System
s710	Structure of Head and Neck Region

Activities and Participation

d315	Communicating with — Receiving — Nonverbal Messages
d330	Speaking
d335	Producing Nonverbal Messages
d360	Using Communication Devices and Techniques
d410	Changing Basic Body Position
d415	Maintaining a Body Position
d420	Transferring Oneself
d440	Fine Hand Use
d445	Hand and Arm Use
d465	Moving Around Using Equipment
d510	Washing Oneself
d520	Caring for Body Parts
d530	Toileting
d540	Dressing
d550	Eating
d560	Drinking
d760	Family Relationships
d940	Human Rights

Environmental Factors

e110	Products or Substances for Personal Consumption
e115	Products and Technology for Personal Use in Daily Living
e120	Products and Technology for Personal Indoor and Outdoor Mobility and Transportation
e125	Products and Technology for Communication
e150	Design, Construction, and Building Products and Technology of Buildings for Public Use
e240	Light
e250	Sound
e310	Immediate Family
e315	Extended Family
e320	Friends
e355	Health Professionals
e360	Other Professionals
e410	Individual Attitudes of Immediate Family Members
e415	Individual Attitudes of Extended Family Members
e420	Individual Attitudes of Friends
e450	Individual Attitudes of Health Professionals
e455	Individual Attitudes of Health-Related Professionals
e465	Social Norms, Practices, and Ideologies
e550	Legal Services, Systems, and Policies
e570	Social Security Services, Systems, and Policies
e580	Health Services, Systems, and Policies

Comprehensive ICF Core Set for Neurological Conditions for Post Acute Care

Body Functions

b110	Consciousness Functions
b114	Orientation Functions
b126	Temperament and Personality Functions
b130	Energy and Drive Functions
b134	Sleep Functions
b140	Attention Functions
b144	Memory Functions
b147	Psychomotor Functions
b152	Emotional Functions
b156	Perceptual Functions
b160	Thought Functions
b164	Higher-Level Cognitive Functions
b167	Mental Functions of Language
b176	Mental Functions of Sequencing Complex Movements
b180	Experience of Self and Time Functions
b210	Seeing Functions
b215	Functions of Structures Adjoining the Eye
b230	Hearing Functions
b235	Vestibular Functions
b240	Sensations Associated with Hearing and Vestibular Functions
b260	Proprioceptive Function
b265	Touch Function
b270	Sensory Functions Related to Temperature and Other Stimuli
b280	Sensation of Pain
b310	Voice Functions
b320	Articulation Functions
b340	Alternative Vocalization Functions
b410	Heart Functions
b415	Blood Vessel Functions
b420	Blood Pressure Functions
b430	Hematological System Functions
b435	Immunological System Functions
b440	Respiration Functions
b450	Additional Respiratory Functions
b455	Exercise Tolerance Functions
b510	Ingestion Functions
b515	Digestive Functions

b525	Defecation Functions
b530	Weight Maintenance Functions
b535	Sensations Associated with the Digestive System
b540	General Metabolic Functions
b545	Water, Mineral, and Electrolyte Balance Functions
b550	Thermoregulatory Functions
b620	Urination Functions
b630	Sensations Associated with Urinary Functions
b710	Mobility of Joint Functions
b715	Stability of Joint Functions
b730	Muscle Power Functions
b735	Muscle Tone Functions
b740	Muscle Endurance Functions
b755	Involuntary Movement Reaction Functions
b760	Control of Voluntary Movement Functions
b770	Gait Pattern Functions
b810	Protective Functions of the Skin

Body Structures

s110	Structure of Brain
s120	Spinal Cord and Related Structures
s130	Structure of Meninges
s410	Structure of Cardiovascular System
s430	Structure of Respiratory System
s530	Structure of Stomach
s710	Structure of Head and Neck Region
s720	Structure of Shoulder Region
s730	Structure of Upper Extremity
s750	Structure of Lower Extremity
s810	Structure of Areas of Skin

Activities & Participation

d110	Watching
d115	Listening
d120	Other Purposeful Sensing
d130	Copying
d135	Rehearsing
d155	Acquiring Skills
d160	Focusing Attention
d166	Reading
d170	Writing
d175	Solving Problems
d177	Making Decisions
d310	Communicating with — Receiving — Spoken Messages
d315	Communicating with — Receiving — Nonverbal Messages
d330	Speaking
d335	Producing Nonverbal Messages
d350	Conversation
d360	Using Communication Devices and Techniques
d410	Changing Basic Body Position
d415	Maintaining a Body Position
d420	Transferring Oneself
d430	Lifting and Carrying Objects
d440	Fine Hand Use
d445	Hand and Arm Use
d450	Walking
d460	Moving Around in Different Locations
d465	Moving Around Using Equipment
d510	Washing Oneself
d520	Caring for Body Parts
d530	Toileting
d540	Dressing
d550	Eating
d560	Drinking
d760	Family Relationships

d930	Religion and Spirituality

Environmental Factors

e110	Products or Substances for Personal Consumption
e115	Products and Technology for Personal Use in Daily Living
e120	Products and Technology for Personal Indoor and Outdoor Mobility and Transportation
e125	Products and Technology for Communication
e310	Immediate Family
e315	Extended Family
e320	Friends
e355	Health Professionals
e360	Other Professionals
e410	Individual Attitudes of Immediate Family Members
e415	Individual Attitudes of Extended Family Members
e420	Individual Attitudes of Friends
e450	Individual Attitudes of Health Professionals
e465	Social Norms, Practices, and Ideologies
e550	Legal Services, Systems, and Policies
e570	Social Security Services, Systems, and Policies
e580	Health Services, Systems, and Policies

Obesity

Stucki, Daansen, et al. (2004)

Brief ICF Core Set for Obesity

Body Functions

b130	Energy and Drive Functions
b530	Weight Maintenance Functions

Activities & Participation

d240	Handling Stress and Other Psychological Demands
d450	Walking
d455	Moving Around
d570	Looking After One's Health

Environmental Factors

e110	Products or Substances for Personal Consumption
e310	Immediate Family

Comprehensive ICF Core Set for Obesity

Body Functions

b126	Temperament and Personality Functions
b130	Energy and Drive Functions
b134	Sleep Functions
b152	Emotional Functions
b180	Experience of Self and Time Functions
b1801	Body Image
b280	Sensation of Pain
b410	Heart Functions
b415	Blood Vessel Functions
b420	Blood Pressure Functions
b430	Hematological System Functions
b435	Immunological System Functions
b440	Respiration Functions
b455	Exercise Tolerance Functions
b510	Ingestion Functions
b515	Digestive Functions
b520	Assimilation Functions
b530	Weight Maintenance Functions
b535	Sensations Associated with the Digestive System

b540	General Metabolic Functions
b545	Water, Mineral, and Electrolyte Balance Functions
b555	Endocrine Gland Functions
b610	Urinary Excretory Functions
b620	Urination Functions
b640	Sexual Functions
b650	Menstruation Functions
b660	Procreation Functions
b710	Mobility of Joint Functions
b820	Repair Functions of the Skin
b830	Other Functions of the Skin

Body Structures

s110	Structure of Brain
s140	Structure of Sympathetic Nervous System
s150	Structure of Parasympathetic Nervous System
s410	Structure of Cardiovascular System
s420	Structure of Immune System
s430	Structure of Respiratory System
s520	Structure of Esophagus
s530	Structure of Stomach
s550	Structure of Pancreas
s560	Structure of Liver
s570	Structure of Gall Bladder and Ducts
s580	Structure of Endocrine Glands
s630	Structure of Reproductive System
s710	Structure of Head and Neck Region
s750	Structure of Lower Extremity
s760	Structure of Trunk
s770	Additional Musculoskeletal Structures Related to Movement
s810	Structure of Areas of Skin

Activities & Participation

d240	Handling Stress and Other Psychological Demands
d410	Changing Basic Body Position
d415	Maintaining a Body Position
d430	Lifting and Carrying Objects
d450	Walking
d455	Moving Around
d465	Moving Around Using Equipment
d470	Using Transportation
d475	Driving
d510	Washing Oneself
d520	Caring for Body Parts
d530	Toileting
d540	Dressing
d570	Looking After One's Health
d620	Acquisition of Goods and Services
d640	Doing Housework
d660	Assisting Others
d710	Basic Interpersonal Interactions
d750	Informal Social Relationships
d760	Family Relationships
d770	Intimate Relationships
d820	School Education
d830	Higher Education
d845	Acquiring, Keeping, and Terminating a Job
d850	Remunerative Employment
d870	Economic Self-Sufficiency
d910	Community Life
d920	Recreation and Leisure

Environmental Factors

e110	Products or Substances for Personal Consumption
e115	Products and Technology for Personal Use in Daily Living
e120	Products and Technology for Personal Indoor and Outdoor Mobility and Transportation
e125	Products and Technology for Communication
e140	Products and Technology for Culture, Recreation, and Sport
e150	Design, Construction, and Building Products and Technology of Buildings for Public Use
e155	Design, Construction, and Building Products and Technology of Buildings for Private Use
e225	Climate
e310	Immediate Family
e320	Friends
e325	Acquaintances, Peers, Colleagues, Neighbors, and Community Members
e330	People in Positions of Authority
e340	Personal Care Providers and Personal Assistants
e355	Health Professionals
e360	Other Professionals
e410	Individual Attitudes of Immediate Family Members
e420	Individual Attitudes of Friends
e425	Individual Attitudes of Acquaintances, Peers, Colleagues, Neighbors, and Community Members
e440	Individual Attitudes of Personal Care Providers and Personal Assistants
e450	Individual Attitudes of Health Professionals
e455	Individual Attitudes of Health-Related Professionals
e460	Societal Attitudes
e465	Social Norms, Practices, and Ideologies
e510	Services, Systems, and Policies for the Production of Consumer Goods
e525	Housing Services, Systems, and Policies
e535	Communication Services, Systems, and Policies
e540	Transportation Services, Systems, and Policies
e560	Media Services, Systems, and Policies
e570	Social Security Services, Systems, and Policies
e575	General Social Support Services, Systems, and Policies
e580	Health Services, Systems, and Policies
e585	Education and Training Services, Systems, and Policies
e590	Labor and Employment Services, Systems, and Policies

Obstructive Pulmonary Diseases

Stucki, Stoll, et al. (2004)

Brief ICF Core Set for Obstructive Pulmonary Diseases

Body Functions

b440	Respiration Functions
b450	Additional Respiratory Functions
b455	Exercise Tolerance Functions
b460	Sensations Associated with Cardiovascular and Respiratory Functions

Body Structures

s410	Structure of Cardiovascular System
s430	Structure of Respiratory System

Activities & Participation

d230	Carrying Out Daily Routine
d450	Walking
d455	Moving Around
d640	Doing Housework

Environmental Factors

e110	Products or Substances for Personal Consumption
e115	Products and Technology for Personal Use in Daily Living
e225	Climate
e260	Air Quality

Comprehensive ICF Core Set for Obstructive Pulmonary Diseases

Body Functions

b130	Energy and Drive Functions
b134	Sleep Functions
b152	Emotional Functions
b1522	Range of Emotion
b280	Sensation of Pain
b2801	Pain in Body Part
b310	Voice Functions
b410	Heart Functions
b430	Hematological System Functions
b435	Immunological System Functions
b440	Respiration Functions
b445	Respiratory Muscle Functions
b450	Additional Respiratory Functions
b455	Exercise Tolerance Functions
b460	Sensations Associated with Cardiovascular and Respiratory Functions
b530	Weight Maintenance Functions
b730	Muscle Power Functions
b740	Muscle Endurance Functions
b780	Sensations Related to Muscles and Movement Functions

Body Structures

s410	Structure of Cardiovascular System
s430	Structure of Respiratory System
s710	Structure of Head and Neck Region
s720	Structure of Shoulder Region
s760	Structure of Trunk

Activities & Participation

d230	Carrying Out Daily Routine
d240	Handling Stress and Other Psychological Demands
d330	Speaking
d410	Changing Basic Body Position
d430	Lifting and Carrying Objects
d450	Walking
d455	Moving Around
d460	Moving Around in Different Locations
d465	Moving Around Using Equipment
d470	Using Transportation
d475	Driving
d4750	Driving Human-Powered Transportation
d510	Washing Oneself
d540	Dressing
d570	Looking After One's Health
d620	Acquisition of Goods and Services
d640	Doing Housework
d650	Caring for Household Objects
d660	Assisting Others
d770	Intimate Relationships
d845	Acquiring, Keeping, and Terminating a Job
d850	Remunerative Employment
d910	Community Life
d920	Recreation and Leisure

Environmental Factors

e110	Products or Substances for Personal Consumption
e115	Products and Technology for Personal Use in Daily Living
e120	Products and Technology for Personal Indoor and Outdoor Mobility and Transportation
e150	Design, Construction, and Building Products and Technology of Buildings for Public Use
e155	Design, Construction, and Building Products and Technology of Buildings for Private Use
e225	Climate
e245	Time-Related Changes
e2450	Day/Night Cycles
e260	Air Quality
e310	Immediate Family
e320	Friends
e340	Personal Care Providers and Personal Assistants
e355	Health Professionals
e410	Individual Attitudes of Immediate Family Members
e420	Individual Attitudes of Friends
e450	Individual Attitudes of Health Professionals
e460	Societal Attitudes
e540	Transportation Services, Systems, and Policies
e555	Associations and Organizational Services, Systems, and Policies
e575	General Social Support Services, Systems, and Policies
e580	Health Services, Systems, and Policies
e585	Education and Training Services, Systems, and Policies
e590	Labor and Employment Services, Systems, and Policies

Osteoarthritis

Dreinhofer et al. (2004)

Brief ICF Core Set for Osteoarthritis

Body Functions

b280	Sensation of Pain
b710	Mobility of Joint Functions
b730	Muscle Power Functions

Body Structures

s730	Structure of Upper Extremity
s750	Structure of Lower Extremity
s770	Additional Musculoskeletal Structures Related to Movement

Activities & Participation

d445	Hand and Arm Use
d450	Walking
d540	Dressing

Environmental Factors

e115	Products and Technology for Personal Use in Daily Living
e150	Design, Construction, and Building Products and Technology of Buildings for Public Use
e310	Immediate Family
e580	Health Services, Systems, and Policies

Comprehensive ICF Core Set for Osteoarthritis

Body Functions

b130	Energy and Drive Functions
b134	Sleep Functions

b152	Emotional Functions
b280	Sensation of Pain
b710	Mobility of Joint Functions
b715	Stability of Joint Functions
b720	Mobility of Bone Functions
b730	Muscle Power Functions
b735	Muscle Tone Functions
b740	Muscle Endurance Functions
b760	Control of Voluntary Movement Functions
b770	Gait Pattern Functions
b780	Sensations Related to Muscles and Movement Functions

Body Structures

s720	Structure of Shoulder Region
s730	Structure of Upper Extremity
s740	Structure of Pelvic Region
s750	Structure of Lower Extremity
s770	Additional Musculoskeletal Structures Related to Movement
s799	Structures Related to Movement, Unspecified

Activities & Participation

d410	Changing Basic Body Position
d415	Maintaining a Body Position
d430	Lifting and Carrying Objects
d440	Fine Hand Use
d445	Hand and Arm Use
d450	Walking
d455	Moving Around
d470	Using Transportation
d475	Driving
d510	Washing Oneself
d530	Toileting
d540	Dressing
d620	Acquisition of Goods and Services
d640	Doing Housework
d660	Assisting Others
d770	Intimate Relationships
d850	Remunerative Employment
d910	Community Life
d920	Recreation and Leisure

Environmental Factors

e110	Products or Substances for Personal Consumption
e115	Products and Technology for Personal Use in Daily Living
e120	Products and Technology for Personal Indoor and Outdoor Mobility and Transportation
e135	Products and Technology for Employment
e150	Design, Construction, and Building Products and Technology of Buildings for Public Use
e155	Design, Construction, and Building Products and Technology of Buildings for Private Use
e225	Climate
e310	Immediate Family
e320	Friends
e340	Personal Care Providers and Personal Assistants
e355	Health Professionals
e410	Individual Attitudes of Immediate Family Members
e450	Individual Attitudes of Health Professionals
e460	Societal Attitudes
e540	Transportation Services, Systems, and Policies
e575	General Social Support Services, Systems, and Policies
e580	Health Services, Systems, and Policies

Osteoporosis

Cieza, Schwarzkopf, et al. (2004)

Brief ICF Core Set for Osteoporosis

Body Functions

b152	Emotional Functions
b280	Sensation of Pain
b710	Mobility of Joint Functions
b730	Muscle Power Functions

Body Structures

s750	Structure of Lower Extremity
s760	Structure of Trunk

Activities & Participation

d430	Lifting and Carrying Objects
d450	Walking
d920	Recreation and Leisure

Environmental Factors

e110	Products or Substances for Personal Consumption
e355	Health Professionals
e580	Health Services, Systems, and Policies

Comprehensive ICF Core Set for Osteoporosis

Body Functions

b134	Sleep Functions
b152	Emotional Functions
b1801	Body Image
b280	Sensation of Pain
b440	Respiration Functions
b455	Exercise Tolerance Functions
b545	Water, Mineral, and Electrolyte Balance Functions
b6202	Urinary Continence
b710	Mobility of Joint Functions
b730	Muscle Power Functions
b740	Muscle Endurance Functions
b755	Involuntary Movement Reaction Functions
b765	Involuntary Movement Functions
b770	Gait Pattern Functions
b780	Sensations Related to Muscles and Movement Functions

Body Structures

s430	Structure of Respiratory System
s720	Structure of Shoulder Region
s730	Structure of Upper Extremity
s740	Structure of Pelvic Region
s750	Structure of Lower Extremity
s760	Structure of Trunk
s770	Additional Musculoskeletal Structures Related to Movement

Activities & Participation

d410	Changing Basic Body Position
d415	Maintaining a Body Position
d430	Lifting and Carrying Objects
d445	Hand and Arm Use
d450	Walking
d455	Moving Around
d465	Moving Around Using Equipment
d470	Using Transportation

d475	Driving
d510	Washing Oneself
d540	Dressing
d620	Acquisition of Goods and Services
d630	Preparing Meals
d640	Doing Housework
d710	Basic Interpersonal Interactions
d770	Intimate Relationships
d850	Remunerative Employment
d855	Non-Remunerative Employment
d859	Work and Employment, Other Specified and Unspecified
d910	Community Life
d920	Recreation and Leisure

Environmental Factors

e110	Products or Substances for Personal Consumption
e115	Products and Technology for Personal Use in Daily Living
e120	Products and Technology for Personal Indoor and Outdoor Mobility and Transportation
e135	Products and Technology for Employment
e150	Design, Construction, and Building Products and Technology of Buildings for Public Use
e155	Design, Construction, and Building Products and Technology of Buildings for Private Use
e225	Climate
e240	Light
e310	Immediate Family
e320	Friends
e325	Acquaintances, Peers, Colleagues, Neighbors, and Community Members
e340	Personal Care Providers and Personal Assistants
e355	Health Professionals
e360	Other Professionals
e410	Individual Attitudes of Immediate Family Members
e420	Individual Attitudes of Friends
e430	Individual Attitudes of People in Positions of Authority
e440	Individual Attitudes of Personal Care Providers and Personal Assistants
e450	Individual Attitudes of Health Professionals
e455	Individual Attitudes of Health-Related Professionals
e460	Societal Attitudes
e535	Communication Services, Systems, and Policies
e540	Transportation Services, Systems, and Policies
e570	Social Security Services, Systems, and Policies
e575	General Social Support Services, Systems, and Policies
e580	Health Services, Systems, and Policies

Rheumatoid Arthritis

Stucki, Cieza, et al. (2004)

Brief ICF Core Set for Rheumatoid Arthritis

Body Functions

b280	Sensation of Pain
b455	Exercise Tolerance Functions
b710	Mobility of Joint Functions
b730	Muscle Power Functions
b780	Sensations Related to Muscles and Movement Functions

Body Structures

s710	Structure of Head and Neck Region
s720	Structure of Shoulder Region

s730	Structure of Upper Extremity
s750	Structure of Lower Extremity

Activities & Participation

d230	Carrying Out Daily Routine
d410	Changing Basic Body Position
d440	Fine Hand Use
d445	Hand and Arm Use
d450	Walking
d850	Remunerative Employment

Environmental Factors

e115	Products and Technology for Personal Use in Daily Living
e310	Immediate Family
e355	Health Professionals
e570	Social Security Services, Systems, and Policies
e580	Health Services, Systems, and Policies

Comprehensive ICF Core Set for Rheumatoid Arthritis

Body Functions

b130	Energy and Drive Functions
b134	Sleep Functions
b152	Emotional Functions
b180	Experience of Self and Time Functions
b1801	Body Image
b280	Sensation of Pain
b2800	Generalized Pain
b2801	Pain in Body Part
b28010	Pain in Head and Neck
b28013	Pain in Back
b28014	Pain in Upper Limb
b28015	Pain in Lower limb
b28016	Pain in Joints
b430	Hematological System Functions
b455	Exercise Tolerance Functions
b510	Ingestion Functions
b640	Sexual Functions
b710	Mobility of Joint Functions
b7102	Mobility of Joints Generalized
b715	Stability of Joint Functions
b730	Muscle Power Functions
b740	Muscle Endurance Functions
b770	Gait Pattern Functions
b780	Sensations Related to Muscles and Movement Functions
b7800	Sensation of Muscle Stiffness

Body Structures

s299	Eye, Ear and Related Structures, Unspecified
s710	Structure of Head and Neck Region
s720	Structure of Shoulder Region
s730	Structure of Upper Extremity
s73001	Elbow Joint
s73011	Wrist Joint
s7302	Structure of Hand
s73021	Joints of Hand and Fingers
s73022	Muscles of Hand
s750	Structure of Lower Extremity
s75001	Hip Joint
s75011	Knee Joint
s7502	Structure of Ankle and Foot
s760	Structure of Trunk

s7600   Structure of Vertebral Column
s76000   Cervical Vertebral Column
s770   Additional Musculoskeletal Structures Related to
          Movement
s810   Structure of Areas of Skin

Activities & Participation

d170   Writing
d230   Carrying Out Daily Routine
d360   Using Communication Devices and Techniques
d410   Changing Basic Body Position
d415   Maintaining a Body Position
d430   Lifting and Carrying Objects
d440   Fine Hand Use
d445   Hand and Arm Use
d449   Carrying, Moving, and Handling Objects, Other
          Specified and Unspecified
d450   Walking
d455   Moving Around
d460   Moving Around in Different Locations
d465   Moving Around Using Equipment
d470   Using Transportation
d475   Driving
d510   Washing Oneself
d520   Caring for Body Parts
d530   Toileting
d540   Dressing
d550   Eating
d560   Drinking
d570   Looking After One's Health
d620   Acquisition of Goods and Services
d630   Preparing Meals
d640   Doing Housework
d660   Assisting Others
d760   Family Relationships
d770   Intimate Relationships
d850   Remunerative Employment
d859   Work and Employment, Other Specified and
          Unspecified
d910   Community Life
d920   Recreation and Leisure

Environmental Factors

e110   Products or Substances for Personal Consumption
e115   Products and Technology for Personal Use in Daily
          Living
e120   Products and Technology for Personal Indoor and
          Outdoor Mobility and Transportation
e125   Products and Technology for Communication
e135   Products and Technology for Employment
e150   Design, Construction, and Building Products and
          Technology of Buildings for Public Use
e155   Design, Construction, and Building Products and
          Technology of Buildings for Private Use
e225   Climate
e310   Immediate Family
e320   Friends
e340   Personal Care Providers and Personal Assistants
e355   Health Professionals
e360   Other Professionals
e410   Individual Attitudes of Immediate Family Members
e420   Individual Attitudes of Friends
e425   Individual Attitudes of Acquaintances, Peers,
          Colleagues, Neighbors, and Community Members
e450   Individual Attitudes of Health Professionals
e460   Societal Attitudes

e540   Transportation Services, Systems, and Policies
e570   Social Security Services, Systems, and Policies
e580   Health Services, Systems, and Policies

Spinal Cord Injury

Kirchberger et al. (2010) and Cieza, Kirchberger, et al. (2010)

Brief ICF Core Set for Spinal Cord Injury — Early post-acute situation

Body Functions

b152   Emotional Functions
b280   Sensation of Pain
b440   Respiration Functions
b525   Defecation Functions
b620   Urination Functions
b730   Muscle Power Functions
b735   Muscle Tone Functions
b810   Protective Functions of the Skin

Body Structures

s120   Spinal Cord and Related Structures
s430   Structure of Respiratory System
s610   Structure of Urinary System

Activities & Participation

d410   Changing Basic Body Position
d420   Transferring Oneself
d445   Hand and Arm Use
d450   Walking
d510   Washing Oneself
d530   Toileting
d540   Dressing
d550   Eating
d560   Drinking

Environmental Factors

e115   Products and Technology for Personal Use in Daily
          Living
e120   Products and Technology for Personal Indoor and
          Outdoor Mobility and Transportation
e310   Immediate Family
e340   Personal Care Providers and Personal Assistants
e355   Health Professionals

Brief ICF Core Set for Spinal Cord Injury — Chronic Situation

Body Functions

b152   Emotional Functions
b280   Sensation of Pain
b525   Defecation Functions
b620   Urination Functions
b640   Sexual Functions
b710   Mobility of Joint Functions
b730   Muscle Power Functions
b735   Muscle Tone Functions
b810   Protective Functions of the Skin

Body Structures

s120   Spinal Cord and Related Structures
s430   Structure of Respiratory System
s610   Structure of Urinary System
s810   Structure of Areas of Skin

Activities & Participation

d230	Carrying Out Daily Routine
d240	Handling Stress and Other Psychological Demands
d410	Changing Basic Body Position
d420	Transferring Oneself
d445	Hand and Arm Use
d455	Moving Around
d465	Moving Around Using Equipment
d470	Using Transportation
d520	Caring for Body Parts
d530	Toileting
d550	Eating

Environmental Factors

e110	Products or Substances for Personal Consumption
e115	Products and Technology for Personal Use in Daily Living
e120	Products and Technology for Personal Indoor and Outdoor Mobility and Transportation
e150	Design, Construction, and Building Products and Technology of Buildings for Public Use
e155	Design, Construction, and Building Products and Technology of Buildings for Private Use
e310	Immediate Family
e340	Personal Care Providers and Personal Assistants
e355	Health Professionals
e580	Health Services, Systems, and Policies

Comprehensive ICF Core Set for Spinal Cord Injury — Early post-acute situation

Body Functions

b126	Temperament and Personality Functions
b130	Energy and Drive Functions
b134	Sleep Functions
b152	Emotional Functions
b260	Proprioceptive Function
b265	Touch Function
b270	Sensory Functions Related to Temperature and Other Stimuli
b2800	Generalized Pain
b28010	Pain in Head and Neck
b28013	Pain in Back
b28014	Pain in Upper Limb
b28015	Pain in Lower limb
b28016	Pain in Joints
b2803	Radiating Pain in a Dermatome
b2804	Radiating Pain in a Segment or Region
b310	Voice Functions
b410	Heart Functions
b415	Blood Vessel Functions
b4200	Increased Blood Pressure
b4201	Decreased Blood Pressure
b4202	Maintenance of Blood Pressure
b430	Hematological System Functions
b440	Respiration Functions
b445	Respiratory Muscle Functions
b450	Additional Respiratory Functions
b455	Exercise Tolerance Functions
b510	Ingestion Functions
b515	Digestive Functions
b5250	Elimination of Feces
b5251	Fecal Consistency
b5252	Frequency of Defecation
b5253	Fecal Continence

b5254	Flatulence
b530	Weight Maintenance Functions
b550	Thermoregulatory Functions
b610	Urinary Excretory Functions
b6200	Urination
b6201	Frequency of Urination
b6202	Urinary Continence
b630	Sensations Associated with Urinary Functions
b640	Sexual Functions
b670	Sensations Associated with Genital and Reproductive Functions
b710	Mobility of Joint Functions
b715	Stability of Joint Functions
b7300	Power of Isolated Muscles and Muscle Groups
b7302	Power of Muscles of One Side of the Body
b7303	Power of Muscles in Lower Half of the Body
b7304	Power of Muscles of All Limbs
b7305	Power of Muscles of the Trunk
b7353	Tone of Muscles of Lower Half of Body
b7354	Tone of Muscles of All Limbs
b7355	Tone of Muscles of Trunk
b740	Muscle Endurance Functions
b750	Motor Reflex Functions
b755	Involuntary Movement Reaction Functions
b760	Control of Voluntary Movement Functions
b765	Involuntary Movement Functions
b770	Gait Pattern Functions
b780	Sensations Related to Muscles and Movement Functions
b810	Protective Functions of the Skin
b820	Repair Functions of the Skin
b830	Other Functions of the Skin
b840	Sensation Related to the Skin

Body Structures

s12000	Cervical Spinal Cord
s12001	Thoracic Spinal Cord
s12002	Lumbosacral Spinal Cord
s12003	Cauda Equina
s1201	Spinal Nerves
s430	Structure of Respiratory System
s610	Structure of Urinary System
s710	Structure of Head and Neck Region
s720	Structure of Shoulder Region
s730	Structure of Upper Extremity
s740	Structure of Pelvic Region
s750	Structure of Lower Extremity
s760	Structure of Trunk
s810	Structure of Areas of Skin

Activities & Participation

d230	Carrying Out Daily Routine
d240	Handling Stress and Other Psychological Demands
d360	Using Communication Devices and Techniques
d4100	Lying Down
d4103	Sitting
d4104	Standing
d4105	Bending
d4106	Shifting the Body's Center of Gravity
d4153	Maintaining a Sitting Position
d4154	Maintaining a Standing Position
d420	Transferring Oneself
d430	Lifting and Carrying Objects
d435	Moving Objects with Lower Extremities
d4400	Picking Up
d4401	Grasping

d4402	Manipulating
d4403	Releasing
d4450	Pulling
d4451	Pushing
d4452	Reaching
d4453	Turning or Twisting the Hands or Arms
d4455	Catching
d4500	Walking Short Distances
d4501	Walking Long Distances
d4502	Walking on Different Surfaces
d4503	Walking around Obstacles
d455	Moving Around
d4600	Moving Around within the Home
d4601	Moving Around within Buildings Other Than Home
d4602	Moving Around outside the Home and Other Buildings
d465	Moving Around Using Equipment
d470	Using Transportation
d475	Driving
d510	Washing Oneself
d520	Caring for Body Parts
d5300	Regulating Urination
d5301	Regulating Defecation
d5302	Menstrual Care
d540	Dressing
d550	Eating
d560	Drinking
d570	Looking After One's Health
d610	Acquiring a Place to Live
d620	Acquisition of Goods and Services
d630	Preparing Meals
d640	Doing Housework
d660	Assisting Others
d760	Family Relationships
d770	Intimate Relationships
d850	Remunerative Employment
d870	Economic Self-Sufficiency
d920	Recreation and Leisure
d930	Religion and Spirituality

Environmental Factors

e110	Products or Substances for Personal Consumption
e115	Products and Technology for Personal Use in Daily Living
e120	Products and Technology for Personal Indoor and Outdoor Mobility and Transportation
e125	Products and Technology for Communication
e130	Products and Technology for Education
e135	Products and Technology for Employment
e140	Products and Technology for Culture, Recreation, and Sport
e150	Design, Construction, and Building Products and Technology of Buildings for Public Use
e155	Design, Construction, and Building Products and Technology of Buildings for Private Use
e165	Assets
e310	Immediate Family
e315	Extended Family
e320	Friends
e325	Acquaintances, Peers, Colleagues, Neighbors, and Community Members
e330	People in Positions of Authority
e340	Personal Care Providers and Personal Assistants
e355	Health Professionals
e360	Other Professionals
e410	Individual Attitudes of Immediate Family Members
e415	Individual Attitudes of Extended Family Members

e420	Individual Attitudes of Friends
e425	Individual Attitudes of Acquaintances, Peers, Colleagues, Neighbors, and Community Members
e440	Individual Attitudes of Personal Care Providers and Personal Assistants
e450	Individual Attitudes of Health Professionals
e460	Societal Attitudes
e515	Architecture and Construction Services, Systems, and Policies
e525	Housing Services, Systems, and Policies
e540	Transportation Services, Systems, and Policies
e555	Associations and Organizational Services, Systems, and Policies
e570	Social Security Services, Systems, and Policies
e575	General Social Support Services, Systems, and Policies
e580	Health Services, Systems, and Policies

Comprehensive ICF Core Set for Spinal Cord Injury — Chronic Situation

Body Functions

b126	Temperament and Personality Functions
b130	Energy and Drive Functions
b134	Sleep Functions
b152	Emotional Functions
b260	Proprioceptive Function
b265	Touch Function
b270	Sensory Functions Related to Temperature and Other Stimuli
b28010	Pain in Head and Neck
b28011	Pain in Chest
b28012	Pain in Stomach or Abdomen
b28013	Pain in Back
b28014	Pain in Upper Limb
b28015	Pain in Lower limb
b28016	Pain in Joints
b2803	Radiating Pain in a Dermatome
b2804	Radiating Pain in a Segment or Region
b420	Blood Pressure Functions
b440	Respiration Functions
b445	Respiratory Muscle Functions
b455	Exercise Tolerance Functions
b525	Defecation Functions
b530	Weight Maintenance Functions
b550	Thermoregulatory Functions
b610	Urinary Excretory Functions
b6200	Urination
b6201	Frequency of Urination
b6202	Urinary Continence
b640	Sexual Functions
b660	Procreation Functions
b670	Sensations Associated with Genital and Reproductive Functions
b710	Mobility of Joint Functions
b715	Stability of Joint Functions
b720	Mobility of Bone Functions
b730	Muscle Power Functions
b735	Muscle Tone Functions
b740	Muscle Endurance Functions
b750	Motor Reflex Functions
b760	Control of Voluntary Movement Functions
b770	Gait Pattern Functions
b780	Sensations Related to Muscles and Movement Functions
b810	Protective Functions of the Skin

b820	Repair Functions of the Skin		d550	Eating
b830	Other Functions of the Skin		d560	Drinking
b840	Sensation Related to the Skin		d570	Looking After One's Health
			d610	Acquiring a Place to Live

Body Structures

			d620	Acquisition of Goods and Services
s12000	Cervical Spinal Cord		d630	Preparing Meals
s12001	Thoracic Spinal Cord		d640	Doing Housework
s12002	Lumbosacral Spinal Cord		d650	Caring for Household Objects
s12003	Cauda Equina		d660	Assisting Others
s1201	Spinal Nerves		d720	Complex Interpersonal Interactions
s430	Structure of Respiratory System		d750	Informal Social Relationships
s610	Structure of Urinary System		d760	Family Relationships
s720	Structure of Shoulder Region		d770	Intimate Relationships
s7300	Structure of Upper Arm		d810	Informal Education
s7301	Structure of Forearm		d820	School Education
s7302	Structure of Hand		d825	Vocational Training
s7500	Structure of Thigh		d830	Higher Education
s7501	Structure of Lower Leg		d840	Apprenticeship (Work Preparation)
s7502	Structure of Ankle and Foot		d845	Acquiring, Keeping, and Terminating a Job
s760	Structure of Trunk		d850	Remunerative Employment
s8102	Skin of Upper Extremity		d870	Economic Self-Sufficiency
s8103	Skin of Pelvic Region		d910	Community Life
s8104	Skin of Lower Extremity		d920	Recreation and Leisure
s8105	Skin of Trunk and Back		d940	Human Rights

Activities & Participation

Environmental Factors

d155	Acquiring Skills		e110	Products or Substances for Personal Consumption
d230	Carrying Out Daily Routine		e115	Products and Technology for Personal Use in Daily Living
d240	Handling Stress and Other Psychological Demands			
d345	Writing Messages		e120	Products and Technology for Personal Indoor and Outdoor Mobility and Transportation
d360	Using Communication Devices and Techniques			
d4100	Lying Down		e125	Products and Technology for Communication
d4102	Kneeling		e130	Products and Technology for Education
d4103	Sitting		e135	Products and Technology for Employment
d4104	Standing		e140	Products and Technology for Culture, Recreation, and Sport
d4105	Bending			
d4106	Shifting the Body's Center of Gravity		e150	Design, Construction, and Building Products and Technology of Buildings for Public Use
d415	Maintaining a Body Position			
d420	Transferring Oneself		e155	Design, Construction, and Building Products and Technology of Buildings for Private Use
d430	Lifting and Carrying Objects			
d4400	Picking Up		e160	Products and Technology of Land Development
d4401	Grasping		e165	Assets
d4402	Manipulating		e310	Immediate Family
d4403	Releasing		e315	Extended Family
d4450	Pulling		e320	Friends
d4451	Pushing		e325	Acquaintances, Peers, Colleagues, Neighbors, and Community Members
d4452	Reaching			
d4453	Turning or Twisting the Hands or Arms		e330	People in Positions of Authority
d4454	Throwing		e340	Personal Care Providers and Personal Assistants
d4500	Walking Short Distances		e355	Health Professionals
d4501	Walking Long Distances		e360	Other Professionals
d4502	Walking on Different Surfaces		e410	Individual Attitudes of Immediate Family Members
d4503	Walking around Obstacles		e415	Individual Attitudes of Extended Family Members
d455	Moving Around		e420	Individual Attitudes of Friends
d4600	Moving Around within the Home		e425	Individual Attitudes of Acquaintances, Peers, Colleagues, Neighbors, and Community Members
d4601	Moving Around within Buildings Other Than Home			
d4602	Moving Around outside the Home and Other Buildings		e440	Individual Attitudes of Personal Care Providers and Personal Assistants
d465	Moving Around Using Equipment			
d470	Using Transportation		e450	Individual Attitudes of Health Professionals
d475	Driving		e455	Individual Attitudes of Health-Related Professionals
d510	Washing Oneself		e460	Societal Attitudes
d520	Caring for Body Parts		e465	Social Norms, Practices, and Ideologies
d5300	Regulating Urination		e510	Services, Systems, and Policies for the Production of Consumer Goods
d5301	Regulating Defecation			
d5302	Menstrual Care		e515	Architecture and Construction Services, Systems, and Policies
d540	Dressing			

e525	Housing Services, Systems, and Policies
e530	Utilities Services, Systems and Policies
e535	Communication Services, Systems, and Policies
e540	Transportation Services, Systems, and Policies
e550	Legal Services, Systems, and Policies
e555	Associations and Organizational Services, Systems, and Policies
e570	Social Security Services, Systems, and Policies
e575	General Social Support Services, Systems, and Policies
e580	Health Services, Systems, and Policies
e585	Education and Training Services, Systems, and Policies
e590	Labor and Employment Services, Systems, and Policies

Sleep Disorders

Gradinger et al. (2011)

Brief ICF Core Set for Sleep Disorders

Body Functions
b110	Consciousness Functions
b130	Energy and Drive Functions
b134	Sleep Functions
b140	Attention Functions
b440	Respiration Functions

Body Structures
s110	Structure of Brain
s330	Structure of Pharynx
s430	Structure of Respiratory System

Activities & Participation
d160	Focusing Attention
d230	Carrying Out Daily Routine
d240	Handling Stress and Other Psychological Demands
d475	Driving

Environmental Factors
e310	Immediate Family
e355	Health Professionals
e580	Health Services, Systems, and Policies

Comprehensive ICF Core Set for Sleep Disorders

Body Functions
b110	Consciousness Functions
b1100	State of Consciousness
b1101	Continuity of Consciousness
b1102	Quality of Consciousness
b114	Orientation Functions
b117	Intellectual Functions
b126	Temperament and Personality Functions
b1300	Energy Level
b1301	Motivation
b1302	Appetite
b1303	Craving
b1304	Impulse Control
b1340	Amount of Sleep
b1341	Onset of Sleep
b1342	Maintenance of Sleep
b1343	Quality of Sleep
b1344	Functions Involving the Sleep Cycle
b1348	Sleep Functions, Other Specified
b140	Attention Functions
b144	Memory Functions

b147	Psychomotor Functions
b152	Emotional Functions
b156	Perceptual Functions
b160	Thought Functions
b164	Higher-Level Cognitive Functions
b180	Experience of Self and Time Functions
b270	Sensory Functions Related to Temperature and Other Stimuli
b280	Sensation of Pain
b410	Heart Functions
b420	Blood Pressure Functions
b435	Immunological System Functions
b440	Respiration Functions
b445	Respiratory Muscle Functions
b450	Additional Respiratory Functions
b455	Exercise Tolerance Functions
b460	Sensations Associated with Cardiovascular and Respiratory Functions
b530	Weight Maintenance Functions
b540	General Metabolic Functions
b550	Thermoregulatory Functions
b555	Endocrine Gland Functions
b620	Urination Functions
b640	Sexual Functions
b735	Muscle Tone Functions
b7650	Involuntary Contractions of Muscles
b7652	Tics and Mannerisms
b7653	Stereotypies and Motor Perseveration
b7658	Involuntary Movement Functions, Other Specified
b780	Sensations Related to Muscles and Movement Functions
b840	Sensation Related to the Skin

Body Structures
s110	Structure of Brain
s310	Structure of Nose
s320	Structure of Mouth
s330	Structure of Pharynx
s410	Structure of Cardiovascular System
s430	Structure of Respiratory System
s580	Structure of Endocrine Glands
s710	Structure of Head and Neck Region

Activity & Participation
d155	Acquiring Skills
d160	Focusing Attention
d166	Reading
d175	Solving Problems
d177	Making Decisions
d220	Undertaking Multiple Tasks
d230	Carrying Out Daily Routine
d240	Handling Stress and Other Psychological Demands
d350	Conversation
d415	Maintaining a Body Position
d470	Using Transportation
d475	Driving
d5700	Ensuring One's Physical Comfort
d5701	Managing Diet and Fitness
d5702	Maintaining One's Health
d640	Doing Housework
d660	Assisting Others
d710	Basic Interpersonal Interactions
d720	Complex Interpersonal Interactions
d740	Formal Relationships
d750	Informal Social Relationships
d760	Family Relationships

d770	Intimate Relationships
d820	School Education
d825	Vocational Training
d830	Higher Education
d845	Acquiring, Keeping, and Terminating a Job
d850	Remunerative Employment
d855	Non-Remunerative Employment
d910	Community Life
d920	Recreation and Leisure

Environmental Factors

e1100	Food
e1101	Drugs
e1150	General Products and Technology for Personal Use in Daily Living
e1151	Assistive Products and Technology for Personal Use in Daily Living
e165	Assets
e215	Population
e225	Climate
e235	Human-Caused Events
e240	Light
e245	Time-Related Changes
e250	Sound
e260	Air Quality
e310	Immediate Family
e315	Extended Family
e325	Acquaintances, Peers, Colleagues, Neighbors, and Community Members
e330	People in Positions of Authority
e355	Health Professionals
e410	Individual Attitudes of Immediate Family Members
e425	Individual Attitudes of Acquaintances, Peers, Colleagues, Neighbors, and Community Members
e430	Individual Attitudes of People in Positions of Authority
e440	Individual Attitudes of Personal Care Providers and Personal Assistants
e450	Individual Attitudes of Health Professionals
e455	Individual Attitudes of Health-Related Professionals
e460	Societal Attitudes
e465	Social Norms, Practices, and Ideologies
e540	Transportation Services, Systems, and Policies
e550	Legal Services, Systems, and Policies
e555	Associations and Organizational Services, Systems, and Policies
e570	Social Security Services, Systems, and Policies
e580	Health Services, Systems, and Policies
e585	Education and Training Services, Systems, and Policies
e590	Labor and Employment Services, Systems, and Policies

Traumatic Brain Injury

Bernabeu et al. (2009)

Brief ICF Core Set for Traumatic Brain Injury

Body Functions

b110	Consciousness Functions
b130	Energy and Drive Functions
b140	Attention Functions
b144	Memory Functions
b152	Emotional Functions
b164	Higher-Level Cognitive Functions
b280	Sensation of Pain
b760	Control of Voluntary Movement Functions

Body Structures

s110	Structure of Brain

Activities & Participation

d230	Carrying Out Daily Routine
d350	Conversation
d450	Walking
d5	Self-Care
d720	Complex Interpersonal Interactions
d845	Acquiring, Keeping, and Terminating a Job
d920	Recreation and Leisure
d760	Family Relationships

Environmental Factors

e115	Products and Technology for Personal Use in Daily Living
e120	Products and Technology for Personal Indoor and Outdoor Mobility and Transportation
e310	Immediate Family
e320	Friends
e580	Health Services, Systems, and Policies
e570	Social Security Services, Systems, and Policies

Comprehensive ICF Core Set for Traumatic Brain Injury

Body Functions

b110	Consciousness Functions
b114	Orientation Functions
b126	Temperament and Personality Functions
b130	Energy and Drive Functions
b134	Sleep Functions
b140	Attention Functions
b144	Memory Functions
b147	Psychomotor Functions
b152	Emotional Functions
b156	Perceptual Functions
b160	Thought Functions
b164	Higher-Level Cognitive Functions
b167	Mental Functions of Language
b210	Seeing Functions
b215	Functions of Structures Adjoining the Eye
b235	Vestibular Functions
b240	Sensations Associated with Hearing and Vestibular Functions
b255	Smell Function
b260	Proprioceptive Function
b280	Sensation of Pain
b310	Voice Functions
b320	Articulation Functions
b330	Fluency and Rhythm of Speech Functions
b420	Blood Pressure Functions
b455	Exercise Tolerance Functions
b510	Ingestion Functions
b525	Defecation Functions
b555	Endocrine Gland Functions
b620	Urination Functions
b640	Sexual Functions
b710	Mobility of Joint Functions
b730	Muscle Power Functions
b735	Muscle Tone Functions
b755	Involuntary Movement Reaction Functions
b760	Control of Voluntary Movement Functions
b765	Involuntary Movement Functions
b770	Gait Pattern Functions

Body Structures

s110 Structure of Brain
s710 Structure of Head and Neck Region

Activities & Participation

d110 Watching
d115 Listening
d155 Acquiring Skills
d160 Focusing Attention
d163 Thinking
d166 Reading
d170 Writing
d175 Solving Problems
d177 Making Decisions
d210 Undertaking a Single Task
d220 Undertaking Multiple Tasks
d230 Carrying Out Daily Routine
d240 Handling Stress and Other Psychological Demands
d310 Communicating with — Receiving — Spoken Messages
d315 Communicating with — Receiving — Nonverbal Messages
d330 Speaking
d335 Producing Nonverbal Messages
d345 Writing Messages
d350 Conversation
d360 Using Communication Devices and Techniques
d410 Changing Basic Body Position
d415 Maintaining a Body Position
d420 Transferring Oneself
d430 Lifting and Carrying Objects
d440 Fine Hand Use
d445 Hand and Arm Use
d450 Walking
d455 Moving Around
d465 Moving Around Using Equipment
d470 Using Transportation
d475 Driving
d510 Washing Oneself
d520 Caring for Body Parts
d530 Toileting
d540 Dressing
d550 Eating
d560 Drinking
d570 Looking After One's Health
d620 Acquisition of Goods and Services
d630 Preparing Meals
d640 Doing Housework
d660 Assisting Others
d710 Basic Interpersonal Interactions
d720 Complex Interpersonal Interactions
d730 Relating with Strangers
d740 Formal Relationships
d750 Informal Social Relationships
d760 Family Relationships
d770 Intimate Relationships
d825 Vocational Training
d830 Higher Education
d840 Apprenticeship (Work Preparation)
d845 Acquiring, Keeping, and Terminating a Job
d850 Remunerative Employment
d855 Non-Remunerative Employment
d860 Basic Economic Transactions
d865 Complex Economic Transactions
d870 Economic Self-Sufficiency
d910 Community Life
d920 Recreation and Leisure

d930 Religion and Spirituality

Environmental Factors

e1100 Food
e1101 Drugs
e1108 Non-Medicinal Drugs and Alcohol
e115 Products and Technology for Personal Use in Daily Living
e120 Products and Technology for Personal Indoor and Outdoor Mobility and Transportation
e125 Products and Technology for Communication
e135 Products and Technology for Employment
e150 Design, Construction, and Building Products and Technology of Buildings for Public Use
e155 Design, Construction, and Building Products and Technology of Buildings for Private Use
e160 Products and Technology of Land Development
e165 Assets
e210 Physical Geography
e250 Sound
e310 Immediate Family
e315 Extended Family
e320 Friends
e325 Acquaintances, Peers, Colleagues, Neighbors, and Community Members
e330 People in Positions of Authority
e340 Personal Care Providers and Personal Assistants
e355 Health Professionals
e360 Other Professionals
e410 Individual Attitudes of Immediate Family Members
e415 Individual Attitudes of Extended Family Members
e420 Individual Attitudes of Friends
e425 Individual Attitudes of Acquaintances, Peers, Colleagues, Neighbors, and Community Members
e440 Individual Attitudes of Personal Care Providers and Personal Assistants
e450 Individual Attitudes of Health Professionals
e455 Individual Attitudes of Health-Related Professionals
e460 Societal Attitudes
e515 Architecture and Construction Services, Systems, and Policies
e525 Housing Services, Systems, and Policies
e535 Communication Services, Systems, and Policies
e540 Transportation Services, Systems, and Policies
e550 Legal Services, Systems, and Policies
e570 Social Security Services, Systems, and Policies
e575 General Social Support Services, Systems, and Policies
e580 Health Services, Systems, and Policies
e585 Education and Training Services, Systems, and Policies
e590 Labor and Employment Services, Systems, and Policies

Vocational Rehabilitation

Finger et al. (2011)

Brief ICF Core Set for Vocational Rehabilitation

Body Functions

b130 Energy and Drive Functions
b164 Higher-Level Cognitive Functions
b455 Exercise Tolerance Functions

Activities & Participation

d155 Acquiring Skills
d240 Handling Stress and Other Psychological Demands
d720 Complex Interpersonal Interactions

d845	Acquiring, Keeping, and Terminating a Job
d850	Remunerative Employment
d855	Non-Remunerative Employment

Environmental Factors

e310	Immediate Family
e330	People in Positions of Authority
e580	Health Services, Systems, and Policies
e590	Labor and Employment Services, Systems, and Policies

Comprehensive ICF Core Set for Vocational Rehab

Body Functions

b117	Intellectual Functions
b126	Temperament and Personality Functions
b130	Energy and Drive Functions
b134	Sleep Functions
b140	Attention Functions
b144	Memory Functions
b152	Emotional Functions
b160	Thought Functions
b164	Higher-Level Cognitive Functions
b210	Seeing Functions
b230	Hearing Functions
b235	Vestibular Functions
b280	Sensation of Pain
b455	Exercise Tolerance Functions
b730	Muscle Power Functions
b740	Muscle Endurance Functions
b810	Protective Functions of the Skin

Activities & Participation

d155	Acquiring Skills
d160	Focusing Attention
d163	Thinking
d166	Reading
d170	Writing
d172	Calculating
d175	Solving Problems
d177	Making Decisions
d210	Undertaking a Single Task
d220	Undertaking Multiple Tasks
d230	Carrying Out Daily Routine
d240	Handling Stress and Other Psychological Demands
d310	Communicating with — Receiving — Spoken Messages
d315	Communicating with — Receiving — Nonverbal Messages
d350	Conversation
d360	Using Communication Devices and Techniques
d410	Changing Basic Body Position
d415	Maintaining a Body Position
d430	Lifting and Carrying Objects
d440	Fine Hand Use
d445	Hand and Arm Use
d450	Walking
d455	Moving Around
d465	Moving Around Using Equipment
d470	Using Transportation
d475	Driving
d530	Toileting
d540	Dressing
d570	Looking After One's Health
d710	Basic Interpersonal Interactions
d720	Complex Interpersonal Interactions
d740	Formal Relationships

d820	School Education
d825	Vocational Training
d830	Higher Education
d840	Apprenticeship (Work Preparation)
d845	Acquiring, Keeping, and Terminating a Job
d850	Remunerative Employment
d855	Non-Remunerative Employment
d870	Economic Self-Sufficiency

Environmental Factors

e1101	Drugs
e115	Products and Technology for Personal Use in Daily Living
e120	Products and Technology for Personal Indoor and Outdoor Mobility and Transportation
e125	Products and Technology for Communication
e130	Products and Technology for Education
e135	Products and Technology for Employment
e150	Design, Construction, and Building Products and Technology of Buildings for Public Use
e155	Design, Construction, and Building Products and Technology of Buildings for Private Use
e225	Climate
e240	Light
e250	Sound
e260	Air Quality
e310	Immediate Family
e320	Friends
e325	Acquaintances, Peers, Colleagues, Neighbors, and Community Members
e330	People in Positions of Authority
e340	Personal Care Providers and Personal Assistants
e355	Health Professionals
e360	Other Professionals
e430	Individual Attitudes of People in Positions of Authority
e450	Individual Attitudes of Health Professionals
e460	Societal Attitudes
e465	Social Norms, Practices, and Ideologies
e525	Housing Services, Systems, and Policies
e535	Communication Services, Systems, and Policies
e540	Transportation Services, Systems, and Policies
e550	Legal Services, Systems, and Policies
e555	Associations and Organizational Services, Systems, and Policies
e565	Economic Services, Systems, and Policies
e570	Social Security Services, Systems, and Policies
e580	Health Services, Systems, and Policies
e585	Education and Training Services, Systems, and Policies
e590	Labor and Employment Services, Systems, and Policies

References

Bernabeu, M., Laxe, S., Lopez, R., Stucki, G., Ward, A., Barnes, M., Kostanjsek, N., Reed, G., Tate, R., Whyte, J., Zasler, N., & Cieza, A. (2009). Developing core sets for persons with traumatic brain injury based on the international classification of functioning, disability, and health. *Neurorehabil Neural Repair, 23*, 464-7.

Bickenbach, J., Cieza, A., Rauch, A., & Stucki, G. (2012). *ICF core sets: Manual for clinical practice.* Ashland, OH: Hogrefe Publishing.

Boldt, C., Grill, E., Wildner, M., Portenier, L., Wilke, S., Stucki, G., Kostanjsek, N., & Quittan, M. (2005). ICF Core Set for patients with cardiopulmonary conditions in the acute hospital. *Disability and Rehabilitation, 27*, 375-380.

Boonen, A., Braun, J., van der Horst Bruinsma, I. E., Huang, F., Maksymowych, W., Kostanjsek, N., Cieza, A., Stucki, G., &

van der Heijde, D. (2010). ASAS/WHO ICF Core Sets for ankylosing spondylitis (AS): How to classify the impact of AS on functioning and health. *Ann Rheum Dis, 69*, 102-107.

Brach, M., Cieza, A., Stucki, G., Fussl, M., Cole, A., Ellerin, B., Fialka-Moser, V., Kostanjsek, N., & Melvin, J. (2004) ICF Core Sets for breast cancer. *J Rehabil Med, Suppl 44*, 121-127.

Cieza, A., Chatterji, S., Andersen, C., Cantista, P., Herceg, M., Melvin, J., Stucki, G., & de Bie, R. (2004). ICF Core Sets for depression. *J Rehabil Med, Suppl 44*, 128-34.

Cieza, A., Kirchberger, I., Biering-Sorensen, F., Baumberger, M., Charlifue, S., Post, M. W., Campbell, R., Kovindha, A., Ring, H., Sinnott, A., Kostanjsek, N., & Stucki. G. (2010). ICF Core Sets for individuals with spinal cord injury in the long-term context. *Spinal Cord, 48*, 305-312.

Cieza, A., Schwarzkopf, S., Sigl, T., Stucki, G., Melvin, J., Stoll, T., Woolf, A., Kostanjsek, N., & Walsh, N. (2004). ICF Core Sets for osteoporosis. *J Rehabil Med, Suppl 44*, 81-6.

Cieza, A., Stucki, A., Geyh, S., Berteanu, M., Quittan, M., Simon, A., Kostanjsek, N., Stucki, G., & Walsh, N. (2004). ICF Core Sets for chronic ischaemic heart disease. *J Rehabil Med, Suppl 44*, 94-99.

Cieza, A., Stucki, G., Weigl, M., Disler, P., Jackel, W., van der Linden, S., Kostanjsek, N., & de Bie, R. (2004). ICF Core Sets for low back pain. *J Rehabil Med, Suppl 44*, 69-74.

Cieza, A., Stucki, G., Weigl, M., Kullmann, L., Stoll, T., Kamen, L., Kostanjsek, N., & Walsh, N. (2004). ICF Core Sets for chronic widespread pain. *J Rehabil Med, Suppl 44*, 63-68.

Coenen, M., Cieza, A., Freeman, J., Khan, F., Miller, D., Weise, A., & Kesselring, J. (2011). The development of ICF Core Sets for multiple sclerosis: Results of the International Consensus Conference. *J Neurol, 258*(8), 1477-1488

Dreinhofer, K., Stucki, G., Ewert, T., Huber, E., Ebenbichler, G., Gutenbrunner, C., Kostanjsek, N., & Cieza, A. (2004). ICF Core Sets for osteoarthritis. *J Rehabil Med, Suppl 44*, 75-80.

Ewert, T., Grill, E., Bartholomeyczik, S., Finger, M., Mokrusch, T., Kostanjsek, N., & Stucki, G. (2005). ICF Core Set for patients with neurological conditions in the acute hospital. *Disability and Rehabilitation, 27*, 367-73.

Finger, M., Escorpizo, R., Glässel, A., Gmünder, H. P., Lückenkemper, M., Chan, C., Fritz, J., Studer, U., Ekholm, J., Kostanjsek, N., Stucki, G., & Cieza, A. (2012). ICF Core Set for vocational rehabilitation: Results of an international consensus conference. *Disability and Rehabilitation, 34*(5), 429-38.

Geyh, S., Cieza, A., Schouten, J., Dickson, H., Frommelt, P., Omar, Z., Kostanjsek, N., Ring, H., Stucki, G. (2004). ICF Core Sets for stroke. *J Rehabil Med, Suppl 44*, 135-141.

Gradinger, F., Cieza, A., Stucki, A., Michel, F., Bentley, A., Oksenberg, A., Rogers, A. E., Stucki, G., & Partinen, M. (2011). Part 1. International Classification of Functioning, Disability and Health (ICF) Core Sets for persons with sleep disorders: Results of the consensus process integrating evidence from preparatory studies. *Sleep Med, 12*, 92-6.

Grill, E., Ewert, T., Chatterji, S., Kostanjsek, N., & Stucki, G. (2005). ICF Core Sets development for the acute hospital and early post-acute rehabilitation facilities. *Disability and Rehabilitation, 27*, 361-366.

Grill, E., Hermes, R., Swoboda, W., Uzarewicz, C., Kostanjsek, N., & Stucki, G. (2005). ICF Core Set for geriatric patients in early post-acute rehabilitation facilities. *Disability and Rehabilitation, 27*, 411-417.

Grill, E., Quittan, M., Fialka-Moser, V., Muller, M., Strobl, R., Kostanjsek, N., & Stucki, G. (2011). Brief ICF Core Sets for the acute hospital. *J Rehabil Med, 43*, 123-130.

Grill, E., Zochling, J., Stucki, G., Mittrach, R., Scheuringer, M., Liman, W., Kostanjsek, N., & Braun, J. (2007). International Classification of Functioning, Disability and Health (ICF) Core Set for patients with acute arthritis. *Clin Exp Rheumatol, 25*, 252-258.

Kirchberger, I., Cieza, A., Biering-Sorensen, F., Baumberger, M., Charlifue, S., Post, M. W., Campbell, R., Kovindha, A., Ring, H., Sinnott, A., Kostanjsek, N., & Stucki, G. (2010). ICF Core Sets for individuals with spinal cord injury in the early post-acute context. *Spinal Cord, 48*, 297-304.

Peyrin-Biroulet, L., Cieza, A., Sandborn, W. J., Kostanjsek, N., Kamm, M. A., Hibi, T., Lemann, M., Stucki, G., & Colombel, J. F. (2010). Disability in inflammatory bowel diseases: Developing ICF Core Sets for patients with inflammatory bowel diseases based on the International Classification of Functioning, Disability, and Health. *Inflamm Bowel Dis, 16*, 15-22.

Rudolf, K. D., Kus, S., Chung, K. C., Johnston, M., LeBlanc, M., & Cieza, A. (2012). Development of the International Classification of Functioning, Disability and Health core sets for hand conditions — results of the World Health Organization International Consensus process. *Disability and Rehabilitation 34*(8), 681-693.

Ruof, J., Cieza, A., Wolff, B., Angst, F., Ergeletzis, D., Omar, Z., Kostanjsek, N., & Stucki, G. (2004). ICF Core Sets for diabetes mellitus. *J Rehabil Med, Suppl 44*, 100-106.

Scheuringer, M., Stucki, G., Huber, E. O., Brach, M., Schwarzkopf, S. R., Kostanjsek, N., & Stoll, T. (2005). ICF Core Set for patients with musculoskeletal conditions in early post-acute rehabilitation facilities. *Disability and Rehabilitation 27*, 405-410.

Stier-Jarmer, M., Grill, E., Ewert, T., Bartholomeyczik, S., Finger, M., Mokrusch, T., Kostanjsek, N., & Stucki, G. (2005). ICF Core Set for patients with neurological conditions in early post-acute rehabilitation facilities. *Disability and Rehabilitation, 27*, 389-95.

Stoll, T., Brach, M., Huber, E. O., Scheuringer, M., Schwarzkopf, S. R., Konstanjsek, N., & Stucki, G. (2005). ICF Core Set for patients with musculoskeletal conditions in the acute hospital. *Disability and Rehabilitation, 27*, 381-387.

Stucki, G., Cieza, A., Geyh, S., Battistella, L., Lloyd, J., Symmons, D., Kostanjsek, N., & Schouten, J. (2004). ICF Core Sets for rheumatoid arthritis. *J Rehabil Med, Suppl 44*, 87-93.

Stucki, A., Daansen, P., Fuessl, M., Cieza, A., Huber, E., Atkinson, R., Kostanjsek, N., Stucki, G., & Ruof, J. (2004). ICF Core Sets for obesity. *J Rehabil Med, Suppl 44*, 107-113.

Stucki, A., Stoll, T., Cieza, A., Weigl, M., Giardini, A., Wever, D., Kostanjsek, N., & Stucki, G. (2004). ICF Core Sets for obstructive pulmonary diseases. *J Rehabil Med, Suppl 44*, 114-20.

Tschiesner, U., Rogers, S., Dietz, A., Yueh, B., & Cieza, A. (2010). Development of ICF core sets for head and neck cancer. *Head Neck. 32*, 210-220.

Vieta, E., Cieza, A., Stucki, G., Chatterji, S., Nieto, M., Sanchez-Moreno, J., Jaeger, J., Grunze, H., & Ayuso-Mateos, J. L. (2007). Developing core sets for persons with bipolar disorder based on the International Classification of Functioning, Disability and Health. *Bipolar Disord, 9*, 16-24.

Wildner, M., Quittan, M., Portenier, L., Wilke, S., Boldt, C., Stucki, G., Kostanjsek, N., & Grill, E. (2005). ICF Core Set for patients with cardiopulmonary conditions in early post-acute rehabilitation facilities. *Disability and Rehabilitation, 27*, 397-404.

Index